TEXTBOOK OF
MEDICAL PHYSIOLOGY

VOLUME 2:
REGULATORY AND INTEGRATIVE SYSTEMS IN MEDICAL PHYSIOLOGY

Dr. Shipra Chandra

ALLIED
HEALTH
PRESS

Textbook of Medical Physiology

Volume 2: Regulatory and Integrative Systems in Medical Physiology

Author: **Dr. Shipra Chandra**

Allied Health Press
4164 Lakeshore Road
Burlington ON L7L 1A4
Canada
www.alliedhealthpress.com
Email: orders@arclereducation.com

ISBN: 978-1-77956-779-6

ABOUT THE AUTHOR

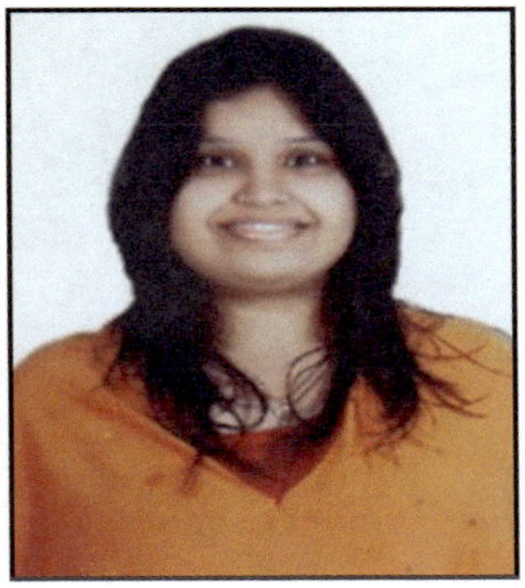

Dr. Shipra Chandra born in Delhi in 1983, completed school from a government school in Delhi in 2001 with First division. Being a science student , took admission in Chemistry Honors at Kirori Mal College, Delhi University. But the wonders of Human Body always fascinated me and I continued preparing for Pre Medical Test (PMT) despite being in a reputed college and course.

By the Grace of God and blessings of my family I secured 5th rank in CPMT 2002 along-with being waitlisted at DPMT and securing rank in AIEEE exam. Joined MBBS on 14/11/2002 at the most prestigious King George Medical College, Lucknow, U.P. Completed MBBS in First division in 2008 and joined AIIMS, New Delhi Department of Emergency Medicine for work experience in 2009 but continued the preparation for Post Graduation Entrance Test and cracked the UP-PGME in 2010 and was allotted MD Physiology from King George Medical University.

After completing the MD in 2013, I again cleared AIIMS, New Delhi entrance test for Senior Residency. Learned a lot during my 3 year tenure from 2013 to 2016 at AIIMS. Following which I joined Fortis Hospital Shalimar Bagh and continued search for a Government Job. Gave the interview at U.P. Public Service Commission in 2017, cracked it and joined as Assistant Professor at Sarojini Naidu Medical College, Agra in 2017. I have 7 research publications , one book chapter and guided 3 MD students during my tenure. Promoted to the post of Associate Professor in 2022 and currently working in the same capacity.

Brief Table of Contents

Getting Started with This Book

Chapter Openers

A list of Chapter Outline is presented providing a brief Introduction to what will be covered in the chapter.

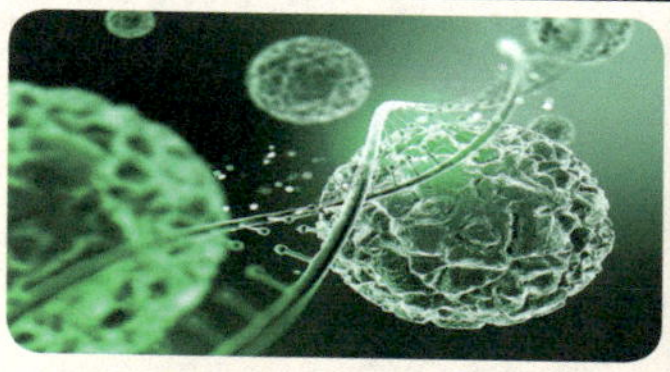

LEARNING OBJECTIVES

After studying this chapter, you will be able to:

1. Discuss the scientific method in biology;
2. Explain the cell theory;
3. Discuss the genetics and heredity;
4. Evolution and natural selection;
5. Focus on ecology and ecosystems;
6. Learn about human biology;
7. Evaluate the plant biology;
8. Explain the microbiology;
9. Focus on current trends in biology.

Introduction

Often referred to as the science of life, biology is a broad field of study aimed at comprehending the several kinds of life on Earth, from tiny creatures to sophisticated multicellular entities. Comprising several subfields, including molecular biology, ecology, and evolutionary biology, each of which advances our knowledge of living systems, this field clarifies the mechanisms controlling life events, including development, reproduction, and interaction with the surroundings, which is the central goal of biology. Moreover, biology fills in the void between the natural sciences and medicine by offering a necessary understanding of health, illness, and the interactions between organisms and their environments. Dealing with urgent global issues such as climate change, biodiversity loss, and new diseases depends on an awareness of these complex biological interactions, therefore highlighting the critical part biology plays in modern civilization. Fundamentally, biology explores and tests ideas about the living world using the scientific method. Through methodical observation and experimentation,

1.1. The Scientific Method in Biology

Learning Outcome

1. Describe the steps of the scientific method;
2. Focus on hypothesis formation;
3. Learn about experimental design.

Learning Outcomes

The beginning of each section of every chapter contains a set of Learning Outcomes that inform students of concepts they should understand. These outcomes help students understand what they should be able to do if they have mastered the material in that section.

Test Your Knowledge

Throughout each chapter, Test Your Knowledge cues you to note which topics have been covered and to self-test your understanding of the material presented.

Test Your Knowledge

1. Explain why correlation does not imply causation in scientific experiments.
2. How does the scientific method help reduce the influence of personal opinions in research?

Chapter Summary

The Summary Section appear at the end of each chapter and summarize main concepts covered throughout the chapter. These points provide key concepts in an engaging and meaningful way.

Summary

The investigation of biological principles highlights the importance of a comprehensive view of life by reflecting the intricate interactions that occur within living systems. The complexity of biology goes beyond individual species or systems, as this essay highlights; it also includes the interactions that mold ecosystems and affect biodiversity. Researchers can conduct in-depth analyses of metabolomic data using sophisticated technologies like MetaboAnalyst, which offer insights into the molecular mechanisms underlying these interactions. As demonstrated by the developments in MetaboAnalyst, for example, the integration of diverse omics data promotes a thorough understanding of metabolic pathways and helps identify important biological markers necessary for research on development and disease (Chong et al., 2018). Additionally, the phenomenon of ecological invasions is a key component of biological research and a vital field of study. The introduction of non-native species into unfamiliar habitats has significant ramifications and calls for multidisciplinary management strategies. Examining the origins and effects of these biological incursions, invasion science has become a crucial field that highlights the need to comprehend ecological dynamics and community interactions. As interest in biological invasions increases, new findings are emerging that put conventional ecological theories and practices to the test. The importance of incorporating various scientific viewpoints is shown by this developing discipline, which also highlights how invasive species shape ecosystems and advances our knowledge of ecological resilience (David et al., 2013). When taken as a whole, these discoveries from invasion science and metabolomics highlight the value of multidisciplinary biology research. Fostering cross-disciplinary collaboration and utilizing technological breakthroughs to improve our comprehension of intricate biological interactions are crucial as we look to the future of biological research. In addition to deepening our understanding of the complexities of life, this method lays the groundwork for tackling urgent environmental issues. Future studies can ensure the continued relevance of biology in a world that is constantly changing by acknowledging the interconnection of biological systems and opening the door to creative solutions that support sustainability and biodiversity conservation. We might imagine a thorough comprehension of life that serves both academia and society at large through ongoing investigation and integration of scientific knowledge.

Knowledge Assessment

The chapter includes material designed to review and reinforce each content. It includes Critical Thinking Questions to help test of your understanding of information presented in the chapter and Short answer Questions to review your understanding of the key concepts presented in the chapter.

Critical Thinking Questions

1. **Who is known as the "Father of Modern Biology"?**
   a. Aristotle
   b. Charles Darwin
   c. Gregor Mendel
   d. Louis Pasteur
2. **What is the basic unit of life?**
   a. Atom
   b. Molecule
   c. Cell
   d. Organism
3. **Which branch of biology studies the interaction of organisms with their environment?**
   a. Genetics
   b. Ecology
   c. Physiology
   d. Botany
4. **Which macromolecule is the main source of energy for living organisms?**
   a. Proteins
   b. Lipids
   c. Carbohydrates
   d. Nucleic acids
5. **DNA is primarily responsible for which function in living organisms?**
   a. Energy production
   b. Protein synthesis
   c. Storing genetic information
   d. Regulating body temperature

Short Answer Questions

1. What is biology, and why is it important to study biology?
2. What are the three main domains of life, and how are they different from one another?
3. Define homeostasis and give an example of how it works in living organisms.
4. What is the cell theory, and why is it fundamental to biology?
5. How do autotrophs and heterotrophs differ in the way they obtain energy?
6. What is the scientific method, and how is it applied in biological research?
7. Discuss how biology helps address global challenges such as climate change, disease, and food security.
8. Explain the levels of biological organization from the smallest unit to the largest. Provide examples at each level.
9. Describe the relationship between structure and function in biology, giving specific examples from cells or organs.
10. How has the discovery of genetics shaped our understanding of inheritance and variation among organisms?

Supplementary Materials

Key Terms: A list of key terms is given for quick reference

KEY TERMS FROM THIS CHAPTER

Annotation enrichment analysis	Biological structure	Cell
Cell theory	Cellular structure	Ecology
Ecosystems	Genetics	Human biology
Microbiology	Natural selection	Organism
Plant biology		

Further Resources: Recommendations for additional readings, websites, and multimedia resources.

References

1. Argelaguet, R., Velten, B., Arnol, D., Dietrich, S., Zenz, T., Marioni, J. C., Buettner, F., et al. (2018). Multi-omics factor analysis—A framework for unsupervised integration of multi-omics data sets. *Molecular Systems Biology, 14*. https://doi.org/10.15252/msb.20178124.
2. Bacher, S., Blackburn, T. M., Essl, F., & Genovesi, P. (2017). *Socio-Economic Impact Classification of Alien Taxa (SEICAT)*. https://core.ac.uk/download/286567949.pdf (accessed on 8th March 2025).
3. Barnett, R., Brace, S., Cucchi, T., & Dobney, K. (2013). *Divergent Evolutionary Processes Associated with Colonization of Offshore Islands*. https://core.ac.uk/download/20664364.pdf (accessed on 8th March 2025).

Detailed Table of Contents

CHAPTER 5

Metabolic Physiology and Energy Balance 151

CHAPTER 6

Reproductive Physiology 187

CHAPTER 7

Immunophysiology and Inflammation 225

CHAPTER 8

Thermoregulation and Temperature Control 261

CHAPTER 9

Exercise Physiology and Adaptations 295

CHAPTER 10

Neuroendocrine Integration and Stress Response in Physiology 331

CHAPTER 11

Sleep Physiology and Circadian Rhythms 369

CHAPTER 12

Developmental Physiology and Aging 405

Index 443

LIST OF FIGURES

PREFACE

To understand the complex processes that allow the human body to survive is one of the grand purposes of physiology. From the function of electrolytes within kidney tubules to the regulation of hormone release, the human body is a remarkable biological machine that must constantly adapt to internal and external changes. Physiology examines how individual organ systems perform their special tasks and are tightly integrated with the overall function of the body. They work dynamically through an impressive set of regulatory systems, feedback mechanisms, chemical messengers, and structural arrangements. Each of these capabilities enables the body to maintain things in equilibrium and adapt to such stresses as growth, stress, injury, and exercise.

With advancing scientific knowledge and clinical requirements becoming ever more specific, there is a need for students and practitioners to focus on physiology not as an aggregation of biological facts but as a science in application. The knowledge gained from the study of physiology has direct relevance to medicine, nursing, and allied health sciences. Physiology aids in the precision of diagnosis, guides treatment planning, and offers feedback on the evaluation of interventions. Whether the management of chronic disease, resolution of acute conditions, or provision of preventive medicine, physiological principles bridge theory and practice. Through appreciation of how organ systems operate in health and disease, practitioners can solve clinical dilemmas with clarity and specificity.

Textbook of Medical Physiology – Volume 2 picks up where the first volume ended, going entirely into human physiological functions. The second volume consists of sophisticated and organ-specific physiological concepts for a full understanding of internal body functions. The content is structured in a way that approximates the complexity of the integrative process concerned with the kidneys, endocrine glands, gastrointestinal tract, metabolism, reproductive organs, immune mechanisms, and neuroendocrine networks. The book is written to include theoretical learning and pragmatic comprehension, serving as a sourcebook for health and medical science students and practitioners. Each chapter represents a development from simple concepts into the mechanisms that perpetuate body function in various circumstances, such as physical exercise, sleep, environmental temperature, and aging.

Chapter 1 describes the physiology of renal tubular function and fluid balance. The chapter discusses mechanisms of reabsorption and secretion of substances in different parts of the nephron, the transporters and channels involved, and fluid volume and electrolyte levels maintenance. It also discusses hormonal control of renal function and how it contributes to systemic homeostasis.

Chapter 2 is dedicated to acid-base physiology. It describes the sources of hydrogen ion production, blood and tissue buffering mechanisms, and the functions of the lungs and kidneys in regulating pH balance. Compensation mechanisms of acid-base disorders and clinical assessment measures, including arterial blood gas analysis, are outlined.

Chapter 3 is on gastrointestinal physiology. Problems addressed include gut secretions regulation, motility patterns, nutrient absorption, and the enteric nervous system. The chapter also has a strong emphasis on the integration of neural, hormonal, and local factors that regulate gastrointestinal function from the mouth to the colon.

Chapter 4 addresses the physiology of endocrinology in the form of synthesis, secretion, transport, and receptor interaction of hormones. It introduces the mechanisms of control for major endocrine glands like the pituitary, thyroid, adrenal, and pancreas. Disruptions in the balance of hormones are also introduced to illustrate the interruption of physiology.

Chapter 5 provides metabolic physiology and energy balance information. Chapter 5 describes metabolic pathways such as glycolysis, lipolysis, and protein metabolism, and the action of hormones such as insulin and glucagon. Regulation of energy intake, storage, and expenditure is explored, along with determinants of body weight and nutritional physiology.

Chapter 6 deals with reproductive physiology. Chapter 6 covers the hormonal control of male and female reproductive organs, gametogenesis, the menstrual cycle, pregnancy, and parturition. Chapter 6 also deals with regulatory mechanisms and feedback control of reproductive hormones and fertility.

Chapter 7 addresses immunophysiology and inflammation. It describes the relationship between innate and adaptive immunity, the body functions of immune cells and cytokines, acute and chronic inflammation, and relates these concepts to disease mechanisms such as infection, allergy, and autoimmunity.

Chapter 8 addresses the topics of thermoregulation and temperature regulation. It addresses mechanisms of heat production and dissipation, how the hypothalamus works, and the physiological reactions to cold and heat stress. The importance of maintaining core body temperature for enzymatic and cellular function is emphasized.

Chapter 9 is exercise physiology and adaptations. It discusses how the cardiovascular, respiratory, muscular, and metabolic systems adapt to exercise. Acute and chronic adaptations are explained in the chapter, and it also provides details about exercise prescriptions for rehabilitation and health.

Chapter 10 considers neuroendocrine integration and stress response. It considers how the hypothalamic-pituitary axis coordinates responses to internal and external stimuli. It considers how stress hormones interface with other body systems and the mechanisms that regulate acute and chronic stress.

Chapter 11 covers sleep physiology and circadian rhythms. The chapter explains the sleep stages, their physiological significance, and the neural mechanisms. The chapter covers biological clocks, melatonin secretion, and how circadian rhythm disturbances affect health and mental function.

Chapter 12 addresses developmental physiology and aging. It traces physiological development from fetal development to childhood, adulthood, and old age. The chapter outlines how body systems become modified in a person during his/her lifetime, why they deteriorate, and the implications for managing health in aging populations.

This book is intended for undergraduate and postgraduate medical, dental, nursing, and allied health sciences students who require a broad and applied understanding of human physiology. It also helps clinicians, teachers, and scientists who require a reliable reference that ties the relationship between physiological facts and clinical relevance. The clear format, conceptual maturity, and practical utility make it worthy of being taught at the academic level, self-taught, and used in the clinic. Readers are presumed to have an elementary knowledge of biology and human anatomy, as this book is founded upon principles to facilitate advancement in specialized areas of physiology.

RENAL PHYSIOLOGY: FUNCTION AND FLUID BALANCE

1

LEARNING OBJECTIVES

After studying this chapter, you will be able to:

1. Understand the anatomy of the kidney functions.
2. Explain the reabsorption mechanisms.
3. Discuss the secretion in renal physiology.
4. Focus on the regulation of fluid balance.
5. Learn about electrolyte balance.
6. Evaluate the acid-base homeostasis.
7. State the pathophysiology of renal function.

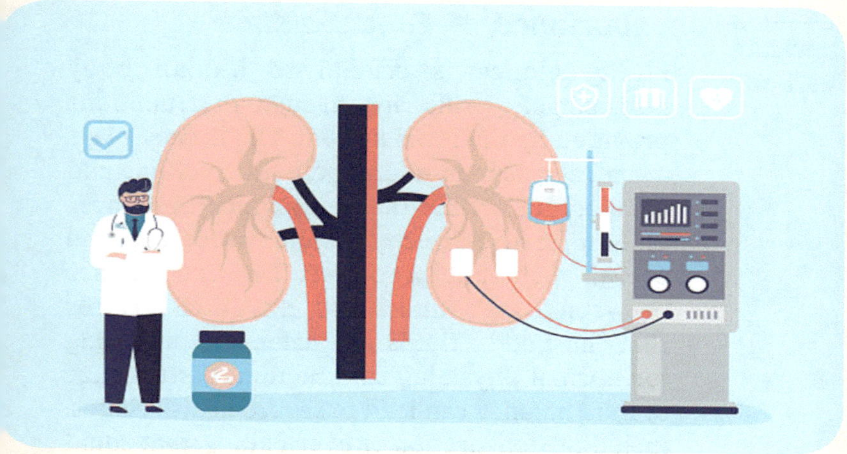

Introduction

The renal system plays a vital role in maintaining homeostasis in the human body primarily through control of fluid balance and electrolyte levels. The kidneys are essential organs that filter blood, eliminate waste, and keep fluid levels in check to maintain efficient functioning of body systems. Renal physiology complexity defines the coordination between various mechanisms responsible for controlling kidney function, such as glomerular filtration, tubular reabsorption, and secretory functions. Understanding the diverse functions of the kidneys not only informs us about their function in fluid balance but also reflects the significance of maintaining renal health to prevent systemic imbalances that can lead to severe health disorders. Further, the kidneys possess remarkable adaptive functions that allow them to accommodate changes in hydration status and food intake, as demonstrated by dehydration and rehydration experiments. Research has shown that under dehydration, there is a significant reduction in kidney solute loads, illustrating the kidneys' ability to pre-sustain water proactively. A case in point is research on adult dromedary camels that demonstrated that extended dehydration periods resulted in reduced plasma and tubular burdens of a number of solutes, illustrating the kidneys' adaptive mechanisms to preserve water but decrease the excretion of solutes (Kataria et al., 2007). These findings not only increase our understanding of renal function during extreme conditions but also illuminate the evolutionary mechanisms that enable survival under situations of limited availability of water. The kidneys are also charged with regulating the body's acid-base status through intricate physiological mechanisms in numerous body systems.

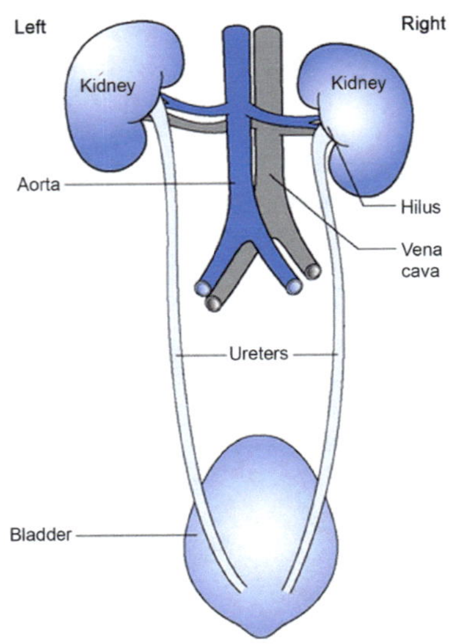

Figure 1.1. Fluid balance and the urinary system.

Source: https://nursekey.com/wp-content/uploads/2016/07/B9780702043581000229_f22-03-9780702043581.jpg.

The coordination between the renal system, the lungs, and buffer systems is essential in the maintenance of pH levels within a very narrow range, as required for cell function and general metabolic activities. This coordination provides for the rapid correction of any acid-base disturbances, allowing the body to efficiently attain homeostasis (White, 2025). The integration of these regulatory systems illustrates the kidney's function in addition to fluid balance, as they have a key function in coordinating metabolic processes. As renal physiology evolves, a greater insight into the kidneys' multifaceted roles will enhance clinical approaches to renal-related disease treatment and guide targeted therapy design (Figure 1.1).

Importance of Fluid Balance

Fluid balance is crucial to human body homeostasis, primarily through the functions provided by the renal system. The kidney plays a central role in regulating the fluid volume and composition within the body, which influences blood pressure directly, cellular processes, and overall metabolic processes. The fine balance between water intake and excretion ensures that the body's fluids are balanced, providing for normal physiological function. Disturbance of fluid balance can lead to severe health issues, including dehydration or overloading, that could significantly affect the activity of the kidneys. Normally, kidneys need to adapt, controlling the reabsorption of water and electrolytes in a way that maintains fluid balance, highlighting the kidneys' key role in disease and health. Maintenance of fluid balance involves a close relationship with other hormonal stimuli controlling renal function. Hormones such as antidiuretic hormone (ADH) and aldosterone transmit important messages to the kidneys, controlling water reabsorption and sodium retention. For instance, ADH increases the permeability of renal tubules for enhanced water reabsorption, particularly during dehydration. Aldosterone, on the other hand, promotes sodium reabsorption, promoting water retention and maintaining blood pressure. This complex hormonal regulation emphasizes the kidneys' responsiveness to body fluid needs and their role in homeostatic mechanisms. As outlined in recent studies, the balance of natriuretic and anti-natriuretic factors is critical, and the interaction between angiotensin II and atrial natriuretic peptide demonstrates the kidneys' multifactorial regulation of fluid balance. Moreover, pathophysiologic characteristics of fluid balance connote its role in the regulation of renal health.

Diseases such as nephrotic syndrome and hypertension disrupt homeostasis controlled by renal mechanisms, often causing deranged sodium excretion and over fluid loading. The atrial natriuretic peptide and the renal dopaminergic system play a significant role in such diseases, acting alongside the renin-angiotensin system to counteract oxidative stress while maintaining renal function (Leonardet al., 1975). Clinically, fluid balance can be maintained by appropriate intervention measures, preventing such diseases' complications. Consequently, the integration of modern monitoring methods with fluid levels and renal function is essential since it enhances better patient care through early adjustments in treatment protocols in order to maintain an optimal fluid balance level (Leonard et al., 2025). The integration of these elements indicates the significance of fluid balance in renal physiology.

Overview of Kidney Functions

The kidneys are central to the body's homeostasis through the performance of a variety of important functions. Maintenance of blood pressure through the renin-angiotensin-aldosterone system is one of their significant roles. The complex system of hormones is activated with reduced blood volume or blood pressure, and the kidneys release renin. To this, angiotensin II is formed, which constricts blood vessels and prompts aldosterone release. Aldosterone increases the reabsorption of sodium from the tubules in the kidneys and therefore water is retained, together with an increase in blood pressure and volume. In this manner, then, the kidneys play a role in keeping the blood pressure steady under various states of physiology, marking them as playing a central role in fluid and electrolyte balance in the body. Another crucial function of the kidneys is the regulation of electrolyte balance, such as sodium, potassium, and calcium levels. Through intricate processes of filtration, reabsorption, and secretion, the kidneys can maintain the delicate balance of these electrolytes within the blood. For instance, while sodium reabsorption is hormone-controlled, such as by aldosterone, potassium excretion is regulated antagonistically; whereas sodium is reabsorbed, excess potassium is secreted into the renal tubules for elimination.

This fine-tuned balance prevents the complexities of hyperkalemia or hypokalemia, both of which carry serious health implications. Because the kidneys not just control how much but also what type of electrolytes there are in the blood, their ultimate role in fluid balance is achieved, synthesizing a number of physiological systems required for well-being. Along with this role, the kidneys participate in acid-base homeostasis, an integral component of physiological equilibrium. The renal system regulates blood acidity by reabsorbing bicarbonate from urine and secreting hydrogen ions so that the body can neutralize acids produced during metabolism. This buffering effect is important in order to avoid fluctuations in the pH of blood that can be detrimental to other biological processes. The complexity of this role is aggravated by the role of renal collecting ducts, which possess a typical epithelial barrier regulated by tight junctions, and have profound effects on reabsorption and solute transport (Leiz ., & Schmidt-Ott, 2019). Failure in these functions could lead to diseases such as metabolic acidosis or alkalosis, vindicating the role of the kidney not only in fluid regulation but also in the entire spectrum of biochemical stability in the organism (Figure 1.2).

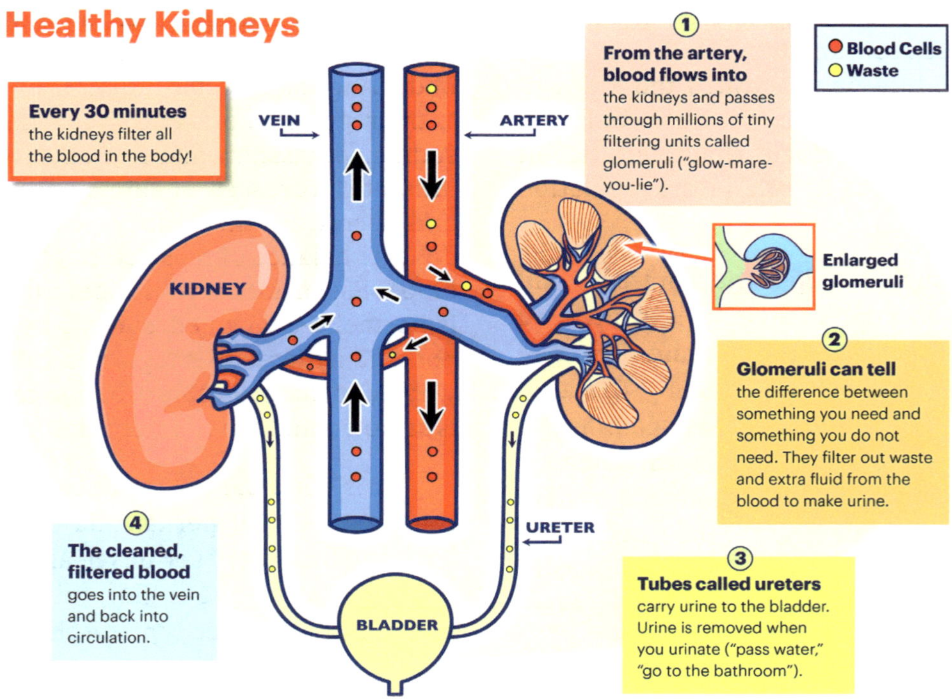

Figure 1.2. Kidneys work.

Source: https://www.kidney.org/sites/default/files/2024-10/11-10-0101_GBH_LearnAboutKidneys_4-5%20%281%29.png.

1.1. Anatomy of the Kidney Functions

Learning Outcome

1. Describe the structure of the kidney;
2. Focus on nephron: the functional unit;
3. Learn about blood supply to the kidneys.

The anatomy of the kidney is well planned so that it can carry out its primary functions like filtration, reabsorption, and secretion. There are three broad regions in a single kidney: outer cortex, inner medulla, and renal pelvis. The cortex consists of the renal corpuscles that cover the glomeruli, where filtration starts. Following the initial filtration, the filtrate flows into the medulla, which consists of renal pyramids containing the nephrons loop and collecting ducts. This structured arrangement enables the kidneys to efficiently concentrate urine and obtain homeostasis through fluid balance and electrolyte regulation. Because the nephron plays a central role in these mechanisms, familiarity with its anatomy is significant in the assessment of renal function and consequences of kidney disease, which may disrupt such finely tuned mechanisms (Lory, 1993). In addition to the nephron, the kidneys are also perfused with blood by an arborescent network of arteries and veins, with a rich blood supply required for filtration and nutrient exchange. The renal artery branches off from the aorta to provide oxygenated blood to the kidneys, and the renal vein returns deoxygenated blood to the inferior vena cava. This double vascular system emphasizes the kidneys' important role in systemic blood pressure and fluid regulation. Besides, special renal features like the juxtaglomerular apparatus are key to the kidney's capacity to adapt to changes in blood flow and composition, regulating the release of renin to control blood pressure. Elucidation of these vascular features enhances our knowledge of renal physiology and shows intervention targets in cases of hypertension and chronic kidney disease (Vu et al., 2015). Admiration of renal variation within the kidneys across species gives profound insights into renal evolution and function. The comparative approach gives a dramatic contrast in kidney architecture between vertebrates and invertebrates, highlighting adaptive fluid handling and waste disposal mechanisms. For instance, studies show that the elementary mechanisms of ultrafiltration and flow modulation are retained across species despite anatomical structure differences. This highlights the universal applicability of these mechanisms to homeostasis. Innovative models, such as using planarians, create new avenues for experimentation to explore underlying pathologies of kidney disease and potentially lead to a paradigm shift in treatment. With continued investigation, this cross-species understanding of renal anatomy will increasingly inform and add sophistication to our interpretation of renal physiology and its application to disease and health (Vu et al., 2015) (Figure 1.3).

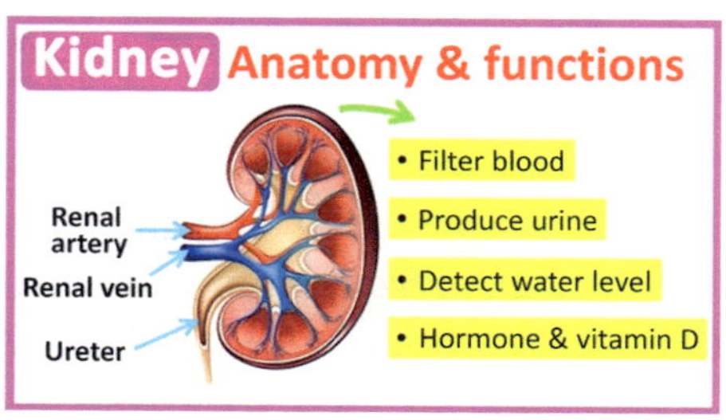

Figure 1.3. Anatomy of the kidney functions.

Source: https://i.ytimg.com/vi/cjz_rCsH0JU/hq720.jpg?sqp=-oaymwEhCK4FEIIDSFryq4qpAxMIARUAAAAAGAElAADIQj0AgKJD&rs=AOn4CLBfRVd_wNS6ld1kHTssu4vd-OBNlA.

1.1.1. Structure of the Kidney

The kidneys' intricate structure is a significant determinant of its fundamental roles of filtration, reabsorption, and secretion, all of which are requisite in the formation of fluid balance and homeostasis. A single kidney is composed of approximately one million functional units known as nephrons, each further divided into independent segments: glomerulus, proximal tubule, loop of Henle, distal convoluted tubule, and collecting duct. The glomerulus initiates the process of filtration by allowing the passage of water and solutes from the blood to the Bowman's capsule, resulting in the generation of filtrate. With the progress of filtrate through the nephron, various reabsorption and secretion processes are performed, exactly regulating the composition of urine as well as assisting in fluid as well as electrolyte balance, thus emphasizing the kidneys' function in renal physiology. Interestingly, the collecting duct is an ideal model of the kidney's dynamic and adaptive structure, particularly in the regulation of sodium and chloride ion reabsorption. It is composed of principal and intercalated cells, both with distinctive roles in acid-base balance and sodium homeostasis. Current research has highlighted that type B intercalated cells can mediate electroneutral NaCl reabsorption both through Na-dependent and Na-independent mechanisms, contradicting previous assumptions with a spotlight on principal cells alone for sodium transport. Type A intercalated cells have also been implicated in NaCl secretion via a bumetanide-sensitive mechanism, showing the heterogeneity and complexity of sodium transport in the collecting duct. These considerations underscore ionic transport mechanisms' interdependence and the requirement for ongoing research into renal physiology, particularly on the determinants of fluid balance (Edwards & Crambert, 2017). Kidneys' structure also enables regulation of systemic blood pressure, rather than a simplistic filtration function. Chronic conditions such as hypertension can be caused by unusual sodium reabsorption in different segments of the nephron, but more predominantly in the thick ascending limb of the loop of Henle. With hypertension, the persistent rise in sodium reabsorption is harmful to sodium balance and results in elevated blood pressure. Understanding the structural component of the nephrons and the specific segments responsible for sodium handling is vital in comprehending the pathophysiology that accounts for salt-sensitive hypertension. This emphasizes the role of the kidney not only in the regulation of fluid homeostasis but also in its ramifications in cardiovascular physiology, revealing the intricate interrelationship of renal function and body physiological processes (Graham et al., 2017).

1.1.2. Nephron: The Functional Unit

The nephron, or the functional unit of renal function, is the key to homeostasis by its intricate mechanisms of fluid and electrolyte balance. With numerous segments, including the glomerulus, proximal tubule, loop of Henle, distal tubule, and collecting duct, each segment has specialized functions that compensate for the total efficiency of the nephron. The glomerulus initiates the filtration process, which will allow the selective passage of water and solutes but not the larger protein molecules. Throughout the transit of the filtrate through the nephron, reabsorptions occur to bring back essential substances to the blood so that fluid and electrolyte balance necessary for normal cellular function is maintained. An increase in nephron workload, particularly following injury or loss of renal mass, initiates significant adaptive responses to maintain physiological equilibrium. Following nephrectomy, the surviving nephrons exhibit an increase in single-nephron glomerular filtration rate (SNGFR) and tubular hypertrophy, compensation to restore excretion with a decrease in the number of nephrons. Experiments have shown that while these adaptations contribute to the maintenance of homeostasis, they are by themselves not enough to absolutely guarantee salt balance, and this is an indication of the complex interaction of nephron adaptations under altered functional demands. Here, computational models have revealed the dynamics of solute transport and illustrated that though filtered load and the capacity for transport by kidneys increase, other alterations in sodium and potassium handling should occur to remain balanced within the nephron population (Edwards & Layton, 2017).

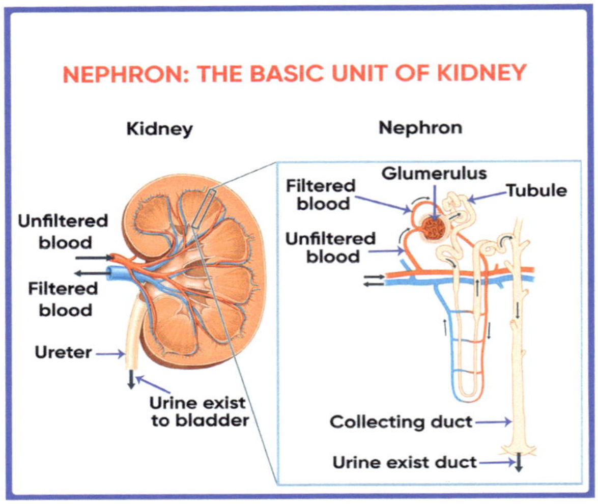

Figure 1.4. Nephron: the functional unit.

Source: https://cdn.teachoo.com/large/fa10836d-5f5e-42e9-911e-a46d52b2b1ef/nephron---the-basic-unit-of-kidney-01.jpg.

The cortical collecting duct (CCD) becomes a central issue as a key mediator of NaCl transport and acid-base status regulation in the nephron system. Groundbreaking research has dismantled previous assumptions that confined Na transport primarily to principal cells, now acknowledging major functions of intercalated cells for NaCl reabsorption and secretion. For instance, type B intercalated cells were identified as mediators of electroneutral NaCl reabsorption, accentuating the energy dynamics engaged by basolateral vacuolar H-ATPase pumps. Type A intercalated cells are also engaged in NaCl secretion, accentuating intricate cross-talk processes that optimize sodium and chloride transport. This functional utility underlines the importance of the CCD in the nephron, validating its role in electrolyte and fluid balance, which is critical to renal physiology (Edwards & Crambert, 2017) (Figure 1.4).

1.1.3. Blood Supply to the Kidneys

Blood supply to the kidneys is crucial in their role to facilitate homeostasis of the body, particularly fluid and electrolyte balance. The renal artery, a direct branch of the abdominal aorta, furnishes each kidney with its blood supply with sufficient oxygenated blood to facilitate filtration. Renal arteries further ramify into smaller arteries and arterioles and lead ultimately to the glomeruli, where filtration of blood occurs. This particular system not only facilitates clearance of the waste products but also controls blood pressure through the renin-angiotensin-aldosterone system. Perfusion is important and should be in good condition; reduced blood supply can lead to ischemia, impaired filtration, and consequent renal impairment, having a direct influence on fluid balance and renal physiology as a whole. With progressing renal blood flow, consideration should be taken of the adaptive renal mechanisms in different physiological states. For instance, studies have demonstrated that a reduction in nephron number, like in models including uninephrectomized rats, leads to significant changes in the kidney structure and function. The remaining nephrons develop an increase in single-nephron glomerular filtration rate (SNGFR) and hypertrophy, suggesting an adaptive response for managing increased workload and maintenance of homeostasis of water and salt. The renal anatomy facilitates this response by optimizing the selective reabsorption and secretion activities along different segments of nephrons. With adaptations, though, it is found through research that such physiological changes are not enough to totally compensate for the loss of nephron mass, showing the complexity of the renal response to altered blood supply (Edwards & Layton, 2017). The evolutionary perspective on renal function offers further insight into the significance of blood supply to renal physiology. As discussed by Homer Smith, renal structural development in more advanced forms, such as the loop of Henle, is contemporaneous with terrestrial lifestyles and the demands for enhanced fluid conservation. The evolutionary enhancement of arterial blood supply and glomerular filtration rates was pivotal in the adaptation of kidneys to varying environments, facilitating successful renal processes in varying vertebrate organisms. Perceptual knowledge of these mechanisms of evolution underscores the importance of the regulation of blood flow in the kidneys, highlighting the ways in which physiological adaptations have developed their function over time. Hence, the intricate interaction between renal perfusion and fluid homeostasis is still a fundamental characteristic of renal physiology that is deserving of study in evolutionary and clinical settings (Natochin, 1996).

Test Your Knowledge

1. How does the structure of the nephron support its function in filtration and reabsorption?
2. Which part of the kidney collects urine before it passes to the ureter?

1.2. Reabsorption Mechanisms

Learning Outcome

1. Explain the proximal tubule reabsorption;
2. Define the loop of Henle functions;
3. Discuss the distal convoluted tubule and collecting duct.

The renal system plays a critical role in the regulation of fluids and the upkeep of electrolyte balance through intricate reabsorptive processes. In the nephron, various sites are involved in the selective reabsorption of various solutes, which directly affect overall renal function. The proximal convoluted tubule (PCT) is the primary site for the reabsorption of water and sodium (Na^+), in which approximately 65-70% of filtered Na^+ is reabsorbed. This process is illustrated for the most part by active transport mechanisms that utilize the action of sodium-potassium ATPase pumps to allow secondary active transport of other solutes. Inasmuch as endothelial and epithelial interactions control such transport systems, derangements in this reabsorption process can have significant clinical repercussions, such as fluid overload or electrolyte imbalances, eventually affecting systemic health as well as blood pressure regulation.

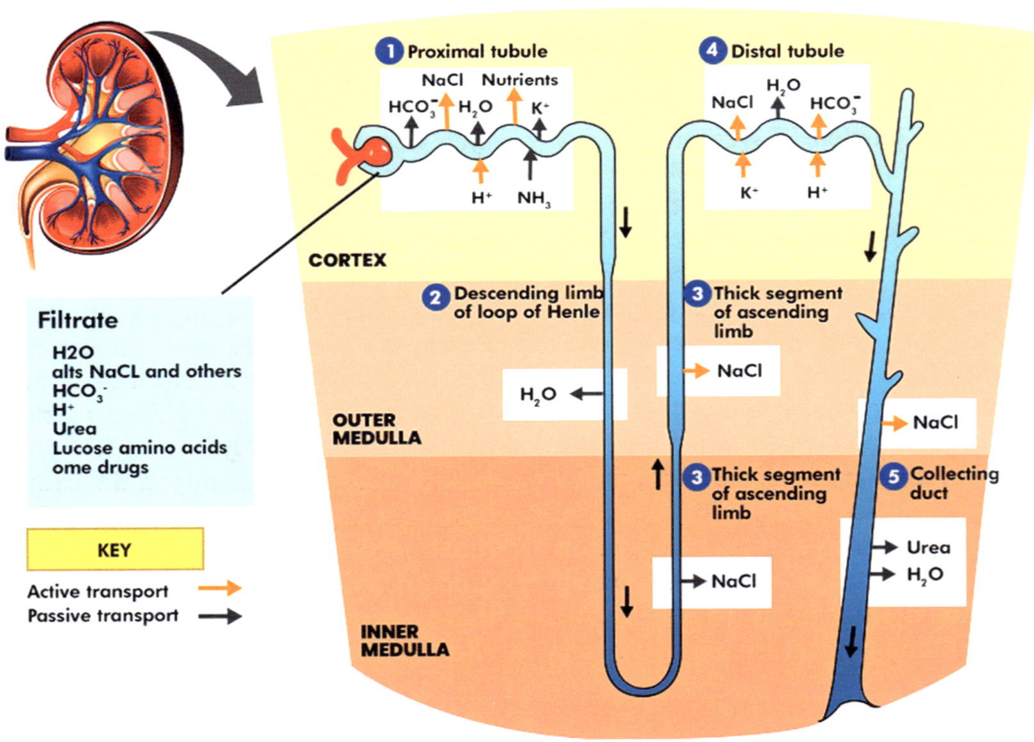

Figure 1.5. Reabsorption-in-kidney.

Source: https://media.geeksforgeeks.org/wp-content/uploads/20221228104632/Reabsorption-in-Kidney.png.

In the cortical collecting duct (CCD), reabsorption becomes more specialized in involving specific cell types with independent functions for sodium and chloride transport. New evidence suggests that type B intercalated cells are able to mediate electroneutral NaCl reabsorption through a mechanism involving both sodium-dependent and sodium-independent processes, implying a dynamic and multifunctional role for these cells within the nephron. Furthermore, the established function of intercalated cells in acid-base homeostasis shows their role in maintaining general fluid balance. Cross-talk between cell types in the CCD has been found to have a major influence on Na^+ and Cl^- reabsorption, with an indication of the intricate interdependence between renal processes maintaining homeostasis in fluctuating physiological states (Edwards & Crambert, 2017). The thick ascending limb of the loop of Henle (TAL) is another critical area in which reabsorption is crucial for sodium management and control of blood pressure. The portion of the nephron employs a distinct Na^+ resorptive process via the Na-K-2Cl cotransporter (NKCC2), and it becomes a critical element with increased dietary salt load. When the TAL's sodium resorptive function is compromised, it can be linked with pathological effects in Na^+ balance and therefore lead to diseases such as hypertension. Sodium reabsorption kinetics by this nephron segment exemplify the complexity of managing blood pressure and highlight salt sensitivity as an important area of study in renal physiology. More research into TAL function not only enhances our understanding of renal function but also offers prospective therapeutic options for the management of salt-sensitive hypertension and concomitant disease (Graham et al., 2017) (Figure 1.5).

1.2.1. Proximal Tubule Reabsorption

The proximal tubule of the nephron is where the reabsorption of essential components of the filtrate takes place, representing approximately 65-70% of glomerular filtrate volume. This serves a purpose of homeostasis in the sense that it reabsorbs water, electrolytes, glucose, and amino acids selectively while allowing the wasteful excretion. Through active transport mechanisms, such as the sodium-hydrogen exchanger (NHE3), the proximal tubule facilitates bicarbonate (HCO_3^-) reabsorption necessary for acid-base balance. Such mechanisms are supported by intricate cellular signaling pathways, where Exchange proteins directly activated by cAMP (Epac) play a significant role. Research has confirmed that Epac isoform deletion dramatically reduces NHE3 activity and illustrates how cellular signaling complexities regulate proximal tubule function, with concomitant influence on global renal acid-base homeostasis (Pyrshev et al., 2024). This confirms the dual role of the proximal tubules in reabsorption and acid-base regulation. Furthermore, proximal tubule reabsorption effectiveness is inextricably linked with renal function as well as fluid balance. Some drugs, such as SGLT2 inhibitors, have been seen to indirectly influence the Na^+ reabsorption in the proximal tubule, causing renal protection through reduced ATP demand and overall tubular cell workload. By reducing sodium reabsorption, the inhibitors maintain glomerular filtration rates and prevent renal injury. In a study of opossum kidney proximal tubule cells, SGLT2 inhibitors were identified to inhibit fluid transport and albumin uptake, displaying how drug intervention may be used to regulate the function of the proximal tubule (Albalawy et al., 2024). Through advancing the understanding of these processes, therapeutic strategies can be better developed, addressing many renal pathologies with increased efficacy while promoting fluid balance and kidney well-being. The complex interplay of many of the mechanisms of the proximal tubule establishes its significance in renal physiology and fluid balance. The most delicate balance must exist for optimal health, with disturbances in reabsorptive processes leading to imbalance. The latter comes in the form of metabolic acidosis or fluid overload. This is best observed on examination of adaptive responses to acid loads in the diet, in which loss of proximal tubule mechanisms, e.g., bicarbonate reabsorption, manifests as clinical disease. The investigation into the molecular signaling role has illuminated pathways that, when disrupted, result in defective renal adaptation to stress such as acid-base imbalance, pointing towards the importance of ongoing research here (Pyrshev et al., 2024). Ultimately, understanding the mechanisms regulating proximal tubule reabsorption not only serves to increase our appreciation for renal physiology but also forms a key component of crafting targeted interventions that improve patient outcomes (Figure 1.6).

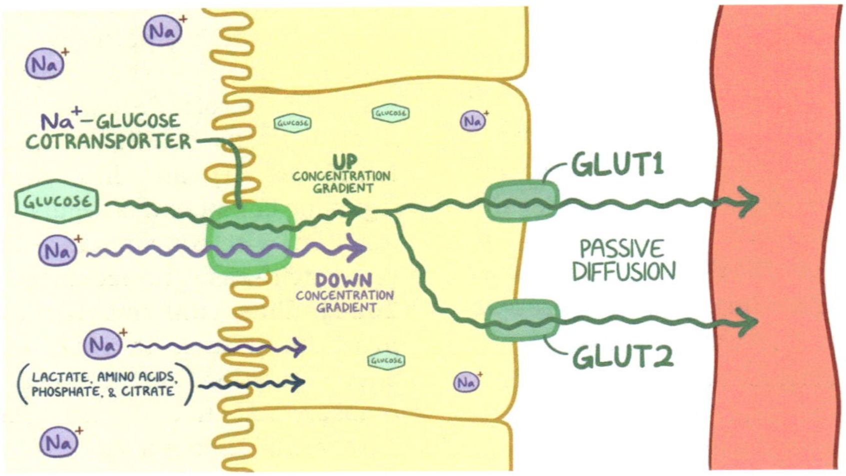

Figure 1.6. Proximal convoluted tubule.

Source: https://d16qt3wv6xm098.cloudfront.net/XkK0yO9jT3egEqpojRcY6qXqTP6q61Xs/_.jpg.

1.2.2. Loop of Henle Functions

The Loop of Henle is a central function in renal physiology, primarily because it generates a gradient of concentration in the renal medulla. Divided into the descending and ascending limbs, this structure allows for the concentration of solutes in a counter-current fashion, significantly influencing kidney function and fluid balance. Descending limb is water permeable but not solute permeable, thus allowing for passive reabsorption of water along with the concentration of sodium and chloride in the tubular fluid. This serves not only for hydration purposes but also in creating an osmotic gradient for water reabsorption in the collecting ducts later on. The unique design of the Loop of Henle thus effectively aids in the concentration of urine, one of the kidneys' significant functions that enables the body to adapt to varying levels of hydration and solute intake. Furthermore, the ascending limb of the Loop of Henle is very crucial in the reabsorption of vital ions, i.e., sodium, potassium, and chloride. Unlike the descending limb, this section is impermeable to water but allows for active transport of such electrolytes from the tubular fluid into the interstitium around the tube. Active transport of such electrolytes helps in achieving electrolyte balance and overall fluid homeostasis within the body. Reabsorbed ions also contribute to the osmotic gradient created by the descending limb, which increases the kidneys' ability to produce concentrated urine. If renal function is impaired, for instance, in conditions such as obesity and hypertension, the normal regulation of these electrolytes is compromised, and imbalances may be induced that need medical intervention (Hall et al., 2015). Therefore, the Loop of Henle is not just a critical structure but a critical component of physiological processes necessary for fluid balance. In addition, the processes within the Loop of Henle play a significant role in the control of the calcium, phosphate, and magnesium content of the body. These ions, vital to numerous biological processes, are controlled by the kidneys in an exquisite balance of glomerular filtration and tubular reabsorption. The tubular sections, like that of the Loop of Henle, ensure regulation of reabsorption of these multivalent cations in response to the body's current demands, keeping their plasma levels steady. Through periods of poor dietary intake, renal regulatory mechanisms compensate by enhancing reabsorption and reducing excretion, thus stabilizing homeostasis (Blaine et al., 2014). This intricate association identifies the importance of the Loop of Henle not only in fluid control but also in the overall scenario of mineral homeostasis, highlighting its multifaceted function in the context of renal physiology and fluid dynamics (Figure 1.7).

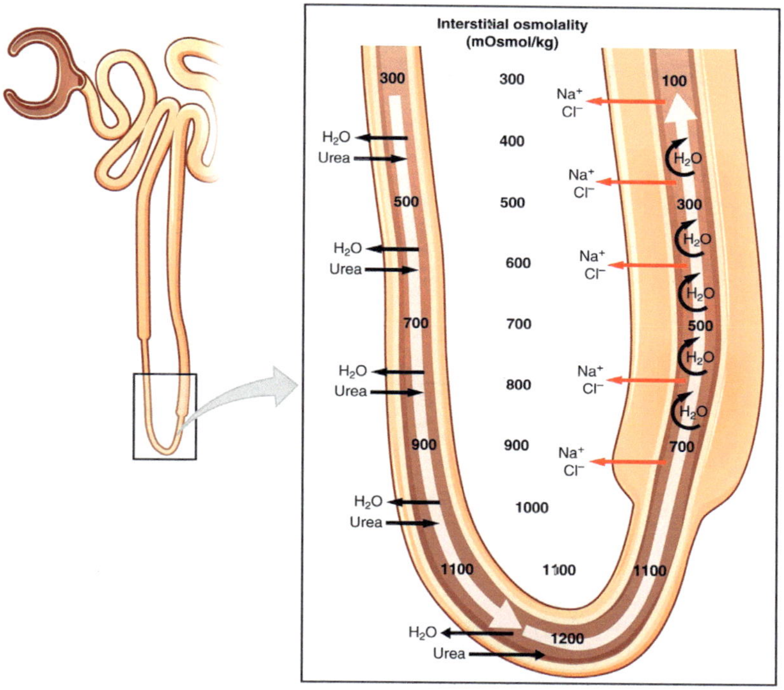

Figure 1.7. Diagram showing ion and water reabsorption within the Loop of Henle.

Source: https://teachmephysiology.com/urinary-system/nephron/loop-henle/.

1.2.3. Distal Convoluted Tubule and Collecting Duct

The distal convoluted tubule (DCT) plays a significant role in sodium and potassium balance and in general fluid homeostasis in the organism. It is positioned downstream of the loop of Henle and is specifically adapted for sodium reabsorption and chloride ion reabsorption, largely through sodium-chloride cotransporter (NCC) activity. This active transport mechanism not only aids in the maintenance of electrolyte balance but is also crucial in the regulation of blood pressure. Current studies highlight how hormones, such as aldosterone, influence NCC expression and function, thereby influencing sodium reabsorption and consequently blood pressure and volume.

In addition, beta-adrenergic receptors are also postulated to regulate NCC function, accounting for the complex relationships between renal processes and neural stimuli that underlie the body's fluid status (Suh et al., 2022). In parallel with the DCT, the collecting duct is essential for the final regulation of urine concentration and volume. The principal cells of the collecting duct are engaged primarily with water and sodium reabsorption, which is strongly influenced by antidiuretic hormone (ADH) and aldosterone. ADH leads to the insertion of aquaporin-2 channels into the apical membrane to enable the collecting duct to modulate water reabsorption based on the body's hydration state. Therefore, this mechanism is activated in acute fluid balance regulation, which focuses the urine and prevents dehydration. Moreover, the collecting duct has intercalated cells that play an important role in acid-base homeostasis, depicting the significant role this renal section has in attaining physiological equilibrium (Arthur et al., 2021). Both the DCT and collecting duct are key to understanding renal physiology and fluid balance, their individual functions having widespread implications for cardiovascular health. Alteration of the transport processes occurring within these tubules can generate a myriad of pathophysiologic states, such as hypertension and electrolyte imbalance. Our understanding of how these segments are regulated by hormones and renal compensation is continually being filled in by research. For instance, the role of the prorenin receptor in mediating fluid homeostasis and blood pressure regulation, particularly in the collecting duct, underscores the delicate interplay between renal function and structure. As we push further in this direction, elucidation of these cellular mechanisms holds promise for solving clinical problems concerning fluid and electrolyte derangements (Arthur et al., 2021; Suh et al., 2022).

Test Your Knowledge

1. What type of transport mechanisms are involved in tubular reabsorption?
2. How does sodium reabsorption drive the reabsorption of water and other solutes?

1.3. Secretion in Renal Physiology

Learning Outcome

1. Explain the importance of tubular secretion;
2. Define the substances secreted by the nephron;
3. Describe the regulation of acid-base balance.

Secretion in renal physiology plays a crucial role in the regulation of homeostasis, particularly through electrolyte and metabolic waste control. The nephron, with various segments such as the proximal convoluted tubule and cortical collecting duct, is key to this process. Secretion is made up of the active transport of substances from the peritubular capillaries to the tubular lumen for waste products, toxins, and excess ion excretion. Specifically, the cortical collecting duct (CCD) exhibits phenomenal plasticity in terms of sodium chloride transport mechanisms, as demonstrated by recent research, which has shown that principal cells and intercalated cells can mediate NaCl reabsorption and secretion. This contradicts the traditional notion that some transport activities are limited to specific cell types, thus highlighting the complex interaction between secretion and reabsorption in the maintenance of renal function and overall body fluid balance (Edwards & Crambert, 2017). Among all the renal units, the majority of water and solute secretion is carried out by the proximal convoluted tubule (PCT). Not only does this segment reabsorb glucose, amino acids, and bicarbonate, but it also secretes organic anions and cations, which are vital for the clearance of drugs and metabolic byproducts. Novel modeling of PCT cell dynamics revealed mechanisms for regulatory volume decrease (RVD) relevant to the regulation of cell volume in osmotic stress. Most notably in hyposmotic exposure, Na^+ HCO_3^- cotransporters have been found to be more effective in preserving intracellular osmolality compared to other channels. Such a regulatory process is essential as it preserves net transcellular Na^+ reabsorption stability and most optimally controls secretion rates to preserve fluid balance in the body (Edwards & Layton, 2017).

Renal physiology is also made more complex by endocrine control and feedback mechanisms to preserve the body's balance of electrolytes as well as blood pressure. Hormones such as aldosterone affect the CCD to boost sodium reabsorption and potassium excretion, with a fine-tuning of electrolyte balance compared to the body's physiological state. Moreover, intercellular cross-talk in the CCD illustrates a sophisticated network in which different cell types can influence each other's transport functions, illustrating the dynamic nature of renal function. Such dependence is needed for effective fluid and electrolyte management so that the kidneys can address shifting physiological demands. Therefore, understanding of these intricate mechanisms of secretion is paramount to an understanding of renal homeostasis and physiology in the human body (Edwards & Crambert, 2017) (Figure 1.8).

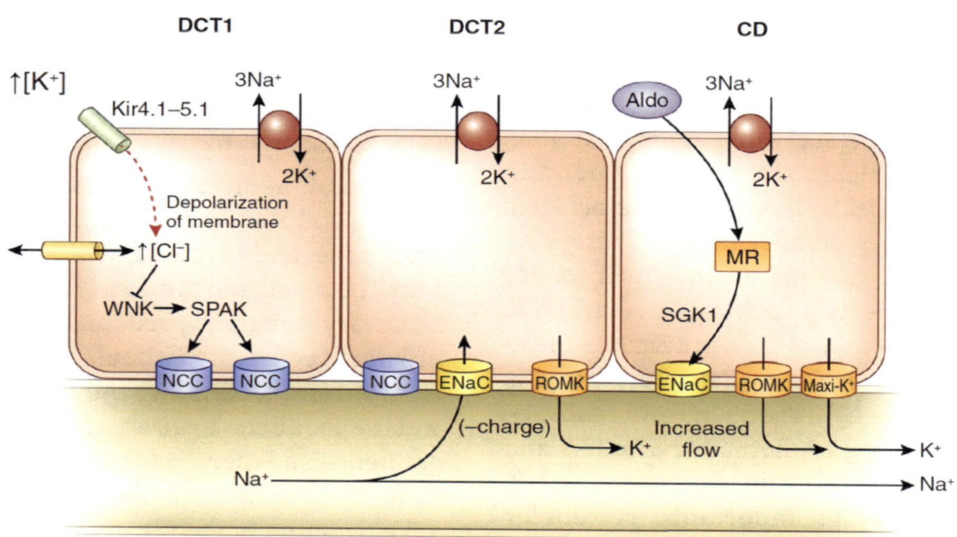

Figure 1.8. Kidney nephron secretion.

Source: https://www.researchgate.net/profile/Catherine-Clase/publication/336433937/figure/fig1/AS:831712204435457@1575307050092/Mechanisms-of-potassium-secretion-by-the-distal-nephron-showing-distal-convoluted.png.

1.3.1. Importance of Tubular Secretion

Tubular secretion is a vital renal physiological process that facilitates the excretion of some substances from the blood into tubular fluid. Tubular secretion occurs primarily in the renal tubules, where various solutes like ions, organic acids, and drugs are secreted into urine. Tubular secretion helps to establish homeostasis in the body by ensuring the body's electrolyte balance and acid-base equilibrium. Furthermore, it offers a means of excretion of waste products that do not get filtered by the glomerulus initially, such as certain drugs, as well as metabolic end products. The secretory process not only serves detoxification but also protects the kidney from getting damaged due to the presence of excess amounts of toxins. Hence, the ability to comprehend tubular secretion mechanisms is paramount in an effort to comprehend renal function in general as well as its impact on fluid balance within the body. Beyond its role in waste elimination, tubular secretion also plays a crucial role in acid-base regulation, particularly with the involvement of intercalated cells within the collecting tubules. These particular cells play a key role in secreting hydrogen ions and reabsorbing bicarbonate, thus influencing blood and urine pH. When metabolic acidosis occurs, the kidneys compensate by increasing proton secretion and increasing bicarbonate reabsorption, thereby achieving acid-base balance. Disregulation of this process can lead to distal renal tubular acidosis, where there is a failure to excrete hydrogen ions and reabsorb bicarbonate, leading to metabolic acidosis and electrolyte imbalance (Mungara et al., 2024). This underscores the importance of tubular secretion not only in eliminating waste but also in maintaining the exact balance of body fluids and acid-base status for optimal health. In addition, the significance of tubular secretion transcends simple renal function to affect broader physiological and clinical environments. Abnormalities in the process can have a major effect on the excretion and metabolism of drugs, since the majority of drugs rely on tubular secretion for their removal from the body. Information on mechanisms of tubular secretion affects pharmacological therapy, as inefficiency in the process may lead to drug toxicity or the failure of therapy. For instance, certain genetic mutations involving tubular transporters have been related to altered responses to drugs and increased susceptibility to renal disease. The union of tubular secretion and drug treatment signifies the central position of renal physiology in clinical application (Edwards & Crambert, 2017). Thus, the comprehension of tubular secretion not only enhances the knowledge of kidney function but also allows for the formulation of an effective treatment plan for various renal as well as systemic diseases.

1.3.2. Substances Secreted by the Nephron

The nephron, as the functional unit of the kidney, plays a significant role in maintaining fluid and electrolyte balance in the body. Among its many functions, the nephron is responsible for secreting a wide array of substances that have direct implications for renal physiology and overall homeostasis. Such constituents are waste products of metabolism , such as urea, creatinine, and uric acid, which are filtered out from the blood and ultimately found in the urine. Secretory functions predominantly occur in the proximal convoluted tubule (PCT), with some transporters facilitating the movement of such waste products against their concentration gradients, and thereby for their effective removal from the circulation. This not only performs a very important role in detoxification but also assists in controlling the body's overall level of hydration and balance of electrolytes. Another significant role that the nephron has is concerning the secretion of ions , such as potassium and hydrogen ions, both of which are required for the sake of acid-base homeostasis. The body's collecting duct and distal convoluted tubule of the nephrons are particularly involved in the fine-tuning of the secretion of these ions according to the body's physiological needs. The hormonal control, particularly by aldosterone, which stimulates sodium reabsorption and potassium secretion, is the main mechanism involved in this process. The fragile balance of these ion transport mechanisms not only contributes to the overall electrolyte balance but also plays a role in the modulation of blood volume and pressure. Disruption of maintaining this balance can result in extreme pathophysiological conditions, which highlights the nephron's singular position in fluid homeostasis. Finally, the nephron also secretes various endocrine messages and bioactive substances that have far-reaching action on renal and systemic physiology. Among these are hormones and peptides , such as erythropoietin and renin, which are secreted upon a change in the level of oxygen or blood pressure. They play crucial roles in erythropoiesis and initiation of the renin-angiotensin-aldosterone system (RAAS), respectively, which thus regulate blood pressure and water retention. In addition, studies of peptide hormones like tachykinins within the insect kidney have also enlightened the conserved excretory regulatory mechanisms in species that indicate evolutionary adaptations to fluid balance under varied environmental contexts. In this regard, understanding the full spectrum of substances being excreted by the nephron not only deepens our knowledge of renal physiology but also places it in the perspective of how its understanding is crucial to maintaining homeostasis and responding to physiological stressors (Agard et al., 2024) (Figure 1.9).

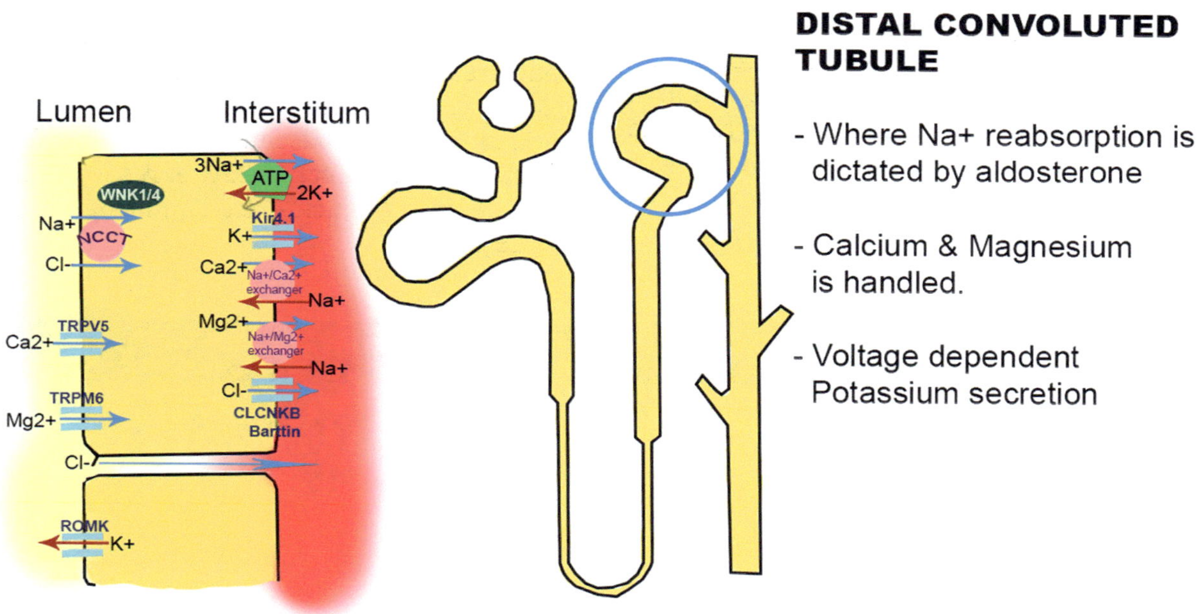

Figure 1.9. Distal convoluted tubule model.

Source: https://external-content.duckduckgo.com/iu/?u=https%3A%2F%2Fimg.stevegallik.org%2Fwhat_is_the_distal_convoluted_tubule_made_up_of.png&f=1&nofb=1&ipt=eabbe47f924de89e5782a8e5c5af2d6a8239448b814ba1463ace36c4f75b563d.

1.3.3. Regulation of Acid-Base Balance

Maintenance of acid-base balance is an essential physiological process that ensures the achievement of homeostasis in the human body. The organism uses a sophisticated mechanism in the form of buffer systems, respiratory regulation, and renal control to manage pH levels effectively. Buffers , such as bicarbonate, phosphate, and proteins act quickly to neutralize excessive acids or bases, and acid-base balance is maintained by the lungs through carbon dioxide (CO_2) regulation. The kidneys are crucial in the long-term regulation by eliminating or retaining hydrogen ions (H^+) and bicarbonate (HCO_3^-) within the body. The intricate process maintains blood pH within the very limited range of 7.35 to 7.45 that is necessary for optimal cellular function and metabolic processes (White, 2025). The kidneys have a direct role in acid-base homeostasis through many mechanisms, including tubular hydrogen ion secretion and reabsorption of renal bicarbonate. A fall in blood pH, indicating acidosis, causes the renal tubules to increase the excretion of H+ with the concomitant preservation of bicarbonate as a buffer. In alkalosis, the kidneys inhibit the secretion of H+ and enhance the secretion of bicarbonate, thereby ensuring the stability of pH. This renal response is slower than the buffering effect of other systems, requiring hours to days to maximize its effect. However, its significance should not be overestimated, as it provides a system of fine-tuning that is crucial for overall acid-base homeostasis (Hassan et al., 2020). The interaction of the various components of the acid-base regulatory systems emphasizes the importance of precise coordination in sustaining physiological balance. Normal pH of the blood is upheld at any price since derangement may lead to significant clinical presentation, for example, CNS dysfunction or metabolic alterations. The relationship between bicarbonate level and tension of carbon dioxide (PCO_2) is pointed out via the Henderson-Hasselbalch equation, which demonstrates how alteration of one will impact the other. An increased anion gap typically reflects metabolic acidosis and must be corrected with appropriate clinical evaluation and treatment. Accurate determination of the anion gap is necessary in order to diagnose and manage acid-base disorders, which further demonstrates the complexity of renal physiology as it pertains to acid-base equilibrium (White, 2025).

Test Your Knowledge

1. What is the primary purpose of tubular secretion in the nephron?
2. Which substances are typically secreted into the renal tubule from the blood?

1.4. Regulation of Fluid Balance

Learning Outcome

1. Identify the role of antidiuretic hormone (ADH);
2. Define the aldosterone and sodium balance;
3. Describe the thirst mechanism and fluid intake.

Regulation of fluid balance is a fundamental renal physiology, as it directly determines the body's general homeostasis. The chief function of the kidneys is to filter blood, reabsorb obligatory solutes, and eliminate waste products. Fluid balance is preserved by the intricate interaction of various mechanisms in the nephron, notably in areas like the glomerulus and the collecting duct. The nephron's ability to dynamically regulate reabsorption of water and electrolytes is significant, enabling the body to maintain its desired blood volume and osmotic pressure. This sensitivity is controlled through hormonal stimulation, with contributors , such as antidiuretic hormone (ADH) playing an important role in stimulating water reabsorption in the collecting ducts. Regulation of fluid excretion is vital, especially under various physiological conditions, so that cells remain well-hydrated and extracellular volumes of fluid are in their normal range. The cortical collecting duct (CCD) is also important in sodium and chloride balance regulation and, hence in the overall fluid homeostasis. Historically, it was believed that the movement of sodium was primarily mediated by principal cells, but recent data indicate the contribution of intercalated cells. Type B intercalated cells, for instance, are now found to mediate electroneutral NaCl reabsorption by Na-dependent and Na-independent Cl/HCO_3 exchange pathways (Edwards & Crambert, 2017). Further, type A intercalated cells are also able to actively mediate NaCl secretion via a bumetanide-sensitive pathway. This emerging understanding highlights the sophisticated interplay between cell types within the CCD that work synergistically to control NaCl balance and, by extension, fluid balance. Through the revelation of these cellular processes, researchers are able to better appreciate how the kidney adapts to physiological needs and maintains fluid stasis in response to variable circumstances. Regulation of fluid balance is also provided by a sophisticated interplay between various signaling pathways , such as natriuretic and anti-natriuretic factors. Hormones , such as atrial natriuretic peptide and angiotensin II have important roles in the interactive network, modulating sodium reabsorption and excretion.

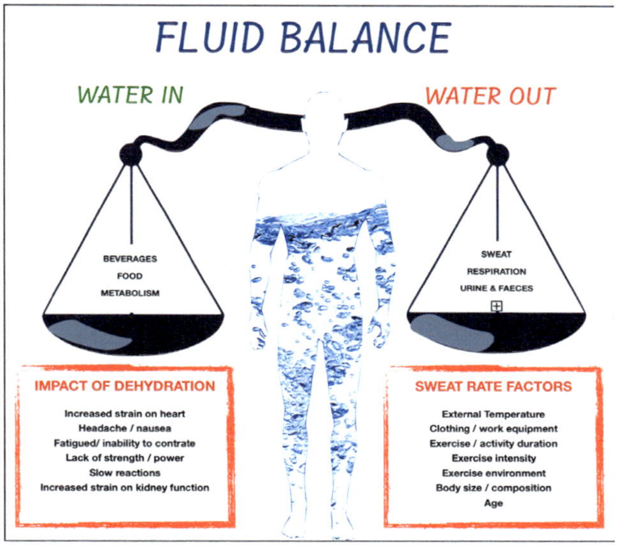

Figure 1.10. Functions of the kidney: fluid balance.

Source: https://leankitchen.org.uk/wp-content/uploads/2023/02/fluidbalance.png.

The delicate balance of these signals is of paramount significance in sustaining homeostasis in the kidney. Dysregulation of this interaction can lead to diseases , such as hypertension or nephrotic syndrome, wherein sodium excretion fails, underlining the pathological implications of impaired fluid balance control (Mikusic et al., 2014). The renal dopaminergic system and atrial natriuretic peptide are an essential counterbalance to the prooxidant effects of the renin-angiotensin system, underscoring the complexity of fluid balance. Understanding of these systems presents avenues for therapeutic intervention in renal disease compromising fluid and electrolyte homeostasis (Figure 1.10).

1.4.1. Role of Antidiuretic Hormone (ADH)

The role of antidiuretic hormone (ADH), or vasopressin, is most important in the regulation of the fluid status of the body and homeostasis. Released by the posterior pituitary gland and secreted from the hypothalamus, ADH regulates primarily the ability of the kidney to concentrate urine. When an increase in plasma osmolality, a sign of dehydration, is sensed by the body's osmoreceptors, ADH is released into the circulation. This hormone then acts on the collecting ducts in the kidneys to enhance reabsorption of water through aquaporin channels. The urine is therefore more concentrated, and excess water is conserved, which is significant in the case of dehydration states or increased plasma osmolality. Understanding the mechanistic action of ADH, particularly in disease when fluid balance becomes compromised, makes it significant in renal physiology. Its effect transcends mere water retention because it is intrinsically linked with sodium balance and extracellular fluid volume. In cases of abnormalities, like renal salt wasting syndrome (RSW), ADH's fine balance ensured by it can be disturbed, complicating clinical outcomes. RSW is also characterized by inappropriately excessive renal loss of sodium with resulting hypovolemia and hyponatremia, circumstances under which ADH secretion can become inappropriately increased (e.g., during the syndrome of inappropriate antidiuretic hormone secretion, or SIADH). Differentiation among these circumstances becomes necessary to optimize patient care algorithms. Particularly in elderly patients or those with neurological compromise, understanding the relationship between ADH and sodium balance will serve healthcare professionals well in the design of good treatment plans, underlining the importance of ADH in broader fields of fluid and electrolyte balance (Corte et al., 2018). In neurology critically ill patients, the regulation of sodium and water balance becomes increasingly complex, particularly in neurology. Central nervous system disorders can disrupt normal ADH release and production to develop SIADH or central diabetes insipidus. For instance, in neurology patients, elevated ADH exacerbates fluid retention, leading to dangerous electrolyte disturbances and plasma sodium level control problems. Early diagnosis of these disturbances is crucial because delayed treatment leads to severe complications , such as cerebral edema. Therefore, understanding the various pathophysiological mechanisms that occur with ADH, along with consequent effective management of such disorders, is still a foundation of renal physiology and fluid management in critical care settings (Crocker et al., 2006) (Figure 1.11).

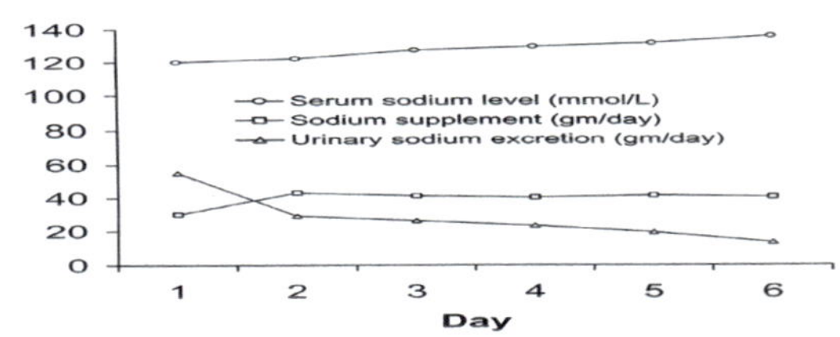

Figure 1.11. Renal salt-wasting syndrome.

Source: https://images.journals.lww.com/amjclinicaloncology/SocialThumb.00000421-200208000-00005.F1-5.jpeg.

1.4.2. Aldosterone and Sodium Balance

Aldosterone plays a central role in sodium balance within the renal system, albeit through its effect on the nephron collecting duct. It is a mineralocorticoid hormone produced in the adrenal cortex, which triggers sodium reabsorption of sodium ions in the cortical collecting duct (CCD) principal cells. As a reaction to increased plasma levels of aldosterone, the sodium channels (ENaC) in the apical membrane of these cells become enhanced, with more sodium reabsorption pathways. Aldosterone increases the activity of sodium-potassium ATPase pumps in the basolateral membrane, which actively transport sodium out of the cell and maintain a beneficial concentration gradient for ongoing reabsorption. Consequently, the increased reabsorption of sodium directly influences extracellular fluid volume and blood pressure, illustrating the linkage between hormonal and renal function. Beyond sodium transport, the new appreciation for the role played by intercalated cells in the CCD has revolutionized the narrative of sodium balance. In the past, these cells were thought of in terms of acid-base homeostasis. But latest studies have established that type B intercalated cells are able to mediate electroneutral NaCl reabsorption efficiently through mechanisms involving bicarbonate and chloride exchange by vacuolar H-ATPase pumps.

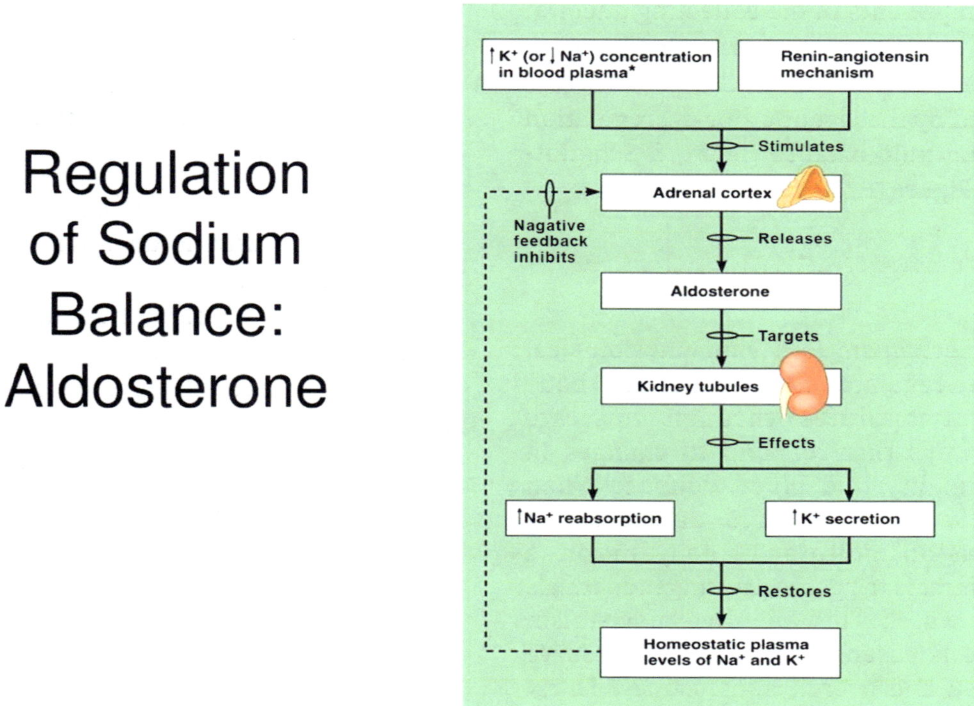

Figure 1.12. Regulation of sodium balance by aldosterone.

Source: https://image1.slideserve.com/3063097/regulation-of-sodium-balance-aldosterone3-l.jpg.

Type A intercalated cells, however, partake in NaCl secretion by a bumetanide-sensitive mechanism driven by apical H, K-ATPase type 2 pumps. This interrelation between principal and intercalated cells illustrates a complex network in the CCD to account for sodium balance while, concurrently, maintaining acid-base balance, revealing the vast versatility of the nephron segment to accommodate physiological needs (Edwards & Crambert, 2017). Moreover, the structure of tight junctions within the collecting duct epithelium plays a crucial role in sodium and fluid balance as a whole. Composed of specific claudin proteins, the tight junctions contribute to the barrier function, which regulates paracellular transport across the epithelium. Claudins like Cldn-3, Cldn-4, Cldn-7, and Cldn-8 found in the collecting duct play a critical function in dictating the extent to which sodium and other solutes can pass through epithelial barriers. Disruption of these tight junctions could lead to drastic physiological abnormalities like impaired blood pressure control and water homeostasis. Thus, understanding the role of tight junctions and their components in the collecting duct not only unveils some renal physiology enigma but also points out that they are such good targets to be targeted by therapeutics for dysregulation of sodium and fluid balance (Leiz ., & Schmidt-Ott, 2019) (Figure 1.12).

1.4.3. Thirst Mechanism and Fluid Intake

The thirst mechanism is a vital physiological function that regulates fluid intake and body hydration. It operates through intricate neural pathways that respond to changes in plasma osmolality and blood volume. When hypothalamic osmoreceptors detect rising osmolality, as an indicator of dehydration, a message of thirst is triggered, causing individuals to consume water. This adaptive mechanism for fluid loss is essential in order to preserve renal function and overall homeostasis. Thirst has been found to be regulated by behavioral as well as environmental factors, further making the argument that hydration is not merely a physiological necessity but a learned behavior based on lifestyle considerations. Understanding this mechanism provides insight into mechanisms of body water conservation and the critical role of fluid balance as a fundamental renal physiology principle (Rowland, 2021). In the clinic, particularly in renal transplant patients, fluid management becomes even more complex. Patients are advised to take large amounts of fluid to prevent dehydration and maintain kidney function. However, very high consumption recommendations, such as, consumption of over three liters per day, do not appear to be based on robust science. This difference implies the necessity for a gap between traditional medical advice and new findings contradicting high levels of fluid consumption among certain populations. Certain research findings are suggesting that thirst drinking may be a more appropriate recommendation than rigid intake instructions, particularly for patients with skewed perceptions of thirst or behavioral constraints in hydration (Mao & Chacko, 2020). It highlights the need for patient-specific strategies for fluid therapy based on the patient's heterogeneity in responding to thirst and fluid needs.

Furthermore, renal physiology connection to hydration status is an intriguing research question. Experiments examining the effects of hydration on renal blood flow and glomerular filtration rates are essential because these are key measures that are central to kidney function. Yet most that has been reported so far has been conducted in animal models, which raises the uncertainty about whether findings can be extrapolated back to human physiology. Particularly in the context of post-renal transplant and chronic kidney disease complications, an awareness of how mechanisms of thirst adjust to fluid consumption patterns can be invaluable when seeking to optimize patient care. Future research should pursue exploring individualized hydration strategies that take into account physiological differences between individuals and possible differential reactions to increased fluid intake (Rowland, 2021). These investigations can provide the basis for creating evidence-based guidelines balancing the danger of dehydration and overhydration in diverse patient populations.

Test Your Knowledge

1. Which hormones are primarily involved in regulating fluid balance in the body?
2. How does the antidiuretic hormone (ADH) influence water reabsorption in the kidneys?

1.5. Electrolyte Balance

Learning Outcome

1. Describe the sodium and potassium regulation;
2. Define the calcium and phosphate homeostasis;
3. Discuss the impact of electrolyte imbalance.

The electrolyte balance is the key to renal physiology since the kidneys play a pivotal role in ensuring homeostasis through the regulation of the various electrolytes within the body. Electrolytes , such as sodium, potassium, calcium, and bicarbonate play vital roles in numerous physiological functions , such as nerve conduction, muscle contraction, and acid-base balance. The kidneys achieve this delicate balance through a range of mechanisms, such as, filtration, reabsorption, and secretion in the nephron, the functional unit of the kidney. Through the precisely controlled functioning of these mechanisms, the kidneys not only control proper electrolyte levels but also control the body's overall fluid status, influencing blood pressure and volume. Any break in this balance has the potential to precipitate severe clinical disorders, so an understanding of renal function is pertinent in the management and diagnosis of electrolyte imbalance, emphasizing the importance of renal physiology to the clinician (Yameny, 2025). One of the most important elements of electrolyte balance is homeostatic regulation of sodium and potassium levels, which is largely under hormonal control. The renin-angiotensin-aldosterone system (RAAS) plays a significant role in sodium retention and potassium excretion. Aldosterone, secreted by the adrenal glands, affects the distal convoluted tubule and collecting ducts of the nephron to increase sodium reabsorption with a stimulation of potassium secretion. This reflects the function of the kidneys to maintain blood volume and pressure and how sodium excretion must be controlled closely in order to obtain overall fluid balance in the body. Besides, in conditions of increased sodium levels, the body can trigger natriuretic peptides that promote sodium excretion. These intricate hormonal mechanisms ensure that even during changes in dietary consumption, the kidneys can respond accordingly to meet the homeostasis of electrolytes and prevent the ill effects of derangements, including hypertension and arrhythmias (Chaudhari et al., 2020). Other than sodium and potassium, calcium and phosphate balance is another critical element of electrolyte balance controlled by the kidneys effectively. The kidneys maintain calcium homeostasis through stimulation of vitamin D and regulation of parathyroid hormone (PTH) levels that influence calcium absorption in the intestines and renal tubular reabsorption. A subtle feedback mechanism inhibits low serum calcium from triggering the release of PTH, which subsequently brings about enhanced reabsorption of calcium accompanied by concomitant excretion of phosphate in order to maintain a maximum calcium-phosphate product necessary for bone mineralization. Furthermore, the renal electrolyte management is adjusted by various inputs including dietary, hormonal signals, and overall health status, exemplifying the adaptive character of the kidneys to maintain balance. Disruption of this regulation results in diseases , such as osteoporosis and kidney stones, underscoring the important role renal physiology plays in controlling the body's electrolyte balance (Yameny, 2025) (Figure 1.13).

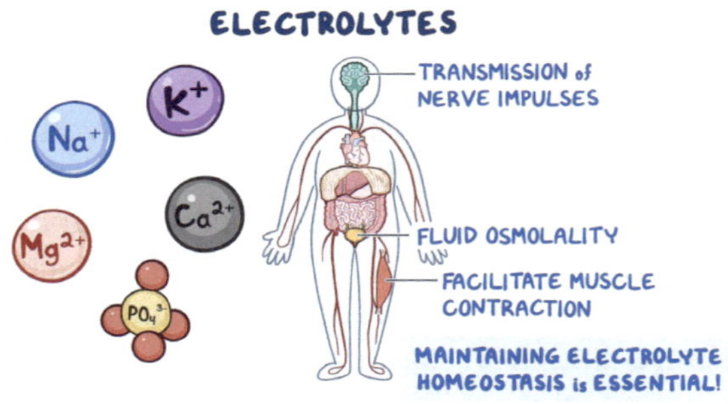

Figure 1.13. Electrolyte balance.

Source: https://external-content.duckduckgo.com/iu/?u=https%3A%2F%2Fosmose-it.s3.amazonaws.com%2FU540jeRATn6H40eKXELeTcM2QkGJAIiP%2F_.jpg&f=1&nofb=1&ipt=593dad6691b04d2e04947d4994025303a9ecb82ffa77599a5b19d06877af516d.

1.5.1. Sodium and Potassium Regulation

Potassium and sodium are critical body electrolytes needed for fluid balance, conduction of nerve impulses, and muscle contraction. The body depends primarily on the kidneys to regulate the electrolyte levels via a highly intricate filtration, reabsorption, and excretion process. Reabsorption of sodium is predominantly performed in the loop of Henle and the proximal convoluted tubule, and reabsorption takes place via numerous various transport processes back into the circulatory system. Conversely, potassium control primarily occurs in the distal convoluted tubule and collecting duct, where it is either reabsorbed or secreted based on the body's needs. This specific regulation is vital since a derangement of the sodium and potassium balance will yield grave medical consequences, such as, hypertension and cardiac arrhythmias. Thus, the kidneys possess a vital role in obtaining homeostasis by controlling such important ions. The balance of sodium and potassium is controlled by a variety of hormones, such as, aldosterone and atrial natriuretic peptide (ANP). Aldosterone, secreted by the adrenal cortex, stimulates reabsorption of sodium and secretion of potassium in the kidneys to maintain the right proportion of these electrolytes. An opposite effect is exerted by ANP, secreted by the heart upon increased blood volume, which results in increased excretion of sodium as well as lowering blood pressure. These hormonal interactions suggest the importance of renal physiology to the overall balance of fluids. In addition, the kidneys are continually monitoring blood levels of electrolytes and adjusting their rate of secretion and reabsorption accordingly, once again highlighting their electrolyte balancing function. Understanding such regulatory mechanisms is essential for the appreciation of the complexity of renal function and its impact on general well-being and health. Changes in the regulation of potassium and sodium can result in severe clinical effects, especially in chronic kidney disease (CKD) and heart failure. In CKD, kidneys increasingly lose their ability to filter blood and therefore sodium and potassium accumulate in the blood. This leads to hypertension and hyperkalemia and extreme effects on cardiovascular status. Additionally, potassium physiology becomes increasingly important in heart failure patients, where potassium levels must be watched very closely so as not to risk potentially fatal dysrhythmias. Thus, a sophisticated awareness of the renal mechanisms of sodium and potassium control is essential for medical professionals. Through cultivating this knowledge, healthcare professionals are better able to prevent and manage electrolyte imbalance, leading ultimately to improved patient outcomes and quality of life (Vale, 2020; Yameny, 2025).

1.5.2. Calcium and Phosphate Homeostasis

Calcium and phosphate homeostasis is critical to renal physiology, especially considering their interdependent roles in many body processes. They are not only crucial to bone strength, but calcium is also required for the contraction of muscles, clotting of blood, and transmission of neurotransmitters. Phosphate, however, is crucial for energy transfer, facilitating ATP and cellular signaling pathway synthesis. The kidneys are key in regulating the balance of these two electrolytes by mechanisms like filtration, reabsorption, and secretion. Between the two, calcium and phosphate balance is most sensitive because any disruption can lead to harmful consequences on health, such as, bone disease and vascular calcification. An appreciation of such relationships provides a perspective on how abnormalities in kidney function can influence systemic health outcomes, thereby augmenting the relevance of renal physiology to overall phosphate and calcium homeostasis (Heron, 2018).

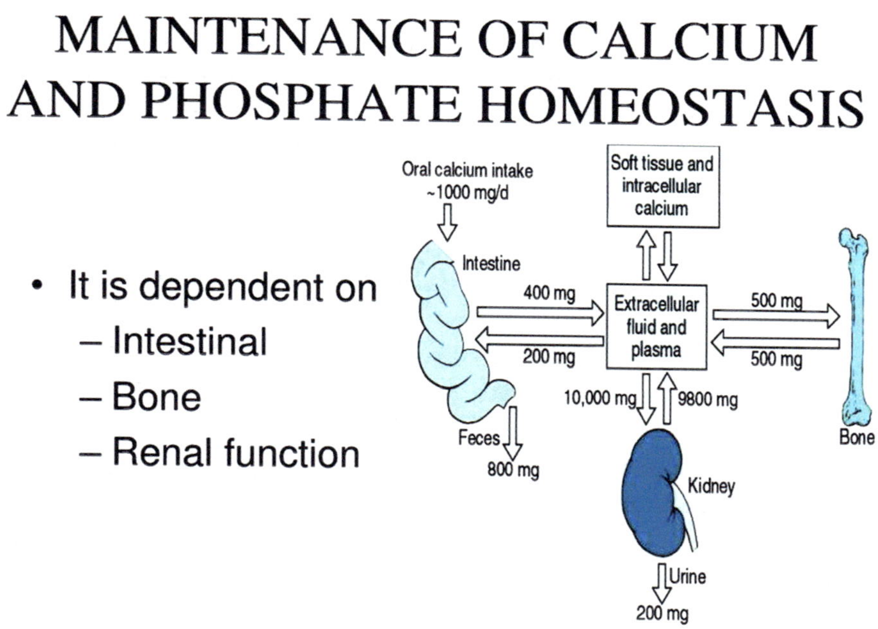

Figure 1.14. Calcium and phosphate homeostasis.

Source: https://image1.slideserve.com/3356849/maintenance-of-calcium-and-phosphate-homeostasis-l.jpg.

To the end of establish proper calcium and phosphate balance, the kidneys employ complex hormonal signaling pathways, with the primary players being parathyroid hormone (PTH) and vitamin D. PTH plays a central role in increasing serum calcium by causing renal tubular reabsorption of calcium and mobilization of phosphate from the bone. Vitamin D, in contrast, controls intestinal absorption of calcium and phosphate and also complements their homeostasis. Besides this, kidneys have specialized transport mechanisms, like sodium-phosphate co-transporters, to facilitate reabsorption of phosphate and regulate its renal excretion. The understanding of these hormonal and cellular interactions is important to clinicians since dysregulation may lead to hyperparathyroidism or renal osteodystrophy. Thus, the interaction among these hormonal controls highlights the significance of maintaining calcium and phosphate homeostasis to prevent catastrophic health outcomes (Bratty et al., 2012). Moreover, renal function in the regulation of calcium and phosphate homeostasis is more than mere reabsorption and filtration and involves a dynamic adaptation to shifting physiological requirements. Renal regulation is modulated by dietary intake and hormonal state. For instance, with excessive phosphate intake or tubular damage, renal excretion of excess phosphate is impaired, leading to hyperphosphatemia. This state can accelerate secondary hyperparathyroidism, further complicating calcium homeostasis. Conversely, hypocalcemia can induce stimulated PTH release, leading to increased phosphate excretion in order to reestablish balance. The kidneys thus serve as an active interface between nutrient inputs and systemic electrolyte homeostasis, which mirrors more general physiological states. A complete understanding of renal function with respect to calcium and phosphate homeostasis is essential to the treatment of clinical disturbances with resultant imbalances, and as such, is a field of significant study and clinical interest (Heron, 2018) (Figure 1.14).

1.5.3. Impact of Electrolyte Imbalance

The impact of electrolyte imbalance on renal physiology is an important factor for the purposes of fluid balance and overall body homeostasis. Electrolytes like sodium, potassium, calcium, and chloride are involved in numerous physiological functions, ranging from muscle contraction to nerve impulse transmission. During an electrolyte imbalance, the kidneys' function is to offset these imbalances. For instance, an increase in serum potassium will activate the kidney to secrete more potassium, thereby attempting to correct normal levels. Yet, chronic imbalances, such as, occur in disease states of chronic kidney disease, lead to deranged renal function. This dysfunction subsequently inhibits the kidneys' ability to regulate fluid and electrolyte balance, leading to additional issues , such as hyperkalemia, which is lethal if not addressed rapidly, representing the overriding role renal physiology has in the regulation of electrolyte balance. In addition, the intricacies of numerous hormonal signals significantly influence the way in which the kidneys respond to the imbalance of electrolytes. The renin-angiotensin-aldosterone system (RAAS) and atrial natriuretic peptide (ANP) are two of the most important components of this regulation. If there is a derangement, then it can upset the fine balance between the natriuretic and antinatriuretic factors, and the fluid balance becomes more complex. Excess angiotensin II, for example, can stimulate sodium retention and thus exacerbate conditions like hypertension and fluid overload. ANP, conversely, promotes natriuresis and counteracts the reabsorptive effect of aldosterone.

The kinetics of such interactions illustrate the delicate balance maintained by the renal system and how its derangement can lead to pathologies, in line with findings indicating the involvement of renal dopaminergic systems in maintaining the oxidant-antioxidant balance for optimal renal function (Mikusic et al., 2014). The impact of electrolyte disturbances has widespread implications extending beyond the kidneys and affecting overall systemic health and producing many pathologies. In diseases like nephrotic syndrome, when sodium excretion is impaired, renal impairment can lead to fluid accumulation and hypertension. These pathologies can form a cycle of vicious causation in which severe electrolyte disturbances result in renal stress and damage, further complicating the treatment. Electrolytes must be checked routinely, particularly in patients with underlying renal disorders, since this enables early treatment before fatal complications set in. Modeling, including the Guyton model of circulatory and fluid regulation, illustrates the interdependence and complexity of these physiological systems and why it is so critical to understand electrolyte dynamics in terms of renal physiology for health and to minimize the dangers inherent in imbalances (Leonard, 1985).

Test Your Knowledge

1. Which electrolytes are most commonly regulated by the kidneys?
2. How does aldosterone influence sodium and potassium balance?

1.6. Acid-Base Homeostasis

Learning Outcome

1. Describe the mechanisms of acid-base regulation;
2. Define the role of the kidneys in pH balance;
3. Identify the clinical implications of acid-base disorders.

Acid-base homeostasis is essential for the maintenance of metabolic processes and overall physiological equilibrium in the human body. The homeostatic balance is maintained by the kidneys through the regulation of blood pH and extracellular fluid pH. The kidneys preserve the balance by excreting hydrogen ions (H^+) and reabsorbing bicarbonate (HCO_3^-), and this action has a direct effect on acid-base balance in the body. This regulation is particularly critical in the renal tubules, where specific mechanisms are employed to ensure that the plasma pH lies within the critical range necessary for optimal cellular function. Consequent to this, derangement of these regulatory mechanisms can lead to metabolic acidosis or alkalosis, pointing towards the role of renal function in maintaining acid-base homeostasis (White, 2025). The complexity of acid-base regulation by the kidneys can be further dissected through the functioning of the cortical collecting duct (CCD). This is the segment of the nephron critical for bicarbonate and sodium transport, whereby distinct cell types in the CCD work together in an attempt to establish acid-base balance. Recent evidence has revealed that type B intercalated cells, previously thought to have a function only in acid secretion, also participate in NaCl reabsorption by mechanisms involving Na-dependent and Na-independent Cl/HCO_3^- exchange. This discovery highlights the coupling between NaCl and acid-base transport mechanisms in the CCD and suggests a more complex interaction than was initially recognized. Understanding these mechanisms explains clearly how the kidneys regulate electrolyte balance and body pH finely (Edwards & Crambert, 2017). Acid-base homeostasis is an active process that involves the participation of multiple organ systems, the respiratory and renal systems in particular, that interact and adapt to a variety of physiological states. The lungs contribute to such a balance by regulating carbon dioxide (CO_2) levels through ventilation and, therefore, impacting carbonic acid concentration in blood. Such interdependent action within the system enables any fluctuation in acid-base status to be aptly reversed because such a sensitive relationship between the renal and respiratory systems is critical in blunting disturbances. Moreover, when such imbalances as respiratory alkalosis or metabolic acidosis occur, feedback mechanisms take action to restore homeostasis, underlining the role played by renal function as well as by fluid balance in ensuring a constant internal environment for the body's cells (White, 2025) (Figure 1.15).

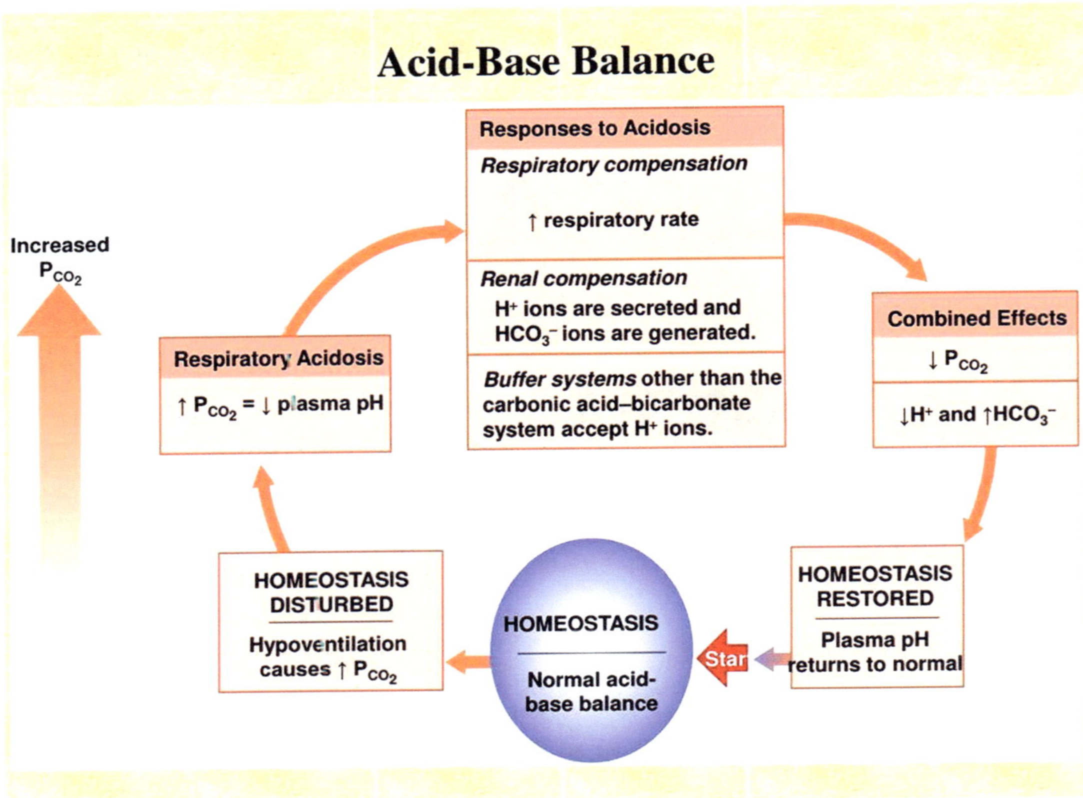

Figure 1.15. Homeostasis acid-base balance.

Source: https://image.slideserve.com/1447148/acid-base-balance1-l.jpg

1.6.1. Mechanisms of Acid-Base Regulation

The acid-base regulating mechanisms are directly related to the renal system's ability to attain homeostasis. The function of the kidneys is pivotal in the regulation of the hydrogen ion (H^+) and bicarbonate (HCO_3^-) equilibrium of the blood. At the center of this is the cortical collecting duct (CCD), which is an important area for NaCl balance and acid-base status regulation. Recent studies have challenged traditional assumptions about Na transport, with the demonstration that both type A and type B intercalated cells of the CCD have crucial roles in acid-base homeostasis. Type A intercalated cells are involved in H+ secretion, while type B intercalated cells secrete bicarbonate. This dynamic interaction not only maintains acid-base homeostasis but also determines the variability of the transport mechanism, hence demonstrating a complex regulatory system inherent in renal physiology needed in overall fluid homeostasis and metabolic balance (Edwards & Crambert, 2017). Besides cellular processes of the collecting duct, renal regulation of acid-base homeostasis is more than immediate ion transport. Acid-base homeostasis is a synchronized process involving multiple systems, including extracellular and intracellular buffers, respiratory, and renal systems, in conjunction. This is provided by the lungs in the form of a rapid response through excretion of CO_2, affecting the pH levels of the blood. However, kidneys provide a slow but longer regulatory response in the form of modification of the excretion or reabsorption of hydrogen ions and bicarbonate. This intricate relationship brings into focus the necessity of understanding acid-base regulation from the perspective of systemic health. Disruption of this regulatory equilibrium can have monumental clinical consequences, which highlights the kidneys role as not only regulators of electrolyte balance but also key players in acid-base homeostasis (White, 2025). The challenge of maintaining acid-base balance is particularly evident in disease states, where renal physiology could be compromised. Diabetes mellitus, diabetic acidosis, and metabolic alkalosis all demonstrate how the delicate equilibrium of acid and base can be disturbed and the need for an understanding of the underlying processes involved in the kidneys' function in these disorders. The emergent functions of the different cell types within the nephron, particularly in the collecting duct, suggest the complexity of controls in operation. As research continues to unveil the interactions of various transport mechanisms, it also becomes increasingly evident that the nephron's environment is no longer a mere filter but an active metabolic regulator. Having these mechanisms identified will not only increase our knowledge about renal physiology but also inform clinical approaches to diagnose and manage acid-base disturbances (Edwards & Crambert, 2017) (Figure 1.16).

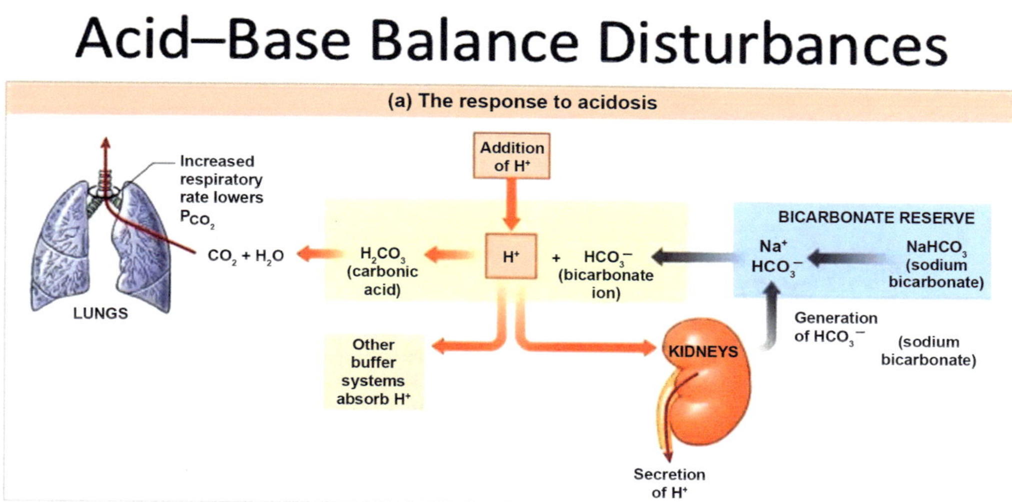

Figure 1.16. Mechanisms of acid-base regulation.

Source: https://image.slidesharecdn.com/acidbasebalancefinal-120325203702-phpapp02/95/acid-base-balance-23-728.jpg?cb=1333516481.

1.6.2. Role of the Kidneys in pH Balance

The kidneys play a vital role in the acid-base balance of the body's homeostasis. The balance is regulated primarily by the excretion of acids and the reabsorption of bicarbonate from urine. When the blood becomes acidic, the kidneys increase the elimination of hydrogen ions, concurrently reabsorbing bicarbonate ions to counteract acidity. Conversely, during alkalosis, the kidneys can absorb hydrogen ions and remove bicarbonate in an effort to revert to normal pH. The efficiency of this biological function is important, as even slight deviations from blood pH become detrimental to metabolic processes and organ function, even more so emphasizing the kidneys' role as central homeostatic regulators of renal physiology. Aquaporins, the specific membrane proteins, are also involved in renal pH balance control. Specific aquaporin isoforms, particularly aquaglyceroporins, facilitate the transport of water and other small molecules, and they play a significant role in renal functions. Their ability to selectively allow passage of water is the basis for the ability of the kidneys to concentrate urine as well as manage fluid balance efficiently, and influence the pH of the body fluids. New studies indicate that aquaglyceroporins found in the kidneys could be crucial in nitrogen balance control, continuing to connect their function to acid-base homeostasis. As we learn more about aquaporins, we can gain a greater sense of how they affect renal health and how intriguing it is to keep the body's pH balanced (Kłek, 2016).

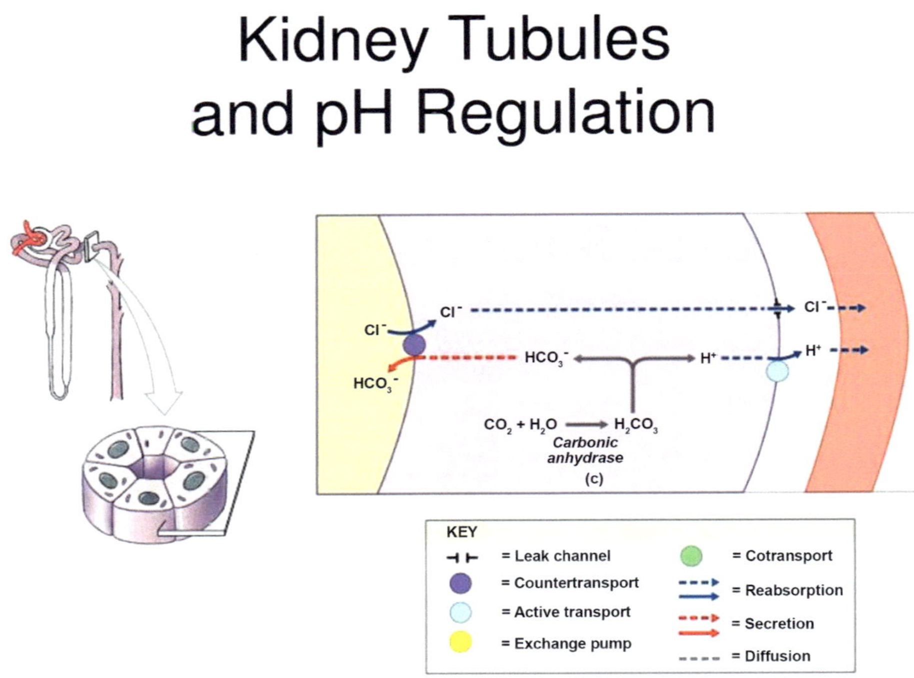

Figure 1.17. Role of the kidneys in pH balance.

Source: https://image1.slideserve.com/2127603/kidney-tubules-and-ph-regulation1-l.jpg.

In addition, the intricate interaction of renal function with environmental stressors cannot be left out, particularly concerning exposure to heavy metals. Heavy metals are of significant health concern because they usually induce renal injury and acid-base disturbance. For instance, metals , such as cadmium and lead will accumulate in the tissues of the body, hindering metabolic functions and worsening oxidative stress, thereby affecting renal function. This interference makes it hard for the kidneys to maintain pH levels appropriately and leads to further complications in the form of metabolic acidosis or alkalosis. Alleviating the effects of heavy metal poisoning is crucial not only for renal function but also for the maintenance of the intricate mechanisms involved in pH balance of the body (Jaishankar et al., 2014). Therefore, the interaction is an active research arena to further understand the dynamics of how environmental exposure interacts with renal physiology (Figure 1.17).

1.6.3. Clinical Implications of Acid-Base Disorders

The management of acid-base disorders is a critical component of clinical practice, particularly within the framework of renal physiology and fluid resuscitation. Acid-base disorders can be caused by numerous different conditions , such as respiratory failure, renal insufficiency, or metabolic disturbances and as such necessitate an advanced understanding of the pathophysiology involved. Specifically, the function of the kidney in maintaining acid-base homeostasis by modulating bicarbonate reabsorption and hydrogen ion secretion cannot be overemphasized. Physicians must be observant in identifying and treating these disorders before causing hazardous complications , such as cardiac arrhythmia or neurologic sequelae. Moreover, knowledge of the way fluid balance is influenced by acid-base imbalances will guide therapeutic measures effectively, highlighting the interconnectedness of renal function and overall well-being. In the perioperative setting, intravenous fluid therapy with hydroxyethyl starch (HES) seems to raise issues regarding acid-base balance and renal function. Studies are put into perspective by literature to highlight methodological shortcomings in those supporting restriction of HES solutions, particularly in high-risk patients , such as critically ill patients. Proper use of such solutions can restore fluid homeostasis and attain hemodynamic optimization, both of which are of critical importance in maintaining acid-base equilibrium in the face of surgery. Notwithstanding this, the danger of adverse effects necessitates a patient-dependent evaluation of factors, such as, existing renal impairment or ongoing acid-base disturbance. As such, an understanding of the nuance of intravenous fluids, particularly that relating to acid-base disorders, is still relevant to the facilitation of patient safety and optimization of outcomes within clinical practice (De Hert & De Baerdemaeker, 2014). In addition, acid-base disorders also have long-term clinical significance that extends beyond immediate treatment for kidney health. Long-term disturbances in acid-base balance can lead to complications in the kidneys , such as renal tubular acidosis or impaired renal function, in populations with higher risk. The monitoring of such disorders in patients with CKD becomes an extremely important factor, considering the worsening of kidney decline caused by accumulated acid. In addition, patient education about the importance of acid-base homeostasis and the ways it can be maintained through diet and hydration habits can empower patients to become actively involved in their own care. As a deeper understanding of acid-base management unfolds, particularly within the context of renal physiology and fluid balance, future studies will prove essential to the evolution of more effective clinical practices and better patient outcomes (Solberg & Pleasant, 1984).

Test Your Knowledge

1. What is the normal pH range of blood, and why is it important to maintain it?
2. How do the kidneys help regulate acid-base balance?

1.7. Pathophysiology of Renal Function

Learning Outcome

1. Understand the common renal disorders;
2. Discuss the impact of diabetes on renal physiology;
3. State the effects of hypertension on kidney function.

The renal pathophysiology is key to the knowledge of how the kidneys obtain homeostasis, particularly of fluid and electrolyte balance. The kidneys first filter blood, regulate the extracellular volume of fluid, levels of electrolytes, and remove metabolic waste products. In renal disease, these mechanisms can be compromised, triggering a cascade of physiological derangements. Chronic Renal Failure (CRF) is such an impairment that is characterized by a progressive loss of the glomerular filtration rate (GFR) and the inability of the body to regulate normal metabolic and fluid balance. As a result, patients may experience signs of uremia that indicate the accumulation of waste products in the blood. Identification of three recent cases where CRF was confirmed has generated increased interest in mechanisms of CRF and therapy approaches, with an imperative for new therapeutic interventions to enhance renal function and quality of life in affected patients (White, 2025). Fluid balance, particularly the ability of the kidneys to accommodate changes in hydration status and blood volume, is closely related to renal function.

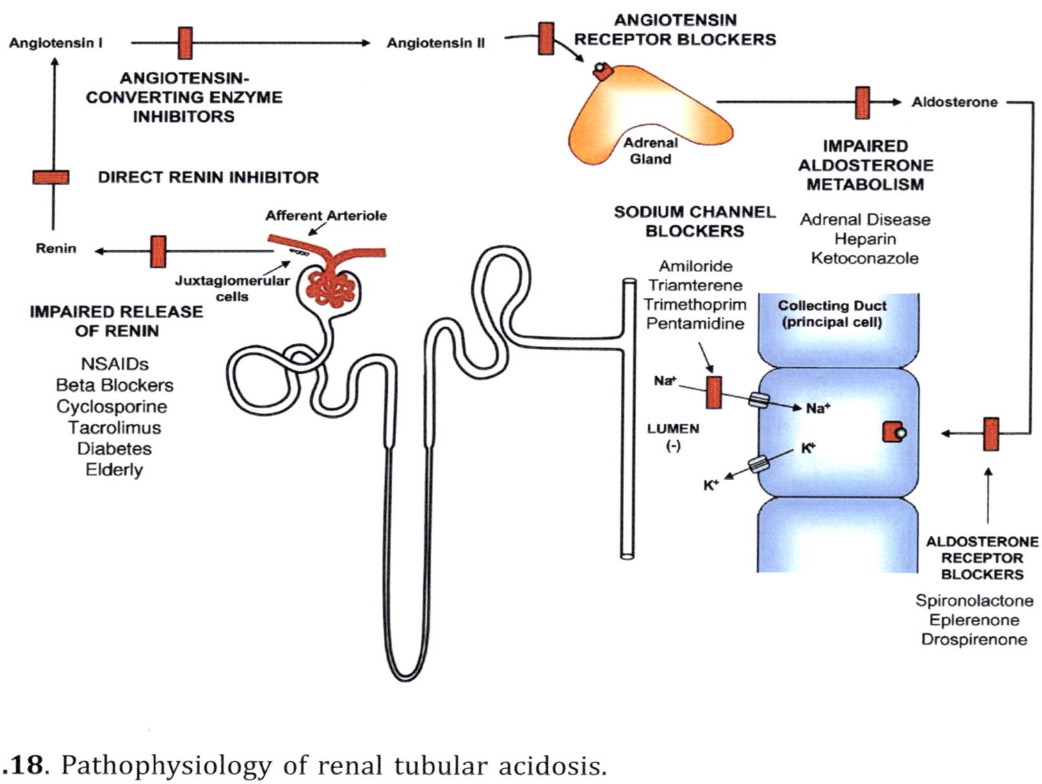

Figure 1.18. Pathophysiology of renal tubular acidosis.

Source: https://els-jbs-prod-cdn.jbs.elsevierhealth.com/cms/attachment/d8c68e17-40e8-465f-b897-4af8c7a20d34/gr6_lrg.jpg.

This dynamic relationship is accentuated by the role of renal blood flow (RBF) in glomerular filtration. Overload or overhydration from excessive fluid intake can predispose to conditions like fluid overload, which adversely affects the cardiovascular system and favors complications. Portal vein pulsatility index has been a crucial marker of fluid status, illustrating the interface between increased circulatory volume and alterations in venous hemodynamics. Changes in these venous indices can reflect volume-induced congestion, impacting renal perfusion and worsening renal dysfunction. Through understanding of the correlation between renal function and fluid dynamics, clinicians can better advance patient care through adequate management of fluids, eventually leading to better outcomes in critically ill patients (Andrei et al., 2024). Renal dysfunction pathophysiological processes are multifactorial and complex and often reflect the impact of underlying systemic illness. Inflammatory processes, oxidative stress, and metabolic dysregulation all play a part in compromised kidney function in diseases , such as diabetes and hypertension. They have the potential to lead to glomerulosclerosis and fibrosis of the tubulointerstitium, further compromising renal function. As an example, increased renal vascular resistance and decreased GFR can result from ongoing inflammation, setting up a vicious cycle of injury and compromised kidney function. It is significant to comprehend such pathophysiological changes for the development of targeted therapy that does not disrupt renal integrity. With ongoing advancements in the field, research studies to clarify distinct molecular and cellular processes engaged will provide insight into new therapeutic options so that healthcare professionals can prevent or improve the detrimental influences of renal disease on well-being (M S*, 2024) (Figure 1.18).

1.7.1. Common Renal Disorders

General renal disease comprises many illness that modify the normal workings of the kidneys, significantly impacting fluid status, electrolyte balance, and homeostasis in general. Acute kidney injury (AKI) is a general disorder that can be induced by a myriad of etiologies, including ischemia, nephrotoxins, and sepsis. AKI results in an acute decrease in renal function, which is characterized by the inability to effectively excrete waste products and maintain fluid and electrolyte balance. The implications of this decline can be harsh, such as, fluid overload, hyperkalemia, and metabolic acidosis. The early recognition of the indicators and treatment of the underlying cause are responsible for the prevention of permanent kidney injury and the restoration of normal renal physiology. Chronic kidney disease (CKD) is another serious renal condition, with a gradual decline in kidney function in the long term. This disease is often a consequence of long-standing comorbidities , such as diabetes mellitus and hypertension, resulting in progressive loss of nephrons and subsequent reductions in glomerular filtration rate (GFR). The consequences of CKDs extend much beyond the kidney, as it has the potential to trigger systemic complications like cardiovascular disease and bone mineral disorders. Fluid management is particularly difficult in patients with CKD due to their compromised ability to excrete excess water and solutes. A general understanding of the pathophysiology permits specific intervention, which is required for the improvement of outcomes in fluid and electrolyte homeostasis balance preservation. Disorders of sodium and water balance, such as, the syndrome of inappropriate secretion of antidiuretic hormone (SIADH) and cerebral salt wasting syndrome, significantly complicate the treatment of patients suffering from renal disease. SIADH generates inappropriate water retention, resulting in dilutional hyponatremia and potential neurological consequences of cerebral edema. In contrast, cerebral salt wasting syndrome elicits inappropriate renal sodium excretion, aggravating hyponatremia and volume loss. Understanding the pathologically distinct mechanisms of these diseases, especially in critically ill patients, is crucial because normalized sodium and fluid balance are both requisite for maximal patient therapy. Ineffective management strategies should be eschewed, weighing intervention benefits against risks to prevent overtreatment and preserve sufficient hydration (Crocker et al., 2006). Additionally, fluid therapy must be practiced carefully, embracing evidence-based treatment protocols for interventions like hydroxyethyl starches, which have been questioned for their safety in various clinical contexts (De Hert & De Baerdemaeker, 2014).

1.7.2. Impact of Diabetes on Renal Physiology

The impact of diabetes on renal physiology is extremely important and multifaceted, encompassing numerous renal function and fluid balance parameters. Diabetes mellitus with hyperglycemia results in a cascade of pathophysiological changes in the kidneys. Hyperglycemia for a long duration may lead to diabetic nephropathy, a condition with structural and functional abnormalities in the renal glomeruli and tubular elements. Since the kidneys are unable to manage the increased load of glucose, the filtration rate can be compromised, resulting in chronic kidney disease (CKD) and eventually renal failure when not treated. Importantly, diabetic patients are likely to experience poor sodium handling due to altered renal physiology that is likely to exacerbate fluid overload and hypertension, thus making diabetes as well as the management strategies of its systemic complications much harder. From a fluid balance perspective, diabetes directly affects renal tubular function via maladaptive mechanisms for responding to osmotic stimuli. For instance, experiments have demonstrated that regulatory volume decrease (RVD) mechanisms that typically regulate cell volume under osmotic stress can be less effective in diabetic patients. Specifically, the proximal convoluted tubule, important for sodium reabsorption and handling of fluid, may have decreased sensitivity in its regulation of cell volume and electrolyte handling during hyperosmotic conditions. This impairment leads to disruption of sodium and fluid excretion, which contributes to the complications due to diabetes.

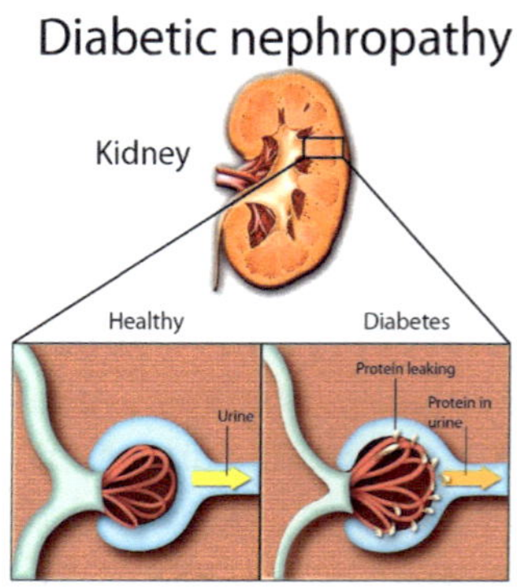

Figure 1.19. Diabetic nephropathy and urine.

Source: https://d2cax41o7ahm5l.cloudfront.net/mi/upload-images/diabetes-conference-2019-23324.jpg.

This points to the requirement for special therapies in order to regain renal function and achieve optimal fluid balance—a crucial aspect in the management of diabetes in the renal environment (Edwards & Layton, 2017). Furthermore, diabetes also impacts the renal microenvironment in that its effect on glomerular filtration rate (GFR) and tubular transport mechanisms is needed to maintain homeostasis. With the onset of diabetic nephropathy, structural changes , such as glomerulosclerosis become exceedingly prevalent, adding complexity to renal function. When tissue in the kidney is being altered, the kidney cannot maintain normal fluid balance, making it more susceptible to acute kidney injury (AKI) during conditions like sepsis and stress. Notably, certain pharmacological interventions, such as, statins, have been shown to be of no significant benefit towards the prevention of AKI disorders in diabetic patients, illustrating the complexity in treating diabetic renal complication (Hsu et al., 2018). Such debates emphasize the intricate interaction between renal physiology and diabetes and emphasize the need for management strategies that integrate both renal protection and glucose control to prevent eventual renal injury and dysfunction (Figure 1.19).

1.7.3. Effects of Hypertension on Kidney Function

The interaction between renal function and high blood pressure is complex but significant. High blood pressure affects renal physiology by disrupting the autoregulatory mechanisms that protect the kidneys from changes in systemic blood pressure. Under normal conditions, the kidneys can maintain a constant glomerular filtration rate (GFR) despite changes in perfusion pressure, but chronic hypertension disrupts this capability. Increased renal vasculature pressure results in glomerular damage and promotes pathological remodeling, ultimately affecting nephron function and lowering the overall efficiency of the kidneys. Such chronic overworking results in nephrosclerosis and may induce a cycle wherein decreased renal function has the sole purpose of elevating hypertension, creating a negative feedback loop that threatens renal health and metabolic stability. The renin-angiotensin-aldosterone system (RAAS) is key to controlling the effect of hypertension on kidney function. As renal perfusion decreases, the kidneys secrete renin, which triggers a cascade culminating in the production of angiotensin II, an extremely potent vasoconstrictor. While needed to assist in lowering blood pressure, excessive activation of RAAS due to chronic hypertension is harmful in inducing vasoconstriction of the renal arteries and sodium retention, which leads to fluid accumulation and elevated pressure. According to Rukavina Mikusic et al., the natriuretic-antinatriuretic imbalance, which also includes factors like atrial natriuretic peptide and renal dopamine, plays a crucial role in this altered state, with an emphasis that coordination of these factors is compromised in hypertensive states, resulting in renal pathophysiology and dysfunction (Mikusic et al., 2014). Additionally, the impact of hypertension extends beyond the momentary operations of the kidneys to additional health effects. Hypertension can result in sustained increases in blood pressure that can cause chronic kidney disease (CKD), which is a condition of progressive kidney dysfunction over time. The interaction of oxidative stress and inflammation is aggravated in hypertensive patients, causing glomerular damage and renal inflammation that accelerates the development of CKD. Recent studies show that sympathoinhibition, particularly after sodium loading, plays a part in blood pressure regulation and renal function, demonstrating a complex interaction with neural activity and fluid balance (Neal et al., 2016). The reality that hypertension produces a cascade of renal problems underscores the importance of early intervention in hypertension treatment to preserve kidney function and overall health.

Test Your Knowledge

1. What are the common causes and consequences of acute kidney injury (AKI)?
2. How does chronic kidney disease (CKD) affect fluid, electrolyte, and waste balance?

SUMMARY

Knowledge of renal physiology and the mechanisms of fluid balance remains vital for advancements in medical science and the provision of effective patient care. The kidneys are not only homeostatic controllers of fluid and electrolyte balance but also dynamic responsive organs to systemic perturbations and alterations. Through intricate mechanisms of filtration, reabsorption, and secretion, the kidneys establish homeostasis along with adjusting to myriad physiological conditions. Thus, dysregulation of these functions can lead to diseases , such as chronic kidney disease and hypertension, and continued research is therefore essential to clarify the mechanisms of renal function and fluid balance. Intermingling molecular and systemic understanding can help researchers develop novel avenues of treatment aimed at preserving renal integrity and diminishing the burden of renal disease. The investigation of renal pathophysiology goes beyond classical knowledge, as recent research proposes that evolutionary models like those using planarians might provide new information on human kidney disease. Research into conserved mechanisms regulating fluid balance across species, as detailed in recent reports, uncovers key links that might guide therapeutic approaches to diseases like chronic kidney disease. As an example, it is revealed by evidence that nephric mechanism disturbances can induce tubular cystogenesis with mimicry of close similarities to vertebrate CKD characteristics, thereby suggesting potential targets for intervention and study. The intricate structure-function relationship in the renal apparatus not only enhances our academic knowledge but also impels the development of new treatment modalities to address particular needs. As these advances and the overall relevance of renal function persist, additional interdisciplinary collaboration will be essential. With insights from genetics, molecular biology, and imaging modalities merging, researchers are increasingly able to tackle the complexities of kidney disease. The central nervous system's contribution to modulating renal response to fluid balance reflects the interaction of systems involved as multifactorial as well. Studies examining mechanisms , such as sympathoinhibition after sodium loading indicate that the regulatory mechanisms are highly intertwined, affecting blood pressure and natriuresis (Neal et al., 2016). Moreover, risk factors for renal diseases need an expansive approach to patient management through lifestyle, genetic predisposition, as well as innovative modalities of treatment. Finally, a deeper appreciation of renal physiology will translate into improved health and a greater understanding of the kidneys' vital role in overall homeostasis.

Renal physiology is the key to understanding how the kidneys control fluid and electrolyte balance in the body. Perhaps the most time-honored description of renal impairment is acute kidney injury (AKI), which can be defined as an abrupt impairment of renal excretory and homeostatic capability. The result is an accumulation of nitrogenous waste products in the bloodstream and the inability of the body to control fluid volume and levels of electrolytes. This illness is not rare; it has been documented in roughly 10% of all acute care hospital stays and in over half of intensive care patients. As such, AKI is a robust marker of physiological stress that is coupled with increasing morbidity, healthcare costs, and mortality. The expert identification of even mild renal impairment as the precursor to adverse outcomes underscores a requirement for careful monitoring and management in the clinic (Gross & Prowle, 2015). AKI is both heterogeneous and variably etiologic, with causes involving nephrotoxins, infection, and ischemia. Ischemic AKI is particularly prevalent in inpatients due to renal underperfusion related to systemic hypotension. It can happen under different medical conditions, including elective procedures , such as coronary artery bypass grafting, wherein the incidence of AKI can be up to 30%. The greatest significance of a greater insight into the pathophysiological mechanisms of ischemic AKI cannot be overstated because AKI onset can result in chronic renal impairment and predispose to chronic kidney disease. Thus, a focus on early detection and preventive strategies should be prioritized to combat the action of renal ischemia as well as its long-term effect on kidney function (Crowley, 2012). Regarding clinical advancement, the establishment of more sensitive biomarkers for AKI is most crucial because traditional markers like serum creatinine typically unveil damage after a lot of renal damage has occurred. Refinements in the detection of new markers that can unveil renal damage earlier will likely broaden the therapeutic field for AKI treatment. For instance, emerging research is exploring the use of noninvasive imaging techniques, such as, ultrasound with molecular contrast agents, to quantify renal perfusion and vascular remodeling during ischemic events. These new approaches can yield crucial insights into AKI pathogenesis and inform future therapeutic strategies. Besides, understanding renal vascular dynamics' interaction with inflammatory processes at the renal endothelium will help to design dedicated treatments aimed at preserving renal function. This development in renal medicine is a radical step towards more effective treatments and improved patient outcomes (Gross & Prowle, 2015).

KEY TERMS FROM THIS CHAPTER

- Acid-base balance
- Antidiuretic hormone (ADH)
- Atrial natriuretic peptide (ANP)
- Detoxification
- Erythropoietin secretion
- Filtration
- Osmoregulation
- Aldosterone
- Aquaporins
- Blood pressure regulation
- Electrolyte regulation
- Excretion
- Medullary osmotic gradient
- Reabsorption

CRITICAL THINKING QUESTIONS

1. **Which hormone is primarily responsible for increasing water reabsorption in the kidneys?**
   a. Aldosterone
   b. Antidiuretic Hormone (ADH)
   c. Renin
   d. Atrial Natriuretic Peptide (ANP)
2. **The juxtaglomerular apparatus regulates which of the following?**
   a. Blood glucose levels
   b. Oxygen saturation
   c. Blood pressure and glomerular filtration rate
   d. Urea reabsorption
3. **What is the main site for sodium reabsorption in the nephron?**
   a. Proximal convoluted tubule
   b. Loop of Henle
   c. Distal convoluted tubule
   d. Collecting duct
4. **Which of the following best describes the function of aldosterone in renal physiology?**
   a. Inhibits sodium reabsorption
   b. Promotes potassium excretion and sodium retention
   c. Increases water excretion
   d. Dilates the afferent arteriole
5. **Which structure in the nephron is most responsible for the concentration of urine?**
   a. Proximal tubule
   b. Glomerulus
   c. Loop of Henle
   d. Bowman's capsule

Short Answer Questions

1. What is the primary function of the nephron?
2. Define glomerular filtration rate (GFR).
3. Name the hormones involved in fluid balance regulation by the kidneys.
4. What role does the loop of Henle play in urine concentration?
5. How does antidiuretic hormone (ADH) affect the kidneys?
6. Discuss the mechanisms of fluid and electrolyte balance controlled by the kidneys.
7. Describe the hormonal regulation of kidney function with reference to ADH, aldosterone, and ANP.
8. Explain how the renin-angiotensin-aldosterone system (RAAS) contributes to blood pressure and fluid balance.
9. Compare and contrast the functions of the proximal and distal convoluted tubules.
10. How does the kidney respond to dehydration and overhydration?

Answers to Critical Thinking Questions

1. (b) 2. (c) 3. (a) 4. (b) 5. (c)

REFERENCES

1. Agard, M. A., Zandawala, M., & Paluzzi, J. (2024). Another fly diuretic hormone: Tachykinins increase fluid and ion transport by adult Drosophila melanogaster Malpighian 'renal' tubules. The Journal of Experimental Biology. https://www.semanticscholar.org/paper/2a2ea58dd6b3ef64efaeb283d9c8a64ceb27ce7e (accessed on 28th June 2025).
2. Al Bratty, M., Chintapalli, V., Davies, S. A., Dow, J. A. T., et al. (2012). Functional correlates of positional and gender-specific renal asymmetry in *Drosophila*. https://core.ac.uk/download/6175807.pdf (accessed on 28th June 2025).
3. Albalawy, W. N., Youm, E. B., Shipman, K. E., Baty, C., Long, K., Rbaibi, Y., & Jurczak, M. (2024). SGLT2-independent effects of gliflozins on proximal tubule function. Physiology. https://www.semanticscholar.org/paper/9c26db4abbdf7c7834a48d81a89a4903f7b737a7 (accessed on 28th June 2025).
4. Thi-Kim Vu, H., Rink, J. C., McKinney, S. A., McClain, M., Lakshmanaperumal, N., Alexander, R., & Sánchez Alvarado, A. (2015). Stem cells and fluid flow drive cyst formation in an invertebrate excretory organ. *eLife*, *4*, e07405. https://doi.org/10.7554/eLife.07405Andrei, S., Longrois, D., Nguyen, M., Bouhemad, B., & Guinot, P. (2024). Portal vein pulsatility is associated with the cumulative fluid balance. European Journal of Anesthesiology, 42, 324–331. https://www.semanticscholar.org/paper/006e60f48adfe9b5b3d1565a4716ca0258a4c5be (accessed on 28th June 2025).
5. Arthur, G., Osborn, J., & Yiannikouris, F. (2021). (Pro)renin receptor in the kidney: Function and significance. *American Journal of Physiology. Regulatory, Integrative and Comparative Physiology*. https://www.semanticscholar.org/paper/3db660583d4bf1d2da47a82167768a25f861c189 (accessed on 28th June 2025).
6. Blaine, J., Chonchol, M., & Levi, M. (2014). Renal control of calcium, phosphate, and magnesium homeostasis. *Clinical Journal of the American Society of Nephrology, 10*, 1257–1272. https://doi.org/10.2215/cjn.09750913 (accessed on 28th June 2025).
7. Chaudhari, S., Mallet, R., Shotorbani, P., Tao, Y., & Ma, R. (2020). Store-operated calcium entry: Pivotal roles in renal physiology and pathophysiology. Experimental Biology and Medicine, 246, 305–316. https://www.semanticscholar.org/paper/2cd39f0370551c08f15a4ff8b20eddadc9cfdf98 (accessed on 28th June 2025).
8. Rukavina Mikusic, N. L., Kravetz, M. C., Kouyoumdzian, N. M., Della Penna, S. L., Rosón, M. I., Fernández, B. E., & Choi, M. R. (2014). Signaling pathways involved in renal oxidative injury: role of the vasoactive peptides and the renal dopaminergic system. *Journal of signal transduction*, *2014*, 731350. https://doi.org/10.1155/2014/731350(accessed on 28th June 2025).
9. Edwards, A., & Crambert, G. (2017). Versatility of NaCl transport mechanisms in the cortical collecting duct. *American journal of physiology. Renal physiology*, *313*(6), F1254–F1263. https://doi.org/10.1152/ajprenal.00369.2017(accessed on 28th June 2025).
10. Crowley, S. (2012). Taking a sound approach to acute kidney injury. American Journal of Physiology. Renal Physiology, 303(11), F1505–F1506. https://www.semanticscholar.org/paper/defcd774a52f1ff7e1e73e2d9641229636db3969 (accessed on 28th June 2025).

11. De Hert, S., & De Baerdemaeker, L. (2014). Why hydroxyethyl starch solutions should NOT be banned from the operating room. *Anaesthesiology intensive therapy*, *46*(5), 336–341. https://doi.org/10.5603/AIT.2014.0057(accessed on 28th June 2025).

12. Della Corte, V., Pecoraro, R., Pinto, A., & Tuttolomondo, A. (2018). Chronic hyponatremia in a patient with renal salt wasting and without cerebral disease: Relationship between RSW, risk of fractures and cognitive impairment. https://core.ac.uk/download/287859289.pdf (accessed on 28th June 2025).

13. Graham, L. A., Dominiczak, A. F., & Ferreri, N. R. (2017). Role of renal transporters and novel regulatory interactions in the TAL that control blood pressure. *Physiological genomics*, *49*(5), 261–276. https://doi.org/10.1152/physiolgenomics.00017.2017(accessed on 28th June 2025).

14. Edwards, A., & Layton, A. T. (2017). Cell Volume Regulation in the Proximal Tubule of Rat Kidney : Proximal Tubule Cell Volume Regulation. *Bulletin of mathematical biology*, *79*(11), 2512–2533. https://doi.org/10.1007/s11538-017-0338-6(accessed on 28th June 2025).

15. J. I. Leonard, Ph.D. S. Furukawa, M.D. P. Van Nordstrand (1975). Systems identification and application systems development for monitoring the physiological and health status of crewmen in space. Study Report Unclas (General Electric Co.) 65 p nc A04/MF A0l GJ/52 22244 https://core.ac.uk/download/pdf/42869637.pdf (accessed on 28th June 2025).

16. Gross, J., & Prowle, J. (2015). Perioperative acute kidney injury. *BJA Education, 15*, 213–218. https://www.semanticscholar.org/paper/cb723eedc4a1d97fbc4797915b37355dc4549c0a (accessed on 28th June 2025).

17. Hall, J. E., do Carmo, J. M., da Silva, A. A., Wang, Z., & Hall, M. E. (2015). Obesity-induced hypertension. *Circulation Research, 116*, 991–1006. https://doi.org/10.1161/circresaha.116.305697 (accessed on 28th June 2025).

18. Hassan, M. M. (2020). Acidosis and anion gap. https://core.ac.uk/download/322580641.pdf (accessed on 28th June 2025).

19. Heron, V. (2018). Calcium, phosphate and magnesium disorders. https://core.ac.uk/download/322439617.pdf (accessed on 28th June 2025).

20. Hsu, R. K., Levitt, J. E., Liu, K. D., Matthay, M. A., et al. (2018). Effect of rosuvastatin on acute kidney injury in sepsis-associated acute respiratory distress syndrome. https://core.ac.uk/download/323062965.pdf (accessed on 28th June 2025).

21. Jaishankar, M., Tseten, T., Anbalagan, N., Mathew, B. B., & Beeregowda, K. N. (2014). Toxicity, mechanism and health effects of some heavy metals. Interdisciplinary Toxicology, 7, 60–72. https://doi.org/10.2478/intox-2014-0009 (accessed on 28th June 2025).

22. Leach, C.S., Johnson, P.C. (1989). Effects of Weightlessness on Human Fluid and Electrolyte Physiology. In: Paganelli, C.V., Farhi, L.E. (eds) Physiological Function in Special Environments. Springer, New York, NY. https://doi.org/10.1007/978-1-4612-3556-9_11(accessed on 28th June 2025).

23. Kataria, A. K., Sahni, M. S., Kataria, N., Garg, S. L., & Agarwal, V. K. (2007). Opterećenje tekućinom i prijenosna sposobnost bubrega u dvogrbe deve u dehidraciji i rehidraciji zimi i ljeti. https://core.ac.uk/download/14397696.pdf (accessed on 28th June 2025).

24. Leiz, J., & Schmidt-Ott, K. M. (2019). Claudins in the Renal Collecting Duct. *International journal of molecular sciences*, *21*(1), 221. https://doi.org/10.3390/ijms21010221(accessed on 28th June 2025).

25. Leonard, J. I. (1985). Description, validation, and modification of the Guyton model for space-flight applications. Part A. *Guyton Model of Circulatory, Fluid and Electrolyte Control.* Part B. *Modification of the Guyton Model for Circulatory, Fluid and Electrolyte Control.* (NASA-CR-171676) D'BCLIFIICN, VAIIDATIC6, N65-i61c'2 AND MCDIEICATICN CF IEF MICE MODLL FCR SFACB-FLIGHT APFIICATICNS. FART A. GUYTCN MODEL OF CIRCULATORY, FLUIC AND ELECTROLYTE Unclae CCNTROL, PART E. (Canagemer.t and Technical G3/52 21223 https://core.ac.uk/download/pdf/42845535.pdf (accessed on 28th June 2025).

26. Lory, P. (1993). Recent advances in the modelling of renal function. https://core.ac.uk/download/11540801.pdf (accessed on 28th June 2025).

27. Mao, C., & Chacko, B. (2020). Fluid intake post renal transplant; drink to thirst or drink to target: Does it matter? *Transplantation*. https://www.semanticscholar.org/paper/73244c9b2e4b326a3202c60d119e482ef9b16349 (accessed on 28th June 2025).

28. Michałek, K. (2016). Aquaglyceroporins in the kidney: Present state of knowledge and prospects. *PubMed, 67*, 185–193.

29. Mungara, P., MacNaughton, K., & Cordat, E. (2024). Investigating the urinary salt losing phenotype in R607H and L919X mutant mice with distal renal tubular acidosis. Physiology. https://www.semanticscholar.org/paper/05f829c6c1be8d85ce89eb154b95da123063abc2 (accessed on 28th June 2025).

30. Natochin, Y. V. (1996). Evolutionary aspects of renal function. https://core.ac.uk/download/pdf/82128875.pdf (accessed on 28th June 2025).

31. Neal, C. M. (2016). Evaluating techniques in tissue clarification using CLARITY imaging and investigating where sodium is sensed in the body. https://core.ac.uk/download/142066226.pdf (accessed on 28th June 2025).

32. Judy L. Solberg and Linda G. Pleasant (1984). Space medicine research publications: 1983–1984. NASA Contractor Report 3860 https://core.ac.uk/download/pdf/42847043.pdf (accessed on 28th June 2025).

33. Pyrshev, K. A., Atamanchuk, A., Kordysh, M., Zaika, O. L., & Pochynyuk, O. (2024). Regulation of renal acid-base balance by Epac isoforms in proximal tubule and collecting duct. *Physiology*. https://www.semanticscholar.org/paper/b125065897700adfc74a92d13813e265895e1139 (accessed on 28th June 2025).

34. Rowland, N. (2021). Thirst and body fluid regulation. https://www.semanticscholar.org/paper/ddb27ad4b1bb9ef689749e8fc7cbd56b56e1523f (accessed on 28th June 2025).

35. Singh, A., Tiwari, A. M., & Mishra, S. (2024). Chronic renal failure—Etiology, pathophysiology, symptoms, diagnosis and its management through electro-homeopathy: An overview. International Journal of Biochemistry & Physiology. https://www.semanticscholar.org/paper/a7975a2d31102f7e64ede2e51c9b1aea269c7d26 (accessed on 28th June 2025).

36. Suh, S. H., Jung, H. J., Wang, W., & Kim, S. (2022). Editorial: Renal regulation of water and sodium in health and disease. Frontiers in Physiology, 13. https://www.semanticscholar.org/paper/a119d411038b04c01360462f7a7ccd72386a77e6 (accessed on 28th June 2025).

37. Vale, H. (2020). Renal and urinary systems/electrolyte balance. *Anesthesiology*. https://www.semanticscholar.org/paper/8620611e8dabbc4827a95108c5f1a01183c86b9b (accessed on 28th June 2025).

38. White, R. J. (2025). Acid-base homeostasis in the human system. https://core.ac.uk/download/pdf/42869639.pdf (accessed on 28th June 2025).

39. Yameny, K. (2025). Understanding kidney health: Physiology, diagnostic markers, and pathological conditions. *Biobacta Journal of Biochemistry and Molecular Biology*. https://www.semanticscholar.org/paper/372d7543076efefb90dea85f2ee266908f074458 (accessed on 28th June 2025).

ACID-BASE PHYSIOLOGY

2

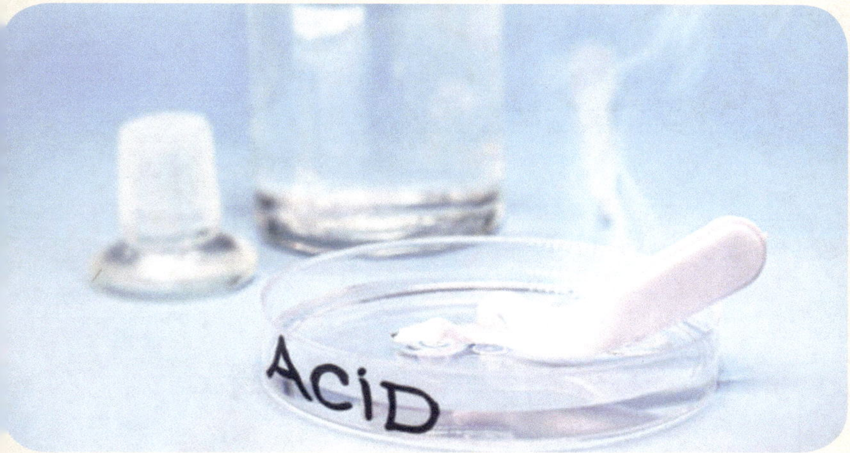

LEARNING OBJECTIVES

After studying this chapter, you will be able to:

1. Discuss the concepts of acids and bases.
2. Explain the role of buffers in the body.
3. Discuss the respiratory regulation of acid-base balance.
4. Focus on renal regulation of acid-base balance.
5. Learn about the clinical implications of acid-base disorders.
6. Evaluate the acid-base physiology in special populations.

Introduction

Acid-base physiology is a fundamental principle in biochemistry and cellular function, the basis of numerous biological processes critical to homeostasis and optimal health. Regulation of pH in a narrow range by the body is crucial for the optimization of enzymatic activity and metabolic processes. Abnormality of this homeostasis will lead to serious physiological derangements, ranging from cell respiration to neurotransmitter action. Understanding acid-base compensation mechanisms involves the study of buffering systems, respiratory, and renal compensation functions. This intricate interplay not only provides evidence of the dynamic nature of human physiology but also underscores the importance of acid-base balance in clinical scenarios, where deviation signals major medical illnesses. Thus, a broad overview of acid-base physiology forms the basis for a more critical examination of its theoretical foundations and clinical utility in medicine and biology. Acid-base physiology consists of several distinct elements, one being the bicarbonate buffering system, which is crucial to the preservation of pH homeostasis.

Bicarbonate is in equilibrium with carbonic acid and hence permits the body to neutralize the excess bases or acids. This buffering mechanism is supplemented by respiratory mechanisms, wherein the body can rapidly correct changes in carbon dioxide by adjusting ventilation. Renal mechanisms also ensure long-term control by removing hydrogen ions and recycling bicarbonate, highlighting the complex controls of acid-base balance.

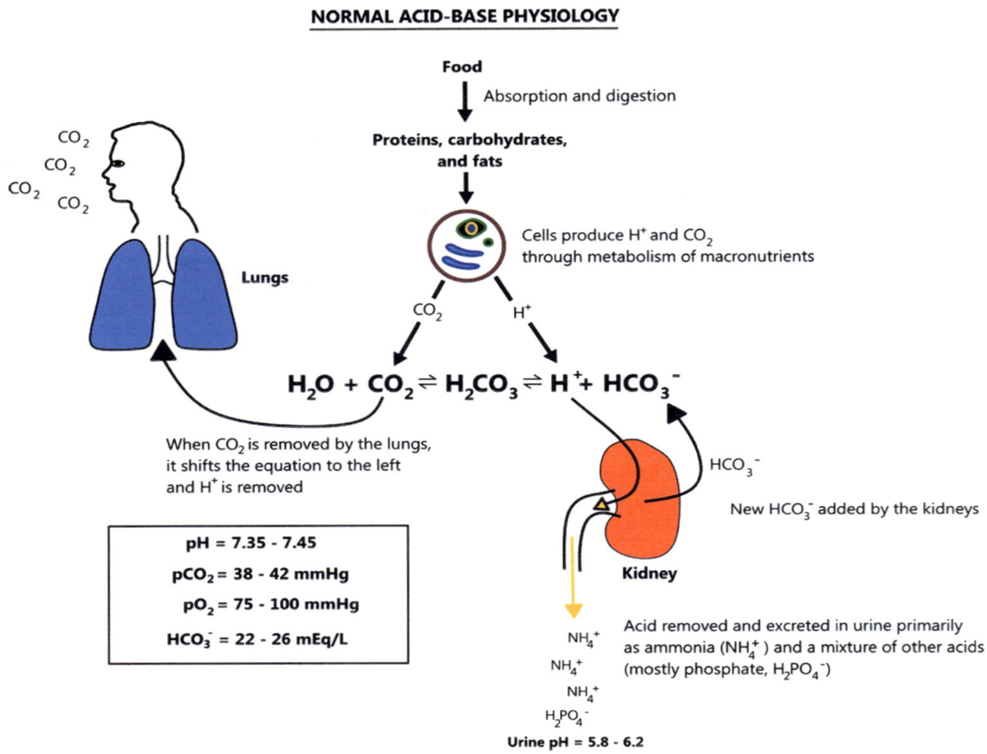

Figure 2.1. Normal acid-base physiology.

Source: https://www.straighthealthcare.com/image/acid-base-normal.png.

The interplay between these mechanisms demonstrates the complexity of homeostasis, as with the situation of metabolic acidosis or alkalosis, which can arise from systemic imbalances. Through their study, the relevance of acid-base physiology grows more apparent, even in disease and in health. Advances over the past few years in the understanding of acid-base physiology have revealed the importance of environmental influences and organism adaptations. For instance, it has been shown how the water chemistry may influence aquatic animals' physiology, particularly through the salinity-dependent modulation of enzyme activity and toxicity to pollutants like copper. The nuances involved in such interactions demonstrate the need to control for extraneous variables when studying acid-base regulation in a broad spectrum of organisms. Such integration of environmental science and physiological mechanisms emphasizes the broad implications of acid-base physiology beyond human health to ecological and environmental contexts (Raju, 2016). Therefore, a proper introduction to acid-base physiology must encompass such far-reaching influences in order to result in a comprehensive exploration that entwines cellular mechanisms with ecological impacts, thereby promoting our knowledge of biology in general (de Polo & Scrimshaw, 2012) (Figure 2.1).

Definition of Acid-Base Physiology

Acid-base physiology is an elementary principle of human biology, concerning the mechanisms by which the body attains a delicate balance between bases and acids. Physiological equilibrium is crucial to a broad spectrum of metabolic processes, cell functions, and organism homeostasis. The body maintains pH within a narrow range, normally 7.35 to 7.45, in order to support maximal enzymatic function, oxygen transport, and metabolism of nutrients. Deviation from this range can produce severe physiological derangements, which produce some pathological states , such as acidosis and alkalosis. Familiarity with the subtlety of acid-base homeostasis allows for a penetrating understanding of an enormous number of health issues, particularly those that concern the respiratory and renal systems, the functioning of which is vital to the maintenance of acid-base homeostasis. At the heart of acid-base physiology is the bicarbonate buffer system, a primary pH controller of extracellular fluid. The bicarbonate buffer system employs the activity of carbonic acid ($H2CO_3$) and bicarbonate ions (HCO_3^-) to minimize shifts in alkalinity or acidity. The catalytic activity of enzymes by carbonic anhydrase maintains the rapid exchange between carbon dioxide, carbonic acid, and bicarbonate, which in reality stabilizes pH. Also, the kidneys contribute to acid-base balance by secreting hydrogen ions in the urine and reabsorbing bicarbonate. The two-pronged regulatory system allows the body to respond immediately to whatever challenge arises, such as, an increase in the levels of metabolic end products following a strenuous exercise session, thereby reinforcing the importance of learning acid-base physiology under health and disease. The acid-base physiology is not merely an intellectual exercise; it carries a lot of clinical significance and patient management impact. Proper management of acid-base disturbances is crucial in most aspects of medicine, particularly in the emergency and critical care settings. By correct interpretation of arterial blood gas analysis, clinicians can diagnose and treat conditions caused by disturbances in acid-base, such as, diabetic ketoacidosis or respiratory failure. In addition, the innovation in therapeutic treatments, including buffer therapy or dialysis, serves to underscore the clinical value of acid-base physiology in managing patients with compromised homeostasis. With advancements in the area of research, it underscores the importance of clinical practitioners possessing a concrete understanding of acid-base principles for optimum patient outcomes and informing clinical decision-making under challenging conditions ((de Polo et al.& Scrimshaw, 2012).

Importance in Human Health

The precarious acid-base physiology is an important determinant of human health, and a departure from the optimal pH can cause severe physiological disturbances. The body maintains its functions within a very narrow pH range of about 7.35 to 7.45, critical for maximal enzyme function, metabolic processes, and cellular activities. When blood pH falls below or increases over this range, as in diseases , such as acidosis or alkalosis, there can be a variety of health effects. For example, acidosis can impair heart function and result in respiratory distress, whereas alkalosis can result in muscle spasms and arrhythmia. Upkeep of this homeostatic balance is essential in order to ensure that biochemical function, such as, nutrient uptake and removal of waste, occurs efficiently, with resultant implications for general well-being and well-being. The gut microbiota also plays an important role in acid-base status and metabolic health. There is current evidence that interactions between the diet and gut microbiota can influence metabolic syndrome and obesity, acid-base derangement-associated diseases. Manipulation of gut microbiota may promote metabolic benefits and thereby enhance the body's ability to maintain acid-base homeostasis. For instance, a study concluded that supplementation of 2-fucosyllactose (2-FL) altered gut microbiota profiles and improved metabolic profiles in high-fat diet-fed mice and proposed potential therapeutic interventions for obesity control with impacts on acid-base balance. These findings highlight the need for the inclusion of nutritional approaches promoting a healthy microbiome into an integrative strategy for maintaining optimal acid-base physiology and overall human health (Barile et al., 2020). Furthermore, the significance of breast milk composition highlights the biochemical intricacy that promotes health during sensitive developmental periods. Evolutionarily fine-tuned nutrients in milk, such as, oligosaccharides, are not only consumed as energy but also as promoters of gut development and microbial diversity among infants. For instance, their highly complex oligosaccharide components, for instance, is globotriose, present in bear milk, have been engaged in the upkeep of developing gastrointestinal physiology among offspring, mirroring processes in human physiology. This particular macronutrient and metabolite balance controls gut microbiota composition and metabolism, setting the trajectory of health in infancy, with this trajectory continuing thereafter. Health professionals are able to treat better metabolic dysregulation and diseases influenced by early nutritional interventions through knowledge of these maternal contributions and their long-lasting effects on metabolic processes, such as, regulation of acid-base balance (Hou et al., 2015) (Figure 2.2).

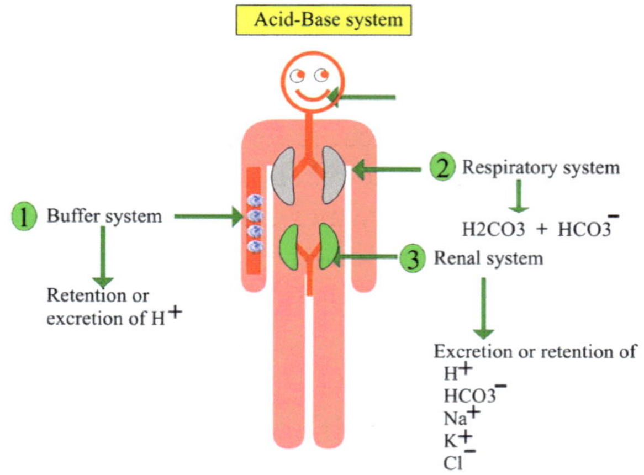

Figure 2.2. Acid-base-maintenance.

Source: https://www.labpedia.net/wp-content/uploads/2020/04/acid-base-maintinance-768x587.jpg.

2.1. Basic Concepts of Acids and Bases

Learning Outcome

1. Describe the acids and bases;
2. Focus on the pH scale and its significance;
3. Learn about strong vs. weak acids and bases.

In acid-base physiology, an understanding of the general principles of acids and bases is the basis for investigating more complicated biochemical interactions. Acids are chemicals that can donate protons (H+) to a solution, thus increasing the hydrogen ion concentration. Bases, on the other hand, are substances that accept protons, thereby lowering the hydrogen ion concentration. This dynamic interaction is essential to provide homeostasis in biological systems, in which the delicate interaction between alkalinity and acidity is essential for enzyme processes and metabolic activities. The pH range from 0 to 14 is a fundamental measure of this balance, in which measurements below 7 are acidic and measurements above 7 are alkaline. Hence, a thorough understanding of acids and bases is crucial in elucidating biological processes that are regulated by pH changes. The deeper we go into acid-base, the clearer the use of buffer systems. Buffers are solutions resistant to pH change upon the addition of tiny amounts of acids or bases. They are typically a weak acid and its conjugate base, or a weak base and its conjugate acid, which work together to stabilize body pH levels. The bicarbonate buffer system, for instance, is essential to maintaining blood pH within a limited range required for proper physiological function. When hydrogen ions are in excess, bicarbonate buffers them to form carbonic acid that can be metabolized to carbon dioxide and expelled from the body by respiration. These processes give an indication of the intricacy of acid-base balance in the human body and the function served by buffers in sustaining life.

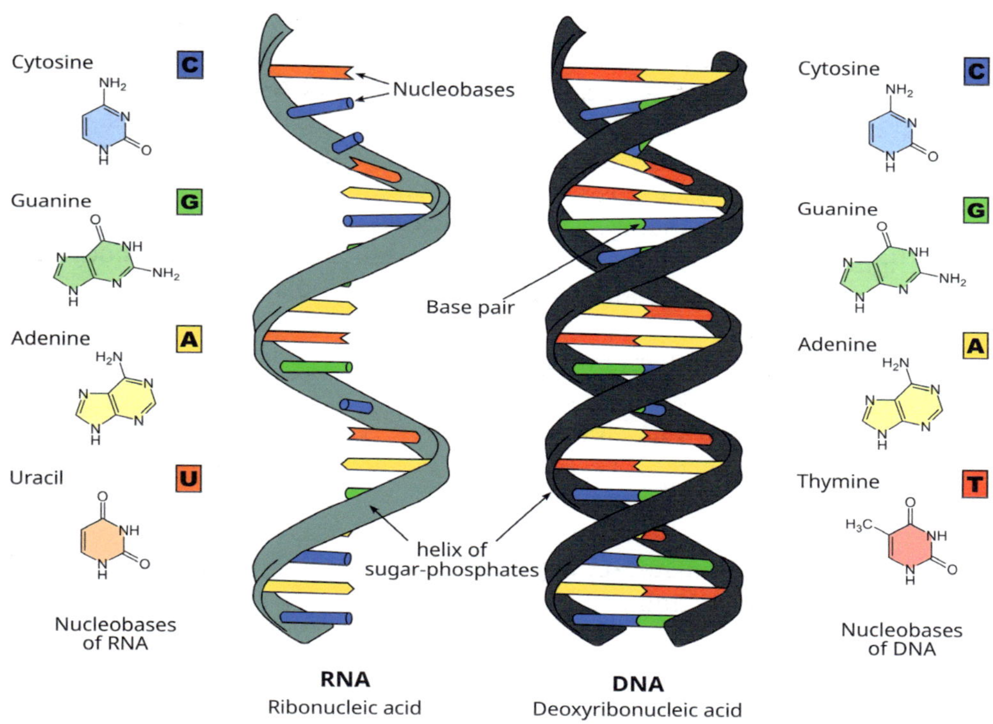

Figure 2.3. Function of nucleic acids.

Source: https://upload.wikimedia.org/wikipedia/commons/thumb/3/37/Difference_DNA_RNA-EN.svg/960px-Difference_DNA_RNA-EN.svg.png.

The definitions of bases and acids also have implications that extend beyond definition to include new biochemical significance, particularly as it pertains to genetic material. Experiments have revealed that changes in the pH level of the environment can affect the conformation and function of nucleic acids, in this case, DNA. Current studies have indicated that fluctuations in acidity regulate the stability of the DNA double helix and, consequently, gene expression. This is particularly significant when considering the accounts of most genetic diseases and mutations. As a case in point, concepts drawn from the study of genetic coding can be adapted to acid-base balance when considering how certain genetic alterations can be contingent on the pH-sensitive character of nucleobases. Explanation of such intricate interactions and mechanisms makes it possible to explore new therapeutic regimes for genetic disease, as seen in the hypotheses of genetic change and their biochemical impact (Sorrivas & Sierra, 2009) (Figure 2.3).

2.1.1. Definition of Acids and Bases

In chemistry, acids and bases are characterized by different theories conceptualized to demonstrate their inherent nature and behaviors. An acid is any compound that increases the concentration of hydrogen ions (H^+) in solution, and a base increases the concentration of hydroxide ions (OH^-), as per the Arrhenius theory. This perspective highlights the role of aqueous solutions in acid-base chemistry, leading to neutralization reactions in which acids and bases react to form water and salts. An understanding of these basics is critical in acid-base physiology because the balance of these ions within biologic systems directly influences cellular processes, enzymatic activity, and metabolic pathways and thus impacts health and well-being. Broadening the Arrhenius definition, the Brønsted-Lowry theory further enhances the definition of acids and bases through emphasizing their roles as proton donors and acceptors, respectively. Such a view broadens acid-base chemistry to chemical environments outside aqueous solution environments so that they can be detected in any chemical environment. For instance, when an acid donates a proton to a base, both create a conjugate acid and a conjugate base, thus enabling the description of compounds in dynamic equilibrium. This perspective is also of great relevance to biological systems, where proton transfer involves a vital function in biochemical reactions , such as cellular respiration and photosynthesis. Moreover, the ability of biologic molecules to have both acidic or basic character (amphoteric activity) adds to their versatility in maintaining homeostasis, a part of acid-base physiology. Lastly, the Lewis definition provides an additional aspect by establishing that acids are electron pair acceptors and bases are electron pair donors. The definition touches more areas of chemical interactions, which can or cannot include protons. In biological systems, it would be particularly applicable when one is observing enzyme-substrate interactions, where electron transfer forms an essential part of catalysis and of control of metabolism. The versatility of acids and bases, as elucidated by these multiple theories, is important in constructing a general picture of acid-base physiology. It facilitates scientists and physicians to comprehend how dysbalances between these chemical species cause the development of diseases , such as acidosis or alkalosis, emphasizing the importance of maintaining body pH levels at the optimum levels (Vaidyanathan, 2004; de Polo & Scrimshaw, 2012) (Figure 2.4).

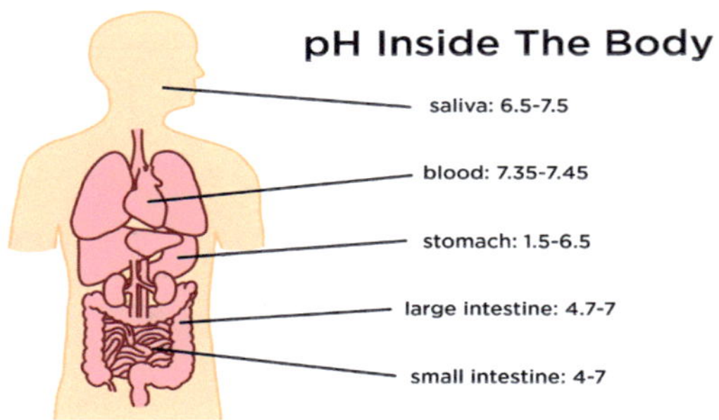

Figure 2.4. Ion balance.

Source: https://d20khd7ddkh5ls.cloudfront.net/ph_inside_the_body.jpg.

2.1.2. The pH Scale and Its Significance

The pH scale is an important tool for understanding acid-base physiology, quantifying the acidity and basicity of biological materials.

The scale is from 0 to 14 and measures hydrogen ion concentration in solution, and the values below 7 denote acidity and above 7 alkalinities. This scale is not only a fundamental principle in chemistry but also of prime importance in applications in biology, particularly in enzymatic reactions and metabolic pathways. The proper physiological pH is key for optimal cell functioning; even slight deviations can influence protein structure as well as their activity and, consequently, overall metabolic pathways. One example is that human blood typically has quite a narrow pH range of 7.35 to 7.45, reflecting the importance of acid-base balance in homeostasis. Any interference in this balance can lead to disorders , such as acidosis or alkalosis, which can tremendously interfere with normal physiological functioning. A nice application of pH measurement can be seen in the studies on various bird species, particularly feral pigeons, that give us an idea of how dietary habits influence the acidity of faces.

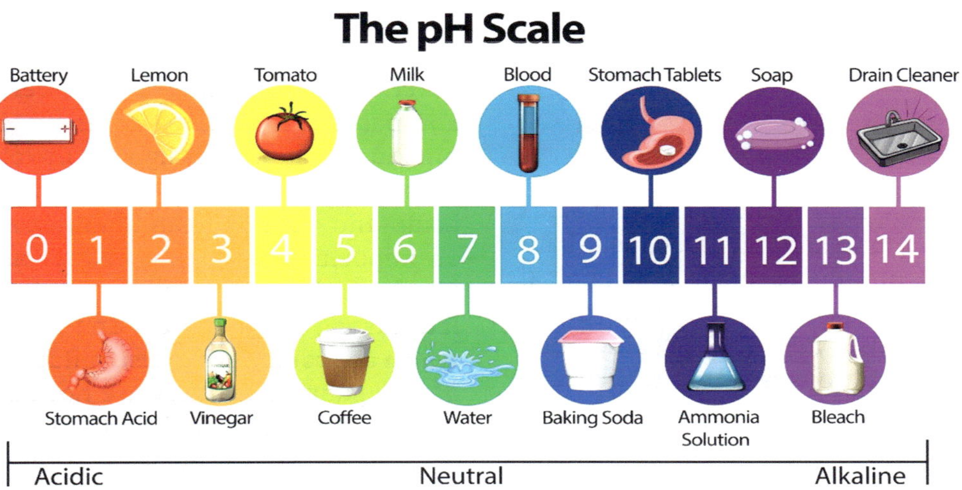

Figure 2.5. pH in water testing.

Source: https://blog.jencoi.com/hubfs/103211917_m.jpg.

Evidence indicates that the urban pigeon's diet, which consists largely of human waste, results in a more acidic fecal output than that of its wild counterpart, the rock dove. This is due in part to their diet quality and increased rate of uric acid synthesis being responsible for the overall acidity of their excreta (Spennemann & Watson, 2017). These findings are a reminder of how environmental and dietary inputs overlap with biochemical mechanisms, thus affecting pH levels in not only avian physiology but also more broadly in ecological contexts. Such relationships assist in resolving human problems pertaining to urban wildlife as well as their public health relevance. The relevance of pH goes beyond physiological relevance, raising questions of comprehension of pathophysiological states. For example, connexin hemichannels in cell membranes are pH-sensitive, and pH changes may alter their function under varying conditions. Under conditions where pH is not within the normal range of physiological pH, subtle changes may lead to leaks in these channels, hence allowing unwanted substances to pass in or out of cells. The pathological consequences uncover therapeutic pathways, such as, targeted treatment modalities with agents , such as abEC1.1, which can facilitate normal channel function through inhibition of hyperactive hemichannels (Buratto et al., 2019). These interventions reflect the significance of pH in more than just physiological integrity, including when considering clinical solutions. Consequently, the pH scale serves as a unifying referent in both interpreting normal biology and managing the subtleties of disease treatment, demonstrating its pivotal position among acid-base physiology (Figure 2.5).

2.1.3. Strong vs. Weak Acids and Bases

The distinction between weak and strong acids and bases forms a fundamental part of acid-base physiology and influences most biochemical processes in living organisms. Strong acids, such as, hydrochloric acid (HCl), completely dissociate upon solution in water to produce a large concentration of hydrogen ions (H^+). Due to total dissociation, there is reduced pH leading to extremely acidic conditions required for certain physiological processes, such as, digestion within the stomach. On the contrary, weak acids like acetic acid (CH_3COOH) ionize to a limited degree to reach equilibrium between undissociated molecules and ions. This property makes weak acids priceless in organismal buffering systems as they can buffer pH alterations and provide homeostasis and thereby their significance in acid-base balance in physiological processes. Similarly, the difference between strong and weak bases suggests their significance in physiological systems. Strong bases, such as, sodium hydroxide (NaOH), dissociate fully to give a high concentration of hydroxide ions (OH^-) in solution, thus raising the pH and making the solution alkaline. This is useful in a number of biological processes, like cellular respiration, where ionic balance is crucial. Weak bases on the other hand, such as, bicarbonate (HCO_3-), exert a more subtle effect by partially dissociating in solution. This property allows weak bases to be a part of buffering systems in order to regulate pH levels within biological fluids, such as, blood. Their capacity to regulate physiological response not only maintains systemic balance but also facilitates reactions that are essential for cellular functioning. The interaction between acids and bases is not limited to their physiological function; they play a significant role in indoor environment quality and health. Various acids and bases, organic and inorganic, play an important role in the indoor air quality of buildings. Primarily, indoor spaces have acids like carbon dioxide (CO_2) and ammonia (NH_3), which are common but also influence the health of occupants when they are not balanced well. Other acids like nitric acid (HNO_3) and sulfuric acid (H_2SO_4) may be present as a result of chemical reactions between consumer products and combustion and influence the air quality. Besides, the separation of the acids and bases between airborne particles, surfaces, and in the gas phase describes their varied interactions in indoor spaces. This is more than just chemistry; understanding these interactions is crucial in improving ambient air quality and sustaining a healthy indoor space for residents, cultural items, and sensitive equipment, as mandated in existing literature (Nazaroff & Weschler, 2020).

Test Your Knowledge

1. What defines a substance as an acid or a base according to the Bronsted-Lowry theory?
2. How is the strength of an acid or base determined?

2.2. The Role of Buffers in the Body

Learning Outcome

1. Explain the function of buffers;
2. Define the major buffer systems in the human body;
3. Learn about the importance of buffers in maintaining pH.

Buffers are essential to the acid-base physiology of the body and are responsible for keeping the pH of body fluids in a very small range. Buffers' main function is to resist gross pH changes when acids or bases are introduced into the system. This process is important to help maintain cellular homeostasis and overall metabolic function since enzymes and biochemical reactions are very sensitive to pH. The buffering systems of the body are primarily bicarbonate, phosphate, and protein buffers, each with a specific role in regulating acid-base control. By neutralizing acids and bases, the buffers ensure that physiological processes can continue unhampered, with a significant contribution to the body's mechanisms for acid-base regulation (White, 2025). The buffering systems, without them, would have detrimental effects even under slight deviation, thus proving their vital role in sustaining physiological welfare. Besides, the interaction of buffers, the respiratory system, and the renal system emphasizes the acid-base regulation of the body as being multifaceted.

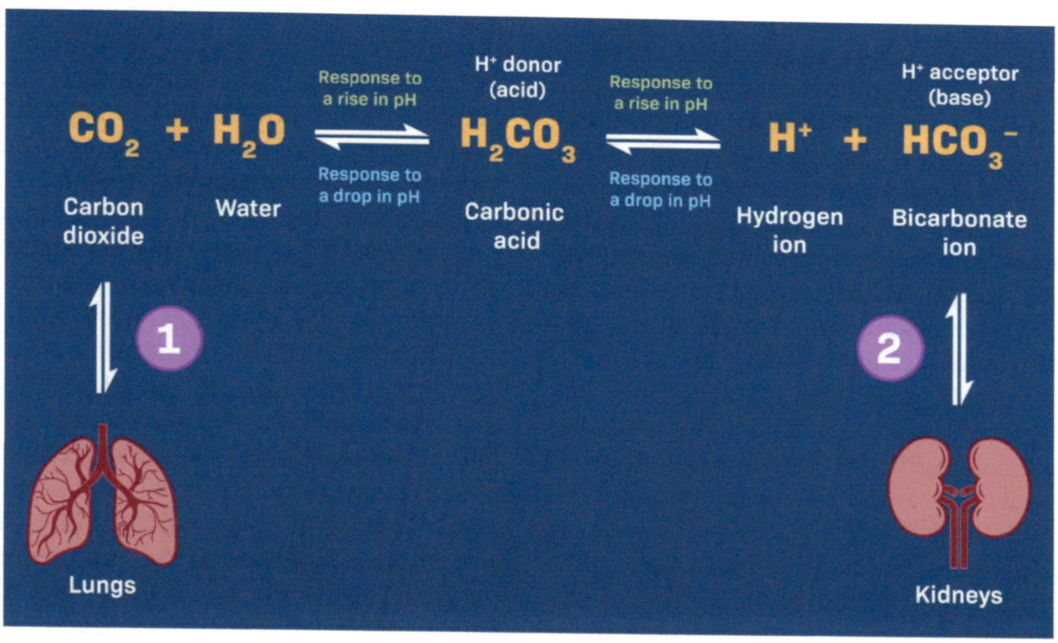

Figure 2.6. Role of buffers in the body.

Source: https://media.labxchange.org/xblocks/lb-LabXchange-a926f7b7-html-1/p111-ap-bio-what-is-a-buffer_21695786230389-d38b7d0f664183237f95fbbb67d5b852.png.

Lungs facilitate rapid pH adjustment by modulation of the quantity of carbon dioxide through respiration, while kidneys assist with water-level regulation in the long run by excretion of hydrogen ions and reabsorption of bicarbonate. This symbiotic process creates a dynamic equilibrium that sustains the body's pH despite changing levels of metabolic acid produced by cellular respiration and exercise. For instance, during strenuous exercise, the accumulation of lactic acid can challenge the body's acid-base balance. The availability of buffers, particularly those found within tissue in the skeletal muscle, such as, carnosine, serves to counteract acidosis during prolonged exercise. Carnosine's capacity as a pH buffer is especially important in sustaining muscle function, thereby illustrating the dual function of buffers in physical and metabolic terms (Derave et al., 2010). Lastly, the functions of buffering agents exceed pH control alone; they play a pivotal role in exercise performance and recovery. For instance, skeletal muscle possesses high concentrations of certain buffers that play an especially critical role in anaerobic metabolism. During intense exercise by muscles, acid metabolites are produced, leading to fatigue and reduced performance. Buffering compounds like carnosine buffer the acids and, thereby, enhance contractile function and general sports performance. Furthermore, it has been found that increasing carnosine content in muscles with supplementation, for example, with beta-alanine, will significantly improve the outcomes of high-intensity exercise. Therefore, again, this emphasizes the dual importance of buffers—both in maintaining acid-base balance and optimizing physiological response during exercise. The role of buffers in complex acid-base control processes provides further confirmation of their essential role both in health and sport (Derave et al., 2010; White, 2025) (Figure 2.6).

2.2.1. Definition and Function of Buffers

Buffers are tasked with acid-base homeostasis regulation in biological systems, particularly human physiology. A buffer, by definition, is a solution that resists the alteration in pH when small amounts of an acid or a base are added. This resistance is primarily due to the presence of the weak acid-base pairs that will donate H+ ions when a base is introduced or accept H^+ ions when an acid is introduced. For example, the bicarbonate buffering system lies at the center of maintaining blood pH under control and is founded on the dynamic equilibrium between carbonic acid and bicarbonate ions. The precise ability of buffers to regulate stable pH values is central to physiological functions because even slight deviations from pH can be injurious to cellular function and metabolic processes, and thus underscores their relevance in acid-base physiology. In critical care and trauma settings, the administration of appropriate fluid resuscitation fluids is central to patient outcomes, particularly about the consequences of metabolic acid-base disturbances. Current studies have indicated that standard intravenous fluids like normal saline can cause harmful metabolic effects, including hyperchloremic acidosis. This undermines the efficiency of saline to function as a buffer in certain clinical settings. Other substances used for buffering, like Lactated Ringer's, are being explored for their efficiency in preserving acid-base balance and enhancing survival rates among trauma patients (Murphy, 2021). These studies bring attention to the function of buffers not only in the maintenance of physiological pH but also to clinical decision making in acute medical interventions. The rigorous management of fluid resuscitation with buffered fluids may be at the heart of improving patient stability in critical conditions. The theoretical underpinnings of acid-base physiology suggest two prevalent strategies: the classic model developed by Ole Siggaard-Andersen and the modern strategy spearheaded by Peter Stewart. Both paradigms offer frameworks for understanding how buffers function in big biology. The traditional one considers predominantly bicarbonate as the major buffer, while the modern one offers a more comprehensive assessment of strong ions and the role they play in acid-base balance, e.g., the activities of proteins and non-volatile acids in plasma (Matoušek, 2013). This integrative information informs clinical interventions on fluid therapy and pH management in patients. As the field progresses, the place of buffer systems in therapy remains at the forefront, serving to illustrate the multifaceted role of buffers in sustaining life and health in the intricate realm of acid-base physiology (Figure 2.7).

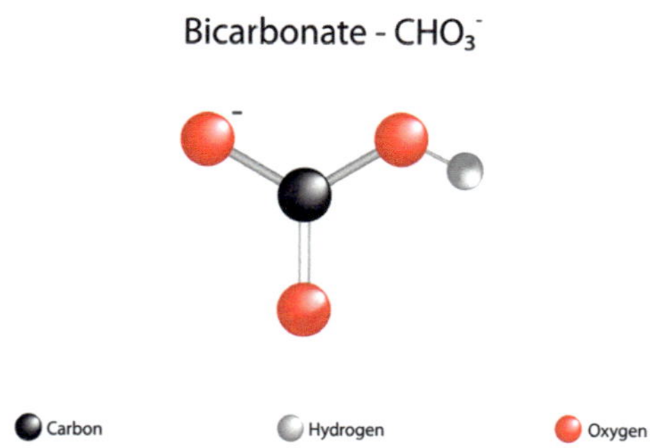

Figure 2.7. Bicarbonate ion.

Source: https://as2.ftcdn.net/v2/jpg/04/74/37/37/1000_F_474373720_gCjxevRwoQ5BmZKIi7GbpVJrgw5X6Mwj.jpg

2.2.2. Major Buffer Systems in the Human Body

The human body controls a delicate balance of pH levels required for normal physiological functions, which is achieved through a series of crucial buffer systems. Of them, the most significant bicarbonate buffer system works primarily in the extracellular fluid. This system uses the equilibrium between carbonic acid ($H2CO_3$) and bicarbonate ions (HCO_3^-) to counteract pH changes. During acidosis, the bicarbonate ions will bind with excess hydrogen ions, and during alkalosis, carbonic acid will break down to give off protons. The dynamic equilibrium provided by this buffer system is a demonstration of the body's excellent capability to maintain acid-base balance using respiratory and renal compensation. Therefore, the understanding of the functioning of the bicarbonate buffer systems provides significant information on general physiological functions, emphasizing its role in maintaining homeostasis of the human body (White, 2025). In addition to the bicarbonate buffer system, proteins are also significant buffers because they exist in huge numbers in the intracellular environment. The amino acids that form proteins have side chains with the ability to accept or donate protons, hence compensating for pH change. This characteristic allows proteins to offer a stable environment within cells, where enzymatic reactions are usually pH-dependent. Moreover, the hemoglobin of red blood cells also acts as a buffer when it carries excess hydrogen ions, facilitating oxygen transport while simultaneously regulating acid-base balance. Such protein buffering highlights the delicate interface between metabolism and body acid-base status, where physiological compensation can impact overall health. Protein buffers' role is vital to biochemical equilibrium as well as preserving the physiological processes that sustain us, demonstrating a stratified complexity to the body's buffering systems (White, 2025).

Phosphate buffers, constituted mainly of dihydrogen phosphate ($H2PO_4^-$) and hydrogen phosphate (HPO^4_{2-}), are particularly important, particularly in intracellular fluids and the renal system. They are all part of cellular metabolism and play a role in pH regulation in both bones and kidneys. While their buffering capacity is less obvious than that of bicarbonate or proteins, phosphates increase in significance in the context of metabolic processes, where they can reverse buffer to eliminate sudden changes in pH. The kidneys actually utilize phosphate buffering when eliminating hydrogen ions, again underlining the interconnectedness of renal function and acid-base homeostasis. Thus, the phosphate buffer system, though not often recognized, is a vital component of the body's intricate mechanisms to respond to metabolic stress, complementing other buffering systems in controlling optimal acid-base physiology (White, 2025) (Figure 2.8).

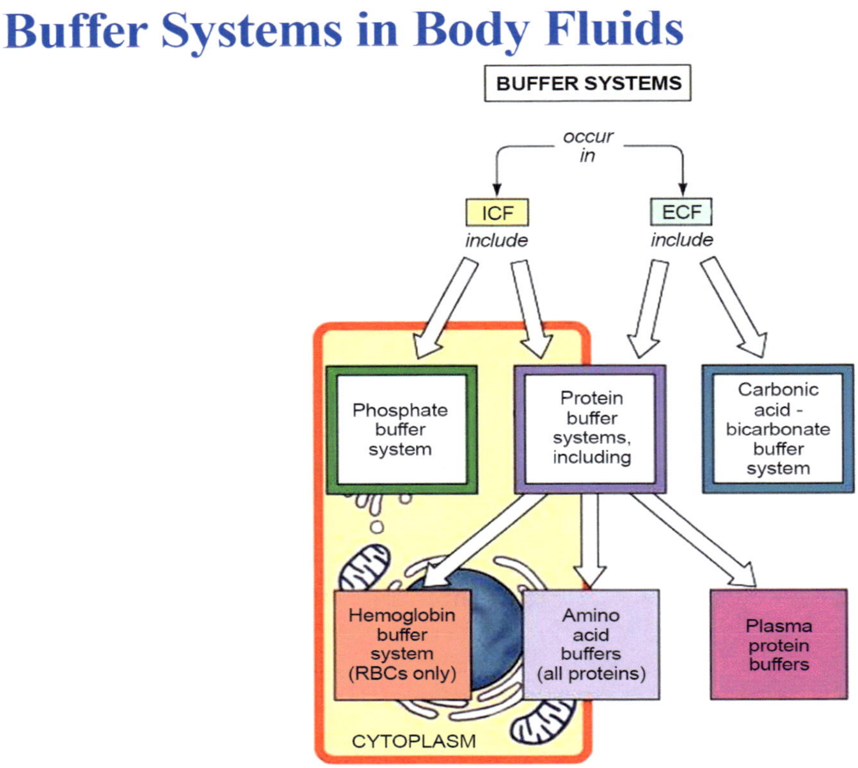

Figure 2.8. Buffer systems in body fluids.

Source: https://image1.slideserve.com/2821926/buffer-systems-in-body-fluids-l.jpg.

2.2.3. Importance of Buffers in Maintaining pH

Purification of small quantities of acid and base within the system is vital to ensure optimal physiological functioning, and buffers play a critical role in regulation and are vital regulators within the process. Buffers are solutions that resist pH changes upon the addition of minute amounts of base or acid, keeping the internal world constant. In biological systems, buffer systems typically consist of a weak acid and its conjugate base, which function together to sequester excess hydrogen ions (H^+) or to release them as needed. This buffering capacity is particularly valuable in numerous tissues and body fluids, including blood, intracellular spaces, and even the aqueous medium of aquatic animals. Since organisms are exposed to varying environmental stressors that can lead to pH changes, there is a need for a proper buffering system to facilitate homeostasis and permit metabolic processes to proceed unabated. Buffers have roles beyond simple stabilization of pH; they facilitate crucial physiological processes that are pH-dependent. Like, enzymes possess optimal performance in a narrow range of pH, and their variation hinders biochemical activities necessary for survival. In the human body, the bicarbonate buffer system is one of the important mechanisms for maintaining blood pH. Elevated levels of CO2 in the blood trigger carbonic acid production, which dissociates to release H^+ ions and lower pH. When CO2 levels drop, bicarbonate can bind to H+, raising pH. This balance is crucial because acid-base derangements can produce states of alkalosis or acidosis with far-reaching health effects and the necessity of re-establishing physiological balance (Stechmiller et al., 2025). Furthermore, some body systems, such as, the respiratory and kidney systems, also work together with buffers to regulate acid-base status effectively. The lungs remove CO2, which is a metabolic byproduct of its immediate effect on blood pH. Meanwhile, the kidneys assist by regulating bicarbonate reserves and removing H+ ions, thus complementing the buffering activity of body fluids. In teleost fish, for instance, the renal system takes on a prominent role in acid-base homeostasis via balancing ammonia and phosphate levels, which are vital against environmental stresses (Takvam et al., 2023). This interesting collaboration between buffers, lungs, and kidneys is a testament to staying in pH balance, as ideal conditions need to be met for life to progress, as well as for proper organism function against many environmental stresses.

Test Your Knowledge

1. What is a buffer, and how does it help maintain pH in biological systems?
2. Which buffer systems are most important in regulating blood pH?

2.3. Respiratory Regulation of Acid-Base Balance

Learning Outcome

1. Explain the mechanism of CO2 regulation;
2. Define the role of the respiratory system in pH balance;
3. Describe the impact of respiratory disorders on acid-base physiology.

Acid-base balance is controlled by the respiratory system, and it is one of the most critical physiological processes which enable the body to establish homeostasis in the face of metabolic changes. Carbon dioxide (CO_2) is constantly exchanged between the body and the environment during respiration. The level of carbonic acid (H2CO_3), which is formed when CO_2 combines with water, is directly influenced by this exchange. An increase in CO_2 concentrations can lead to respiratory acidosis, a process that is characterized by low pH due to increased blood acidity. The respiratory system is hence responsible for compensating for such acidotic conditions; increasing the rate and depth of respiration enables greater excretion of CO_2. Thus, the respiratory system provides a rapid, regulatory mechanism that harmonizes with the other systems, most critically the renal system, to maintain acid-base balance. In aquatic animals, such as, fish, the restriction of their environment contributes significantly to their acid-base physiology. Fish gills are specially modified to extract oxygen from water, allowing effective respiratory function. However, these gills are not very adaptable to the exposure to air, leading to hypoxia and hypercapnia upon removal from water. Gill collapse to air pressure prevents adequate gas exchange, and respiratory acidosis ensues as CO_2 accumulates due to impaired excretion (Odunze, 2005). This situation illustrates the complex interplay of respiratory function and acid-base homeostasis in aquatic organisms. The inherent limitations placed on aquatic animals emphasize the key role of respiratory regulation in managing a stable internal environment, illustrating the broader importance of acid-base balance in diverse habitats. Coordination between the lungs, kidneys, and various buffering mechanisms is required to control acid-base balance adequately in higher organisms. Lungs are the first line of defense against altered blood pH by regulating CO2 through varying respiratory rate. At the same time, renal function contributes to this effect by removing hydrogen ions (H^+) and reabsorbing bicarbonate (HCO_3^-) to stabilize pH on a longer time frame (White, 2025). The interaction between such regulatory processes underlines the complexity of acid-base balance, whereby acute as well as chronic imbalances must be corrected to maintain physiological integrity. A clear understanding of such interactions not only accounts for normal physiological responses but also elucidates the pathophysiologic mechanisms of most diseases capable of disrupting acid-base homeostasis (Figure 2.9).

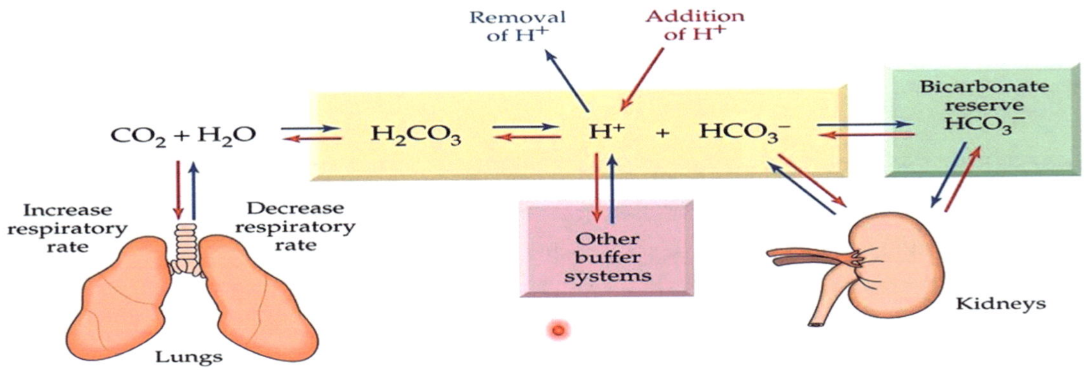

Figure 2.9. Respiratory mechanism for the regulation of pH.

Source: https://i.ytimg.com/vi/GKFxuHKVh10/maxresdefault.jpg.

2.3.1. Mechanism of CO_2 Regulation

Carbon dioxide (CO_2) control in the human body is a critical component of acid-base homeostasis. The interaction between metabolic processes and respiratory function ensures CO_2 is within a preferred range. CO_2 is an end-product of cellular respiration that is generated by cells, and when it dissolves in blood, it can influence the extracellular fluid pH. The principal mechanism of CO_2 control is through the bicarbonate buffering system, wherein there exists a dynamic equilibrium between carbon dioxide (CO_2), bicarbonate (HCO_3^-), and carbonic acid (H_2CO_3). The lungs and kidneys also work together to control CO_2 concentration through respiration and renal excretion. Enhanced ventilation can improve the removal of CO_2, while reduced rates of respiration lead to its accumulation. Thus, an understanding of these mechanisms is essential to an appreciation of the overall dynamics of acid-base physiology, where pathways are interdependent and produce systemic pH homeostasis (White, 2025). In aquatic animals, CO2 regulation is particularly difficult, particularly in fish, which rely on gills for respiration. Fish gills close in air, substantially impairing their ability to expel CO_2 and cope with concurrent respiratory acidosis upon air exposure. This disparity highlights the necessity for adjustments to their water environment, where CO2 elimination is a continuous process. Failure in CO_2 regulation leads to dangerous conditions , such as hypoxia and hypercapnia, thus complicating acid-base balance in these organisms. Fish display remarkable physiological mechanisms that allow them to adjust to altered environmental conditions, but the built-in limit of their respiratory system is behind the necessity of CO_2 regulation to survive in an aquatic environment (Odunze, 2005). The interaction between such regulatory systems in human beings or aquatic animals depicts the fundamental role of CO_2 management for the maintenance of acid-base balance. In human beings, as exercise increases, so does the production of CO_2, necessitating higher rates of respiration to eliminate excess gas. Under alkalosis or acidosis conditions, nevertheless, the kidneys play a pivotal role in compensatory bicarbonate reabsorption or excretion and therefore in the maintenance of blood pH levels. Such dynamic adaptations reflect the interdependent relationship between the renal and respiratory systems in acid-base regulation. So, the mechanisms of CO_2 regulation are not only stabilizing pH in an immediate way but also revealing a subtle yet intricate physiological architecture that allows for life in a variety of organisms. All this intricate relationship makes it clear why these processes are imperative for understanding acid-base physiology (White, 2025) (Figure 2.10).

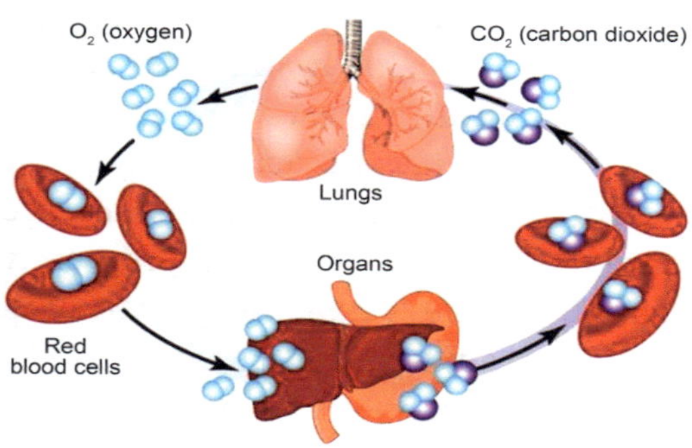

Figure 2.10. Oxygen-and-carbon-dioxide-transported-in-human.

Source: https://classnotes123.com/wp-content/uploads/2021/07/oxygen-and-carbon-dioxide-transported-in-human-beings.jpg.

2.3.2. Role of the Respiratory System in pH Balance

The respiratory system plays a very significant role in the acid-base equilibrium of the human body by controlling the level of carbon dioxide (CO_2) in the body. When formed in cellular metabolism, CO2 goes into solution in blood, where it reacts with water to form carbonic acid ($H2CO_3$). The acid further decomposes to bicarbonate (HCO_3^-) and hydrogen ions (H^+), hence reducing pH and increasing acidity. The lungs achieve this stability by regulating the rate and depth of breathing; increased breathing eliminates more CO2, leading to a pH increase, while decreased ventilation allows for accumulation of CO2, later decreasing pH. This regulation is necessary to prevent conditions like alkalosis or acidosis, hence supporting the truth that respiratory physiology forms part of homeostasis in acid-base physiology (Bahr et al., 2015). Furthermore, the buffering ability of blood is predominantly regulated by the respiratory system's ability to maintain CO_2 levels. Respiratory function is closely related to the bicarbonate buffer system, the simplest mechanism of pH regulation. When the pH value departs from its standard, the respiratory system reacts accordingly to eliminate these differences. For instance, in metabolic acidosis, when pH falls, the rate of respiration may increase to expel CO2 and thus regain equilibrium. In metabolic alkalosis, decreased ventilation retains CO_2 to allow pH to become normal once more. This exchange emphasizes the importance of the respiratory system as more than just a facilitator of gas exchange but also as an essential acid-base regulator through its buffering action and changes in CO_2 concentrations (Leonard et al., 1975). The integrative function of the respiratory system in pH regulation is also demonstrated during exercise, as well as other pathophysiological conditions. Increased muscle activity produces more CO_2 and lactic acid, which also alters the blood pH. This leads to the respiratory system enhancing ventilation to eliminate CO_2 more efficiently and thus showing an immediate physiological response to maintain acid-base balance. This also holds true in diseases , such as chronic obstructive pulmonary disease (COPD), where the impaired ventilation capacity can cause respiratory acidosis, emphasizing the role of respiratory dysfunction on pH equilibrium. Hence, any derogation in respiratory function would have important implications for the entire acid-base status in the body, with great focus given to the respiratory systems role as an integral component of acid-base physiology (Bahr et al., 2015) (Figure 2.11).

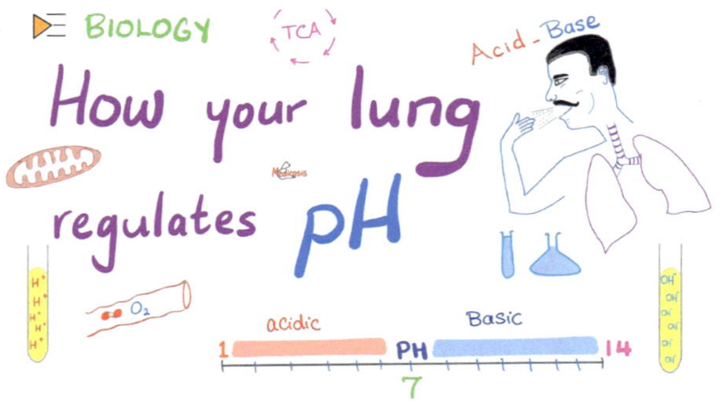

Figure 2.11. Role of the respiratory system in pH balance.

Source: https://i.ytimg.com/vi/FWQHBjE0i-k/maxresdefault.jpg.

2.3.3. Impact of Respiratory Disorders on Acid-Base Physiology

This is significant because any respiratory dysfunction can lead to serious imbalances of the acid-base status of the body. Respiratory disorders , such as asthma and COPD, frequently impair the lungs' ability to exchange gases effectively. The impairment leads to hypoventilation and the accumulation of carbon dioxide, a condition known as hypercapnia. The subsequent elevation in concentration of carbon dioxide further lowers the blood pH, leading to respiratory acidosis. Through compensatory mechanisms in the body, renal mechanisms can be provoked to excrete more hydrogen ions and reabsorb bicarbonate, exemplifying the complex physiological mechanisms involved. Knowledge of these mechanisms is relevant in that neglect of the impact of respiratory disease on acid-base homeostasis can aggravate patient outcomes and simplify management plans. In addition to respiratory acidosis, respiratory disease is also able to result in metabolic derangement, further complicated by acid-base physiology. For instance, severe attacks of asthma can cause such respiratory alkalosis due to hyperventilation, but also result in a state of metabolic acidosis due to the generation of lactic acid from oxygen deficiency. Both of these disturbances create a challenge in classifying the particular acid-base state of patients, hence necessitating careful scrutiny of blood gases.

Further, the involved respiratory dysfunction in these patients can generate a self-perpetuating vicious cycle; with worsening acidosis or alkalosis, the consequent additional respiratory distress and maladaptive physiological adaptation can be initiated. This dynamic feedback cycle underscores the necessity of aggressive treatment protocols that address both the underlying respiratory disease and the resulting acid-base disturbance to promote patient prognosis and quality of life. New data highlights the broader relevance of environmental factors in respiratory diseases and the latter's accompanying acid-base disturbances. Air pollution, allergens, and occupational exposures are progressively implicated in the respiratory pathologies that enhance acid-base disturbances. More specifically, environmental exposure has been associated with epigenetic marker changes that may affect the severity and course of respiratory disease. For example, mounting evidence illustrates how DNA methylation alterations can be involved in mediating the impact of environmental stressors on respiratory health, ultimately affecting acid-base physiology through mechanisms , such as inflammation and altered gas exchange mechanisms. It is essential to understand these intricate relationships as they can direct certain interventions to reverse the impact of environmental exposure on populations vulnerable to respiratory disease, hence improving overall clinical acid-base management (Zhu et al., 2020).

Test Your Knowledge

1. How does the respiratory system regulate blood pH through CO_2 levels?
2. What happens to blood pH during hypoventilation and hyperventilation?

2.4. Renal Regulation of Acid-Base Balance

Learning Outcome

1. Identify the mechanisms of renal acid-base regulation;
2. Define the role of the kidneys in bicarbonate reabsorption;
3. Describe the effects of renal dysfunction on acid-base status.

The kidneys play an important function in the acid-base homeostasis of the body, a task necessary for homeostasis. The mechanism involves the filtration of blood plasma, which is utilized to remove hydrogen ions (H^+) and reabsorb bicarbonate (HCO_3^-), acting as a buffer in the blood. The glomeruli filter the blood so that the renal tubules actively engage in secreting excess H+ and reabsorbing bicarbonate. This fine balance enables the kidneys to counteract acid level variations, adapting to metabolic and dietary conditions. Furthermore, the renal reaction to acid-base imbalance is not constant; it is associated with complex interactions with many hormones and neurotransmitters that adapt renal function to the needs of the body. It is necessary to keep this fine balance to prevent the occurrence of acidosis and alkalosis, the impact of which could prove detrimental to cellular activity. Besides these primary mechanisms, renal regulation of acid-base balance also shows diurnal variation, which is indicative of an advanced chronobiological process. As characterized in studies, kidneys exhibit 24-hour periodicity regulated by circadian rhythms, which affect renal filtration and H+ and bicarbonate reabsorption rates. The physiological changes regulated by these rhythms are accompanied by hormonal fluctuations that regulate renal function at different points throughout the day. As an example, hormone secretion , such as the release of aldosterone and cortisol, can regulate the kidneys' reaction to changes in acid-base composition in order to align renal function with the body's total physiological requirements (Bonny et al., 2013). It is important to understand this temporal aspect of renal physiology, particularly in a clinical setting where timing is a major factor influencing intervention outcomes. Besides, integration of renal function with global systemic health also gives precedence to the kidneys' role in acid-base homeostasis in broader biological contexts. Disturbances in this balance have the potential to trigger a number of pathophysiological states, which include metabolic disease and chronic kidney disease. The cross-relation between diurnal variation and renal activity suggests that extrinsic forces , such as lifestyle and environmental change, have a significant bearing on the efficiency of the kidneys in sustaining acid-base balance. Research shows that circadian rhythm disturbances, often as a result of alterations in environmental factors or lifestyles, can lead to misregulation of renal functions with subsequent long-term health issues (Skotnicka et al., 2007). Understanding deeper into the renal regulation of acid-base balance in both physiological and temporal aspects is therefore important to develop holistic treatment solutions for related health disorders (Figure 2.12).

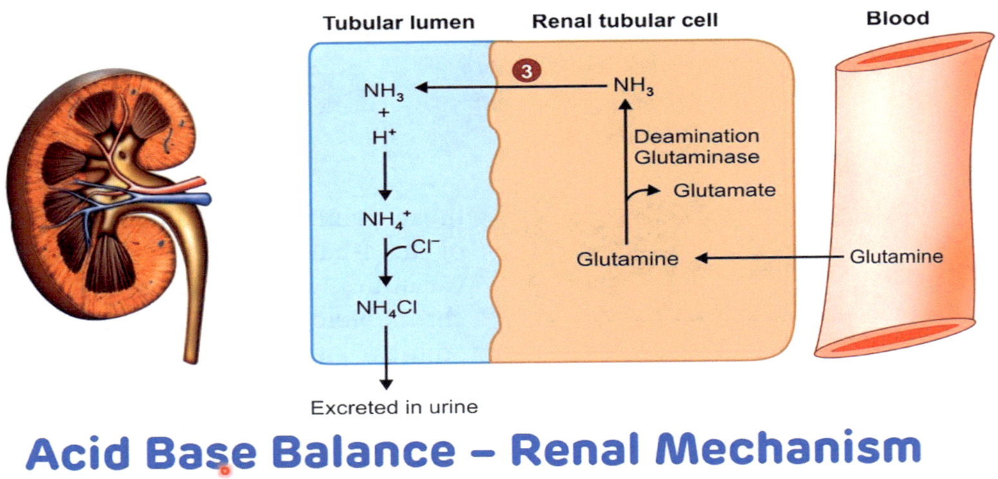

Figure 2.12. Renal regulation of acid-base balance.

Source: https://i.ytimg.com/vi/gUe2J400ULo/maxresdefault.jpg.

2.4.1. Mechanisms of Renal Acid-Base Regulation

Renal acid-base regulatory mechanisms play a pivotal role in ensuring homeostasis in the human body. The kidneys are at the heart of this process in that they cleanse blood and adjust the excretion or the process of reabsorbing various ions like hydrogen ions (H^+) and bicarbonate (HCO_3^-). Renal tubular organizations allow for such regulation by incorporating complex transport activities that adjust the pH of blood and body fluids. Of particular interest are the nephron segments, i.e., the proximal convoluted tubule and the cortical collecting duct, which are equipped with special cells with a dynamic ability to respond to metabolic conditions. Such function of these cells to secrete acids or reclaim bicarbonate is of prime significance in counteracting states of acidosis or alkalosis and therefore plays a vital role in the organism's overall acid-base status. Notably, acid-base homeostasis regulation is not just a static process but also exhibits circadian rhythmic modulation. The kidney undergoes diurnal alterations in function that reflect the body's overall circadian rhythms and are controlled by the light-dark cycle.

This periodicity affects how renal functions , such as acid-base regulation and electrolyte balance, perform over the day. Disruptions of these rhythmic events may cause internal inconsistencies and, hence a range of pathophysiological states. More information about the interweaving of circadian mechanisms with renal physiology can give clues to how the pathology underlying diseases , such as hypertension and metabolic syndrome might arise and also direct potential therapeutic interventions for increasing renal function by timing therapies in concert with the body's own internal rhythms (Bonny et al., 2013). The cortical collecting duct (CCD) is the central site of acid-base homeostasis regulation that has revealed the intricacy of mechanisms employed by the kidneys. Recent studies have unraveled the involvement of principal and intercalated cells of the duct, where there is an intricate interaction of transport mechanisms. Traditionally, intercalated cells were considered to be mainly regulators of acid-base status, but recent findings have uncovered the function of these cells in sodium chloride (NaCl) absorption as well. Additionally, type A intercalated cells are currently recognized for their capacity for secretion of NaCl through H,K-ATPase type 2 pump-energized processes. This new perspective emphasizes the masterful versatility of the CCD in the regulation of both salt and acid-base transport. Thus, such renal physiology interactions emphasize the necessity of the kidneys to acid-base balance and highlight the intricacy of renal adaptation to physiological requirements (Edwards & Crambert, 2017) (Figure 2.13).

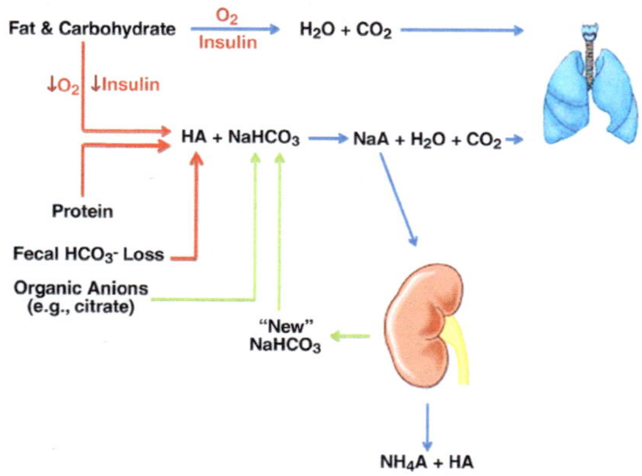

Figure 2.13. Kidney and acid base regulation in physiology.

Source: https://journals.physiology.org/cms/10.1152/advan.00054.2009/asset/images/large/zu10040925570001.jpeg.

2.4.2. Role of Kidneys in Bicarbonate Reabsorption

Kidneys have a central role in acid-base homeostasis in the body through bicarbonate (HCO_3^-) reabsorption. Bicarbonate reabsorption is important for the stability of the pH of the extracellular fluids, especially during metabolic changes. Bicarbonate reabsorption mostly happens in the proximal tubule, where renal tubular cells use different transport processes to recover this critical buffer. Sodium-bicarbonate cotransporters and bicarbonate exchangers are key to the process, allowing for the easy exchange of bicarbonate ions back into the circulation while maintaining sodium equilibrium. The dynamic equilibrium between bicarbonate reabsorption and hydrogen ion secretion is part of the kidneys' function in acid neutralization and hence serves to highlight their role in acid-base physiology as well as overall metabolic health, as later explored in research on renal acid-base regulation (White, 2025). In addition to bicarbonate reabsorption, kidneys also regulate other acid-base equivalents , such as ammonia and phosphate, which act as urinary buffers. Regulation of ammonia by the kidneys demonstrates a clear mechanism for acid removal through its conversion to ammonium ions. It operates in tandem with bicarbonate kinetics to offset excess acidity in cases of metabolic imbalance. Furthermore, the kidneys identify and respond to changes in systemic pH, controlling transport mechanisms to ensure an effective modulation of bicarbonate levels. Such advanced regulatory processes confirm the kidneys' function not only as passive filtration organs but as active mediators of acid-base homeostasis. This is better understood in those species with diverse acidifying and alkalinizing issues, where renal adaptations become essential in maintaining homeostasis (Takvam et al., 2023). Furthermore, the physiological significance of bicarbonate reabsorption extends beyond mere pH homeostasis; it is an expression of the kidney's capacity for adaptation to varying environmental and metabolic conditions. For instance, variations in salt intake in the diet as well as levels of respiratory gas influence bicarbonate handling directly, with kidneys adjusting their rates of reabsorption according to the body's homeostatic requirements. Understanding these regulatory mechanisms is of clinical importance, too, particularly in disorders , such as metabolic acidosis or alkalosis, in which renal bicarbonate regulation can be disrupted. Lastly, an understanding of the kidneys' role in bicarbonate reabsorption sheds light on broader considerations for renal function and disease, bridging elementary physiological processes to potential therapeutic targets in managing acid-base disturbances (White, 2025) (Figure 2.14).

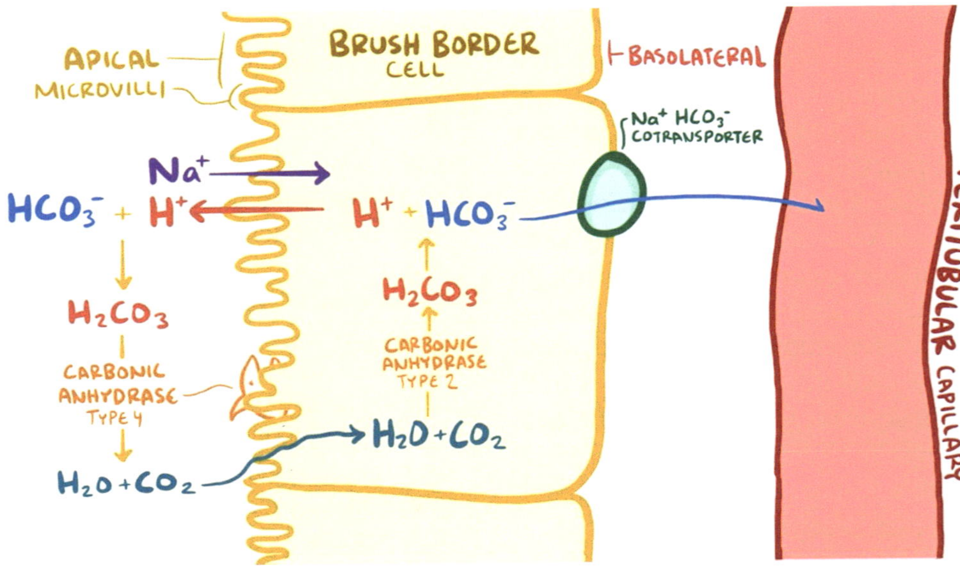

Figure 2.14. The role of the kidney in acid-base balance.

Source: https://osmose-it.s3.amazonaws.com/EapuASmDQb69TQQ5qoZVRUUQR5uZFyGw/_.jpg.

2.4.3. Effects of Renal Dysfunction on Acid-Base Status

The kidneys are central organs involved in the acid-base homeostasis process, managing hydrogen ion excretion and bicarbonate reabsorption. In renal impairment, these processes are severely compromised and cause acids to build up within the body, leading to metabolic acidosis. It is most evident in renal tubular acidosis (RTA), when the kidneys cannot effectively acidify urine, leading to systemic acid-base derangement. Systemic effects of RTA extend beyond mere physiological alterations; it influences cardiovascular function and can lead to complications of hypertension and arrhythmias. Knowledge of these dysfunctions is pivotal in allowing healthcare providers to utilize targeted interventions that not only address renal well-being but also the systemic effects of acid-base imbalance, hence promoting comprehensive patient care and improved outcomes (Coral, 2024). This interrelationship is further complicated by extrarenal conditions like dietary habits and associated diseases. For instance, patients with eating disorders like anorexia nervosa and bulimia nervosa may present with profound renal impairment due to reasons like dehydration and electrolyte imbalance. Such malnutrition not only compromises renal perfusion but also precipitates acute kidney injury (AKI), which further escalates acid-base disturbance. As indicated in recent literature, renal function in patients with eating disorders must be controlled carefully, considering that these patients are prone to sharp fluctuations in blood urea nitrogen, serum creatinine, and glomerular filtration rates. Correction of such fluctuations is essential in the process of restoring acid-base balance, emphasizing the importance of a multi-assertive approach in treating kidney status and nutritional rehabilitation (Burlaka & Mityuryayeva, 2024). In managing renal dysfunction and its impact on acid-base balance, both the short-term and long-term interventions need to be attended to. Effective management of metabolic acidosis is often achieved through fluid rehydration and the correction of electrolyte balance, which may be particularly significant in patients with a history of eating disorders. Re-establishing normal fluid volumes not only sustains renal function but also enhances the kidneys' ability to maintain acid-base balance. As more research unmasked the complexity of acid-base physiology in renal well-being, follow-up studies should give top priority to the establishment of new therapeutic strategies tailored to individual patient profiles. These include the combination of pharmacologic therapy and diet supplementation to optimize the function of the kidneys as well as protection against the formation of acute acid-base disturbances, thereby improving patient care and quality of life (Burlaka & Mityuryayeva, 2024; Coral, 2024).

Test Your Knowledge

1. What role do the kidneys play in maintaining acid-base balance?
2. How do the kidneys regulate blood pH?

2.5. Clinical Implications of Acid-Base Disorders

Learning Outcome

1. Identify the common acid-base disorders (acidosis and alkalosis);
2. Define the symptoms and diagnosis of acid-base imbalances;
3. Describe the treatment options for acid-base disorders.

The clinical importance of acid-base disorders is more than a reductionist response to blood pH. In intensive care, acid-base balance is critical because derangement in it can have huge impacts on patient outcomes. Chloride, as the principal extracellular anion, plays a crucial but frequently underestimated part in these conditions. The abnormal levels of chloride can be caused by multiple interventions, but particularly fluid therapy, hence adding to the complex clinical picture. Recent studies have proposed that familiarity with the implications of chloride levels can also refine our strategy in acid-base physiology and reveal that changes in chloremia can have a direct bearing on organ function and patient stability during intensive therapy. As such, analysis of acid-base status should incorporate chlorides into the assessment in addition to the conventional parameters of bicarbonate levels and blood pH for effective management planning. It is essential for clinicians to identify the multifactorial pathogenesis of acid-base disturbances because acid-base disturbances may lead to serious complications in different populations of patients. Acidosis or alkalosis may be caused by respiratory illness, metabolic illness, or combined etiology and, therefore, require individually tailored intervention measures. It should be noted that acid-base disturbances may have pronounced effects on cardiovascular stability, respiratory status, and metabolism and, hence, require careful monitoring. For instance, metabolic acidosis, which is frequent in such disorders as diabetic ketoacidosis or renal insufficiency, can aggravate cardiovascular collapse, while respiratory alkalosis can lead to cerebral hypoperfusion. Therapy thus must be precision-based and address not only the immediate cause of the disorder but also the mechanisms of metabolic compensation employed by the body. Owing to the complex interplay between electrolyte abnormalities and acid-base abnormalities, effective treatment necessitates an interdisciplinary approach. Physicians must keep in mind monitoring and correcting chloride and other electrolyte abnormalities throughout therapy. In intensive care units, where there may be abrupt changes, physicians should use advanced diagnostic techniques and algorithms to guide interventions appropriately. This approach not only increases knowledge of the individualized needs of the patient but can also direct intravenous fluid choice, an aspect intended to maximize acid-base balance and hydration without exacerbating concurrent disorders. Accordingly, increased awareness of the function of chlorides along with other electrolytes can lead to better outcomes and less morbidity in patients who present with critical acid-base disorders, ultimately leading to more targeted care in acute medical practice (Figure 2.15).

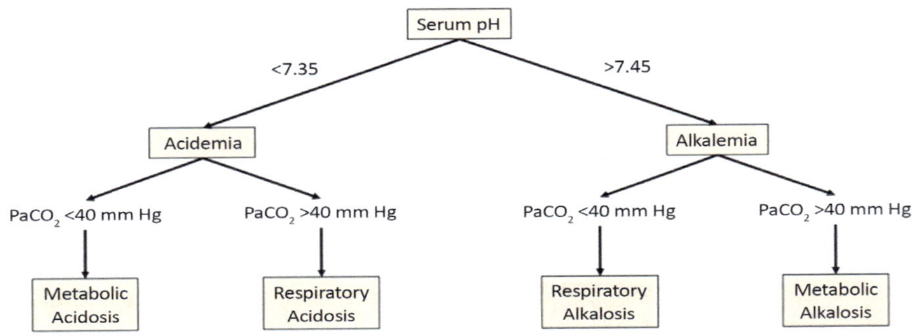

Figure 2.15. Acid-base disorders.

Source: https://media.springernature.com/lw685/springer-static/image/chp%3A10.1007%2F978-3-031-77335-8_27/MediaObjects/602737_1_En_27_Fig1_HTML.png.

2.5.1. Common Acid-Base Disorders (Acidosis and Alkalosis)

The pH of the body is an unstable balance by virtue of many physiological mechanisms, and disruption of these mechanisms is the cause of the typical acidosis and alkalosis in terms of acid-base disturbances. Acidosis is a decrease in blood pH secondary to increased acid production or bicarbonate loss. The two general categories of acidosis are respiratory and metabolic. Respiratory acidosis is likely to occur due to hypoventilation, which leads to the retention of carbon dioxide and therefore to the rise in hydrogen ion concentration. Metabolic acidosis, on the other hand, can be caused by disorders , such as chronic renal failure or diabetic ketoacidosis, in which the body either generates excess acids or fails to eliminate them in the right manner. Understanding these mechanisms is vital in the diagnosis and proper management of patients with evidence of acid-base imbalances, as the clinical outcome would be disastrous if they were not noticed and treated. In contrast to acidosis, alkalosis is characterized by elevated blood pH, with significant types being respiratory and metabolic alkalosis. Respiratory alkalosis is most often a result of hyperventilation, most often a consequence of anxiety, pain, or pulmonary disorders, which lead to excessive loss of carbon dioxide with a resultant decrease in acidity. Metabolic alkalosis may be due to hyperemesis, diuretic administration, or excessive bicarbonate intake, all resulting in an excess of bicarbonate or loss of hydrogen ions.

The physiological abnormalities associated with alkalosis can include muscle spasm, cardiac arrhythmias, and impaired tissue oxygen supply, emphasizing the necessity for early detection and intervention. As medical practitioners, differential diagnosis of acid-base disorders forms a systematic approach involving patient history, clinical examination, and investigations to identify the underlying causative factor and direct appropriate treatment interventions. All areas of healthcare must work together in the treatment of acid-base disorders, particularly when mixed disturbances are present in complicated cases. For instance, individuals with chronic obstructive pulmonary disease will become precipitously acidotic, respiratory complications, and a secondary metabolic alkalosis resulting from compensation mechanisms that further complicate their clinical condition and complicate therapy (Bruno & Valenti, 2012). Similarly, in diabetic ketoacidosis, dominance by high anion gap metabolic acidosis may occur along with other respiratory or metabolic disturbances, and hence accurate diagnosis is critical to successful treatment (Duarte et al., 2012). Understanding the interactions between these disorders not only potentially optimizes individual patient results but also widespread clinical developments in acid-base physiology. Thus, the detection and treatment of both acidosis and alkalosis in a holistic manner remains a pillar of medical practice, emphasizing the utmost importance of ongoing education and collaboration in addressing these conditions of profound significance (Figure 2.16).

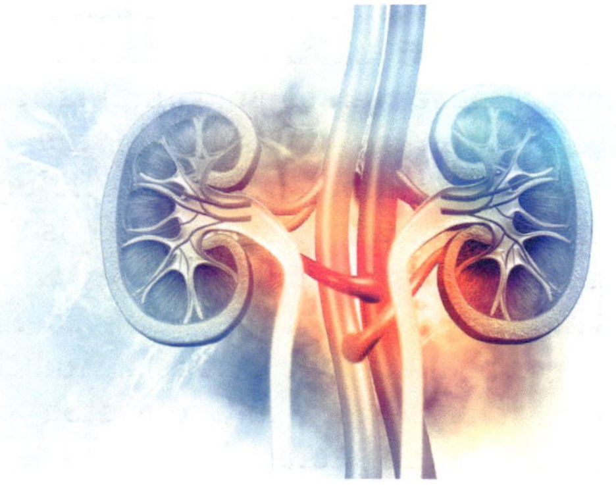

Figure 2.16. Acidosis and alkalosis.

Source: https://pathologytestsexplained.org.au/content/summaryimages/kidneys.jpg.

2.5.2. Symptoms and Diagnosis of Acid-Base Imbalances

The manifestations of acid-base derangements may be very diverse depending on the disorder—either metabolic acidosis, metabolic alkalosis, respiratory acidosis, or respiratory alkalosis. Metabolic acidosis is presented in patients who have labored respirations, confusion, and somnolence due to the accumulation of acids in the bloodstream. Metabolic alkalosis can manifest as muscle fasciculations, hand tremors, or seizures due to the disturbance of the body's electrolyte balance. Respiratory disorders also contribute significantly; respiratory acidosis is typically accompanied by dyspnea and confusion due to carbon dioxide retention, whereas respiratory alkalosis results in dizziness, light-headedness, and palpitations owing to excessive loss of carbon dioxide. Detection and correction in early stages are critical for treating the conditions and therefore the importance of clinical assessment in acid-base physiology. Acid-base imbalance diagnosis is predominantly by blood gas tests, with arterial blood gas (ABG) tests being particularly common. Blood gas tests monitor essential parameters , such as arterial pH, partial pressure of carbon dioxide (pCO_2), and bicarbonate (HCO_3^-) level. A pH value less than 7.35 can indicate acidosis, while greater than 7.45 indicates alkalosis. Physicians interpret these values in combination with clinical symptoms to ascertain the precise nature of the imbalance and etiology. For instance, low pH with elevated pCO_2 is typically indicative of respiratory acidosis, while low pH with either normal or decreased HCO_3^- is indicative of metabolic acidosis. Additionally, elevated bicarbonate and elevated pH are characteristic of metabolic alkalosis, while decreased pH with decreased pCO_2 is indicative of respiratory alkalosis. Thus, accurate diagnosis hinges on an exhaustive understanding of these parameters to institute appropriate therapeutic plans. Because of the complexity of acid-base disturbances, differential diagnosis involves many conditions that can lead to imbalances. For instance, metabolic acidosis is caused by disorders , such as renal failure, diabetic ketoacidosis, or profound diarrhea, all of which alter the body's acid-base homeostasis.

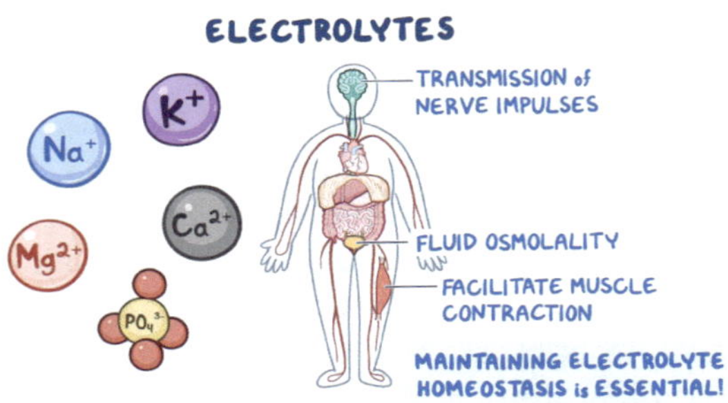

Figure 2.17. Electrolyte balance.

Source: https://d16qt3wv6xm098.cloudfront.net/U540jeRATn6H40eKXELeTcM2QkGJAIiP/_.jpg.

Respiratory acidosis, however, can be due to chronic obstructive pulmonary disease (COPD) or acute respiratory distress, both of which result in excessive retention of carbon dioxide. It is imperative that clinicians integrate patient history, clinical presentation, and laboratory findings to develop a clear clinical picture. An understanding of possible underlying pathology is required for successful management. In addition, continued research continues to illuminate the genetic and molecular basis of these disorders, holding promise for new therapeutic options. Greater understanding of these intricate interactions will certainly form the basis of clinical practice in acid-base physiology, ultimately resulting in improved patient outcomes (Figure 2.17).

2.5.3. Treatment Options for Acid-Base Disorders

Treatment of acid-base disturbances is dependent on a profound understanding of pathophysiology to allow clinicians to properly modify the treatment modalities. The cornerstone of the treatment of such disturbances is determination of the specific type—respiratory acidosis, metabolic acidosis, respiratory alkalosis, or metabolic alkalosis—with its individual etiologic causes and outcomes. In respiratory acidosis, as an example, therapy often addresses optimizing ventilation in an attempt to increase carbon dioxide removal, perhaps with bronchodilators or mechanical ventilation in severe illness. In metabolic acidosis, perhaps caused by diabetic ketoacidosis or renal failure, bicarbonate infusion or, in some instances, treating the primary cause directly may be employed. Thus, a thoughtful approach that treats both the acid-base status and the pathophysiology itself is crucial to the effective treatment of these conditions. Recent improvements in acid-base physiology have provided insights into new therapies outside the realm of traditional interventions. For example, it has been shown that custom-tailored bicarbonate infusion will reverse the effects of chronic metabolic acidosis in renally compromised patients. Also, certain dietary interventions, such as, increased intake of alkali-rich foods, are suggested to be employed as adjuvant treatments to counteract excessive acid accumulation in the body. The most pivotal therapy in diuretic-induced hypokalemic metabolic alkalosis patients is the replacement of electrolytes, as they address the drug-induced ionic disproportion directly. This flexibility of treatment highlights the demand for tailored therapy that responds to patients' unique biochemical terrain to achieve optimal efficacy and safety. Additionally, current literature cites the unification of therapeutic technologies with enhanced treatments in acid-base disorders. For instance, innovation in continuous renal replacement therapy can be particularly beneficial in critically ill patients who exhibit sudden disturbances in acid-base balance. New approaches also include new drug therapies that target specific metabolic pathways implicated in acid-base derangements, just as it is currently becoming apparent that next-generation sequencing is a new method for detecting genetic factors that shape these conditions. Still, as so frequently happens with medicine, it remains necessary to couple these new treatments with good, old-fashioned clinical practice. Its multidisciplinary nature not only guarantees effective management but also draws upon applied uses of research developments in the branch. As seen in recent publications, the search for new avenues of treatment continues to characterize the way acid-base disorder management is directed, with hopes for improved patient outcomes to come.

Test Your Knowledge

1. What are the clinical signs of metabolic acidosis?
2. How does respiratory alkalosis affect serum calcium levels?
3. Why is arterial blood gas (ABG) analysis important in diagnosing acid-base disorders?

2.6. Acid-Base Physiology in Special Populations

Learning Outcome

1. Describe the acid-base balance in infants and children;
2. Define the considerations in elderly patients;
3. Discuss the impact of pregnancy on acid-base physiology.

In acid-base physiology, there are some populations , such as neonates and the elderly, that react differently and have to be approached with caution in research. Neonates, for instance, have immature renal function and altered respiratory mechanics, which impact their ability to correct acid-base derangements optimally. Their altered metabolic demands and impaired capacity to reabsorb bicarbonate mean that small alterations in acid-base balance can have major clinical consequences. It is important for clinicians to recognize the physiological alterations at this age to develop plans for monitoring and treating illnesses like metabolic acidosis or alkalosis. Effective intervention can significantly improve results for critically ill newborns, and that makes individualized therapeutic care so important in this vulnerable group. Similarly, the elderly are a complex mix of factors that control acid-base balance. Renal deterioration with age, along with comorbidities and polypharmacy, affects the body's homeostatic mechanisms. Age-induced loss of the capacity to excrete hydrogen and reabsorb bicarbonate predisposes older individuals to acid-base derangements, particularly in the context of acute illness or hospitalization. Additionally, the physiological alterations that accompany aging—e.g., diminished muscle mass and altered respiratory function—render it increasingly difficult to maintain acid-base equilibrium. With these aspects in mind, healthcare providers must be keen when assessing acid-base status among older adults since early intervention can prevent adverse effects on health outcomes. The role of dietary factors and intestinal well-being in acid-base physiology has gained increasing attention, with significant implications for special populations. For instance, dietary non-starch polysaccharides (NSP) are extensively documented to exert considerable effects on gastrointestinal function and microbial counts, which were demonstrated to alter metabolic acidosis or alkalosis in healthy humans as well as in patients with some medical conditions. The proportion and solubility of NSP in diets have been reported to affect organic matter digestibility and the overall gut environment, thus altering the production of organic acids and, in turn, systemic pH levels. In species , such as neonatal piglets, where gut health is critical to development and growth, optimizing NSP intake could have therapeutic benefits that can be extrapolated to other species and even humans. A comprehension of how nutrition, gut health, and acid-base balance are intertwined is essential to develop integrative management strategies in special populations (Högberg, 2003; Talling, 2004) (Figure 2.18).

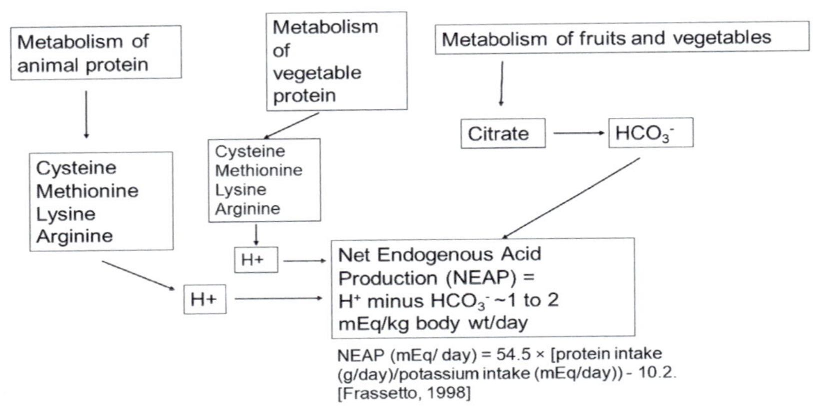

Figure 2.18. Acid–base metabolism and human physiology.

Source: https://pub.mdpi-res.com/ijms/ijms-25-02420/article_deploy/html/images/ijms-25-02420-g001-550.jpg?1708339048.

2.6.1. Acid-Base Balance in Infants and Children

It is important to learn about acid-base balance in children and infants due to their unique physiological characteristics. The immature respiratory and renal machinery of young patients results in the failure to maintain acid-base homeostasis as effectively as adults. Owing to increased body surface area relative to volume, infants lose more insensible water and hence add more to acid-base disturbances. They also have increased metabolic rates and hence yield an increased amount of metabolic acids. Consequently, situations , such as acidosis or alkalosis can arise faster than in adults. Serum bicarbonate and electrolytes must be monitored closely on any clinical assessment to maintain adequate acid-base balance and prevent significant clinical presentations in this vulnerable group. Diarrhea is a prevalent disorder that has a significant impact on acid-base status in children, especially infants in resource-poor settings. This category is at greatest risk for dehydration and electrolyte imbalance due to their high metabolic needs and low reserves. Management of acute diarrheal disease is largely dependent on effective rehydration procedures aimed at restoring fluid and electrolyte balance. Where diarrhea leads to metabolic acidosis, early rehydration interventions can cut short the risk of morbidity from the disease (Nweji, 1988). Appreciation of the complexities of such interventions is crucial to medical professionals as they endeavor to stabilize the affected children so that any reduction in acid-base status can be rapidly rectified. In addition, respiratory infections are also capable of complicating acid-base status in pediatric patients. These infections tend to impair gas exchange, with a consequent potential accumulation of carbon dioxide and resulting respiratory acidosis. Children and infants may demonstrate somnolence and poor feeding that mask underlying disturbances in acid-base. Early intervention is critical to prevent worsening, as untreated respiratory acidosis has the potential to evolve into severe complications.

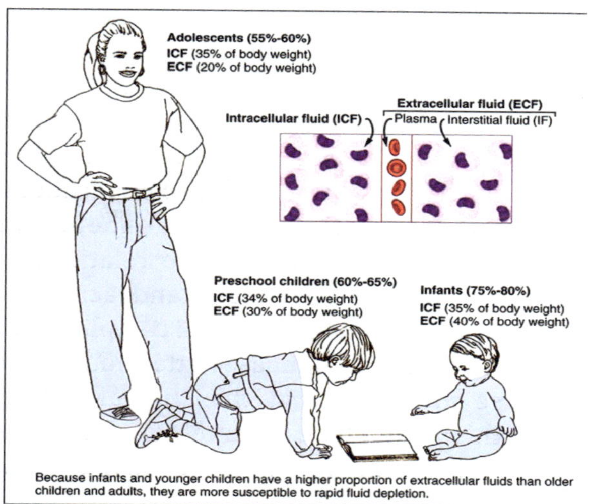

Figure 2.19. The child with a fluid and electrolyte alteration.

Source: https://nursekey.com/wp-content/uploads/2016/10/F00040Xu40-01-9781437727753.jpg.

The close relationship between respiratory function and acid-base state emphasizes the need for close observation in pediatric patients, particularly those with compromised status. Deep understanding of these dynamics assists healthcare professionals in providing holistic care and identifying the optimal outcomes for children suffering from acid-base imbalance (Figure 2.19).

2.6.2. Considerations in Elderly Patients

With the aging of the world's population, physiological considerations of acid-base balance in the elderly patient come into increasing prominence. Aging is also associated with decreased kidney function, leading to impaired acid excretion and susceptibility to metabolic acidosis. This complication can complicate the course of such chronic diseases prevalent among this group as diabetes and cardiovascular disease. In older patients, buffering capacity of acidosis can be lost due to decreased skeletal muscle mass and impaired gastrointestinal absorption. It underlines the need for regular monitoring and evaluation of acid-base status on the part of medical practitioners. Co-morbidities also have a tendency that needs a holistic treatment approach to enable the identification of interrelated conditions, enhance patient outcomes, and enhance quality of life. By identifying these changes, clinicians can formulate individualized treatment plans that consider the acute and chronic conditions of aging patients. Some nutritionally related issues also occur within the context of acid-base physiology among elderly individuals. Older adults may be vulnerable to dietary deficiencies due to insufficient intake or absorption of various vitamins and amino acids, which may further amplify metabolic imbalance. For example, protein deficiencies can be detrimental to muscle metabolism and compromise the body's ability to maintain acid-base homeostasis. Vitamins have also been investigated for their contribution to mediating musculoskeletal healing and musculoskeletal function, and with initial evidence pointing towards benefits in processes of recovery. The importance of appropriate nutrition complemented by the appropriate nutrients is paramount in tipping the physiologic demand in favor of elderly patients. Appreciation of how nutritional alterations can affect not only global health but also the sophisticated mechanisms of acid-base balance emphasizes the worth of thorough nutritional assessment in the elderly (Tack et al., 2018). Knowing about potential complications in elderly patients with acid-base imbalance is also crucial. Elderly subjects have comorbid diseases that may obscure or dominate acid-base disturbances. For instance, COPD patients may develop respiratory acidosis due to impaired gas exchange, and the disorder may be missed if symptoms are attributed to other age-related diseases. The subtle interplay between chronic conditions may influence diagnosis and treatment. Comprehensive evaluation of clinical symptoms, in addition to laboratory investigations, will aid in prompt diagnosis and treatment. Apart from that, symptoms , such as post-concussion syndrome (PCS) may be a reflection of the interrelatedness of physical stability and metabolic status, which shows the complexities in caring for elderly patients (Kaster et al., 2017). Such findings underscore the need for physicians and other healthcare providers to be holistic in caring for the health and well-being of the aged, particularly the physiological response of the aged to treatments and interventions.

2.6.3. Impact of Pregnancy on Acid-Base Physiology

The physiological changes occurring during pregnancy exert a deep impact on acid-base balance in the mother's body, and these are accommodations to make both mother and fetus healthy. Throughout pregnancy, as the metabolic needs rise, ventilation and renal function change. Particularly, the heightened metabolic rate leads to a higher production of carbon dioxide, which tests the respiratory system to compensate by elevating ventilation. This compensatory mechanism enables the condition of respiratory alkalosis, which is characterized by reduced arterial carbon dioxide. In addition, renal accommodation during pregnancy enables bicarbonate excretion, which also contributes to the redistribution of acid-base balance. These mechanisms are important in that they enable the acidic intrauterine milieu of the fetus to be optimally controlled in order to facilitate maximum growth while concurrently enabling the pregnant subject to accommodate the metabolic alterations, thereby enabling global physiological homeostasis. Further, the role of the placenta in acid-base physiology cannot be stressed too much. The placenta is an area for gas exchange where oxygen and carbon dioxide may be exchanged effectively between mother and fetus. Elevated levels of hormones, particularly progesterone, enhance reabsorption of renal tubular bicarbonate and therefore systemic bicarbonate levels during pregnancy. This dynamic feedback mechanism is accountable for a mild alkalotic state, which is essential for maintaining fetal development and ensuring proper delivery of oxygen. In addition, abnormalities in placental function can lead to disturbed acid-base regulation, affecting maternal as well as fetal complications, for instance, in gestational diabetes or preeclampsia. Understanding the relationship between placental physiology and acid-base homeostasis illuminates potential complications during pregnancy and focuses attention on the acid-base monitoring in the clinical setting during this susceptible interval. Furthermore, recent research highlights the contribution of ionic fluctuations to uterine excitability and contractility and links acid-base physiology with labor outcome. Large ion channels, such as, Na^+ leak channel NALCN, have been considered to be involved in controlling myometrial excitability and influencing the timing and effectiveness of contractions during labor. Experiments indicate that NALCN expression varies throughout pregnancy with great significance to mechanisms of parturition. For example, variations in Na^+ conductance can regulate the length and frequency of action potentials in myometrial cells and consequently influence the labor. Thus, information on acid-base mechanisms during pregnancy has the potential to yield substantial information on uterine function and potential intervention to maximize the outcome of labor. These correlations present a strong case for the intricate interaction between acid-base physiology and reproductive health, calling for extensive investigations in this area (Figure 2.20).

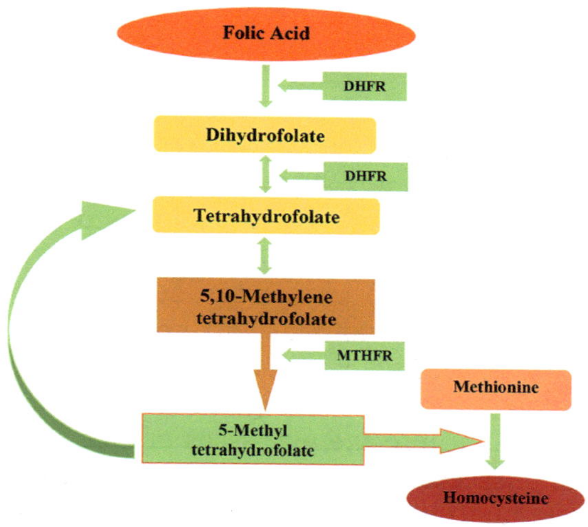

Figure 2.20. Pregnancy on acid-base physiology.

Source: https://www.mdpi.com/biomedicines/biomedicines-11-00272/article_deploy/html/images/biomedicines-11-00272-g001.png.

Test Your Knowledge

1. How does acid-base balance differ in neonates compared to adults?
2. Why are elderly individuals more susceptible to acid-base disturbances?

SUMMARY

The acid-base physiology is paramount in understanding the homeostatic regulation of biological systems. The ability of the body to maintain pH status is proof of its advanced coordination between respiration, metabolism, and renal processes. Disruption of these processes can lead to serious pathological implications, which illustrate the need for an ideal acid-base status. Through means , such as buffer systems, respiratory compensation, and renal responses, the body ensures quick responses to changes in pH, which otherwise would hinder cellular functioning. It is such a fluid balance that is used to illustrate the interconnectedness of metabolic processes and their impact on physiology as a whole. Further research into how many external factors can influence acid-base physiology is required to drive our understanding of this field forward. For instance, there is new evidence that nutrients in diets, e.g., essential oils, can influence cation balance and absorption of electrolytes. Of greater significance, research demonstrates that a blend of essential oils (BEO) not only enhances milk production in lactating cows but also changes plasma levels of essential ions , such as calcium and urea through more efficient mechanisms of absorption (Braun et al., 2019). These observations emphasize the intricate web of relationships between metabolic pathways and emphasize the relevance of acid-base physiology outside traditional contexts, suggesting new avenues for applied investigation in animal and human disease. Acid-base physiology is extended to relevance in a variety of ecological environments where organisms are demonstrated to accommodate their habitats. For instance, learning about the physiological reactions of larval sea lampreys to exercise gives one insight into the processes of metabolic acidosis and ion regulation in aquatic organisms. Upon intense exercise, these organisms demonstrate quick adaptations in oxygen consumption, metabolic fuel kinetics, and acid excretion, which reflect high adaptability (Wilkie et al., 2001). Such physiological reactions reinforce the importance of acid-base balance in survival mechanisms, either as predator avoidance or feeding. Collectively, research in this field reiterates the validity of a diminutive understanding of acid-base physiology, elucidating both its ubiquity in health as well as the broader environmental impact.

Acid-base physiology plays a key role in maintaining homeostasis of the human body, forming the basis for many physiological processes that are essential to life. The basic principle behind this physiology is the balance between acids and bases that is primarily regulated by the respiratory and renal systems. The two systems work together to maintain the pH of body fluids within an extremely narrow range, ideally 7.35-7.45, which is essential for optimal cellular function. Dysregulation of this equilibrium can result in serious health conditions, such as, acidosis or alkalosis, states of hyper-acidity or hyper-alkalinity, respectively. These mechanisms permit holistic diagnosis and management of disorders associated with acid-base imbalance, highlighting the role played by integrated physiologic systems in maintaining life. Discussing the implications of acid-base physiology reveals how metabolic processes and extrinsic forces affect this homeostasis. For instance, exercise alters acid-base states by producing increased carbon dioxide and lactic acid production, wherein renal compensation is needed to normalize. Additionally, chronic obstructive pulmonary disease (COPD) can weaken respiratory capacity, resulting in respiratory acidosis wherein the blood contains excessive carbon dioxide. Such factors must be known to healthcare professionals, who must consider both physiological conditions and environmental conditions while treating acid-base disorders. By embracing this inclusive view that incorporates both the extrinsic and biological influences on acid-base balance, clinicians will be in a position to more effectively tailor their treatments for patients with accompanying health issues. In addition, advances in research indicate the interconnectedness of acid-base physiology with overall health issues like neurodegenerative disease. Research indicates that acid-base disturbance can result in cognitive loss in populations at risk for diseases like dementia. For instance, geriatric delirium may exacerbate prior cognitive impairment, making active management strategies highly relevant. Such strategies can be directed towards efforts to reduce delirium through environmental and psychological support to maintain global health. Synthesis of evidence from different research areas has the further benefit of enhancing acid-base physiology knowledge, which in turn feeds back into effective treatment paradigms. This integrated approach stresses the necessity of constant observation of the worldwide implications of acid-base disturbances in every clinical setting, as is expressed with reference to the significance of integrated systems for health governance (Livingston et al., 2020; Intergovernmental Panel on Climate Change, 2023).

KEY TERMS FROM THIS CHAPTER

- Acidosis
- Alkalosis
- Ammonia buffer system
- Anion gap
- Base excess
- Bicarbonate buffer system
- Bicarbonate ion (HCO_3^-)
- Buffer systems
- Carbon dioxide (CO_2)
- Carbonic acid (H_2CO_3)
- Henderson-hasselbalch equation
- Hydrogen ion (H^+)
- Metabolic acidosis
- Metabolic alkalosis

CRITICAL THINKING QUESTIONS

1. **What is the normal pH range of human arterial blood?**
   a. 6.8 – 7.0
   b. 7.35 – 7.45
   c. 7.5 – 7.8
   d. 6.5 – 7.2
2. **Which of the following acts as the primary buffer system in extracellular fluid?**
   a. Hemoglobin buffer system
   b. Phosphate buffer system
   c. Bicarbonate buffer system
   d. Protein buffer system
3. **What condition is caused by an accumulation of CO_2 due to hypoventilation?**
   a. Respiratory alkalosis
   b. Metabolic acidosis
   c. Metabolic alkalosis
   d. Respiratory acidosis
4. **Which organ is primarily responsible for the long-term regulation of blood pH?**
   a. Lungs
   b. Liver
   c. Kidneys
   d. Heart
5. **In metabolic alkalosis, which of the following is a likely compensatory mechanism?**
   a. Increased renal hydrogen ion secretion
   b. Increased respiratory rate
   c. Decreased respiratory rate
   d. Decreased bicarbonate reabsorption

Short Answer Questions

1. Explain the mechanisms by which the body maintains acid-base homeostasis.
2. Describe the role of the bicarbonate buffer system in detail.
3. Compare and contrast respiratory and metabolic acidosis and alkalosis, including causes and compensations.
4. Discuss the renal regulation of acid-base balance, including bicarbonate reabsorption and hydrogen ion secretion.
5. Explain how blood pH is affected during exercise and how the body compensates.
6. What is the normal pH range of arterial blood?
7. Define acidosis and alkalosis.
8. Name two major buffer systems in the body.
9. What role do the kidneys play in acid-base balance?
10. How does the respiratory system help regulate pH?

Answers to Critical Thinking Questions

1. (b); 2. (c); 3. (d); 4. (c); 5. (c).

REFERENCES

1. Tack, C., Shorthouse, F., & Kass, L. (2018). The Physiological Mechanisms of Effect of Vitamins and Amino Acids on Tendon and Muscle Healing: A Systematic Review. *International journal of sport nutrition and exercise metabolism*, *28*(3), 294–311. https://doi.org/10.1123/ijsnem.2017-0267 (accessed on 28th June 2025).
2. Amazu, C., Bok, R., England, S. K., Hurt, K., et al. (2018). Na^+-leak channel, non-selective (NALCN) regulates myometrial excitability and facilitates successful parturition. https://core.ac.uk/download/212865916.pdf (accessed on 28th June 2025).
3. Atzori, L., Fanos, V., Ferrazzi, E., Makarenko, M., et al. (2013). Metabolomics application in maternal-fetal medicine. https://core.ac.uk/download/pdf/54594438.pdf (accessed on 28th June 2025).
4. Derave, W., Everaert, I., Beeckman, S., & Baguet, A. (2010). Muscle carnosine metabolism and beta-alanine supplementation in relation to exercise and training. *Sports medicine (Auckland, N.Z.)*, *40*(3), 247–263. https://doi.org/10.2165/11530310-000000000-00000 (accessed on 28th June 2025).
5. Bahr, C., Romanini, C. E. B., Berckmans, D., Decuypere, E., Bergoug, H., McGonnell, I. M., Molenaar, R., et al. (2015). Higher levels of CO_2 during late incubation alter the hatch time of chicken embryos. https://core.ac.uk/download/36778323.pdf (accessed on 28th June 2025).
6. Skotnicka, E., Muszczyñski, Z., Dudzinska, W., & Suska, M. (2007). A review of the renal system and diurnal variations of renal activity in livestock. *Irish veterinary journal*, *60*(3), 161–168. https://doi.org/10.1186/2046-0481-60-3-161(accessed on 28th June 2025).
7. Barile, D., Goodson, M., Kalanetra, K., Lee, H., et al. (2020). 2'-Fucosyllactose supplementation improves gut-brain signaling and diet-induced obese phenotype and changes the gut microbiota in high fat-fed mice. https://core.ac.uk/download/323308640.pdf (accessed on 28th June 2025).
8. Barreiro Sorrivas, J. M., & Pazos Sierra, J. (2009). Computing vs. genetics. https://core.ac.uk/download/148655226.pdf (accessed on 28th June 2025).
9. Bellomo, R., Kellum, J., Story, D., Yunos, N., et al. (2010). Bench-to-bedside review: Chloride in critical illness. https://core.ac.uk/download/pdf/8456206.pdf (accessed on 28th June 2025).
10. Bonny, O., Vinciguerra, M., Gumz, M. L., & Mazzoccoli, G. (2013). Molecular bases of circadian rhythmicity in renal physiology and pathology. *Nephrology, dialysis, transplantation : official publication of the European Dialysis and Transplant Association - European Renal Association*, *28*(10), 2421–2431. https://doi.org/10.1093/ndt/gft319on 28th June 2025).
11. Wilkie, M. P., Bradshaw, P. G., Joanis, V., Claude, J. F., & Swindell, S. L. (2001). Rapid metabolic recovery following vigorous exercise in burrow-dwelling larval sea lampreys (Petromyzon marinus). *Physiological and biochemical zoology : PBZ*, *74*(2), 261–272. https://doi.org/10.1086/319656(accessed on 28th June 2025).
12. Braun, H. S., Mahlkow-Nerge, K., Rosendahl, J., Schrapers, K., et al. (2019). Dietary supplementation of essential oils in dairy cows: Evidence for stimulatory effects on nutrient absorption. https://core.ac.uk/download/225124766.pdf (accessed on 28th June 2025).
13. Zhu, T., Brown, A. P., & Ji, H. (2020). The Emerging Role of Ten-Eleven Translocation 1 in Epigenetic Responses to Environmental Exposures. *Epigenetics insights*, *13*, 2516865720910155. https://doi.org/10.1177/2516865720910155(accessed on 28th June 2025).

14. Bruno, C. M., & Valenti, M. (2012). Acid-base disorders in patients with chronic obstructive pulmonary disease: A pathophysiological review. https://core.ac.uk/download/pdf/8697493.pdf (accessed on 28th June 2025).
15. Buratto, D., Carrer, A., Chiani, F., Kuang, Y., et al. (2019). A human-derived monoclonal antibody targeting extracellular connexin domain selectively modulates hemichannel function. https://core.ac.uk/download/220684751.pdf (accessed on 28th June 2025).
16. Burlaka, I., & Mityuryayeva, I. (2024). Episode of renal dysfunction in a child with eating disorder: A case report. Science Rise: Medical Science. https://www.semanticscholar.org/paper/f52050020cb0b15842cc01ece6809f92f17b84f7 (accessed on 28th June 2025).
17. Carson, D. A., Chen, P. P., Kipps, T. J., Tomhave, E., et al. (1988). Autoantibody-associated kappa light chain variable region gene expressed in chronic lymphocytic leukemia with little or no somatic mutation: Implications for etiology and immunotherapy. https://core.ac.uk/download/323078807.pdf (accessed on 28th June 2025).
18. Kaster, Kristen; Kalmar, Jayne M. Ms.; and Cinelli, Michael E. Mr, "Task-dependent Modulation of Cortical Excitability and Balance Control in Individuals with Post-concussion Syndrome" (2017). Theses and Dissertations (Comprehensive). 1983. https://scholars.wlu.ca/etd/1983(accessed on 28th June 2025).
19. Edwards, A., & Crambert, G. (2017). Versatility of NaCl transport mechanisms in the cortical collecting duct. *American journal of physiology. Renal physiology*, *313*(6), F1254–F1263. https://doi.org/10.1152/ajprenal.00369.2017(accessed on 28th June 2025).
20. Anna de Polo, Mark D. Scrimshaw, Challenges for the development of a biotic ligand model predicting copper toxicity in estuaries and seas, Environmental Toxicology and Chemistry, Volume 31, Issue 2, 1 February 2012, Pages 230–238, https://doi.org/10.1002/etc.1705 (accessed on 28th June 2025).
21. Duarte, R., Kanayama, K. K., Kogika, M. M., Simões, D. M., et al. (2012). Acid-base abnormalities in dogs with diabetic ketoacidosis: A prospective study of 60 cases. https://core.ac.uk/download/268256561.pdfs (accessed on 28th June 2025).
22. J. I. Leonard, Ph.D. S. Furukawa, M.D. P. Van Nordstrand (1975). Systems identification and application systems development for monitoring the physiological and health status of crewmen in space. Study Report Unclas (General Electric Co.) 65 p nc AO4/MF A0l GJ/52 22244 (accessed on 28th June 2025).
23. Gomez Coral, M. I. (2024). Beyond the nephron: Exploring systemic implications of renal tubular acidosis. JOJ Urology & Nephrology. https://www.semanticscholar.org/paper/5a6a2e67629bd09cac7bd8821fecf27d1383e3fd (accessed on 28th June 2025).
24. Högberg, A. (2003). Cereal non-starch polysaccharides in pig diets. https://core.ac.uk/download/11694626.pdf (accessed on 28th June 2025).
25. Hou, R., Kennedy, M. W., Loeffler, I. K., Wang, X., et al. (2015). Changes in the milk metabolome of the giant panda (Ailuropoda melanoleuca) with time after birth: Three phases in early lactation and progressive individual differences. https://core.ac.uk/download/42367839.pdf (accessed on 28th June 2025).
26. Imelda, J., & Paulraj, R. (2002). Nutritional deficiency diseases in fish – Winter school on recent advances in diagnosis and management of diseases in mariculture, 7th to 27th

November 2002, Course Manual. https://core.ac.uk/download/33015412.pdf (accessed on 28th June 2025).

27. Intergovernmental Panel on Climate Change. (2023). Climate Change 2022–Impacts, Adaptation and Vulnerability. https://doi.org/10.1017/9781009325844 (accessed on 28th June 2025).

28. Takvam, M., Wood, C. M., Kryvi, H., & Nilsen, T. O. (2023). Role of the kidneys in acid-base regulation and ammonia excretion in freshwater and seawater fish: implications for nephrocalcinosis. *Frontiers in physiology*, *14*, 1226068. https://doi.org/10.3389/fphys.2023.1226068(accessed on 28th June 2025).

29. Livingston, G., Huntley, J., Sommerlad, A., Ames, D., Ballard, C., Banerjee, S., Brayne, C., et al. (2020). Dementia prevention, intervention, and care: 2020 report of the Lancet Commission. The Lancet, 396, 413–446. https://doi.org/10.1016/s0140-6736(20)30367-6 (accessed on 28th June 2025).

30. Machado, R. (2012). The molecular genetics and cellular mechanisms underlying pulmonary arterial hypertension. https://core.ac.uk/download/20320889.pdf (accessed on 28th June 2025).

31. Matoušek, S. (2013). Znovusjednocení popisu acidobazické fyziologie a chemie krevní plazmy. https://core.ac.uk/download/401794831.pdf (accessed on 28th June 2025).

32. Murphy, D. S. (2021). Back to basics: The effects of buffered crystalloids on mortality in the setting of severe trauma. https://core.ac.uk/download/489810519.pdf (accessed on 28th June 2025).

33. Nazaroff, W. W., & Weschler, C. J. (2020). Indoor acids and bases. https://core.ac.uk/download/305124479.pdf (accessed on 28th June 2025).

34. Nweji, A. A. (1988). The use of corn-water-salt solution as an oral rehydration therapy in the management of diarrhea. https://core.ac.uk/download/481678182.pdf (accessed on 28th June 2025).

35. Odunze, F. C. (2005). Environmentally induced physiological responses that determine fish survival and distribution: A review. https://core.ac.uk/download/11019634.pdf (accessed on 28th June 2025).

36. Raju, P. (2016). Homoacetogenesis as an alternative hydrogen sink in the rumen: A thesis presented in partial fulfilment of the requirements for the degree of Doctor of Philosophy in Microbiology and Genetics at Massey University, Palmerston North, New Zealand. https://core.ac.uk/download/148643491.pdf (accessed on 28th June 2025).

37. Spennemann, D. H. R., & Watson, M. J. (2017). Dietary habits of urban pigeons (Columba livia) and implications of excreta pH – A review. https://core.ac.uk/download/286139273.pdf (accessed on 28th June 2025).

38. Talling, J. (2004). The development of freshwater science in Britain, and British contributions abroad, 1900–2000. https://core.ac.uk/download/11020206.pdf (accessed on 28th June 2025).

39. Vaidyanathan, P. P. (2004). Genomics and proteomics: A signal processor's tour. https://core.ac.uk/download/4877225.pdf (accessed on 28th June 2025).

40. White, R. J. (2025). Acid-base homeostasis in the human system. https://core.ac.uk/download/pdf/42869639.pdf (accessed on 28th June 2025).

GASTROINTESTINAL PHYSIOLOGY

3

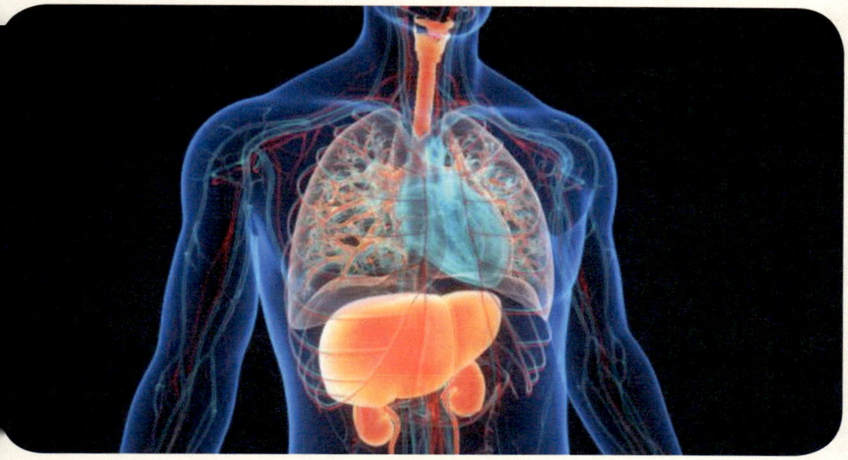

LEARNING OBJECTIVES

After studying this chapter, you will be able to:

1. Understand the anatomy of the gastrointestinal tract.
2. Explain the digestive processes.
3. Discuss the gastrointestinal motility.
4. Focus on gastrointestinal secretions
5. Learn about the role of gut microbiota.
6. Define the disorders of the gastrointestinal system.

Introduction

The gastrointestinal (GI) tract plays a critical role in the delivery of homeostasis by facilitating the digestion and absorption of nutrients. The intricate system consists of varied organs, including the stomach, intestines, liver, and pancreas, which all offer specialized functions that are vital in contributing to health. Ingestion starts the process with food coming into contact with the oral cavity, which leads to enzymatic digestion, which commences with saliva. When food is swallowed and goes into the stomach, gastric juices further disintegrate it, preparing nutrients for absorption. It is not a completely mechanical process because it is also controlled and regulated by complex neural and hormonal stimuli, so that the digestive process is well coordinated with the body's needs. Understanding of the physiological mechanisms behind these processes of digestion is incredibly enlightening in terms of what influence diet, health, and hormonal variations have on overall gastrointestinal function. In addition, the relationship between diet composition and GI physiology has profound implications for animal nutrition and well-being. Diets have been discovered to contain non-starch polysaccharides (NSP) that affect gastrointestinal processes as observed by experiments on pigs. Increased NSP content is linked with decreased digestibility of organic matter, particularly in the small intestine, which highlights the role of dietary fiber in gut health. Moreover, these alterations in diet have the potential to modify gut habitat, for example, organic acid type and microbial populations. Manipulation of these factors provides the potential to modulate feed design for different growth stages of animals for maximum utilization of nutrients and overall welfare. Thus, gastrointestinal physiology not only contributes towards understanding the health of humans but also has significant implications in agricultural technology, indicating its importance across different fields. Apart from nutritional influences, hormonal regulation in the GI system highly impacts gastrointestinal physiology, that is, in relation to conditions , such as Irritable Bowel Syndrome (IBS) and Inflammatory Bowel Disease (IBD). Such conditions show the complexity of how hormonal fluctuations impact gut health, as reflected in the interaction between reproductive hormones like progesterone and intestinal hormones. The oscillatory nature of symptoms characteristic of IBS and IBD shows that fluctuating hormone levels might precipitate episodes of distress, such as, cramping and diarrhea. Understanding such mechanisms informs potential therapeutic targets for improved treatments that treat the underlying causes of these gastrointestinal illnesses, rather than merely the relief of symptoms. Thus, research into where hormonal interaction intersects with gastrointestinal physiology expands understanding of digestive health and potential avenues for improved treatment of GI illness (Figure 3.1).

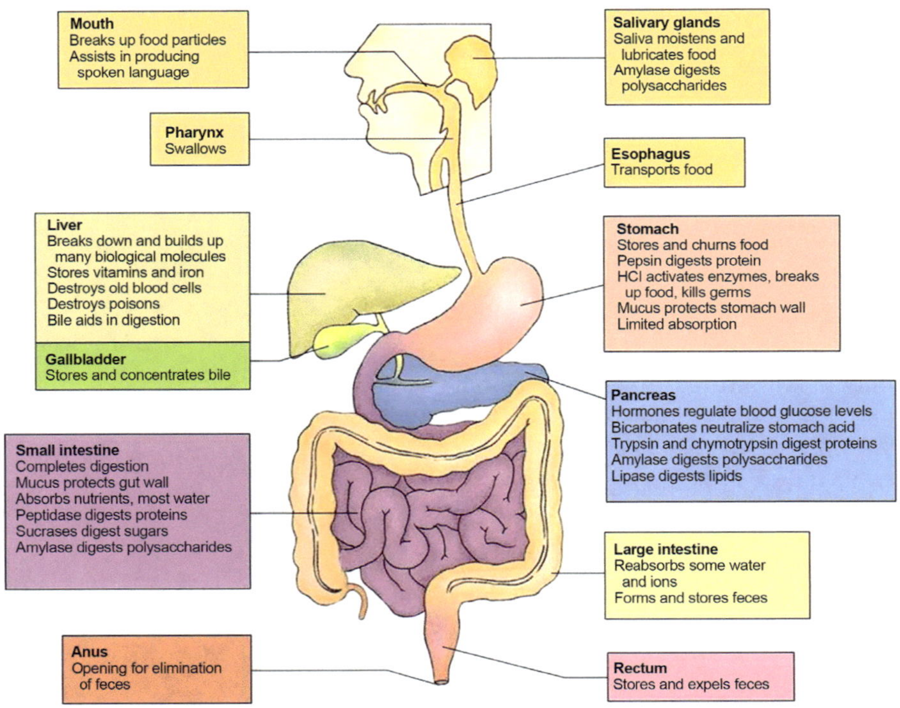

Figure 3.1. Gastrointestinal Function.

https://i2.wp.com/basicmedicalkey.com/wp-content/uploads/2016/09/F000358f35-19-9781455726509.jpg?fit=1026%2C837&ssl=1.

Definition and Importance of Gastrointestinal Physiology

Gastrointestinal physiology refers to the study of the complex mechanisms that regulate the digestive system and its functions, such as, digestion, nutrient uptake, and expulsion of wastes. It is fundamental in grasping body interaction with the food eaten, as well as interaction among various organ systems to maintain homeostasis. The gastrointestinal tract is more than a tube that food flows through; it is a highly organized system of organs that depend on biochemical mechanisms, nervous control, and hormonal signals. This is perhaps most evident in syndromes like Irritable Bowel Syndrome (IBS) and Inflammatory Bowel Disease (IBD), in which hormonal alterations, including spikes in progesterone, can initiate symptoms like cramping and constipation, thereby illustrating the critical interaction between gastrointestinal physiology and hormones (Linson, 2013Linson, 2013). In addition to its rudimentary digestive roles, gastrointestinal physiology also plays a role in overall health outcomes and well-being. Research indicated that a properly functioning gastrointestinal system is necessary for adequate nutrition and could have a crucial function in disease prevention, such as, cardiovascular disease and diabetes. Beyond, it has also been observed that whole-grain consumption benefits digestive health, suggesting that dietary factors could exert potent influences on gut physiology. Higher consumption of whole grains is associated with a lower incidence of chronic diseases, illustrating the impact of gut health on overall well-being. This interconnectivity serves to highlight the need for greater gastrointestinal physiology knowledge not just among clinicians, but across public health systems tasked with delivering dietary advice and promoting healthy consumption (Seal & Brownlee, 2015). Gastrointestinal physiology is key to medical practitioners and scientists as it yields information necessary to formulate therapeutic interventions for gut diseases. By understanding the typical digestive processes and how they are derailed, the practitioners are then in a position to use this knowledge to avert such conditions as IBS and IBD. With studies probing the intricate interaction between diet, hormonal responses, and intestinal function, the potential for discovering new strategies for treatment continues to expand. Correction of the underlying physiological mechanism, however, will not only enhance symptom control but also improve the quality of life of the patient, reinforcing the fundamental significance of gastrointestinal physiology in the clinic and in individual health care (Figure 3.2).

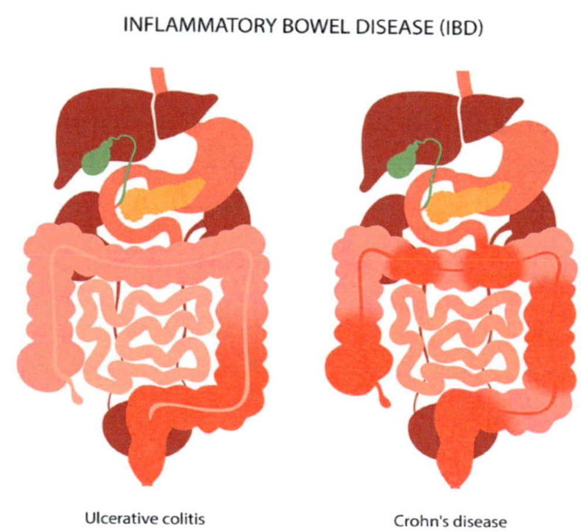

Figure 3.2. Inflammatory bowel disease (IBD).

Source: https://www.hopkinsmedicine.org/-/media/images/health/1_-conditions/stomach-and-gut/inflammatory-bowel-disease-graphic-large.ashx.

Overview of the Gastrointestinal Tract

The gastrointestinal system (GI tract) is a complex and vital system that is an integral part of an organism's physiology. It serves for the ingestion, digestion, assimilation, and excretion of waste food. The GI tract begins in the oral cavity, where food is mechanically broken down by teeth and mixed with saliva, initiating the process of digestion. Following this, food proceeds through the esophagus to the stomach, where gastric acids further disintegrate it. The stomach is a mechanical and chemical digestive organ before the contents are released into the small intestine, where the majority of nutrient absorption occurs. The function and structure of GI tract components play a vital role in maximizing the amount of nutrient absorption and maintaining metabolic homeostasis, as this system's intricate design. After passing through the small intestine, it is again divided into the duodenum, jejunum, and ileum. All of them are utilized for specific purposes in digestion and nutrient absorption. The duodenum is where the majority of enzymatic activity takes place with the help of bile from the liver and digestive enzymes from the pancreas. The jejunum is primarily involved in the absorption of carbohydrates and proteins, while the ileum is involved in vitamin B12 and bile salt absorption. Structural adaptations of the small intestine, like villi and microvilli, greatly increase the surface area, thus the efficiency of nutrient absorption. Understanding these specific functions is crucial in knowing why malabsorption syndromes are produced, which can influence the condition and nutrition of a person. The large intestine or colon serves to support the digestive process through controlling water and electrolyte absorption and enabling the creation and elimination of feces. It consists of the cecum, colon, rectum, and anal canal, where the remaining food material is processed. It is characterized by containing a very large population of microbial communities that play an important function in fermenting undigested carbohydrates and producing short-chain fatty acids that are healthy. These microorganisms also play a central function in maintaining an equilibrated gut environment, which has implications for immune function and overall well-being. Moreover, food content and fiber intake can also influence colonic function, as evidenced is presented through alterations in gut well-being through various levels of non-starch polysaccharide (NSP) in animal feeding stuff formulations (Högberg, 2003). Therefore, the small intestine and large intestine are imperative in supplying the body with sufficient nutrients and eliminating waste material, highlighting their relevance in gut physiology (Figure 3.3).

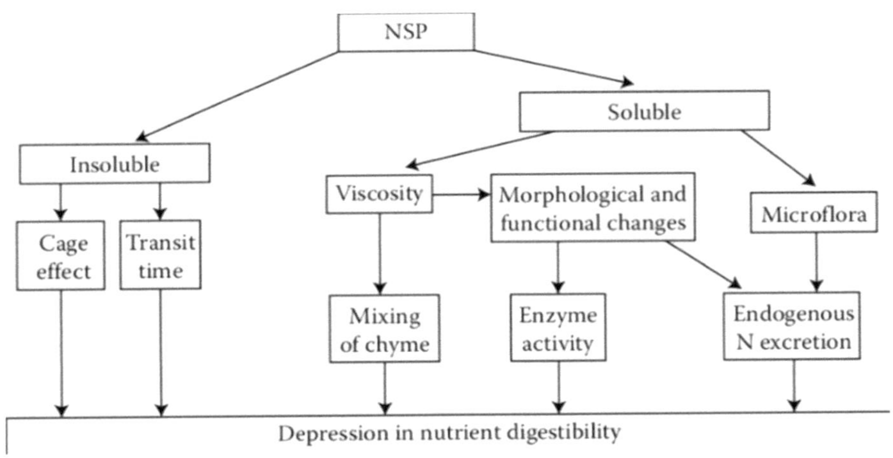

Figure 3.3. Mechanism of action of non-starch polysaccharides.

Source: https://www.researchgate.net/profile/Veronika-Halas/publication/300428696/figure/fig2/AS:510846847512576@1498806787153/Mechanism-of-action-of-nonstarch-polysaccharides-NSP.png.

Key Functions of the Gastrointestinal System

The GI system plays a vital role in the digestion and absorption of nutrients, which are necessary to maintain overall health as well as support energy levels. The process begins in the oral cavity with mechanical digestion when food is chewed, and enzymatic digestion begins when saliva is introduced. When food travels down the esophagus to the stomach, it is still broken down by churning as well as the gastric acids. These collective mechanisms guarantee that macronutrients—proteins, carbohydrates, and fats—are efficiently broken down to tiny molecules. The small intestine, with its large surface area contributed by microvilli and villi, has a major role in nutrient uptake in that it facilitates the movement of digested nutrients into the bloodstream. It is necessary to know the efficiency of such digestive mechanisms, particularly in diseases , such as gastrointestinal disorders, where malabsorption of nutrients may be of great importance to health (Linson, 2013). Apart from digestion and absorption, the GI system also participates in regulating various hormonal and neural responses towards homeostasis. Particularly, the enteric nervous system, usually referred to as the second brain, regulates gut motility and secretion. This complex system of neurons communicates with the central nervous system to enable the GI tract to act appropriately in the presence of food. Apart from this, the secretion of gastrointestinal hormones, such as, gastrin, cholecystokinin, and secretin, controls the digestive processes and appetite control. The communication of the hormones with other body systems, such as, the endocrine system, also shows the multifaceted role of the GI system. Research on the impact of hormonal changes in gastrointestinal disease yields data on potential therapy considering symptom relief and improving quality of life (McRae et al., 2015). Another crucial function of the gastrointestinal tract is its capacity to contribute to immune defense, particularly through interaction with the gut microbiota. The intestine is home to trillions of microorganisms that play a role in digestion but also in defending the body against infection. The mucosal barrier, which is derived from epithelial cells, along with mucins and secretory immunoglobulin A (sIgA), functions as a frontline defense mechanism against colonizing microorganisms. The immune responses stimulated by the gut microbiota can also be capable of altering systemic immunity and general health. Dysbiosis or an imbalance in the gut microbiota has been linked to numerous gastrointestinal diseases, and hence it is very important that microbial equilibrium is maintained. Thus, gastrointestinal immune function is key to both local gut health as well as general immunity to diseases (Linson, 2013).

3.1. Anatomy of the Gastrointestinal Tract

Learning Outcome

1. Describe the structure of the esophagus;
2. Focus on the anatomy of the stomach;
3. Learn about the composition of the small and large intestines.

Gastrointestinal (GI) tract anatomy is a complex structure that plays an important part in the digestion and absorption process. It begins in the oral cavity when mechanical and chemical digestion of food first occurs. The salivary glands produce enzymes like amylase that initiate the breakdown of carbohydrates. It then proceeds through the esophagus and into the stomach, where it is further broken down by acidic gastric secretions. The stomach lining, full of specialized cells, not only secretes hydrochloric acid but also many enzymes essential in digesting proteins. Such a refinement in anatomy highlights the efficient compactness of the GI tract in transforming food into substances that can be absorbed, reinforcing its significance in gastrointestinal physiology. When partially digested food moves from the stomach to the small intestine, anatomy once more presents itself in stunning complexity. The small intestine is segmented into three: the duodenum, the jejunum, and the ileum, which all play a role in enhanced nutrient absorption. The duodenum is supplied with bile and pancreatic secretions to aid in digestion, while the long villi and microvilli of the lining of the jejunum and ileum provide maximum surface area for nutrients to be absorbed into the bloodstream. Such a structure ensures that proteins, fats, and carbohydrates are absorbed efficiently.

Also, the relationship of the small intestinal structure and digestive enzymes is a paradigm of the principles of gastrointestinal physiology, illustrating how anatomy is integrated with function in digestion. The colon's function is equally essential, though anatomically distinct from the small intestine. Functionally, it has the function of water absorption and fecal formation, which accentuates a significant aspect of gastrointestinal physiology. Structurally, it comprises various numbers of segments like the cecum, colon, rectum, and anus, all contributing to the effective removal of waste. The large intestine harbors a rich microbiota that plays significant roles in fermentation and short-chain fatty acid generation, which also influences host metabolism and immune status. Understanding the anatomy of the large intestine, including its muscular coats and disposition of gut flora, enlightens its essential processes. This is supplementary information regarding the understanding of gastrointestinal disease and therapeutic aims in Irritable Bowel Syndrome and Inflammatory Bowel Disease, as proposed by Linson (2013) and Liu et al. (2013) (Figure 3.4).

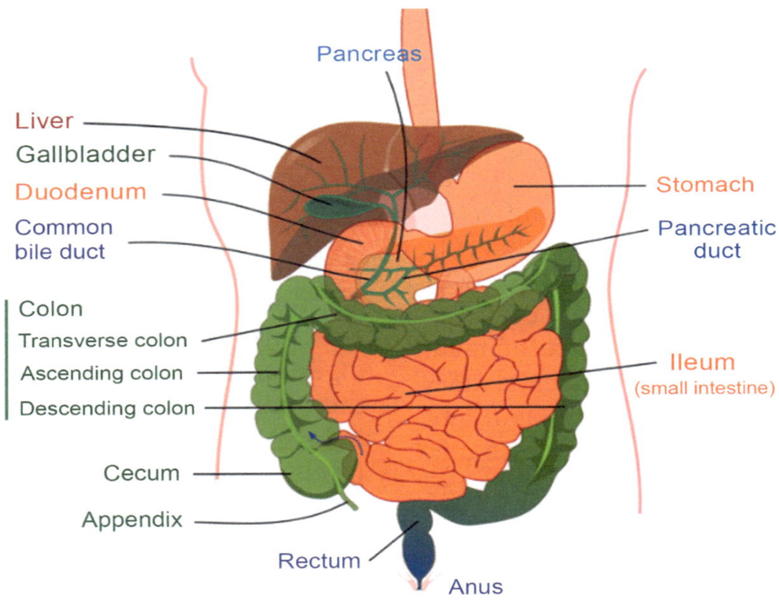

Figure 3.4. Anatomy of the gastrointestinal tract.

Source: https://www.nicepng.com/png/detail/772-7720830_a-diagram-of-the-lower-gastrointestinal-tract-human.png.

3.1.1. Structure of the Esophagus

The esophagus is an essential conduit through the gastrointestinal tract that facilitates the passage of food from the mouth to the stomach. Its anatomy is specialized to accommodate the mechanical stress and varied pressures of swallowing. Composed of four principal layers—the mucosa, submucosa, muscularis, and adventitia—the wall of the esophagus possesses a high degree of organization that allows both resiliency and rigidity. The submucosa contains glands that secrete mucus for the lubrication of the food passage, while the mucosa is lined with stratified squamous epithelium as a protective covering against abrasion. The tiered structure envelopes not only the esophagus's functional demands but also its function in maintaining homeostasis within the larger picture of gastrointestinal physiology (Rosse & Mejino, 2007).

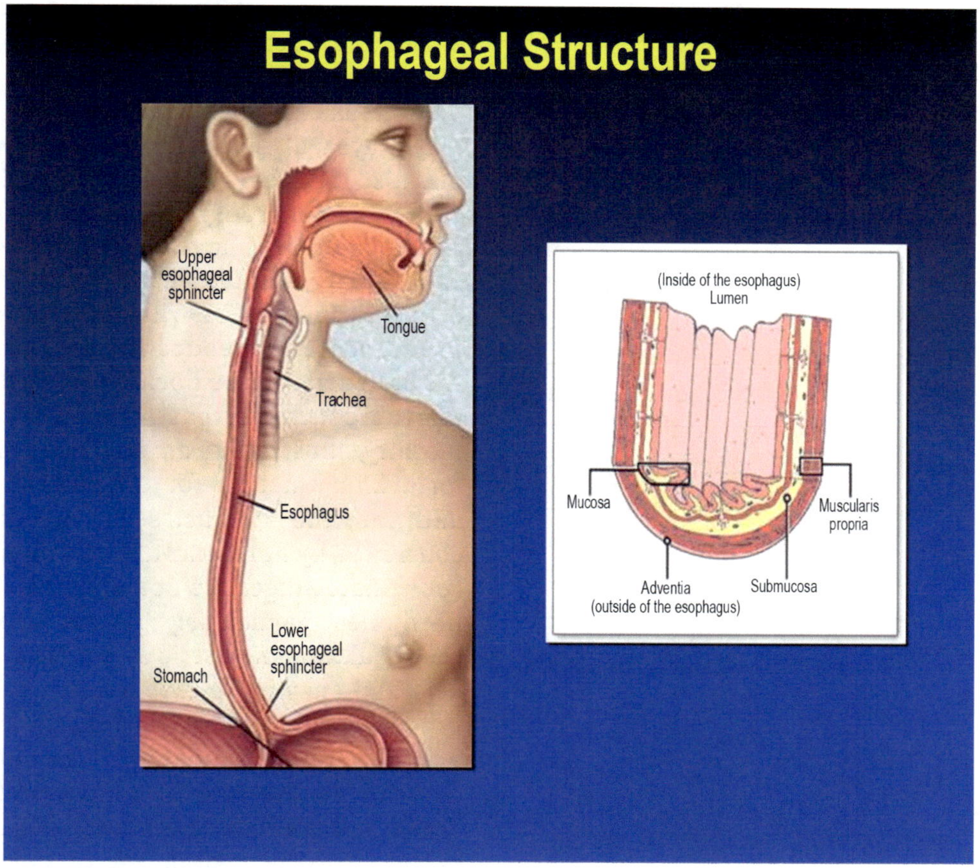

Figure 3.5. Esophageal structure.

Source: https://cf.ppt-online.org/files/slide/1/1sjoIHTJWvMhDfB6R2yxPrQ4c7AV8el3qdKZUL/slide-2.jpg.

One of the most significant academic issues regarding the esophagus is the function of the lower esophageal sphincter (LES) in regulating material flow from the esophagus into the stomach. The LES lies anatomically proximal to the esophageal hiatus, which is formed largely by the right crus of the diaphragm. It has the sphincter-like action that prevents retrograde flow of gastric contents, which is required for the protection of the esophagus against acid exposure. Studies based on high-resolution manometry show that a failure of relaxation of the LES can lead to pathological conditions like gastroesophageal reflux disease. Understanding the physiology and anatomy of the LES is the backbone to appreciating esophageal pathology and its treatment, particularly in the context of the prevalence of hiatal hernias and their impact on esophageal function (Ghahremani et al., 2020). The esophagus further has a distinct pattern of motility necessary for the sequential movement of food. Peristalsis, the wave-like muscular contractions that make this process feasible, is regulated by the intricate interaction of the muscularis layer and the nervous system. The muscular composition of the esophagus changes from the upper third, striated muscle, to the lower two-thirds, smooth muscle, the differing functions and regulation mechanisms being the reason for this. This smooth shifting aids efficacious swallowing and transport of food subsequently. Dysfunction in such motility can result in other clinical symptoms, including dysphagia and chest pain, justifying the importance of being aware of esophageal structure in connection with gastrointestinal wellness and illness (Rosse & Mejino, 2007) (Figure 3.5).

3.1.2. Anatomy of the Stomach

The stomach is a critical organ of the gastrointestinal tract responsible for being a main site for the initial enzymatic breakdown of food. It is anatomically separated into four major sections: the cardia, fundus, body, and pylorus. All of the segments have specialized functions that contribute to the overall process of digestion. Cardia, near the esophagus junction, is a point of entry of food, while the fundus is an intermediate storage area with the facility for gradual emptying of content into the body of the stomach. The extremely precise anatomical positioning facilitates maximum mixing of ingested food with gastric juice consisting of hydrochloric acid and pepsinogen for initiation of protein digestion. Moreover, the pylorus regulates the passage of chyme into the duodenum such that only thoroughly digested material passes through the digestive system. The histological organization of the stomach is also crucial to its role in that the gastric mucosa consists of specialized secretory cells that secrete mucus, hydrochloric acid, and digestive enzymes to create a perfect acidic environment for digestion. Parietal cells within the gastric pits release hydrochloric acid (HCl), which not only plays a digestive function in food digestion but also acts as a barrier protection against pathogenic microorganisms. Chief cells release pepsinogen, an inactive enzyme, which, upon exposure to stomach acid, becomes activated. Synergy of enzymes is vital for protein digestion. In addition, enteroendocrine cells located within the stomach release hormones , such as gastrin for the control of gastric acid secretion and motility, illustrating an advanced harmony of form and function for effective digestion. In addition, the stomach's activity is positively controlled by hormonal and neural input, which coordinates digestive activity. The functions of hormones, particularly gastrin, are pivotal in the regulation of gastric operations, influencing acid and enzyme release according to the food type. Coordination between gastric motility and hormonal stimulation is essential since it determines the rate at which food is broken down and pushed around the gastrointestinal system. Further studies have pointed to the fact that hormonal signaling disruption could lead to gastrointestinal conditions that manifest as abdominal pain and bloating, linking the stomach's anatomical and physiological functions to more general health issues. For instance, understanding how hormones like progesterone could influence symptoms of Irritable Bowel Syndrome (IBS) could uncover new therapeutic opportunities, implying the potential for hormone-based treatments for addressing the underlying causes of gastrointestinal disease (Högberg, 2003; Linson, 2013) (Figure 3.6).

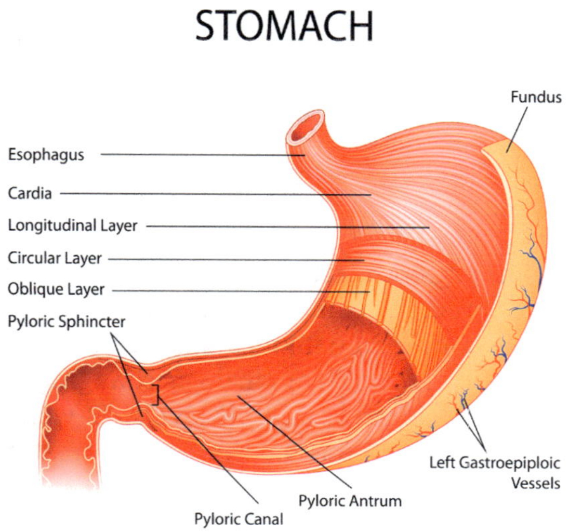

Figure 3.6. Anatomy of the stomach.

Source: https://static.vecteezy.com/system/resources/previews/002/803/165/original/illustration-of-healthcare-and-medical-education-drawing-chart-of-human-stomach-for-science-biology-study-vector.jpg.

3.1.3. Composition of the Small and Large Intestines

The architecture of the small and large intestines is characterized by a high level of interplay between structure and function, which is crucial in digestion and nutrient uptake. The small intestine, composed of three segments in the duodenum, jejunum, and ileum, features specialized structures , such as villi and microvilli that significantly increase surface area. The extremely large surface area enables effective nutrient absorption of carbohydrates, proteins, and lipids. Furthermore, pancreatic secretions and bile from the liver facilitate the emulsification and breakdown of the macromolecules to ease absorption. Conversely, the large intestine's primary focus is on water and electrolyte absorption, whose composition is less focused on nutrient breakdown. It has structural elements like gut flora, which have a crucial role to play in the fermentation of residual undigested food and the production of short-chain fatty acids, pointing towards the multifunctional role of the intestines in gastrointestinal physiology. The gut microbiota, residing predominantly in the large intestine, contributes significantly to digestive health and metabolic function. This microbiota is a symbiotic network of trillions of microbes that assist in numerous functions, such as, the production of essential vitamins and metabolism of dietary fiber. Of particular note is the growing evidence implying a link between the gut microbiota composition and general health, including immunomodulation and pathogen resistance. Modulation of gut microbiota has been linked to numerous diseases, including gastrointestinal disease and metabolic syndrome. The intricate interaction between microbial populations and host cells highlights the importance of maintaining the gut ecosystem in balance, which generally relies upon diet and lifestyle. Notably, the involvement of gut microbiota is not limited to cardiovascular disease pathogenesis, suggesting an obligatory relationship between intestinal functions and physiological activities at the systemic level, and constructing a complex narrative of gastrointestinal physiology (Tousoulis et al., 2022). In addition, knowledge of the intestines' composition requires recognition of the role that dietary constituents play, including possibly toxic components , such as cadmium. Studies show that some infant formulas can provide consumers with elevated cadmium intake, which warrants investigation of food sources within the infant population (Eklund, 2003). Gastrointestinal heavy metal absorption can be quite variable from person to person, especially among infants whose internal gut environment is in the process of maturation. This variability emphasizes the relevance of knowing the food bioavailability of toxic chemicals and how foods influence the enhancement or suppression of metal absorption. As the small and large intestines orchestrate elimination of wastes and nutrient supply, maintaining their integrity and health is critical for both acute digestive function and long-term systemic health and disease prevention.

Test Your Knowledge

1. What is the function of the liver in the GI system?
2. How is the pancreas involved in digestion?

3.2. Digestive Processes

Learning Outcome

1. Explain the mechanical and chemical digestion;
2. Define the absorption of nutrients.

The digestive processes of the human body are multifactorial and complex, involving a series of coordinated physiological processes that occur in the gastrointestinal tract. The processes begin in the mouth, where mechanical digestion in the process of mastication and chemical digestion in the process of saliva initiate the breakdown of food. The food is swallowed and reaches the esophagus before entering the stomach, where acidic gastric juices continue to digest proteins and kill pathogens. The stomach is also a reservoir that regulates the rate at which digested food enters the small intestine. Most of the nutrient absorption here is achieved by pancreatic enzymes and bile of the liver, which emulsifies fats. The digestive functions are thus not just the macromolecule breakdown but also involve a highly controlled function that ensures maximum nutrient absorption. Some new studies on non-starch polysaccharides (NSP) in animals' diet, i.e., pigs, have provided information on the mechanisms of digestion that can further be used in human knowledge too. It was discovered through the research that higher NSP content in the diet leads to a fall in the small intestinal organic matter digestibility, as well as the total tract, in comparison. The differential digestibility observed implies that NSP impinges on the gut environment through changing the level of organic acids and pH levels, as well as microbial populations in the gastrointestinal tract. Supplementation of enzymes also changes the dynamics, highlighting the complex interactions between the diet components and digestive efficiency. These points emphasize the importance of nutritional quality on digestion processes and intestinal well-being with potential implications in maximizing diets in various age ranges of pigs as well as humans (Högberg, 2003).

Much earlier, digestion physiology was comprehended by age-old techniques, e.g., outlined in Ayurveda books, which describe the balance of various systems of the body and their role in digestion. The Annavaha Stotas is the embodiment of the digestive system in this system, tying it to overall concepts of health and homeostasis. Modern physiology, while empirically founded to a large degree, is conceptually analogous to these old ideas, for example, the need for balance within the body's systems for optimal functioning. This holistic approach echoes the integrative nature of processes of digestion, where the relationship between physiological processes, forms of nutrients, and the health of the individual is most crucial. From this comprehension of intricate interrelationship among systems that regulate digestion, our practice of health and nutrition can be enhanced towards greater well-being and avoidance of disease (Patwardhan, 2008) (Figure 3.7).

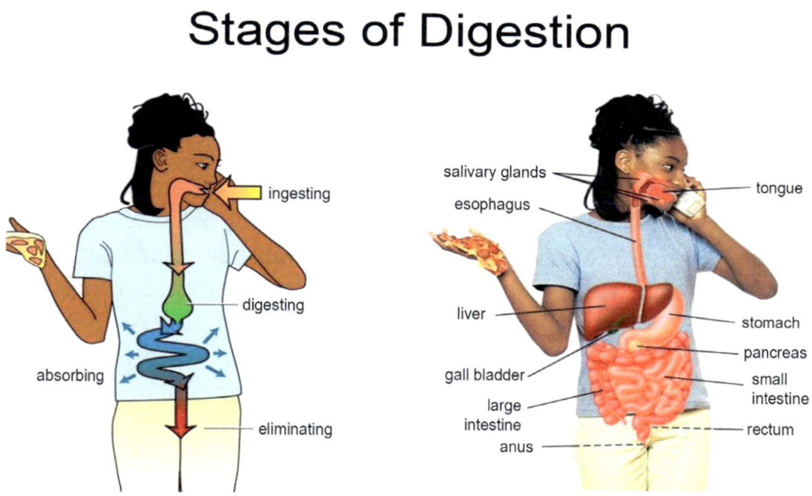

Figure 3.7. Digestive processes in the human body.

Source: https://image.slideserve.com/1182226/stages-of-digestion-l.jpg.

3.2.1. Mechanical Digestion

The mechanical digestion process is a fundamental part of gastrointestinal metabolism and represents the first stage of food breakdown in the digestive system. The process involves physical disruption of food into smaller, more accessible portions for enzymatic digestion. It begins in the oral cavity during mastication and is characterized by synchronized tooth, tongue, and jaw movements. These mechanical actions not only fragment food into smaller pieces but also mix it with saliva, which contains enzymes that trigger carbohydrate digestion. Once food is swallowed and reaches the stomach, gastric contractions again mix the food, combining it with gastric juices. This maximizes food's surface area, exposing its interior in greater quantities to the digestive enzymes present in the gastrointestinal tract, and ultimately leading to better nutrient uptake. Besides, mechanical digestion also contributes significantly to the bio accessibility of nutrients because of food matrix structures. In vegetables, for instance, the cell wall structural complexity is a pivotal element of digestion. Cell wall composition, comprising cellulose and hemicellulose polysaccharides, may limit the availability and release of nutrients. The brute physicality of mechanical digestion helps to break down such structures, thereby facilitating ease of cell wall breakdown with more accessibility to nutrients. As noted, the supramolecular structures differ according to plant tissue type, which can influence how easily the nutrients inside are digested and absorbed. Identification of these dynamics discloses the effect of various types of food on digestive efficacy and nutrient availability and reaffirms the importance of mechanical digestion in the physiology of the gastrointestinal tract (Holland et al., 2020). Finally, the role of mechanical digestion extends beyond food demolition and promotes interconnectedness between body processes. Physiologically, mechanical digestion initiates a reaction cascade of reactions involving the entire digestive apparatus.

Physical perturbation: Food causes physical disruption; it initiates gastric secretions and hormone reactions signaling digestive preparedness and enzyme release. For instance, distension of stomach walls releases hormones influencing appetite and digestion. Ancient Ayurvedic texts, on the contrary, emphasize balance among various bodily systems in maintaining health, much like current knowledge of digestion's complexity. By realizing the subtle interaction between mechanical digestion and overall physiology, it can be appreciated how such activity primes for optimal health and metabolic health (Patwardhan, 2008) (Figure 3.8).

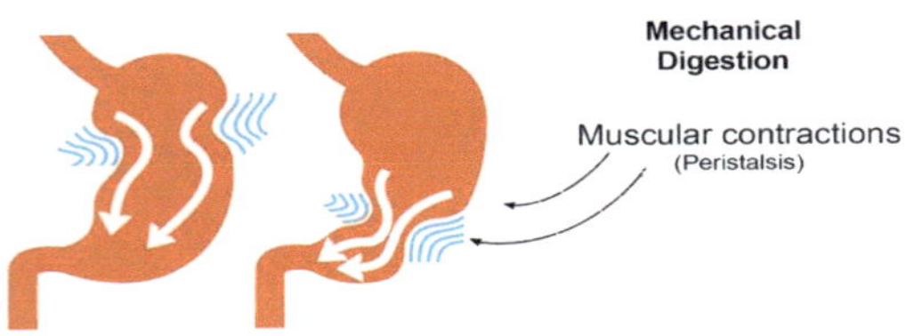

Figure 3.8. Mechanical digestion.

Source: https://external-content.duckduckgo.com/iu/?u=https%3A%2F%2Fwww.organsofthebody.com%2Fimages%2Fmechanical-Digestion-in-Stomach.jpg&f=1&nofb=1&ipt=db758cfc4dd57914f85c56d151c0b5a2cc3b27b0c4e18bfce1a15708be65d38d.

3.2.2. Chemical Digestion

Chemical digestion is a key activity within the gastrointestinal tract, during which food materials are broken down to their molecular structures for the absorption of nutrients. The complex chain of biochemical activities begins in the mouth, where enzymes like amylase initiate the breakdown of carbohydrates. As food descends the esophagus to the stomach, gastric juices containing hydrochloric acid and pepsin further break down proteins to form a semi-liquid material known as chyme. This blend is pivotal in enabling the subsequent stages of absorption that take place within the small intestine, highlighting the complex coordination that must exist amongst different enzymes and digestive secretions within the gastrointestinal tract. How efficiently these processes take place goes a long way to affect the total nutrient bioavailability, making it critical to unravel their biochemical foundations within the frame of gastrointestinal physiology. Chemical digestion is also continuous in the small intestine with the assistance of pancreatic enzymes and bile salts that also play vital functions in emulsifying and digesting fats and further digesting carbohydrates and proteins. The pancreas secretes enzymes , such as lipase, proteases, and amylase into the digestive system lumen, where they hydrolyze food particles into their fundamental components: fatty acids, amino acids, and monosaccharides. This enzymatic activity is facilitated by the presence of bile, which is produced by the liver and concentrated in the gallbladder, that breaks down fats by splitting large lipid globules into diminutive micelles to offer greater access to enzymatic action. The nutrient-rich chyme interacts with the intestinal mucosa, from which nutrients are absorbed. This phase is significant since the efficiency of enzyme activity and nutrient absorption can be very reliant on other processes, for instance, dietary composition and associated gut microbiota. Dietary composition plays a significant role in creating chemical digestion by predominantly through the character of the dietary fiber and plant cell walls. The integrity of these components in the intestine affects their digestibility and the subsequent bioavailability of nutrients. For example, the dietary NSP can interfere with the digestive environment to affect the digestion of organic matter and fiber components in the intestines. Literature has proven that an increased proportion of insoluble NSP can reduce total digestibility, particularly in newly weaned piglets and growing pigs (Högberg, 2003). In addition, cell wall structure within plants can regulate the release of nutrients during digestion and hence their bio accessibility as nutrients (Holland et al., 2020). These observations identify the interrelationship between diet and biochemical processes that govern nutrient digestion within the gastrointestinal tract and illustrate the importance of dietary formulation to the development of optimal digestive health (Figure 3.9).

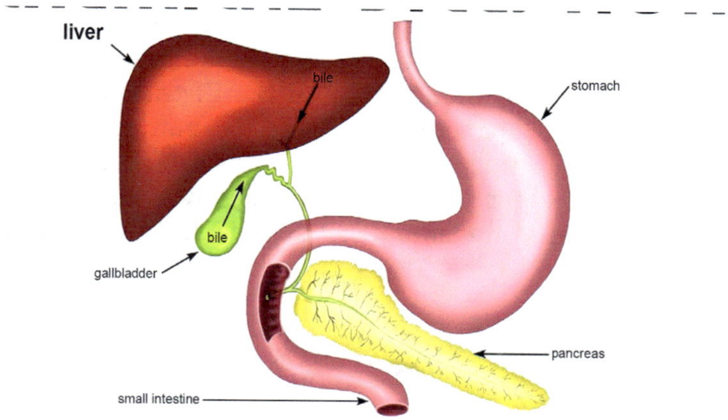

Figure 3.9. Chemical digestion.

Source: https://i.ytimg.com/vi/yyuQMi0V-SE/maxresdefault.jpg.

3.2.3. Absorption of Nutrients

In the intricate landscape of gastrointestinal physiology, nutrient absorption is a prominent process that ensures the body receives building materials for development and maintenance. Absorption begins essentially in the small intestine, where villi and microvilli increase the surface area to facilitate the effective absorption of macromolecules. The presence of carbohydrates, fatty acids, and amino acids within the intestinal lumen causes stimuli to secrete a variety of enzymes and transport proteins, which allow them to be absorbed into the blood. This interaction, in addition to enabling the transport of nutrients, also has a significant influence on the gene expression in the intestine since nutrients have the ability to regulate the synthesis of proteins that are used for digestion and absorption. By adjusting gene expression dynamically according to the availability of nutrients, the gut has an adaptive response mechanism to changes in diet, facilitating both metabolic health and the prevention of gastrointestinal disease (Bauer et al., 2011). In addition, nutrient absorption is directly related to the microbiota of the gastrointestinal tract. These microbial populations are similarly significant in fermenting unused fiber and in the production of short-chain fatty acids (SCFAs), which have been shown to have an impact on host metabolism and immune status. Through metabolism of unrecovered nutrients, the microbiota generate byproducts that can affect intestinal health and efficiency of nutrient uptake and absorption. For instance, SCFAs can enhance mucosal barrier functions and control inflammatory responses, hence supporting intestinal integrity alongside nutrient absorption. Such a mutualistic process underscores the importance of diet components not only for their direct substrate supply for absorption but also in terms of how they modulate the microbial community that catalyzes these processes. Without the mutual interaction between host physiology and microbial metabolism, the full potential of nutrient absorption can go unrealized, resulting in numerous health problems (Patwardhan, 2008). Beyond the biochemical and microbiological parameters that regulate nutrient absorption are the physiological composition of the gastrointestinal system itself. The sequential transit of food through the esophagus, stomach, and small intestine is precisely controlled for optimal release and absorption of nutrients. Stomach mechanical digestion and following pancreatic and small intestine enzymatic digestion ensure that nutrients are effectively digested into absorbable forms. Furthermore, hormonal stimulants , such as gastrin, secretin, and cholecystokinin are released in response to food intake and offer feedback control on digestion. Understanding these processes is crucial for the design of therapeutic interventions for gastrointestinal dysfunctions, particularly when nutrient absorption is compromised. With a detailed discussion of the interactive workings of the GI tract, it would then be realized that effective nutrient absorption is a multifaceted set of physical, chemical, and biological processes ultimately accountable for overall health and disease resistance (Bauer et al., 2011).

Test Your Knowledge

1. How does mechanical digestion differ from chemical digestion?
2. Where does most nutrient absorption occur in the digestive tract?

3.3. Gastrointestinal Motility

Learning Outcome

1. Explain the peristalsis and segmentation;
2. Define the role of smooth muscle;
3. Describe the regulation of motility by the nervous system.

Gastrointestinal motility is a fundamental aspect of gastrointestinal physiology that provides for the movement of food within the gastrointestinal tract and participates in various physiological responses. It consists of regulation by smooth muscle coordinated contractions of the gastrointestinal tract walls under the oversight of intrinsic and extrinsic neural control. The enteric nervous system, or second brain, plays a key role in coordinating such contractions to have the utmost control over patterns of motility depending on food quantity and composition. This finely tuned regulation offers a smooth function of the digestive organs for maximum absorption of nutrients and expulsion of waste. Any disruption in this motility can cause gastrointestinal diseases, and thus the necessity to understand the mechanisms of these complex movements, particularly in disorders like Irritable Bowel Syndrome (IBS) and Inflammatory Bowel Disease (IBD) (Linson, 2013). Recent research has told us something about the impact of hormonal control on gastrointestinal motility, particularly regarding symptomology of IBS and IBD. Hormones , such as progesterone are discovered to be implicated as potential mediators of changes in motility, exacerbating such symptoms as cramping and constipation. The cyclical nature of the aforementioned symptoms in females can be associated with varying levels of hormones, thus suggesting a close interassociation between hormonal fluctuations and motility. By further examining such correlations, investigators are gaining insight into how endocrine imbalances can influence gastrointestinal function and symptomatology. Furthermore, interference with such hormonal pathways presents a therapeutic potential, shifting the focus from mere symptomatic treatment to therapy for the underlying causes of motility disorders, thereby improving the outcomes of the patients in IBS and IBD (Linson, 2013). The enteric nervous system is also influenced by external factors like microbiota composition, nutrition, and aging, further modulating gastrointestinal motility. The gut-brain axis interaction and the enteric nervous system exhibit the complexity of gastrointestinal physiology. Recent studies indicate that gut microbiota can affect motility signaling mechanisms, and thus affect not only digestive but also broader aspects of physiology, behavior, and immunity. This plasticity of gastrointestinal innervation reinforces adaptive responses to varied stimuli, dictating the general health of an individual. Hence, understanding how the extrinsic factors are going to interact with the intrinsic motility mechanisms can help in designing improved interventions for gastrointestinal disease, ultimately leading to more advanced therapeutic solutions for patients suffering from motility-related diseases (Figure 3.10).

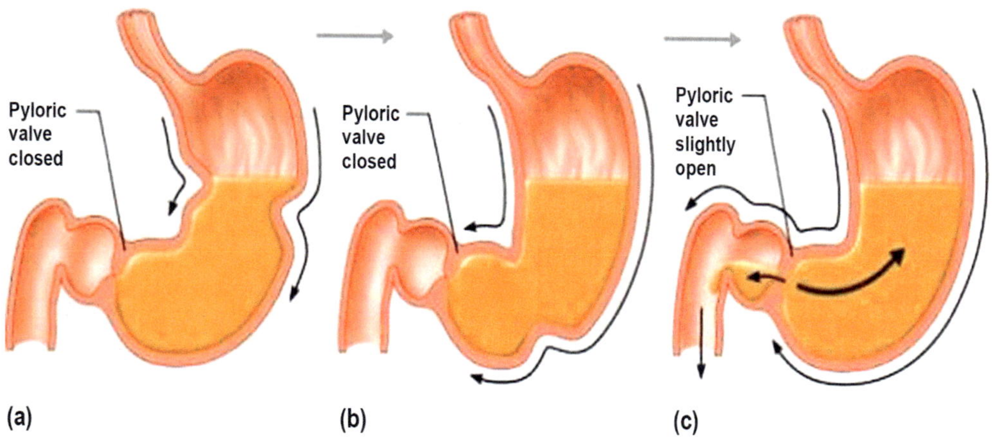

Figure 3.10. Gastrointestinal Motility.

Source: https://external-content.duckduckgo.com/iu/?u=https%3A%2F%2Fi2.wp.com%2Fmedicoapps.org%2Fwp-content%2Fuploads%2F2018%2F07%2FGASTROINTESTINAL-MOTILITY.jpg%3Fresize%3D600%252C315%26ssl%3D1&f=1&nofb=1&ipt=f573a3f5c74c10df4b4ce12c63a4269a70f63cb18d8686815cde77669a2bb941.

3.3.1. Peristalsis and Segmentation

The GI tract motor activity is generally explained by two mechanisms, which are peristalsis and segmentation. Peristalsis refers to a wave-like muscular contraction that propels food through the digestive tract and enables transportation from the esophagus to the rectum in an efficient manner. It is an involuntary process that depends on coordinated contraction and relaxation of circular and longitudinal muscle layers, which produce a peristaltic wave. There is such a mechanism that not only serves the transportation of food but also prevents backflow in the digestive tract. Peristalsis acquires importance in the event of gastrointestinal obstruction, where compromised peristaltic function will lead to severe complications. Familiarity with the nuances of peristalsis provides insight into the overall efficiency of digestive activity and illustrates the relevance of smooth muscle function in the physiology of the gastrointestinal tract. Segmentation, as compared to peristalsis, is characterized by spasmodic contractions that mix and churn the content of the intestines rather than moving it forward. It is primarily performed in the small intestine, where it plays a vital role in the digestion and absorption process. The circular muscle fibers of smooth muscle contract in a rhythmic manner, fragmenting the intestinal contents into segments, which are appropriately mixed by the activity of these contractions. The significance of segmentation is that it has the capacity to enable digestion due to increased exposure of food particles to digestive enzymes and absorptive surfaces. As emphasized in recent studies, segmentation is the process that contributes not only to mechanical mixing but also concurrently facilitates chyme transport by causing regular propagating contractions, thereby enabling efficient absorption of nutrients along the intestine (Avvari, 2019). The interplay between peristalsis and segmentation exemplifies the complexity of gastrointestinal physiology and underscores the importance of mechanical forces in digestion. Both mechanisms are required for effective breaking down, mixing, and transport of food that ultimately affects nutrient assimilation. The mechanical dynamics at play are based on a variety of factors that include patterns of contractility in the muscularis mucosae as well as rheological characteristics of luminal contents. Abnormalities of viscera in either peristalsis or segmentation are reported to result in digestive disorders, thereby implying that a very specific balance must be maintained. Research continues to investigate how variations in these contractions affect flow rates, mixing volumes, and ultimately digestion efficiency. Such continued research also suggests the intricate relationship between mechanical contractility and the resulting physiological effect in the gastrointestinal tract, supporting the necessity of understanding these processes in the big picture of digestive well-being (Valls-Bellés, 2024) (Figure 3.11).

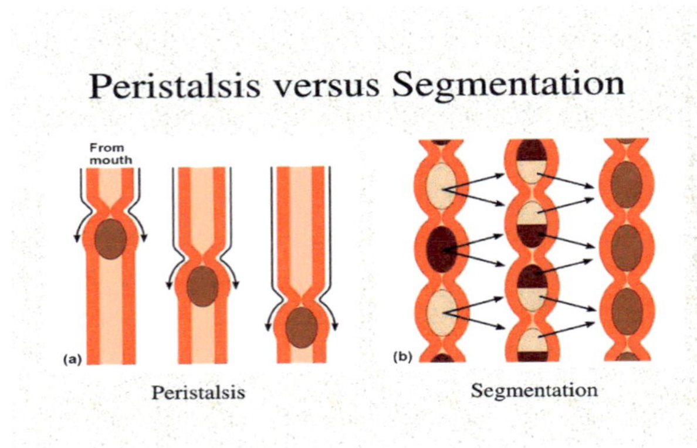

Figure 3.11. Peristalsis-versus-segmentation.

Source: https://image.slideserve.com/1418318/peristalsis-versus-segmentation-l.jpg.

3.3.2. Role of Smooth Muscle

Smooth muscle is also a vital aspect of gastrointestinal physiology, primarily through its ability to contract and facilitate the propulsion of food material through the digestive tract. Smooth muscle is most prevalent in hollow organs , such as the stomach and intestines, and is actively in operation involuntarily, reacting to physiological stimuli rather than conscious control. This peculiar muscular organization allows for peristalsis—a synchronized sequence of muscle contractions that move contents through the digestive tract. Rhythmic contractions not only aid in transport but also in blending food with digestive juices and thereby maximizing the biochemical decomposition of nutrients. This unconscious regulation is necessary for the support of the digestive processes going on continuously, regardless of outside needs. Smooth muscle activity is tightly controlled by the enteric nervous system (ENS), an advanced network of neurons contained within the gut wall. The ENS, or brain-in-the-gut, consists of two main plexuses—the myenteric and submucosal plexuses—that communicate to regulate not only smooth muscle contractions but also the circulation of blood through the gut and mucosal secretion (Serio et al., 2011). This ability to control both motility and secretory functions demonstrates the fundamental role in managing homeostasis of the gastrointestinal tract. The extensive range of neurotransmitters and signaling mechanisms utilized by enteric neurons further demonstrates the sophisticated regulation of smooth muscle function, such that the digestion process remains efficient and reactive. Furthermore, pathophysiologic conditions have the capability of significantly impacting smooth muscle function, resulting in many disorders of the gastrointestinal tract. Conditions like achalasia and irritable bowel syndrome demonstrate how dysfunctional smooth muscle contraction can disrupt normal digestive function, resulting in abdominal pain and dysphagia. Understanding the function of smooth muscles in such conditions can be used to explain potential therapeutic interventions in restoring normal function.

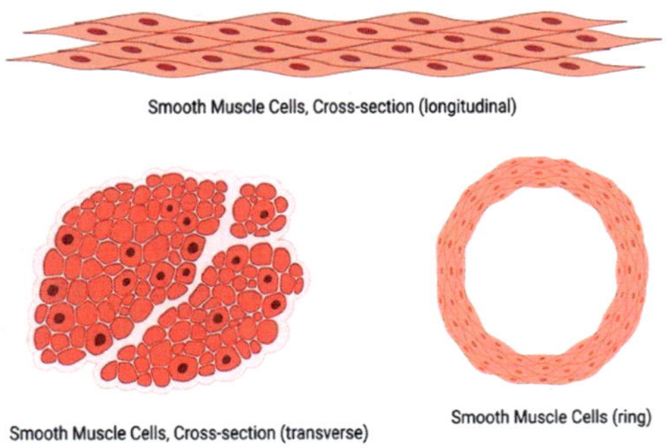

Figure 3.12. Smooth muscle.

Source: https://researchtweet.com/wp-content/uploads/2021/09/Smooth-Muscle-1-Smooth-Muscle-Tissue-Smooth-Muscle-Function-Where-is-Smooth-Muscle-Found.jpg.

The capacity of ENS to maintain gut motility in the presence of interference testifies to the function of smooth muscle in gastrointestinal health. Through an extensive study of the interplay of smooth muscle function, neural control, and related pathologies, scientists can formulate more efficient treatment options for gastrointestinal disorders, finally enhancing patient outcomes (Serio et al., 2011) (Figure 3.12).

3.3.3. Regulation of Motility by the Nervous System

Gastrointestinal motility is controlled primarily by the ENS, an extremely intricate neural system capable of independent function within the gut. This sophisticated system appears as two large ganglionated plexuses, the submucosal and myenteric plexuses. These interact to control smooth muscle contractility, mucosal secretion, and intestinal blood flow. The ENS is unique in having an equal number of neurons to the spinal cord, demonstrating a highly developed state of organization and functional diversity akin to that of the central nervous system. Its high ability has been nicknamed brain-in-the-gut, highlighting its purpose of maintaining gut motility and ensuring coordinated transport of food along the digestive tract (Serio et al., 2011). In addition, the ENS operates by complex coordination of excitatory and inhibitory information provided by multiple neurotransmitters. Neurotransmitters , such as acetylcholine, serotonin, and nitric oxide play crucial roles in regulating segmental and peristaltic contraction of the gut. These signals can initiate contractions to propel contents along the intestinal lumen or relaxation of the gut to accommodate new food. In addition, sensory neurons of the ENS are mechanoreceptive and chemoreceptive, and these stimuli give rise to feedback employed in coordinating motility patterns. The ability of the ENS to autonomously control such processes ensures gastrointestinal motility is efficient even without extrinsic input from the CNS, placing it at the central location in gastrointestinal physiology (Serio et al., 2011). Interestingly, communication between the enteric and central nervous systems is significant in controlling motility. While the ENS can autonomously control most gut function mechanisms, it can also be modulated by extrinsic parasympathetic and sympathetic nervous inputs. The parasympathetic nervous system would stimulate motility and secretion and facilitate digestion and nutrient absorption. Sympathetic input would generally inhibit motility and reallocate energy into more critical functions under stress conditions. This close control between the intrinsic and extrinsic systems is able to dynamically adjust gut motility according to various physiological states and stimuli. The understanding of the interactions is crucial to that of gastrointestinal disorders, in which motility dysfunction often represents the key aspect of clinical presentation, prompting the demand for selective therapeutic strategies (Serio et al., 2011).

Test Your Knowledge

1. What is gastrointestinal motility?
2. What is the role of peristalsis in the GI tract?

3.4. Gastrointestinal Secretions

Learning Outcome

1. Identify the salivary glands and their secretions;
2. Define the gastric juice composition;
3. Describe the pancreatic and biliary secretions.

Gastrointestinal secretions are pivotal to the overall physiology of the digestive system since they facilitate the breakdown and absorption of the nutrients. The important secretions include saliva, gastric juices, bile, pancreatic secretions, and intestinal secretions. Saliva, which is produced by salivary glands, starts digestion, transmitting enzymes , such as amylase that initiate the digestion of carbohydrates while preparing the food for swallowing. Gastric juice, secreted by the lining of the stomach, consists of hydrochloric acid, pepsinogen, and intrinsic factor, the latter being essential for the absorption of vitamin B12. In addition, neural and hormonal stimuli regulate the intricate coordination of these secretions so that the compartment of digestion remains in the most advantageous state for enzyme function and nutrient absorption. A system like this displays the complexity of gastrointestinal physiology, where fine-tuning for proper digestion and absorption is most critical. Moreover, the ENS is also a central driving force behind the regulation of gastrointestinal secretions. This extensive neural plexus, alternatively referred to as the brain-in-the-gut, regulates many physiological occurrences, including the regulation of secretory function along the gastrointestinal tract. The ENS operates independently of the central nervous system to govern exocrine secretion in mucosa and smooth muscle function, suggestive of a large degree of functionality similar to the spinal cord (Serio et al., 2011). Besides, ENS and gastrointestinal mucosal secretory cells' interactions are also a good example of the regulation of digestion, where stimuli , such as ingestion, trigger intricate neuronal mechanisms that lead to specific secretions. Therefore, the understanding of the ENS's function provides important information on how digestive secretions are precisely coordinated to facilitate digestion. The interaction among hormones has a significant function in the secretions of the gastrointestinal system and also in the creation of gastrointestinal disease. Various intestinal hormones regulate the secretion of digestive juices and enzymes based on the various phases of digestion. For instance, CCK induces the release of bile and pancreatic enzyme secretion following the entry of fats into the duodenum. Hormonal fluctuations can impact secretory processes, leading to disorders , such as Irritable Bowel Syndrome (IBS) and Inflammatory Bowel Disease (IBD) with a complex array of debilitating symptoms from abdominal pain to altered bowel habits (Linson, 2013). The potential role of hormones, such as, progesterone, in their deterioration suggests that understanding the hormonal effects on the gastrointestinal secretions can offer therapeutic possibilities in the treatment of such often chronic diseases and hence enhance patient care in gastrointestinal health (Figure 3.13).

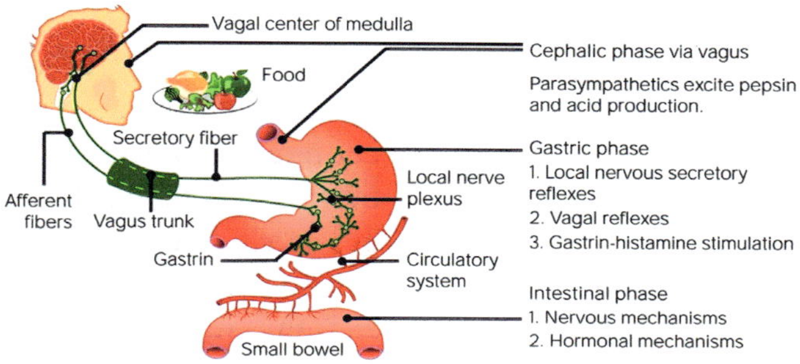

Figure 3.13. Gastrointestinal secretions.

Source: https://cdn.lecturio.com/assets/Phases-of-digestion-with-their-functional-components.jpg.

3.4.1. Salivary Glands and Their Secretions

Salivary glands play an important role in gastrointestinal tract physiology, as their primary function is to assist in digestion and oral health. The exocrine parotid, submandibular, and sublingual glands help secrete saliva, a composition of water, electrolytes, enzymes, and antimicrobial substances. Saliva stimulates the digestion process by breaking down starches with enzymes like alpha-amylase. Besides, mucin in saliva contributes to lubrication, which helps to create a cohesive bolus that makes swallowing possible. Salivary gland functions are physiologically more than just digestive; they contribute significantly to mucosal health and defense of the oral environment against infection. Salivary gland secretions are controlled by a number of factors, including taste, odor, and even mastication. On stimulation by these stimuli, the autonomic nervous system triggers secretion of saliva that varies in constitution according to the physiological state of the body. For instance, during active coping conditions , such as an anxiety memory test, sympathetic activity is significantly heightened, which is accompanied by increased secretion of MUC7 and lactoferrin proteins. Conversely, passive coping strategies, such as, viewing surgical procedures in a video, have a different autonomic impact, wherein cardiovascular reactivity is associated with increased secretion of proteins. The heterogeneity demonstrates the flexibility of the salivary glands to respond to environmental and psychological stimuli, thereby demonstrating their complex role in general gastrointestinal function and health (Bosch et al., 2000). Aside from their role in digestion, salivary secretions offer a first defense against oral pathogens, highlighting the significance of saliva in gastrointestinal physiology. Salivary gland secreted proteins , such as protective molecules including immunoglobulins and antimicrobial peptides, play a role in inhibiting microbial colonization as well as keeping the oral microbiome in balance. A robust profile of secretion can be influenced by psychological stress; a stressful situation, for example, often leads to an increase in the overall secretory protein production of saliva. This response demonstrates the dynamic interaction between stress, salivary gland function, and gut health. Besides, the study of these glands not only enhances the understanding of the digestive process but also sheds light on the larger implications of immune function and oral health, pointing to the interconnectedness of the body's physiological systems (Valls-Bellés, 2024) (Figure 3.14).

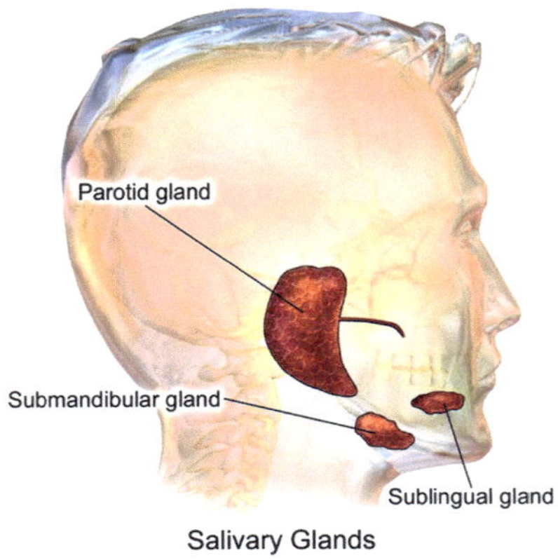

Figure 3.14. Saliva and salivary glands.

Source: https://images.saymedia-content.com/.image/t_share/MTc0NjQxNzM2MDQ3NTM2MDcz/interesting-facts-about-saliva-and-salivary-glands.jpg.

3.4.2. Gastric Juice Composition

The composition of gastric juice is vital to the entire physiology of gastrointestinal function. Gastric juice consists primarily of hydrochloric acid (HCl), pepsinogen, intrinsic factor, and mucus. The highly acidic pH, ranging from 1.5 to 3.5, achieved through HCl, allows for the denaturation of food proteins to facilitate easier digestion. In addition, pepsinogen, the inactive form of the enzyme pepsin, is activated in this acidic environment, catalyzing protein breakdown into smaller peptides. This first phase of digestion is important, as it not only conditions food for subsequent enzymatic activity in the small intestine but also kills ingested potential pathogens, hence adding to the host's immune defense mechanism. Intrinsic factor, a glycoprotein secreted by gastric parietal cells, is essential for ileal absorption of vitamin B12 and thus the role of gastric juice extends beyond the digestive process.

A deficiency in intrinsic factor leads to pernicious anemia, which demonstrates the connection between gastric secretions and overall well-being. Moreover, the mucus secretion of gastric juice protects the gastric epithelium against the corrosiveness of acid and enzymes and maintains the gastric lining intact. This balancing mechanism of secretion is essential both for digestive purposes as well as to prevent gastric injuries that may result from prolonged contact with acidic environments, maintaining the fine balance of gastrointestinal physiology. Recent studies have also demonstrated how the activity and composition of gastric juice are modulated by food and meals. For instance, the type and amount of fiber in food may alter gastric emptying and thereby gastric juice secretion afterwards. An MRI study illustrated how different meals, such as, whole meal bread and rice pudding, influenced gastric volumes and the kinetics of gastric emptying. The whole meal bread formed a cohesive bolus that prevented gastric sieving, leading to longer gastric emptying times compared with the more rapidly emptied rice pudding meal, highlighting the physiological consequences of meal structure on digestion and absorption (Marciani et al., 2013). These results are important in constructing an understanding of how various habits of eating may influence gastric physiology and overall health (Figure 3.15).

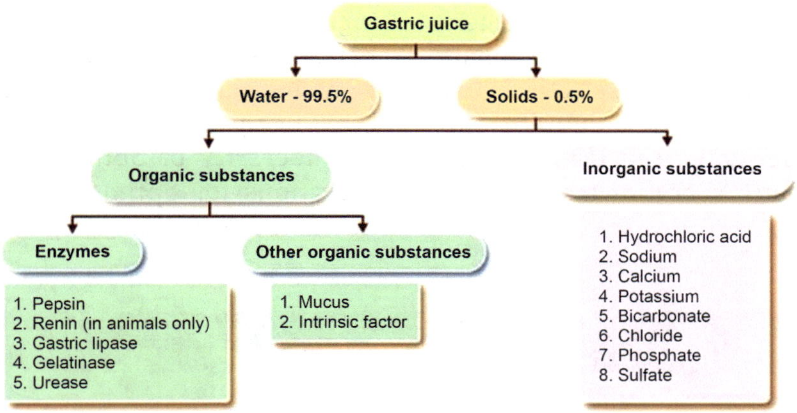

Figure 3.15. Composition of gastric juice and functions.

Source: https://image.slidesharecdn.com/propertiesofgastricjuicecompositionofgastricjuiceandfunctionsofgastricjuice-191104142114/85/properties-of-gastric-juice-composition-of-gastric-juice-and-functions-of-gastric-juice-11-638.jpg?cb=1665786342.

3.4.3. Pancreatic and Biliary Secretions

In the intricate landscape of gastrointestinal physiology, pancreatic and biliary secretions are vital factors in the digestion and absorption of nutrients. The pancreas releases a wide range of enzymes, such as, amylase, lipase, and proteases, into the small intestine to facilitate the digestion of carbohydrates, fats, and proteins. The concentrations of these enzymes are crucial because each is specific for a specific macromolecule and their lack will cause malabsorption that results in nutrient deficiencies. Additionally, the pancreas also secretes bicarbonate ions to neutralize gastric acid entering the duodenum and create a comfortable environment for enzymatic activity. These secretions are stringently regulated by hormonal stimuli, primarily cholecystokinin and secretin, that respond to the presence of food in the gut, and hence optimize the digestion process. Secretions from the bile of the liver are also very important for effective digestion. Bile, containing bile salts, cholesterol, bilirubin, and electrolytes, serves multiple functions, one of which is emulsification of fat, facilitating its absorption in the intestines. The process of bile secretion encompasses production at the hepatocytes and storage and concentration by the gallbladder until triggered by digestive needs. Interestingly, hormones like secretin also stimulate secretion of bicarbonate-containing fluid from bile duct cholangiocytes, an activity critical to the alkalinity and functional role of bile within the duodenum. The interaction between these secretions offers an ideal setting for the action of the digestive enzymes to occur while optimizing effective lipid digestion and absorption, thereby emphasizing the pivotal symbiosis of pancreatic and biliary physiology in gastrointestinal physiology. The coordination and regulation of pancreatic and biliary secretions emphasize the complexity of gastrointestinal physiology. Once food is transferred to the small intestine, the secretion of hormones , such as glucagon and secretin elevates the secretion of bicarbonate to further facilitate the digestion process (Valls-Bellés, 2024). The bicarbonate-rich secretions facilitate a process known as hydrocholeretic, whereby the osmotic pressures drive water movement along with electrolytes , such as bicarbonate and chloride ions (Banales et al., 2006). This dynamic interaction not only maintains pH balance but also facilitates the transmission of bile and pancreatic secretions, important for emulsification and efficient digestion of ingested fat. By complex mechanisms involving hormone-receptor interfaces and intracellular signaling pathways, the GI tract is the model of a highly integrated system, demonstrating the necessity of both pancreatic and biliary secretions for optimum digestive health and nutrient absorption.

Test Your Knowledge

1. What is the role of hydrochloric acid in the stomach?
2. Which cells in the stomach secrete pepsinogen?

3.5. Role of Gut Microbiota

Learning Outcome

1. Describe the composition of gut microbiota;
2. Define the functions of gut microbiota in digestion;
3. Discuss the impact of gut microbiota on health.

The gut microbiota plays a significant role in gastrointestinal physiology because it facilitates the digestion process, vitamin production, and maintenance of intestinal mucosa barrier integrity. This ecosystem of microbes is vital for nutrient absorption and metabolism, particularly the fermentation of fiber in the diet. For instance, some types of dietary fiber, such as, chicory, influence the activity and composition of gut microbiota and hence enhance nutrient utilization and gut health. Research emphasizes the connection between fiber intake and diversity of microbiota, as well as how some gut bacteria influence the host's digestive function and immune system. Through triggering good balance in the microbiome, dietary fibers may improve gut morphology, which subsequently results in increased digestion and nutrient absorption and hence validate the function of diet in gut microbiota dynamics and functionality (Liu, 2013). In addition to that, the effects of environmental factors on gut microbiota composition cannot be underestimated, particularly climate change. For example, in the research, it has been established that elevated carbon dioxide levels can induce dysbiosis among aquatic animals , such as fish. Under high exposure to CO_2, sea bream's intestinal microbiota altered significantly, as indicated by a considerable reduction in Firmicutes and the rise in Proteobacteria. Such alteration could have efficient effects on the hosts' health, altering digestive efficiency, immunity, and disease susceptibility. This mechanism illustrates how environmental stressors disrupt the delicately balanced equilibrium of gut microbiota, bringing into focus the importance of gaining profound knowledge about environmental factors' influence on gastrointestinal physiology. The intricate interaction between the environment of an organism and its gut microbiota also emphasizes the dynamic nature of such microbial communities (Fonseca et al., 2019). In short, the polyvalent activity of gut microbiota constitutes the foundation of gastrointestinal physiology, influencing not just nutrient absorption but also immune response and general health. Dietetic preferences as well as external environmental factors determine microbiota diversity, proving the necessity for individualization in dietetic intervention and health interventions. The communication between the host's physiology and gut microbiome also underscores the necessity of maintaining a healthy microbiota through a balanced diet and awareness of external stimuli. As the search continues to find correlations between diet, gut microbiota, and health endpoints, care must be taken to integrate these findings into clinical practice to facilitate better health promotion strategies and better comprehension of gastrointestinal physiology. The study of gut microbiota is a promising field of overlap among nutrition, health, and environmental science that ultimately results in more holistic methods of sustaining health and avoiding disease (Figure 3.16).

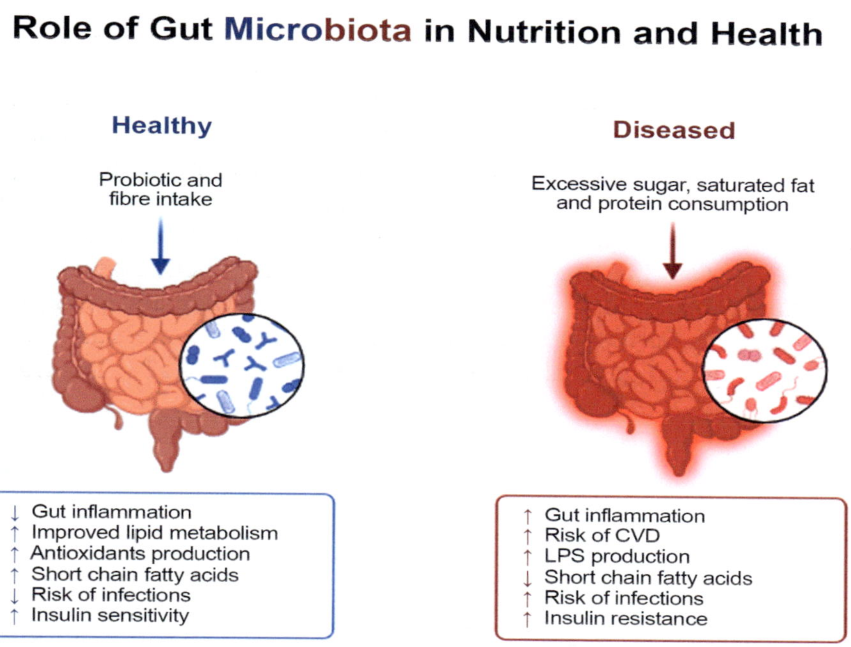

Figure 3.16. Role of Gut Microbiota in Nutrition and Health.

Source: https://cdn.prod.website-files.com/621e95f9ac30687a56e4297e/64a8d6aedebdf69e121bb29e_V2_1675789562952_ce4f2191-a069-47f5-a7e0-19e1f00c258a.png.

3.5.1. Composition of Gut Microbiota

The gut microbiota is a highly complex group of microorganisms that live in the gastrointestinal tract and play roles in human health and disease. The community is constituted primarily of bacteria, but also includes archaea, viruses, and fungi, with the latter being highly influenced by varied factors like diet, genetics, and exposures to the environment. Research has proven that the microbial populations are quite different between individuals and can exhibit temporal variability, which reflects the dynamic nature of gut ecosystems. For example, gut microbiota from chimpanzees was found to exhibit obvious differences within communities, suggesting a balance between environmental pressures and host genetics in shaping microbial diversity. This implies that it is vital in gastrointestinal physiology to understand the determinants of gut microbiota composition, as the microorganisms are involved in metabolic function, immunity, and health (Degnan et al., 2012). Among the most significant determinants of gut microbiota composition is diet. Some fiber-rich foods, such as, those from chicory, have been reported to balance the population of gut microbes, thereby enhancing digestive and immune functions. Experimental studies in animals with dietary chicory show alterations in gut anatomy and populations of health-promoting microbes , such as lactic acid bacteria. Enhanced utilization of nutrients and gut environment is the outcome of such mechanisms. The effect of fiber on the microbiota indicates the interaction between nutrition and gut microbial community, influencing not just gut health but systemic immune responses as well. This kind of dynamic between food components and gut microbiota underlines the significance of understanding dietary interventions as a way to promote optimal gut health and avoid gastrointestinal disease (Liu, 2013). Aside from digestion, the significance of gut microbiota composition extends beyond the gut since it is actively interacting with the host's immune system. The presence of some bacterial species can stimulate the production of protective proteins like heat shock proteins, which play a crucial role in cell protection and stress response. This host-microbiota association is essential to preserve gut barrier function and prevent dysbiosis, a characteristic that is frequently associated with disease states like inflammatory bowel disease and metabolic disease. Understanding the organization of gut microbiota and its physiologic roles in host function is vital since it has the potential to open up therapeutic possibilities to manipulate microbial communities in order to preserve health. With the study ever coming to light, it more and more appears that gut microbiota structure is implicated in numerous aspects in elucidating gastrointestinal physiology and general well-being (Degnan et al., 2012; Liu, 2013) (Figure 3.17).

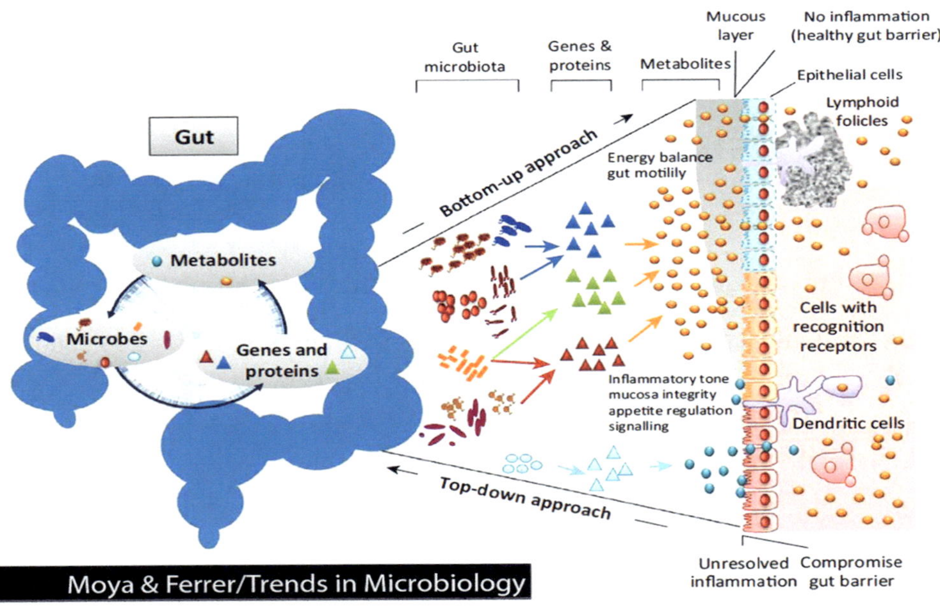

Figure 3.17. Composition of gut microbiota.

Source: https://www.gutmicrobiotaforhealth.com/wp-content/uploads/2016/04/gut_microbiote_is_stable_or_ever_changing.jpg.

3.5.2. Functions of Gut Microbiota in Digestion

The human gastrointestinal system contains an enormous community of different microorganisms, called the gut microbiota, which is crucial for digestion as well as health. The complex ecosystem facilitates fiber and other non-digestible substances digestion and supports the uptake of nutrients. Particularly, certain gut microbes are involved in the fermentation of complex carbs into short-chain fatty acids (SCFAs), an energy source for colon cells and systemically advantageous for , such as the suppression of inflammation. A good balance of the gut microbiota is thus required for optimizing digestive function, not merely the delivery of nutrients but also the maintenance of intestinal barrier integrity. Disruptions of this microbiota, caused by antibiotics or unhealthy diets, lead to gastrointestinal illnesses, which underscore the symbiotic interplay between diet, gut health, and microbiota activity. Aside from the digestion of nutrients, gut microbiota has an impact on gastrointestinal physiology through the modulation of immune function. This microbiome can communicate with the host's immune system to produce healthy antibodies and regulate inflammatory responses. For instance, certain lactic acid bacterial strains trigger heat shock protein production, which is a protective protein during stress and enhances the gut's barrier function against pathogenic microorganisms (Liu, 2013). Such interactions lie at the core of microbiota's mechanism of action in not causing illness that is related to dysbiosis, or an imbalance of microbes. Apart from that, the presence of diverse microbial communities is linked with increased immunological resistance of the gut because they can occupy space and compete for resources with pathogens, making infection less likely.

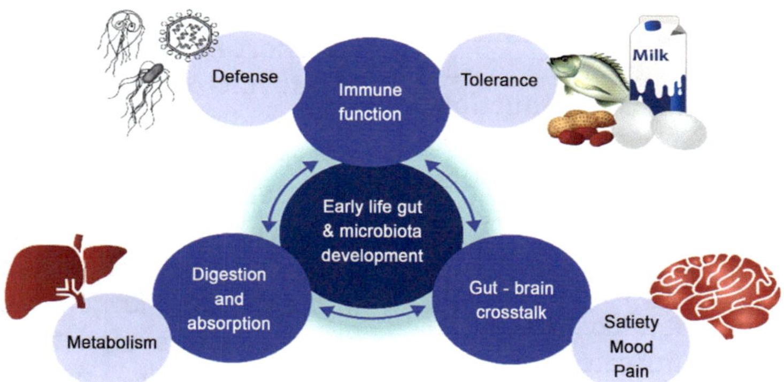

Figure 3.18. The central role of the gut.

Source: https://external-content.duckduckgo.com/iu/?u=https%3A%2F%2Fwww.nutriciaresearch.com%2Fwp-content%2Fuploads%2F2017%2F08%2FGut-Microbiota-triangle-functions-1.png&f=1&nofb=1&ipt=d0175fbf63a2b2eed1f37c4571cbd3e7e4f2b7b6a78de671ca4ccaea3203261d.

This shows the multiple functions of gut microbiota not only in digestion but also in immune status. The new research has also uncovered the involvement of gut microbiota in the overall metabolic processes of the host organism. For example, variation in microbial content can regulate the extraction of energy from the diet, regulating body weight and susceptibility to metabolic syndrome. It has been shown that the changes of gut microbiota that come with dietary modifications, i.e., increased consumption of dietary fiber , such as chicory, can enhance nutrient uptake and regulate energy use in animal models like pigs and chickens (Liu, 2013). Also, environmental factors , such as high atmospheric CO_2 and related stressors, including ocean acidification, are shown to modify the microbial composition in aquatic animals, potentially hinting at downstream effects on fish digestion and nutrient uptake. Such results enhance the significance of maintaining a healthy gut microbiota for effective digestion and general metabolic state and highlight its prominence in the field of gastrointestinal physiology (Figure 3.18).

3.5.3. Impact of Gut Microbiota on Health

The role of gut microbiota goes far beyond mere digestion, affecting many aspects of human physiology fundamental to the understanding of gastrointestinal function. The complex population of microorganisms inhabiting the gastrointestinal tract is involved in the absorption of nutrients, vitamin production, and metabolism of energy. Perhaps more significantly, it is responsible for modulating the host's immune response and the level of inflammation. These are the age, eating habits, and antibiotic use, which play a significant role in determining the gut microbiota composition and hence health status. The intricate interaction between body functions and gut microbiota is particularly impressive; an imbalance in this microbiota is responsible for diseases , such as inflammatory bowel disease, obesity, and metabolic syndrome, all of which emphasize the necessity of a healthy balance in the gut community for maintaining physiological well-being (Shatakshi et al., 2024). Furthermore, the role of gut microbiota also extends to mental wellbeing, revealing the profound effect that our diet and gut can have on mental health. The gut-brain axis, a hunger communication system between the brain and the gut, demonstrates the way that gut microbiota have the ability to influence mood and cognition. Current evidence indicates shifts in gut microbiota could play a role in psychiatric illnesses , such as depression and anxiety. Administration of certain probiotics has been shown to potentially reconstitute normal gut microbiota, which in turn can enhance depression symptoms and emotional well-being. This is a new field of study that emphasizes the relevance of health in the gut, not only in the physical but also in mental and emotional processes, suggesting more integrated health care with the inclusion of dietary and psychological dimensions (Tang et al., 2024). The consequences of gut microbiota research presented in both sports and general health contexts pinpoint the intricate impact of such microorganisms on human physiology. For sport individuals, for instance, a high level of gut microbiota diversity is associated with increased energy utilization, immune function, and recovery following exercise. The interaction between exercise, dietary behaviors, and the structure of gut microbiota is critical in optimizing performance and health outcomes in sports. On a large scale, knowing how daily lifestyle factors impact the well-being of the gut can give valuable insights into the prevention of disease and the maintenance of health among the wider population. The current research on gut microbiota and health outcomes reemphasizes the necessity of a holistic understanding of gastrointestinal physiology, suggesting that a healthy gut may form the foundation for overall health and functioning in all aspects of life (Shatakshi et al., 2024).

Test Your Knowledge

1. What is the function of gut microbiota in digestion?
2. How does gut microbiota influence the immune system?

3.6. Disorders of the Gastrointestinal System

Learning Outcome

1. Describe the common gastrointestinal disorders;
2. Define the impact of lifestyle on gastrointestinal health;
3. Describe the diagnostic approaches for gastrointestinal disorders.

The gastrointestinal conditions, particularly Irritable Bowel Syndrome (IBS) and Inflammatory Bowel Disease (IBD), have gained increasing attention both in clinical settings and in scientific studies. Both of them are not only somatically diagnosed through symptoms , such as abdominal pain, bloating, and changes in bowel habits; they also have complex dynamics among physiological and psychosocial processes. Studies have indicated that psychological status accounts for a significant contribution to the etiology of these disorders. For instance, patients with IBD are found to have inconsistent autonomic nervous system (ANS) responses based on their emotional state, thereby showing the role of affective adaptation in disease presentation and symptom management. The interaction of psychological forces with gastrointestinal physiology highlights the requirement of an integrative treatment strategy involving physical as well as emotional well-being, creating a more integrated model of these gastrointestinal diseases (Pellissier et al., 2010). In addition, the endocrine impact on gastrointestinal illness is a critical field of study. Estrogen and progesterone have been put forward as playing a significant role in the symptomatology of IBS and IBD. Endocrine fluctuations have been found to be associated with the episodic nature of symptoms in patients and have been proposed as possible mediators of disease symptoms. Specifically, sudden surges in the rate of progesterone may lead to cramping and constipation, which are common symptoms of IBS. These observations on the hormonal etiology of gastrointestinal dysfunction offer the possibility of targeted treatment therapies that address underlying pathologies rather than merely suppressing symptoms, thus transforming the therapy of these disabling diseases (Linson, 2013). The ANS dysregulation also has important implications for understanding gastrointestinal disease. In one study of patients with Crohn's disease, ulcerative colitis, and IBS, there were measurable changes in sympatho-vagal balance that were related to affective states. Positive affectivity patients, for instance, exhibited signs of adaptive sympathetic activity in Crohn's disease, while ulcerative colitis patients exhibited parasympathetic blunting during negative emotions. On the other hand, the IBS patients had dysautonomia with increased sympathetic and decreased parasympathetic tone regardless of emotional status. This also indicates the potential impact of both psychological as well as physiological factors on disease progression and presentation, which advocates for an integrated approach to comprehending the complicated interrelation between emotional well-being and gastrointestinal function for treatment of such disorders (Pellissier et al., 2010) (Figure 3.19).

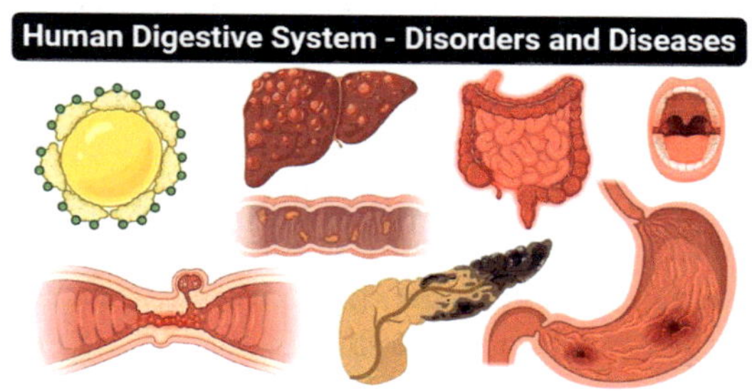

Figure 3.19.

Source: https://external-content.duckduckgo.com/iu/?u=https%3A%2F%2Fmicrobenotes.com%2Fwp-content%2Fuploads%2F2019%2F03%2FDisorders-and-Diseases-of-the-Human-Digestive-System.jpeg&f=1&nofb=1&ipt=953d436a8426d0c2b1e4778d5e725f7d567b0676d5a2f37dd37ebdff59060e84.

3.6.1. Common Gastrointestinal Disorders

Gastrointestinal disease encompasses a wide range of conditions affecting normal digestive function. GERD, IBS, and peptic ulcers are examples of such diseases, each placing specific physiological demands. GERD is characterized by the retrograde movement of gastric contents into the esophagus, with resultant symptoms of heartburn and regurgitation. This syndrome is generally caused by a dysfunctional lower esophageal sphincter, highlighting the importance of muscular regulation in intestinal physiology. IBS, on the other hand, is an immutable gastrointestinal disorder with the features of cyclic abdominal discomfort, bloating, and bowel habit alterations. Its pathogenesis is complex and involves dysregulation of gut movement and enteric nervous system hyperresponsiveness, with the underlying theme being the complexity of communication between physiological mechanisms and patient symptomology.

These disorders are known to be valuable information, as they are associated with anatomical and functional features of gastrointestinal physiology. Peptic ulcers, another extremely prevalent gastrointestinal condition, are mucosal breakage in the stomach or duodenum, and owe their origin primarily to Helicobacter pylori infection and long-term NSAID use. Peptic pathophysiology involves an imbalance between protective and aggressive elements, including gastric acid secretion, and mucosal bicarbonate and mucus secretion. Notably, the enteric nervous system (ENS) plays a crucial role in the balance and influences smooth muscle function, secretory function, and gastrointestinal tract blood flow (Serio et al., 2011). When protective elements are overcome and aggressive secretions predominate, ulceration will follow. This emphasizes the important overlap between disease expression and digestive physiology, as each ulcer is a local failure in a general regulatory framework. In addition, optimal therapy for gastrointestinal disorders often entails a multidisciplinary approach, including pharmacologic treatments, dietary adjustment, and adjustment of lifestyle. For GERD, for instance, therapy could include proton pump inhibitors to reduce acid secretion and lifestyle adjustments to reduce distress. For IBS, dietary modifications, such as, the low-FODMAP diet, can be highly beneficial in symptom alleviation through diet sensitivity control and improvement in gut health. Apart from this, studies on rehabilitation exercises to strengthen pharyngeal muscles have been found to be beneficial in enhancing the efficacy of swallowing, particularly in dysphagia, a common complication of most gastrointestinal illnesses (Shaker et al., 2016). These therapeutic interventions accentuate the ever-changing state of gastrointestinal physiology and the ongoing demand for new means in treatment, aimed at the re-establishment of the tenuous balance of digestive health (Figure 3.20).

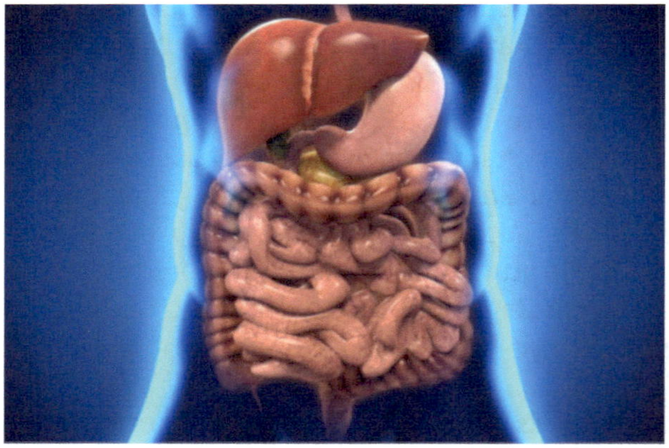

Figure 3.20. Gastrointestinal disorders.

Source: https://external-content.duckduckgo.com/iu/?u=https%3A%2F%2Fwww.rheumatologyadvisor.com%2Fwp-content%2Fuploads%2Fsites%2F18%2F2019%2F02%2Fdigestivesystemsh193293677_1517908.jpg&f=1&nofb=1&ipt=db59fbc749fd38161408446fd8dda0eedf1d0addb36bbc856f9304334facbda3.

3.6.2. Impact of Lifestyle on Gastrointestinal Health

Gastrointestinal (GI) health is directly associated with various determinants of lifestyle, including diet, physical inactivity, and psychosocial issues. Proper diet with dietary fiber from fruits, vegetables, and whole grains has been associated with healthy gut flora, which is essential for digestion and overall health. The composition of gut microbiota is decided by dietary choice, and a rich diet in fiber has been found to enhance microbiome diversity, enabling more effective nutrient capture as well as improved immune function. In contrast, processed food and sugar-based diets are found to kill the microbiome, leading to dysbiosis, which is associated with gastrointestinal disorders , such as irritable bowel syndrome (IBS) and inflammatory bowel disease (IBD). In addition, understanding how exercise influences GI health is also significant; regular exercise has been found to enhance gut motility and reduce the risk of constipation, hence underscoring the importance of including favorable life choices into daily habits (Shatakshi et al., 2024). More importantly, the connection between obesity and gastrointestinal health cannot be overstated. Obesity has been linked with a large array of gastrointestinal disorders, including gastroesophageal reflux disease and Barrett's esophagus, which is a condition of metaplasia involving escalating the risk for adenocarcinoma of the esophagus. The pathogenesis of this relationship is multifactorial; obesity can lead to increased intra-abdominal pressure, exacerbating reflux symptoms. Lifestyle habits, for example, physical inactivity and an unhealthy diet, contribute significantly to the causation of the burden of obesity and hence have an effect on GI health. Furthermore, genetic risk in this interaction is multifactorial, which implies that intervention via lifestyle can counteract some hereditary risks (Palmese, 2016). The multifactorial etiology of obesity highlights the need for comprehensive lifestyle interventions for GI health and the prevention of associated diseases. Lastly, psychosocial factors, including stress and mental health, are significant in gastrointestinal health. Stress has been shown to affect gut function adversely, leading to depression and anxiety symptoms, which also help cause gastrointestinal disorders. The gut-brain axis, a complex network of communication between the GI tract and central nervous system, illustrates that emotional well-being is as vital as physical well-being in maintaining gastrointestinal function. Moreover, lifestyles that are health-conscious and stress-decreasing, such as, meditation and yoga, can be beneficial to GI health. By acknowledging the interconnectedness of lifestyle factors—nutrition, level of activity, and state of mind—health care professionals can more holistically heal and prevent gastrointestinal illness. Such an interaction highlights the importance of individuals adopting lifestyle changes that promote the maintenance of gastrointestinal health and well-being (Shatakshi et al., 2024) (Figure 3.21).

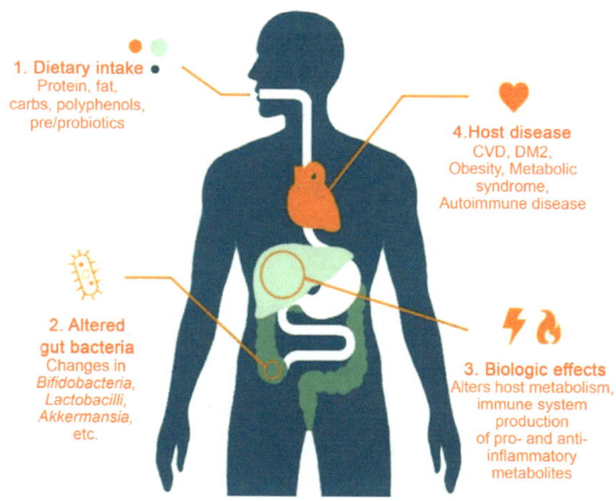

Figure 3.21. Impact of diet on the gut microbiome and human health.

Source: https://www.researchgate.net/publication/315978151/figure/fig1/AS:963516475383820@1606731637652/Impact-of-diet-on-the-gut-microbiome-and-human-health.gif.

3.6.3. Diagnostic Approaches for Gastrointestinal Disorders

Diagnosis of gastrointestinal illness is an involved process involving a good understanding of both symptomatology and related physiological underpinnings. Initial assessment commonly includes detailed patient history and physical exam to identify pertinent symptoms , such as abdominal pain, bloating, or bowel habit change. According to these observations, physicians would prescribe ancillary testing like imaging studies or blood work to assess organ structure and function. An example would be the performance of serological tests that identify certain antibodies in diseases like celiac disease, which differentiates it from other gastrointestinal diseases. A credible diagnostic pathway is therefore necessary for customized treatment protocols, with this eventually leading to better patient outcomes in gastrointestinal physiology. Additionally, endoscopic techniques have revolutionized the diagnosis of gastrointestinal disease. Endoscopic techniques facilitate the direct visualization of the gastrointestinal tract and permit the gastroenterologist to identify abnormalities , such as inflammation, ulceration, or neoplastic lesions. Histological details on biopsy specimens taken during endoscopy are extremely valuable for confirming or ruling out particular conditions. Additionally, sophisticated imaging modalities like MRI and CT scans offer non-invasive techniques for assessing structural changes associated with gastrointestinal disease. The use of such technologies in combination not only offers improved diagnosis but also monitoring of disease progression and therapeutic response, making advanced diagnostics' contribution to gastrointestinal physiology very significant. In recent years, there has been a center of focus on the interaction between the gut microbiome and various gastrointestinal disease conditions, which has encouraged new diagnostic approaches. More recent evidence suggests that disturbances in gut microbiota may be the cause of diseases , such as irritable bowel syndrome (IBS) and inflammatory bowel disease (IBD). Fecal microbiota analysis holds promise to identify dysbiosis and putative microbial markers for certain diseases. In addition, novel immunologic tests, e.g., immune-mediated response measurement, can clarify ailments like non-celiac gluten intolerance, where Thomas (2020) points out the need to distinguish it from celiac disease to avoid misdiagnosis. If these new diagnostic techniques are embraced, practitioners will better understand gastrointestinal physiology and develop successful, patient-centered therapies, and eventually redefine gastrointestinal disease treatment.

Test Your Knowledge

1. What are the common symptoms of irritable bowel syndrome (IBS)?
2. How does gastroesophageal reflux disease (GERD) occur?

SUMMARY

A physiology of gastrointestinal physiology, it is imperative to understand the intricate relationship among various physiological processes involved in digestion and how dysregulation impacts overall health. The gastrointestinal system not only permits the mechanical and chemical breakdown of food but also has a significant role in nutrient absorption and the expulsion of waste. Improvements in understanding muscular control of the pharynx, for instance, show the potential for rehabilitative exercises to maximize pharyngeal function. As noted in prior research, experimentation with activities like resistive swallowing can cause muscle fatigue, therefore potentially enhancing pharyngeal contractile capacity (Shaker et al., 2016). Such observations highlight the dynamic nature of gastrointestinal function, with a clear imperative for ongoing research in the identification of therapeutic interventions to maximize digestive function. In addition, this discussion is extended to the effects of neurological pathology on gut function, particularly in the case of spinal-injured patients. The interplay between spinal injury and dysfunctional autonomic control underlines the urgent need to understand vascular responses to diet modification. In thoracic spinal-level injury, for example, decreased blood flow in the superior mesenteric artery leads to adverse gastrointestinal effects, such as, inflammation and dysmotility (Besecker et al., 2016). Investigating such physiological disturbances not only sheds light on the fundamental mechanisms at play but also brings with it the possibility of potential clinical interventions aimed at preventing such challenges. This is, thus, a presentation of the necessity of interdisciplinary interventions to address the multidimensionality of gastrointestinal health. Lastly, the conclusion drawn from this examination of gastrointestinal physiology is the identification of its complexity and the necessity of homeostasis for optimal functioning. Interactions of neuromuscular dynamics, vascular control, and physiological responses to external stimuli result in a system that necessitates intense study and practical understanding. Novel techniques for pharyngeal strength measurement and the effects of spinal trauma provide a foundation for further therapeutic advancement. It will be crucial for future research to maintain a broad brush of gastrointestinal physiology, particularly as we work to enhance the quality of life in those with gastrointestinal illness. By continued use of what is learned from both basic and translational science, the subspecialty can progress toward more effective interventions and improved health outcomes.

The intricate interplay of gastrointestinal physiology is vital to the understanding of many pathologies, particularly the regulatory mechanisms in parasitic infections. One of the best candidates is Giardia lamblia, a common protistan parasite that produces so much gastrointestinal distress worldwide. The life cycle of Giardia is marked by the reversibility of form between cyst and trophozoite, and conversion following ingestion with colonization of the proximal small intestine. Recent advances using bioluminescent imaging (BLI) have enhanced the understanding of Giardia's infectious patterns, revealing that trophozoites create high-density foci during colonization, thereby affecting encystation processes. The concentration of parasites in a focal area not only causes damage to the intestinal epithelium but also reconfigures the host's response to infection, highlighting the parasite's adaptive tactics within the gastrointestinal tract, as illustrated in the examination of its temporospatial dynamics (Barash et al., 2017). Of equal concern in the gut ecosystem is the prevalence of constipation, particularly in the long-term care setting. Constipation can have a profound negative effect on an individual's quality of life and, if not treated, may have more acute health consequences. Prompt identification of constipation is crucial since intervention becomes more complex and costly with the passage of time. Effective management is founded upon a full understanding of the multiple lifestyle factors that lead to constipation, including dietary patterns, fluid intake, and physical activity levels. Early detection and prevention measures are reduced to simple-to-implement guidelines that are advantageous to nurses and caregivers. A properly constructed red flag table is a valuable instrument in the identification of constipation as a potential red flag for underlying accompanying health conditions, thereby guaranteeing prompt intervention and the overall well-being of residents (Lee et al., 2016). To summarize, the multifaceted elements of gastrointestinal physiology, it is apparent that parasitic infestations and conditions like constipation play central roles in determining health outcomes. The Giardia lamblia research sheds light on the host-parasite relationship complexities, and the emphasis on constipation highlights the systemic effects of gastrointestinal function, particularly in vulnerable individuals. Both of these issues highlight the necessity of continuing research and education about gastrointestinal physiology so that health care practitioners are able to treat both common and uncommon conditions of this system effectively. By combining evidence from research on parasitic dynamics and the management of constipation, we can formulate a more holistic understanding of gastrointestinal health, enabling more effective treatment that incorporates prevention and active treatment in clinical practice (Lee et al., 2016; Barash et al., 2017).

KEY TERMS FROM THIS CHAPTER

- Absorption
- Chyme
- Enzymes
- Gastric juice
- Hydrochloric acid (HCl)
- Large intestine
- Motility
- Bile
- Digestion
- Gallbladder
- Gastrointestinal hormone
- Ingestion
- Liver
- Pancreatic juic

CRITICAL THINKING QUESTIONS

1. **Which hormone is primarily responsible for stimulating the secretion of gastric acid in the stomach?**
   a. Secretin
   b. Gastrin
   c. Cholecystokinin (CCK)
   d. Motilin
2. **What is the primary function of bile in digestion?**
   a. Breakdown of proteins
   b. Neutralization of gastric acid
   c. Emulsification of fats
   d. Activation of pepsinogen
3. **Which part of the gastrointestinal tract is mainly responsible for nutrient absorption?**
   a. Stomach
   b. Large intestine
   c. Duodenum
   d. Small intestine
4. **What triggers the release of cholecystokinin (CCK)?**
   a. Presence of carbohydrates in the stomach
   b. Presence of fat and protein in the duodenum
   c. High levels of hydrochloric acid
   d. Emptying of the rectum
5. **Which of the following best describes the migrating motor complex (MMC)?**
   a. Continuous contraction of the colon
   b. Periodic waves of activity during fasting that clear the stomach and small intestine
   c. Contractions that occur only during vomiting
   d. Muscle activity that occurs during defecation

Short Answer Questions

1. Define peristalsis and its role in the gastrointestinal tract.
2. What is the function of the enteric nervous system?
3. List the major gastrointestinal hormones and their primary actions.
4. What is the role of secretin in digestion?
5. How is hydrochloric acid (HCl) secreted by parietal cells in the stomach?
6. What is the significance of the ileocecal valve?
7. Differentiate between segmentation and peristalsis.
8. Name two functions of the liver related to digestion.
9. Explain the role of bile salts in fat digestion.
10. What are the phases of gastric secretion?

Answers to Critical Thinking Questions

1. (b); 2. (c); 3. (d); 4. (b); 5. (b).

REFERENCES

1. McRae, K. M., Stear, M. J., Good, B., & Keane, O. M. (2015). The host immune response to gastrointestinal nematode infection in sheep. *Parasite immunology*, *37*(12), 605–613. https://doi.org/10.1111/pim.12290(accessed on 28th June 2025).
2. Marciani, L., Pritchard, S. E., Hellier-Woods, C., Costigan, C., Hoad, C. L., Gowland, P. A., & Spiller, R. C. (2013). Delayed gastric emptying and reduced postprandial small bowel water content of equicaloric whole meal bread versus rice meals in healthy subjects: novel MRI insights. *European journal of clinical nutrition*, *67*(7), 754–758. https://doi.org/10.1038/ejcn.2013.78 (accessed on 28th June 2025).
3. Ameku, T., Beckwith, H., Blackie, L., Miguel-Aliaga, I., et al. (2019). Food, microbes, sex and old age: On the plasticity of gastrointestinal innervation. https://core.ac.uk/download/287580141.pdf (accessed on 28th June 2025).
4. Tousoulis, D., Guzik, T., Padro, T., Duncker, D. J., De Luca, G., Eringa, E., Vavlukis, M., Antonopoulos, A. S., Katsimichas, T., Cenko, E., Djordjevic-Dikic, A., Fleming, I., Manfrini, O., Trifunovic, D., Antoniades, C., & Crea, F. (2022). Mechanisms, therapeutic implications, and methodological challenges of gut microbiota and cardiovascular diseases: a position paper by the ESC Working Group on Coronary Pathophysiology and Microcirculation. *Cardiovascular research*, *118*(16), 3171–3182. https://doi.org/10.1093/cvr/cvac057 (accessed on 28th June 2025).
5. Avvari, R. K. (2019). Biomechanics of the small intestinal contractions. https://core.ac.uk/download/322443183.pdf (accessed on 28th June 2025).
6. Shaker, R., Sanvanson, P., Balasubramanian, G., Kern, M., Wuerl, A., & Hyngstrom, A. (2016). Effects of laryngeal restriction on pharyngeal peristalsis and biomechanics: Clinical implications. *American journal of physiology. Gastrointestinal and liver physiology*, *310*(11), G1036–G1043. https://doi.org/10.1152/ajpgi.00010.2016(accessed on 28th June 2025).
7. Banales, J. M., Medina, J. F., & Prieto, J. (2006). Cholangiocyte anion exchange and biliary bicarbonate excretion. https://core.ac.uk/download/83571233.pdf (accessed on 28th June 2025).
8. Fonseca F, Cerqueira R and Fuentes J (2019) Impact of Ocean Acidification on the Intestinal Microbiota of the Marine Sea Bream (Sparus aurata L.). Front. Physiol. 10:1446. doi: 10.3389/fphys.2019.01446 (accessed on 28th June 2025).
9. Barash, N. R., Dawson, S. C., Gourguechon, S., McCarthy-Sinclair, T., et al. (2017). *Giardia* colonizes and encysts in high-density foci in the murine small intestine. https://core.ac.uk/download/323069052.pdf (accessed on 28th June 2025).
10. Bauer, E., Metzler-Zebeli, B. U., Mosenthin, R., Verstegen, M. W. A., et al. (2011). Intestinal gene expression in pigs: Effects of reduced feed intake during weaning and potential impact of dietary components. https://core.ac.uk/download/pdf/29230036.pdf (accessed on 28th June 2025).
11. Besecker, E. S., Cooper, T. K., Deiter, G. M., Holmes, R., et al. (2016). Mesenteric vascular dysregulation and intestinal inflammation accompanies experimental spinal cord injury. https://cupola.gettysburg.edu/cgi/viewcontent.cgi?article=1073&context=healthfac (accessed on 28th June 2025).

12. Pellissier, S., Dantzer, C., Canini, F., Mathieu, N., & Bonaz, B. (2010). Psychological adjustment and autonomic disturbances in inflammatory bowel diseases and irritable bowel syndrome. *Psychoneuroendocrinology*, *35*(5), 653–662. https://doi.org/10.1016/j.psyneuen.2009.10.004(accessed on 28th June 2025).

13. Bosch, J. A., de Geus, E. J. C., Hoogstraten, J., Nieuw Amerongen, A. V., et al. (2000). Innate secretory immunity in response to laboratory stressors that evoke distinct patterns of cardiac autonomic activity. https://core.ac.uk/download/pdf/15457442.pdf (accessed on 28th June 2025).

14. Seal, C. J., & Brownlee, I. A. (2015). Whole-grain foods and chronic disease: evidence from epidemiological and intervention studies. *The Proceedings of the Nutrition Society*, *74*(3), 313–319. https://doi.org/10.1017/S0029665115002104(accessed on 28th June 2025).

15. Holland, C., Ryden, P., Edwards, C. H., & Grundy, M. M. (2020). Plant Cell Walls: Impact on Nutrient Bioaccessibility and Digestibility. *Foods (Basel, Switzerland)*, *9*(2), 201. https://doi.org/10.3390/foods9020201(accessed on 28th June 2025).

16. Eklund, G. (2003). Cadmium in newborns. https://core.ac.uk/download/11694662.pdf (accessed on 28th June 2025).

17. Tang, E.-K., Loo, K.-Y., Thye, A. Y.-K., Law, J. W.-F., Tan, L. T.-H., Selvaraja, M., Thurairajasingam, S., Lee, L.-H., & Letchumanan, V. (2024). The Impact of Antidepressants on Gut Microbiome and Depression Management. *Progress In Microbes & Molecular Biology*, *7*(1). https://doi.org/10.36877/pmmb.a0000446 (accessed on 28th June 2025).

18. Ghahremani, G., Horgan, S., Kumar, D., Kunkel, J., et al. (2020). Morphology of the esophageal hiatus: Is it different in 3 types of hiatus hernias? https://core.ac.uk/download/323065805.pdf (accessed on 28th June 2025).

19. Greenwood, I. A., Tribe, R. M., Selyanko, A. A., & Taggart, M. J. (2013). Kv7 and Kv11 channels in myometrial regulation. https://core.ac.uk/download/29469426.pdf (accessed on 28th June 2025).

20. Högberg, A. (2003). Cereal non-starch polysaccharides in pig diets. https://core.ac.uk/download/11694626.pdf (accessed on 28th June 2025).

21. Dr. Shatakshi, Dipanshu Kumar, Saloni Arora, Murugalatha. N.(2024). Examining the relationship between gut microbiota and sports performance: A narrative review. https://core.ac.uk/download/603898113.pdf (accessed on 28th June 2025).

22. Lee, A. (2016). Identifying and managing constipation in older people. https://core.ac.uk/download/151161179.pdf (accessed on 28th June 2025).

23. Linson, E. A. (2013). The interplay between hormones and irritable bowel disease. https://open.bu.edu/bitstream/2144/12149/6/Linson_Elyse_2013_nosig_nocv.pdf (accessed on 28th June 2025).

24. Liu, H. (2013). Interactions between dietary chicory, gut microbiota and immune responses. https://core.ac.uk/download/11698989.pdf (accessed on 28th June 2025).

25. Rosse, C., Mejino, J.L.V. (2008). The Foundational Model of Anatomy Ontology. In: Burger, A., Davidson, D., Baldock, R. (eds) Anatomy Ontologies for Bioinformatics. Computational Biology, vol 6. Springer, London. https://doi.org/10.1007/978-1-84628-885-2_4(accessed on 28th June 2025).

26. Palmese, S. J. (2016). An investigation of the progression from Barrett's esophagus to adenocarcinoma. https://open.bu.edu/bitstream/2144/16178/1/Palmese_bu_0017N_11143.pdf (accessed on 28th June 2025).
27. Patwardhan, K. (2008). Concepts of human physiology in Ayurveda. https://core.ac.uk/download/pdf/87482.pdf (accessed on 28th June 2025).
28. Degnan, P. H., Pusey, A. E., Lonsdorf, E. V., Goodall, J., Wroblewski, E. E., Wilson, M. L., Rudicell, R. S., Hahn, B. H., & Ochman, H. (2012). Factors associated with the diversification of the gut microbial communities within chimpanzees from Gombe National Park. *Proceedings of the National Academy of Sciences of the United States of America*, *109*(32), 13034–13039. https://doi.org/10.1073/pnas.1110994109 (accessed on 28th June 2025).
29. Thomas, V. (2020). Comparisons of celiac disease and non-celiac gluten sensitivity. https://core.ac.uk/download/322851056.pdf (accessed on 28th June 2025).
30. Valls-Bellés, V. (2024). The biochemistry of digestion. https://core.ac.uk/download/614526814.pdf (accessed on 28th June 2025).
31. Rosa Serio, Maria Garzia Zizzo, Mariangela Mastropaolo (2011). The enteric nervous system: New developments and emerging concepts. Malta Medical Journal Volume 23 Issue 03 2011 https://core.ac.uk/download/46602300.pdf (accessed on 28th June 2025).

ENDOCRINE PHYSIOLOGY: HORMONES AND THEIR MECHANISMS

4

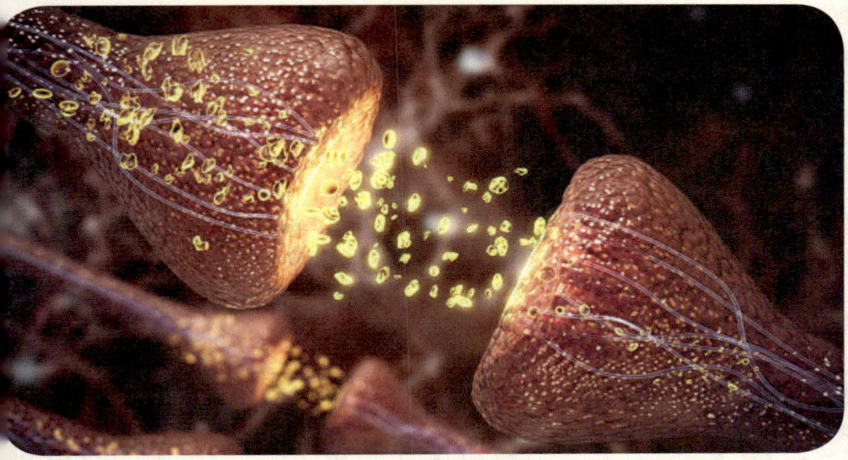

LEARNING OBJECTIVES

After studying this chapter, you will be able to:

1. Discuss the types of hormones.
2. Explain the hormone synthesis and secretion.
3. Discuss the hormone transport in the blood.
4. Focus on hormone receptors and signal transduction.
5. Learn about the effects of hormones on target tissues.
6. Evaluate the disorders of the endocrine system.

Introduction

Endocrine physiology is a field of study of hormones, their origin, release, and the very complex mechanisms through which they cause their effects on the processes in the body. Underlying this information is the axiom that hormones are chemical messengers that facilitate the mediation of communication between different systems and organs in the body. They regulate an extensive range of processes, including metabolism, growth, development, and reproductive processes. Hormones , such as insulin, glucagon, and estrogen are the quintessence of this regulatory role, influencing metabolic function and reproductive health. As advancing knowledge continues, it is increasingly necessary to unravel the complex mechanisms of signaling behind hormone action as these dictate the physiological actions needed for homeostasis and adaptation to environmental change. One special area of concern in endocrine physiology is hormonal regulation of reproductive behavior, particularly in domestic farm breeds , such as dairy cattle. The estrous cycle, regulated by hormones like estradiol and progesterone, shows the relationship between endocrine signaling and behavior. Elevated milk production in dairy cows has been linked to decreased fertility, illustrating the impact of metabolic stress on hormonal homeostasis and reproductive success. This link emphasizes the significance of a proper comprehension of the endocrine regulation of estrous behavior. The present work emphasizes that gene expression modifications related to hormone modifications can have a significant role in influencing reproductive performances, and hence the role of endocrine signaling as well as genetic factors. These results suggest potential ways of stimulating fertility in high-performance dairy cows through intervention in a specific way. Moreover, the employment of systems biology in endocrine physiology is a new approach to understanding complex biological interactions. Mathematical modeling has the capability of combining physiological data with genomic data, allowing scientists to predict the multi-dimensional actions of hormones on reproductive behavior and more. The integrated approach is well-suited to uncovering mechanisms by which hormones act upon neuronal networks and behavior, as demonstrated through estrous behavior regulation. For example, estrogen-induced gene expression in the hypothalamus can modify neurotransmitter discharge and neuronal connectivity and therefore change behavioral endpoints. As research continues, the integration of systems biology will improve our understanding of how several parameters, such as, metabolic status and hormonal balance, interact to impact physiological processes, especially in the case of fertility and reproductive disease in farm animals (Gross et al., 2001; Boer et al., 2010) (Figure 4.1).

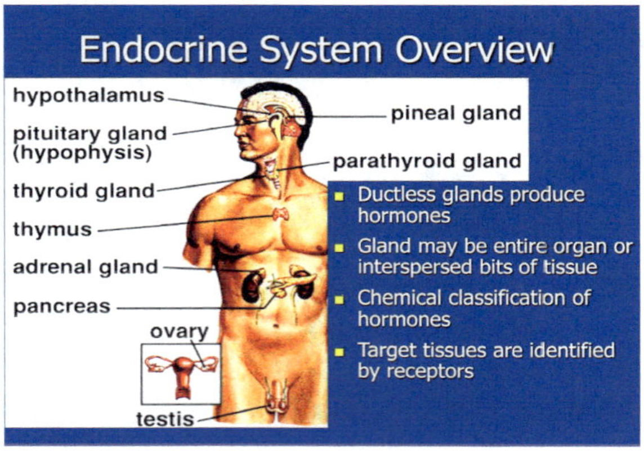

Figure 4.1. Endocrine system.

Source: https://image.slideserve.com/1291034/endocrine-system-overview-l.jpg.

Definition of the endocrine system

The endocrine system is an extremely complex system of glands and organs that secrete, store, and produce hormones directly into the bloodstream. These hormones have vital roles in regulating various body functions, including metabolism, growth, development, and reproductive processes. The major components of the endocrine system include the hypothalamus, pituitary gland, thyroid gland, adrenal glands, and the pancreas, among others. Each gland is responsible for specific hormones with specific functions in maintaining homeostasis and facilitating communication between body systems.

Understanding the definition and function of the endocrine system is paramount to studying how hormones operate their effect because their action extends beyond mere biochemical activity; they also define physiological responses to stimuli and contribute to overall health and wellness. Moreover, the interplay of hormones with other bodily functions highlights the contribution of the endocrine system to human health. Hormones are not static entities; their levels are variable in terms of gender, nutrients, or stress. Such a variability necessitates the integration of knowledge of hormonal activities with sensitivity to gender and sexual distinction. For instance, sex hormones like estrogens and testosterone not only determine sexual characteristics but also mold diverse physiological outcomes, from metabolic rates and therapeutic response, as elucidated in recent research.

These endocrine-gender differences support the importance of individualized practice in medicine, particularly when diagnosing and treating disease involving a specific hormonal factor, such as, that targeting reproductive health (Lauretta et al., 2018). In addition, the clearly defined endocrine actions are noted when it involves certain individual disorders with no identified cause, such as, anorexia nervosa (AN). This mental illness, occurring primarily in young women, demonstrates how disruptions to hormone levels can have far-reaching physiological consequences, including disruption of the hypothalamic-pituitary-ovarian axis. The consequent functional amenorrhea highlights the intricate interplay between psychological and endocrine functioning (Poterasu et al., 2020). Understanding these mechanisms is vital in designing effective treatment strategies that not only address the psychology of AN but also consider the hormonal repercussions that compromise fertility and general reproductive health. Thus, a general understanding of the endocrine system is the foundation both for diagnosing pathologies and developing interventions to restore balance to hormones and thereby enhance the quality of life in individuals affected.

Importance of Hormones in Bodily Functions

Hormones are at the center of regulating a variety of body functions, guiding complex physiological processes to maintain homeostasis. The endocrine system secreted biochemical messengers that coordinate various organs and tissues into communication, enabling the body to respond to internal and external stimuli appropriately. For instance, the interaction between hormones , such as insulin and glucagon is an important factor in glucose metabolism to maintain normal blood sugar levels. Hormones also play a pivotal role in growth and development and influence processes that involve metabolism, reproduction, and response to stress. As referred to under the concept of "Tridosha" in Ayurveda, coordination of these hormonal pathways is essential in achieving complete health, with emphasis on interconnectedness of hormonal harmony in body and mind well-being (Patwardhan, 2008). The significance of hormone regulation even covers reacting to stress, where hormones like cortisol and adrenaline play a key role in the body's reaction to stressors. This hormonal stimulation is not a singular event; rather, it is a reflection of the complex interaction between the immune system and the neuroendocrine system. The stress and hormonal response dynamic is at the center of understanding many states of health and therapy. Based on the literature, in the majority of situations, there is a lack of congruence between health care practices that address the physiological aspect of stress and practices that address the psychological aspect, with the inference being that additional action should be taken in an integrative fashion (DeLisle & Estrine, 2006). Identifying these hormonal pathways allows for a clearer understanding of how the systems of the body collaborate with one another in maintaining a person in good health despite stressful conditions. Further, hormonal control is crucial in certain illnesses where illness as thyroid and hormone cancers, and diabetes are induced by hormonal imbalances. These develop when there is an imbalance between various axes of hormones, showing the importance of homeostasis in hormones. For instance, in diabetes mellitus, an insulin production or response failure enables the blood glucose concentration to rise, resulting in grave systemic consequences if not addressed. This correlation serves to emphasize the importance of early diagnosis and regulation of endocrine disease due to the fact that hormonal balance is crucial not just for short-term body activity but for future health as well. Finally, a good understanding of endocrine mechanisms contributes to the realization of therapeutic targets for treatment to reestablish balance and consequently result in better health outcomes among individuals affected by endocrine disturbances (Patwardhan, 2008) (Figure 4.2).

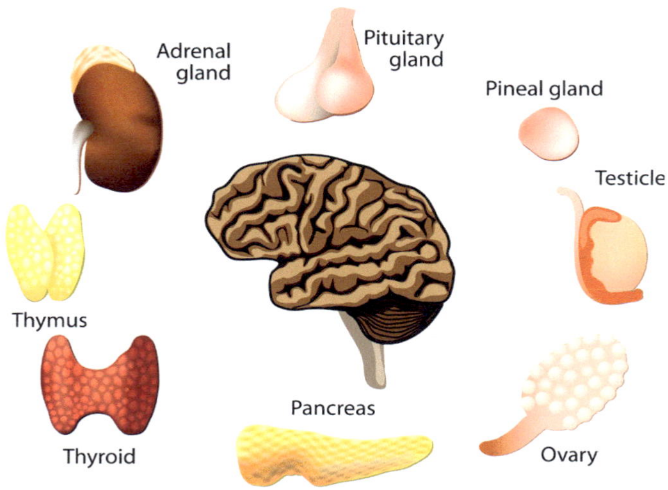

Figure 4.2. Hormones in bodily functions.

Source: https://askthescientists.com/wp-content/uploads/2018/04/AdobeStock_71056506-e1524167131112-1500x1210.png.

Overview of Hormone Classification

An overview of hormone classification begins with the fact that hormones are categorized based on their chemical nature. Mostly, hormones come under three broad categories: peptide hormones, steroid hormones, and amine hormones. Peptide hormones, composed of amino acids, are produced from large precursor proteins and are likely to act by way of cell surface receptors that initiate cascades of signals. Steroid hormones, derived from cholesterol, can pass through cell membranes and affect intracellular receptors, thus leading to changes in gene expression. Amine hormones, derived from tyrosine or tryptophan, are intermediate in nature between steroids and peptides, i.e., hydrophilic and lipophilic, and thus can penetrate cells or act on surface receptors based on some structural characteristics. This classification is vital for the understanding of the varied mechanisms of hormone action in the endocrine system. Additionally, hormones are also classified based on secretion modes. Endocrine hormones are secreted directly into the circulatory system, from where they travel towards the target organs or tissues and cause particular physiological impacts. Paracrine hormones, on the other hand, are localized since they diffuse to neighboring cells to produce their effects, while autocrine hormones influence the same cells that secrete them. These are important distinctions that contribute to explaining the sophistication of hormonal signaling pathways and the mechanism of interaction of various categories of hormones in regulating physiological processes. For instance, the interaction of paracrine signaling in immune response regulation explains how localized hormonal communication matters. Understanding these various modes of secretion gives depth to the study of hormone actions and their mechanistic roles in the regulation of homeostasis in the body. Also, functional classification of hormones is significant, particularly the manner in which they are associated with the physiologic systems that they regulate. Hormones are tropic or non-tropic, and the former stimulate the secretion of other endocrine hormones while the latter work directly on the target tissues. An example of a tropic hormone is the thyroid-stimulating hormone (TSH), which, on acting on the thyroid gland, causes it to secrete thyroid hormones that regulate the body's metabolism. On the other hand, insulin is a non-tropic hormone that stimulates glucose absorption into fat and muscle tissues directly. Determining these functional classifications serves to further characterize the intricate webs of hormone control, validating the theory that hormones are not only signal molecules but part and parcel of larger physiologic systems that control many facets of disease and health. It is through the realization of these categorizations that therapeutic and research options become available, especially where hormonal disturbances lead to health complications , such as endocrine dysfunction, as in anorexia nervosa, which can lead to reproductive dysfunction, as discussed in literature (Poterasu et al., 2020). Moreover, stress response in animals, like fish, has been found to be relieved by understanding the physiological disparity of hormonal response to environmental factors, revealing the intricacy and diversity in categorizing hormones (Herrera et al., 2019).

4.1. Types of Hormones

Learning Outcome

1. Describe the peptide hormones;
2. Focus on steroid hormones;
3. Learn about amine hormones.

The classification of hormones can be broadly categorized into three general classes: peptide hormones, steroid hormones, and amino acid hormones. The peptide hormones, consisting of chains of amino acids, play vital roles in the highly diverse physiological activities , such as growth, metabolism, and the immune system. A few examples are insulin and glucagon which regulate the level of glucose in the blood. On the other hand, steroid hormones, being of cholesterol origin, differ in their mechanism of action by binding intracellular receptors and consequently influencing gene expression and protein synthesis. The hormones have a key reproductive function, such as, testosterone and estrogen, which are pivotal in sexual growth and function. Lastly, amino acid-derived hormones , such as thyroxine and epinephrine are quick in onset to elicit physiological effects and are particularly important in metabolic regulation and the body's response to fight-or-flight. The mechanism of action of hormones varies with the chemical nature and water solubility of the hormone. Peptide hormones, being hydrophilic molecules, typically interact with receptors located on the cell surface, activating second messenger systems to transduce the hormonal signal. This cascade can trigger numerous intracellular events within seconds, illustrating the rapidity of these hormones' activity. Steroid hormones are able to diffuse across the plasma membrane since they are lipophilic, allowing them to bind receptors in the cytoplasm or nucleus. Steroid hormones regulate long-term modification of cellular function by modifying gene expression, for example, regulating growth and metabolism. Hormones derived from amino acids lie between the two extremes, being somewhat water-soluble and possessing a receptor binding mechanism that allows them to act on immediate as well as long-term responses in the target tissue. The biological activity of these hormones determines their importance in homeostasis and health. For instance, the balance of estrogen and testosterone is at the heart not only of reproductive health but also of metabolic development and behavioral outcomes, such as, aggression and caregiving behaviors. Research has described the complex relationship between these hormones and disorders like polycystic ovary syndrome, demonstrating how distortions lead to severe health issues (Zubeldia-Brenner et al., 2016). Additionally, the protective functions performed by some steroids, like progesterone, in neurodegenerative diseases illustrate the widespread effect of such hormones beyond the typical reproductive and metabolic functions (Zubeldia-Brenner et al., 2016). Thus, understanding the diverse types of hormones and their function is critical in appreciating their intricate roles in the endocrine system and how they affect human physiology (Figure 4.3).

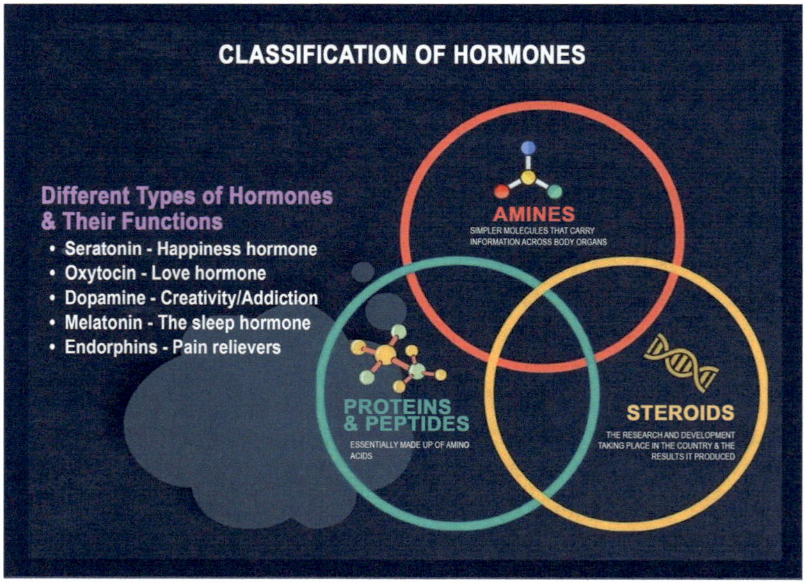

Figure 4.3. Classification of hormones.

Source: https://alignthoughts.com/wp-content/uploads/2020/05/different-types-of-hormones-and-their-functions-alignthoughts.jpg.jpg.

4.1.1. Peptide Hormones

Peptide hormones are a significant group of endocrine system hormones that are characterized by their structure as an amino acid chain. They are synthesized in various organs and tissues like the pancreas, hypothalamus, and pituitary gland. They primarily function to mediate various physiological functions by binding to a specific receptor on target cells, triggering a series of signaling reactions. For instance, insulin, a well-known peptide hormone that is secreted by the pancreas, has a critical function in glucose homeostasis, signaling cells to absorb glucose and thus regulating blood sugar. The sophisticated processes involved in peptide hormone action exhibit the intricacy of endocrine physiology and reinforce their pivotal function in maintaining homeostasis in the body. The mechanism of action of peptide hormones is largely through their interaction with G-protein coupled receptors (GPCRs), which initiates intracellular activity upon activation. This interaction often leads to the generation of second messengers, such as, cyclic AMP (cAMP), that further propagate the signal intracellularly. The significance of these signaling pathways is revealed through their involvement in various physiological responses, including stress adaptation and metabolic regulation.

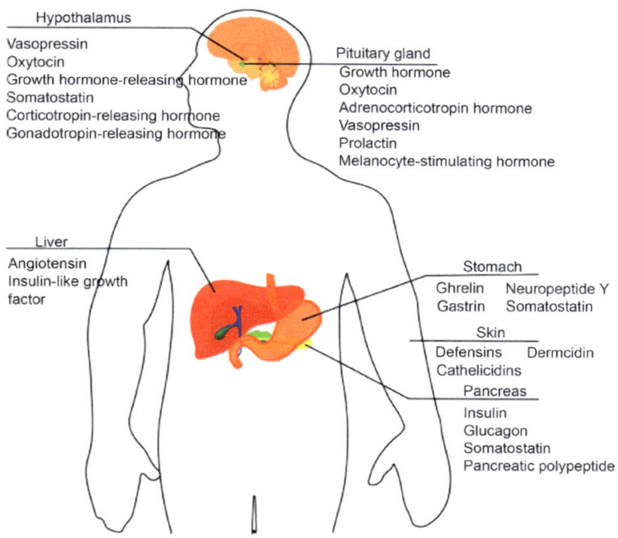

Figure 4.4. Peptide hormone

Source: https://ars.els-cdn.com/content/image/3-s2.0-B9780081007365000089-f08-01-9780081007365.jpg.

Along with that, the effects of these hormones may have consequences that extend beyond acute cellular activity, influencing long-term physiological adaptation and behavior. An example is offered by corticotropin-releasing hormone (CRH) in its role within the hypothalamic-pituitary-adrenal (HPA) axis to mobilize an organism's stress response by the release of adrenocorticotropic hormone (ACTH) and subsequently cortisol, illustrating the ubiquitous nature of peptide hormone signaling within endocrine physiology (Inda et al., 2017). Of interest is the therapeutic potential of peptide hormones, particularly in the management of metabolic disorders , such as Type 2 diabetes mellitus (T2DM). It has been highlighted in more recent studies that glucagon-like peptide-1 receptor agonists (GLP-1RAs), one group of peptide hormones, not only improve glycemic control but may also have favorable skeletal effects. Such an observation suggests a treatment approach with a multi-dimensional focus towards overall health management rather than the mere management of hyperglycemia. The finding of GLP-1RAs illustrates the evolving landscape of peptide hormones, revealing their metabolic control and skeletal activity and affirming the imperative for continued exploration into their mechanisms (Mabilleau et al., 2017). Such an advance reflects the plasticity of endocrine physiology and the central position of peptide hormones in health and disease (Figure 4.4).

4.1.2. Steroid Hormones

The function of steroid hormones in the endocrine system is a multifaceted process involving various physiological mechanisms. Steroid hormones, all cholesterol-derived, comprise androgens, estrogens, and corticosteroids. These hormones play a key role in controlling numerous biological processes , such as metabolism, immune response, and reproduction. Steroid hormone action is mainly controlled by their ability to diffuse through cell membranes and bind intracellular receptors. Once bound, these hormone-receptor complexes translocate to the nucleus, influencing gene expression and evoking a variety of different cellular responses. This paradigm of function is used to highlight the essential role steroid hormones play not only during normal physiology but also during pathological states in which hormone regulation may be disrupted.

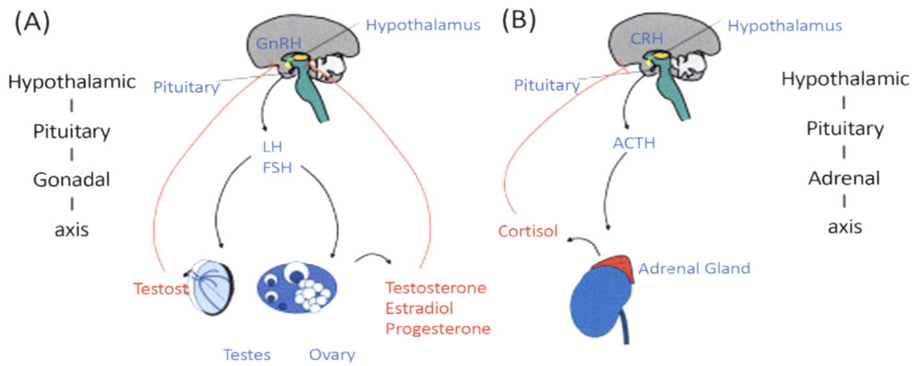

Figure 4.5. Steroid hormones.

Source: https://ars.els-cdn.com/content/image/3-s2.0-B9780323911412000040-f01-01-9780323911412.jpg.

The pathological effects of environmental toxicants like dichlorodiphenyltrichloroethane (DDT) serve to exemplify the precarious balance maintained by steroid hormones within the endocrine system. Exposure to DDT during developmental stages has been discovered to have profound impacts on the synthesis of male sex hormones, with reduced testosterone and androstenedione levels in male rats. These findings indicate that exposure to low concentrations of endocrine disruptors can lead to extreme hormone alteration, especially through disruption of androgen biosynthesis pathways. Specifically, there is increased progesterone synthesis with reduced synthesis of male sex hormones following impaired hydroxylation. Such observations underscore the importance of understanding how exogenous substances interact with hormonal mechanisms, illustrating the vulnerability of endocrine physiology to systemically distributed contaminants (Yaglova et al., 2024). An interesting illustration of control by steroid hormones is the hibernation of brown bears. Apart from the inaction and attendant heavy weight increase of hibernation, bears have metabolic resistance, especially avoiding those conditions that are adverse in humans, such as, type 2 diabetes and cardiovascular disease. Studies indicate that hibernating bears see changes in androgens, such as, testosterone and androstenedione, including a decrease in females and overall increase in males. The role of sex hormone-binding globulin (SHBG) is also highly critical during this period, as its elevated levels can be utilized to control the activity of reproductive hormones when in a relative quiescence. This balance in the hormones offers the needed metabolic support without allowing bears to expend energy by utilizing fat as energy, which demonstrates the intricate adaptations of steroid hormones for the regulation of physiological states (Poterasu et al., 2020) (Figure 4.5).

4.1.3. Amine Hormones

Amine hormones are an important class of endocrine signaling molecules, which are virtually made from the amino acids tryptophan and tyrosine. The hormones include, but are not restricted to, the catecholamines epinephrine and norepinephrine, which are primarily secreted by the adrenal medulla. They are engaged in central functions of the body's stress reaction, facilitating fight or flight by inducing heart rate, muscle perfusion, and energy mobilization. The amine hormones like thyroid hormones, which are tyrosine-derived, are important in metabolic regulation, controlling transcription and expenditure of energy. The effect of such hormones is typically mediated by binding to cognate receptors, which generate rapid-acting cellular responses. It is crucial to grasp amine hormones' diverse behavior in order to comprehend how they function in homeostasis as well as physiological adaptation to environmental changes. During the last decade or so, research has shown complex interactions among amine hormones and other signaling pathways, particularly within the framework of neuroendocrine functions. For instance, the rapid action of corticosteroids, which fall outside of the strict definition of amine hormones and peptide hormones, intersects with the actions of amine hormones , such as dopamine and serotonin. Studies demonstrate that glucocorticoids inhibit monoamine transport via mechanisms involving organic cation transporter 3 (OCT3), a discovery that emphasizes the nuanced regulatory interaction among endocrine structures. These interactions are most relevant to stress disorders, in which the balance of neurotransmitters is upset and can lead to mood disorders. Through it, studying these complex relationships among the hormones sheds light on their collective influence on body functions, showing why an integrated endocrine response is significant. Moreover, amine hormone effects are not merely transient, physiological effects since they also affect long-term developmental trends and actions. The prenatal programming theory caught on, with the notion that being exposed to particular hormonal milieus in the womb has the potential to program neuroendocrine systems across generations. As an example, maternal stress or dietary deficiencies that alter amine hormone levels have been shown to affect the reproductive neuroendocrine axis, demonstrating the flexibility of hormone regulation during key stages of development. It is among the reasons revealed in existing literature that disrupt normal programming and eventually result in transgenerational effects. Understanding how amine hormone synthesis and action are affected by the factors could be crucial because it may uncover mechanisms to result in resilience or susceptibility to subsequent disease, thereby informing preventative interventions to endocrine disease and health.

Test Your Knowledge

1. What is the primary difference in how peptide hormones and steroid hormones interact with target cells?
2. Write the amine hormones.

4.2. Hormone Synthesis and Secretion

Learning Outcome

1. Explain the mechanisms of hormone production;
2. Define the factors influencing hormone release;
3. Learn about the role of feedback mechanisms.

Hormone synthesis and secretion are fundamental processes in the endocrine system that regulate various physiological processes in multiple organ systems. The intricate interaction in hormone production typically initiates in specialized endocrine glands, such as, the pituitary, thyroid, and adrenal glands. They secrete hormones—chemical messengers that regulate processes of metabolism, growth, and homeostasis—through unique biosynthetic pathways. For instance, steroid hormones, which are chemically derived from cholesterol, undergo enzymatic modification to produce biologically active molecules that then gain access to the blood. This is a highly integrated regulatory process in such a way that hormone levels are maintained within the physiological range, thereby preventing excess or deficiency disorders. Notably, the processes of feedback involved in these mechanisms, such as, negative feedback loops, are highly significant in maintaining endocrine balance and responsiveness to internal and external stimuli (Gross et al., 2001). The hormone secretion mechanism is just as significant as the synthesis of hormones, involving complex regulatory cues that stimulate endocrine glands to secrete their products into the circulation. Hormones are secreted in response to varying stimuli, i.e., hormonal, neural, or humoral, illustrating the intercommunication of the endocrine system with other systems of the body. For instance, the pituitary gland is regulated by the hypothalamus through releasing and inhibiting hormones, which regulate downstream glands in turn. A prime example is the GnRH release, which stimulates the anterior pituitary to release LH and FSH. The secretion of these gonadotropins is pivotal in reproductive processes and serves as a good example of how highly interconnected hormonal activities shape fertility as well as reproductive well-being. It is important to understand such relationships as a way to craft effective clinical interventions in case of hormonal dyscrasias (Boer et al., 2010). Greater study of hormone secretion and synthesis still finds evidence of the potential of external pressures, such as, nutritional status and environmental stressors, on hormonal control. Selection in dairy cattle, for example, for higher milk yields have been associated with declines in fertility, and alterations in estrous behavior have been a notable outcome. This experience reflects the interaction of metabolic demands and hormonal signals and necessitates insight into the genetic and physiological foundation of estrous control. Estradiol (E2) and progesterone are key hormones that interact with a number of such metabolic pathways to strongly influence reproductive cycles. Furthermore, recent evidence reveals that gene expression changes in specific brain regions, such as, the hypothalamus, demonstrate that environmental factors can alter endocrine control at the gene level. This is a research area that emphasizes the need to integrate endocrine physiology with overall concepts of biology for a complete appreciation of endocrine interaction in disease and health (Boer et al., 2010) (Figure 4.6).

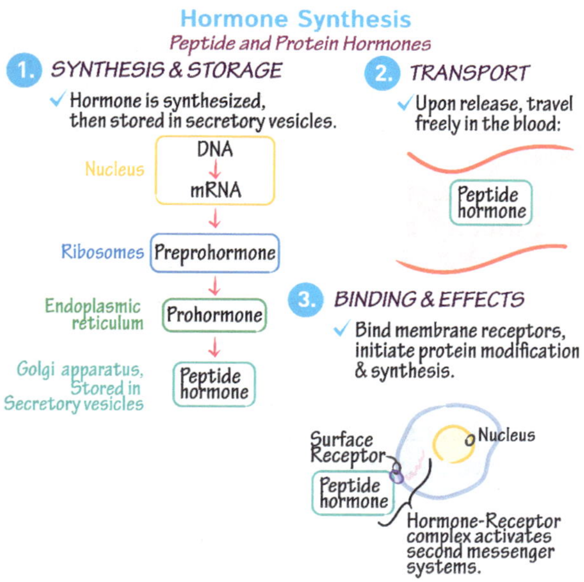

Figure 4.6. Peptide-and-protein-hormone-synthesis.

Source: https://d1j63owfs0b5j3.cloudfront.net/term/images/peptide-and-protein-hormone-synthesis-3397.png.

4.2.1. Mechanisms of Hormone Production

The endocrine system's process of hormone production is intricate and must be utilized to attain homeostasis in the body. Biochemical messengers called hormones are produced and secreted by various glands, including the pituitary, thyroid, adrenal glands, and pancreas. Each gland responds to an intricate combination of physiological stimuli, occasionally by the hypothalamus, which acts as a regulating center. For example, the secretion of gonadotropin-releasing hormone (GnRH) from the hypothalamus stimulates the anterior pituitary to secrete luteinizing hormone (LH) and follicle-stimulating hormone (FSH), which are both involved in reproductive function. The chain of control illustrates the hierarchical mechanism of endocrine signaling whereby higher-level hormone activity controls lower-level responses for precise control of body functions and reactions to environmental stimuli. In this system, some hormones serve pivotal roles in controlling physiological responses. Estradiol (E2), for instance, has been characterized as a central mediator of reproductive behavior, i.e., in the regulation of estrous cycles in animals , such as dairy cows. Synthesis of E2 is subject to tight feedback control using progesterone and other hormones. Hormonal changes can greatly influence behaviors such as estrus, which are critical to reproduction. Recent studies have determined the molecular processes underlying the phenomena, showing how certain gene expression induced by estrogen in brain regions , such as the hypothalamus, affects neuronal circuits critical to such behavioral manifestations. This intersection of gene expression with hormone signaling is an active area of research because it has the potential to explain how metabolic stress affects reproductive fitness, particularly in high-performance dairy cows (Boer et al., 2010).

Systems biology's integration into studies on the production of hormones also has the potential for expanding our knowledge of complex endocrine relationships. Mathematical modeling coupled with physiological and genomic data can improve understanding of hormone regulation, particularly with the plethora of genomic information available. For instance, disruption of signaling cascades by environmental stressors or genetic predisposition can be modeled to understand the effect on the secretion of hormones and overall health. Interdisciplinary approaches like these will play an important role in understanding the intricacies of endocrine illness as well as reproductive dysfunction in high-output livestock. This cross-disciplinary fusion of biology, mathematics, and technology will ultimately lead to enhanced agricultural management strategies and the promotion of fertility in dairy cows as we seek greater insight into the processes behind hormone synthesis and their action (Gross et al., 2001) (Figure 4.7).

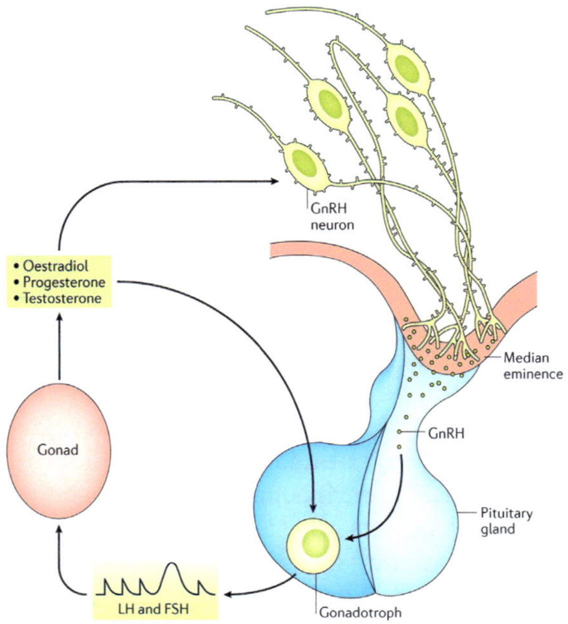

Figure 4.7. Mechanisms of hormone production.

Source: https://media.springernature.com/full/springer-static/image/art%3A10.1038%2Fnrendo.2016.70/MediaObjects/41574_2016_Article_BFnrendo201670_Fig1_HTML.jpg.

4.2.2. Factors Influencing Hormone Release

Hormone discharge is a complex process involving multiple factors, such as, physiological stimuli, environmental stimuli, and intrinsic feedback mechanisms. One of the main elements is the role of the endocrine glands in the production and secretion of hormones in response to specific stimuli. For instance, insulin secretion from the pancreas is regulated largely by blood glucose level; elevated glucose causes the release of insulin so that glucose can be absorbed by cells. The hypothalamus also plays a vital role in regulating hormone secretion via its interaction with the pituitary gland, leading to a series of hormone production, influencing numerous functions of the body. These pathways play a critical role in illustrating the mechanisms of hormone secretion and how they influence overall well-being, therefore indicating the importance of maintaining balance in hormones in homeostasis. Compounding the difficulty of hormone regulation are the extrinsic influences of stress and diet. One instance is that of chronic stress, which activates the hypothalamus-pituitary-adrenal (HPA) axis and the resulting release of the hormone cortisol, a central hormone to the body's response to stress. Elevated levels of cortisol eventually have strong effects on many of the body's metabolic functions, like glucose metabolism and immune function. In addition, food selection may influence hormone release; the intake of certain nutrients can enhance or suppress the release of hormones. For instance, increased protein consumption could stimulate glucagon secretion, and excessive carbohydrate intake could promote insulin release. Hence, it is essential that the interplay of internal physiological states and external environmental stimuli plays a vital role in regulating hormone secretion, stressing the need for keen knowledge of these factors as part of endocrine physiology. Feedback mechanisms are also inherent to regulate the level of hormones in the body, independent of external stimuli. The endocrine system applies mechanisms for negative feedback in order to attain homeostasis through the adjustment of the secretion of hormones based on blood levels. An example of a classic process is that of thyroid hormone regulation. If thyroxine levels are elevated in the blood, the hypothalamus reduces the release of thyrotropin-releasing hormone (TRH), causing decreased release of thyroid-stimulating hormone (TSH) from the pituitary gland. This feedback decreases thyroxine production by the thyroid gland, keeping things in balance. In other instances, in some situations, positive feedback mechanisms can also be involved, as during delivery, with oxytocin release, further augmenting uterine contractions. The fine-tuned control of hormonal discharge through feedback processes underscores the delicacy and precision of hormonal regulation in human biology, inviting further scope for such mechanisms' application in disease and health (Patwardhan, 2008; Zubeldia-Brenner et al., 2016) (Figure 4.8).

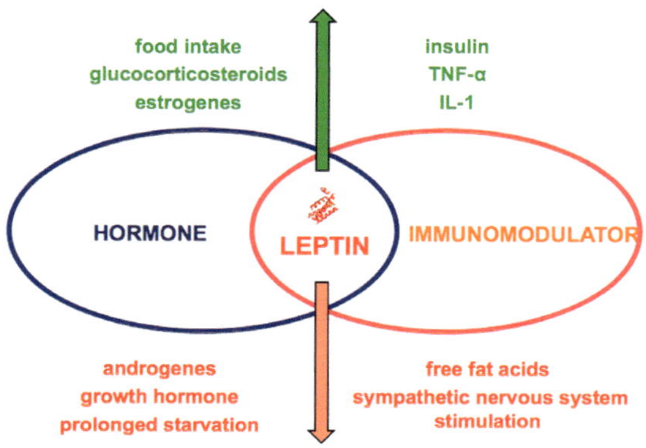

Figure 4.8. Factors affecting serum leptin concentration are either as a hormone.

Source: https://www.researchgate.net/publication/258734616/figure/fig2/AS:297373617147931@1447910803982/Factors-affecting-serum-leptin-concentration-either-as-a-hormone-or-immunomodulator-The.png.

4.2.3. Role of Feedback Mechanisms

The intricacy of feedback mechanisms underlies the control of hormonal activity within the endocrine system, and homeostasis is achieved. Feedback loops fall into two general categories: negative and positive feedback. Negative feedback is most prevalent, wherein an elevation of a specific hormone results in a counter-response to bring about decreased production of the hormone. This form of feedback occurs in the regulation of physiological balance, like in the case of steroid hormones like estrogen and testosterone that have key functions in a wide variety of biological processes like reproductive activity and metabolic programming (Zubeldia-Brenner et al., 2016). Positive feedback mechanisms, though less common, also play critical functions in processes that have a necessity for an absolute result, like luteinizing hormone release during ovulation. Both forms of feedback highlight the capacity of the endocrine system to regulate itself, responding effectively to internal and external stimuli. Peripheral hormones are also central to the mechanism of feedback regulation of energy homeostasis, whereby several hormones coordinate together to govern metabolic functions. Significant hormones, such as, ghrelin and leptin, provide significant feedback to central mechanisms in the hypothalamus that can control appetite and energy use. For instance, leptin, which is secreted from fat tissues, signals the brain about the fat reserves in the body and decreases hunger signals to bring about satiety. Feedback is essential in energy homeostasis because it provides a mechanism to ensure that energy intake is equal to energy expenditure (Bartha et al., 2011). Ghrelin, which is secreted in the stomach, is a hunger-stimulating hormone, and this gives an idea about the contrasting function of the hormones in the feedback system. The subtle interplay between these hormonal messages underscores the advanced regulatory processes of energy homeostasis, so advanced that even the dynamic and complicated nature of endocrine physiology emerges. Besides energy regulation, the impact of feedback is not restricted to physiological activity on a larger scale, such as, reproductive processes and pathologies. Endocrine feedback is important in the development of physiological traits as well as the regulation of the reproductive cycle. For instance, in the female genital tract, estrogen and progesterone feedback control the menstrual cycle to create the appropriate hormonal background for ovulation and preconception (Zubeldia-Brenner et al., 2016). Furthermore, disruption of these feedback mechanisms could be responsible for pathological conditions, such as, polycystic ovary syndrome or pituitary disease, underscoring the importance of feedback mechanisms in endocrinology. The interactions of these hormones not only enable normal biological functions to take place but also demonstrate how disturbances within these systems can lead to significant health complications, thereby emphasizing the importance of learning about endocrine feedback mechanisms comprehensively in both clinical and physiological contexts.

Test Your Knowledge

1. What are the main steps involved in the synthesis of peptide hormones?
2. How do steroid hormones differ in their synthesis compared to peptide hormones?

4.3. Hormone Transport in the Blood

Learning Outcome

1. Explain the binding proteins and their functions;
2. Define the half-life of hormones;
3. Describe the impact of transport on hormone activity.

Hormone transport in the bloodstream is a crucial mechanism in endocrine physiology that influences the action of hormones on target tissues. Hormones are generally divided into two groups according to their water solubility: hydrophilic (water-soluble) hormones, like peptides and catecholamines, and hydrophobic (lipid-soluble) hormones, like steroid hormones and thyroid hormones. Water-soluble hormones tend to travel in the bloodstream dissolved in plasma, allowing rapid distribution and immediate effect on target cells. Lipid-soluble hormones, however, preferentially bind with transport proteins, which increases their blood solubility and modulates their delivery into target organs. Not only is this binding responsible for their increased half-life while in circulation, but it also moderates their release and effect, demonstrating the intricacy of hormonal signaling and transport mechanisms. The physiology of hormone transport is intricately interwoven with various physiological statuses and needs of the organism. An example is that variation in binding protein concentration influences hormone availability to receptors, with a direct bearing on metabolic pathways. Such interaction accentuates the importance of the control mechanisms governing hormone transport and their impact on transport proteins. Significantly, co-injection of particular hormones has been shown to trigger enzymatic activity and stimulate immunity, e.g., upon activation of prophenoloxidase in locusts, demonstrating the complex interaction between hormones and systemic responses (Goldsworthy et al., 2003). This intricate regulation emphasizes the reality that hormone action's effectiveness not only relies on secretion but also on the way hormones travel and interact in the circulatory system. Apart from the biological outcome, understanding of hormone transport in the blood reveals therapeutic avenues for managing endocrine disease. Maltransport of hormones could lead to hormonal resistance or deficiency, needing appropriate interventions. For instance, transport accelerators and modified release preparations are under investigation to improve hormone delivery in the clinic. In addition, results that emerge from research with hormone transport systems provide useful models for designing new treatment protocols. The increasing literature on hormone interactions, transport mechanisms, and therapeutic potential highlights the value of ongoing research on endocrine physiology. With additional discovery of blood navigation by hormones, we can obtain valuable insight pertinent to clinical interventions to optimize endocrine well-being (Gross et al., 2001) (Figure 4.9).

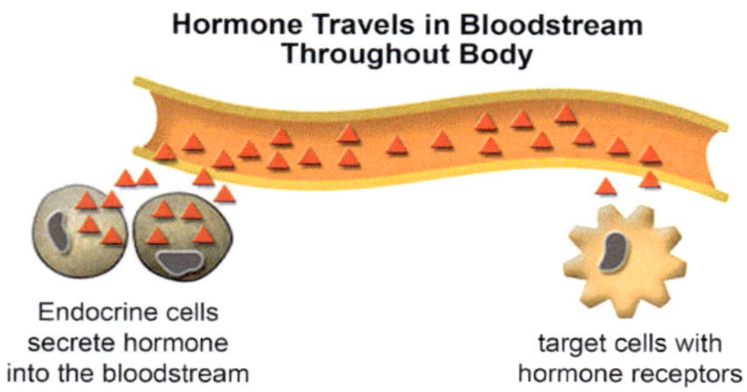

Figure 4.9. Hormone transport in the blood.

Source: https://www.mrgscience.com/uploads/2/0/7/9/20796234/b30-m2-021-l_orig.jpg.

4.3.1. Binding Proteins and Their Functions

Binding proteins are crucial to the endocrine system since they regulate the activity of hormones once in the bloodstream. Proteins primarily function as carriers, binding to hormones and carrying them through the circulatory system. For instance, the thyroid hormones triiodothyronine (T3) and thyroxine (T4) are bound by thyroid hormone-binding globulin (THBG), not only increasing their plasma solubility but also regulating their bioavailability to target tissues. The binding of hormones with binding proteins is a vital interaction since it maintains the levels of the hormone in the optimal ranges, thereby facilitating proper physiological responses. This binding affinity also serves to prolong the half-life of the hormones, which is essential for sustained biological activity, giving rise to a more effective hormonal regulation of many body functions and processes. The binding of the proteins to hormones is not merely passive transport; they actually alter the bioactivity of the hormones themselves. Some of the binding proteins can activate or inhibit hormone function by being conformationally altered when binding to a hormone. For example, sex hormone-binding globulin (SHBG) is a protein that binds to sex hormones like testosterone and estradiol, controlling their bioactivity and affecting their availability for binding to cellular receptors. The same is more specifically applicable in the context of explaining hormonal imbalance-related disorders , such as polycystic ovary syndrome (PCOS) and androgen excess disorders, in which altered levels of binding proteins result in gross clinical manifestations. More and more research illustrates the way changes in levels of such binding proteins could be correlated with reproductive and sexual function alterations, which mirror their function in endocrine physiology (Gross et al., 2001). Also, the intricate interaction between binding proteins and hormonal processes has far-reaching effects on reproductive health. That thyroid hormone receptors exist in reproductive tissues in males and females shows that thyroid hormones exert direct action on reproductive function via binding proteins (Carosa et al., 2018). Evidence from disruptions of fertility in thyroid dysfunction points to the significance of binding proteins in maintaining hormonal balance and reproductive outcome. In an investigation of the action of thyroid hormones on sex function, researchers are beginning to identify the molecular mechanisms by which such interactions occur, emphasizing the merit of a comprehensive understanding of binding proteins in endocrine physiology overall. Not only does such comprehension inform therapeutic management of hormonal disease, but it also provides us with more insight into how endocrine systems interact with other physiological processes (Figure 4.10).

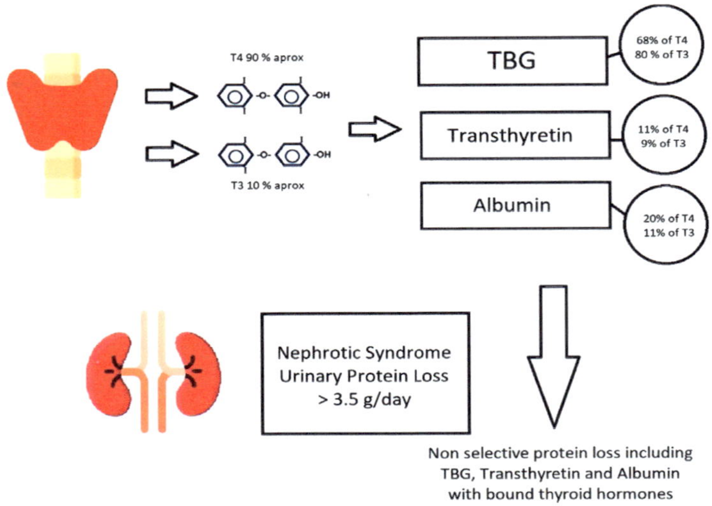

Figure 4.10. Urinary loss of thyroid hormones.

Source: https://static.elsevier.es/multimedia/25300180/0000007000000010/v1_202312071927/S2530018023001749/v1_202312071927/en/main.assets/gr2.jpeg.

4.3.2. Half-Life of Hormones

Half-life of hormones is an important concept to understand in endocrine physiology, as it determines the duration and intensity of hormonal action in the body. Half-life is the time during which the blood level of a hormone falls by half, an important factor in both pharmacologic and physiologic effects. Short half-life hormones , such as epinephrine, are quick-acting but must have quick signaling pathways to deliver instant physiological response, e.g., fight-or-flight response. Other hormones, e.g., thyroid hormones, possess longer half-lives and give long-term results on growth and metabolism. This time aspect of hormonal action is an important determinant of homeostasis, and half-life is an important consideration for predicting the duration that the hormone will be active prior to metabolic clearance. Degradation and clearance processes for hormones are also sophisticated and include enzymic degradation as well as renal or hepatic excretion. Hormones are metabolized by active pathways that inactivate them for final excretion. For instance, peptide hormones generally have shorter half-lives due to their susceptibility to proteolytic enzymes in the blood. Steroid hormones, on the other hand, being lipid-soluble, are typically bound to plasma proteins that protect them from immediate degradation and thus enhance their half-life. The interaction between the biosynthesis of the hormones and their catabolic processes is thus central to physiological homeostasis. Understandings of these dynamics allow scientists to account for the intricate control systems governing the regulation of hormonal signaling, further illustrating their value in the broader field of endocrine physiology. The consequences of anomalous hormone half-lives are notably important in the argument over endocrine-disrupting chemicals (EDCs). EDCs can potentially disrupt normal hormonal action and half-lives, particularly during periods of key development. For instance, evidence is growing that exposure to EDCs during pregnancy or early childhood can lead to permanent disruption of hormone regulation, thereby affecting the course of development of an organism. As such, chemicals act at extremely low concentrations, fine-tuning the half-life of hormones becomes even more critical. The interaction of EDCs, disrupted hormone homeostasis, and subsequent health implications, such as, metabolic dysfunction and thyroid dysfunction, creates a compelling need for further research into the mechanisms of action of these chemicals in disrupting endocrine signaling (Pietro et al., 2023; Koyama et al., 2025). As endocrinology advances, understanding the half-life of hormones remains significant to the development of effective regulatory policies as well as therapeutic interventions (Figure 4.11).

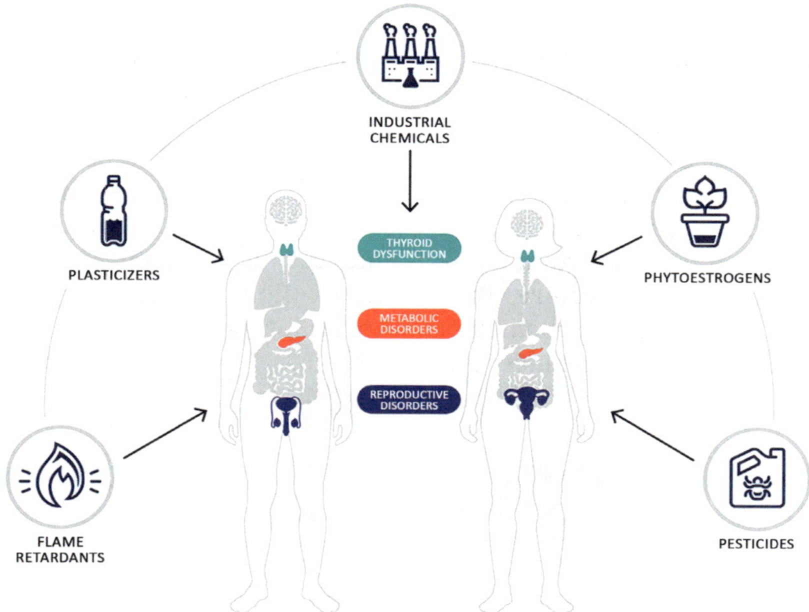

Figure 4.11. Endocrine disrupting chemicals present human and environmental health risks.

Source: https://cdn2.caymanchem.com/cdn/cms/caymanchem/PublishingImages/Lists/NewsItems/AllItems/Endocrine%20Disrupting%20Chemicals.jpg.

4.3.3. Impact of Transport on Hormone Activity

The transport of hormones within the organism plays a significant role in endocrine system performance. Hormones are inclined to be secreted into the blood and travel to target tissues and organs to act upon them. This system of transport is not merely passive, but is under strict control by various factors , such as plasma protein binding, circulation of blood, and vascular organization. For instance, some hormones, like steroid hormones, are lipophilic and require carrier proteins for solubility in the aqueous environment of blood. Such a transport dynamic can have a significant impact on the availability of hormones at target locations, leading to amplification or suppression of physiological responses. The complexity of such interactions serves to underscore the importance of transport in the modulation of endocrine action, settling its place as a vital mechanism in endocrine physiology. Moreover, the efficiency of hormonal transport is pivotal in the regulation of homeostasis and metabolic function. As an instance, hormones , such as insulin, which facilitate the uptake of glucose by tissues, heavily depend on their transport mechanisms of action in order to deliver effective distribution in states of metabolic demand. In pathophysiological contexts, such as, obesity or diabetes, dysfunctions in transport can lead to resistance at cellular levels and therefore contribute to enhanced disease. While as vital as the roles of hormones are in modulating metabolic processes, any disruption in their transport can have spillover effects on health overall. Hormones also possess differential transport mechanisms according to their structure—For example, peptide hormones, unlike their steroid analogs, are water-soluble and freely move in the circulation, reiterating that an understanding of the type of transport can enlighten one on the larger context of hormonal action in endocrine processes. Finally, the process of hormone transport is also influenced by external forces in the form of the impact of pharmacological agents or environmental pollutants that can mimic or interfere with endogenous hormone transport mechanisms. Certain endocrine disruptors, for instance, are recognized to bind hormone carriers, which can alter the bioavailability and transport efficacy of essential hormones. Through studies, it has been found that such bindings play a role in pervasive hormonal disruptions affecting developmental and reproductive health. A key topic of this is the description of signaling pathways and feedback mechanisms, in particular, relative to steroid hormones. One can clearly see that the neuroendocrine axis plays a central role in the potentiation of the effects of such hormones as estrogen and testosterone, sexual orientation, and the programming of metabolism (Zubeldia-Brenner et al., 2016). Understanding the intricacy of transport mechanisms is therefore not a biological curiosity alone but essential to understanding the intricacy of endocrine physiology as a whole (Gross et al., 2001).

Test Your Knowledge

1. What are the differences between free and protein-bound hormone transport in the bloodstream?
2. Explain how binding proteins influence the half-life and bioavailability of hormones.

4.4. Hormone Receptors and Signal Transduction

Learning Outcome

1. Identify the types of hormone receptors;
2. Define the mechanisms of signal transduction;
3. Describe the role of second messengers.

In the complex realm of endocrine physiology, hormone receptors play a central role in signal transduction as the central regulators of hormonal action in target cells. The receptors, which can be divided into two broad categories—membrane-bound and intracellular—exhibit conformational changes upon interaction with hormones and initiate molecular cascades that lead to physiological responses. For instance, membrane-bound receptors might employ second messengers , such as cyclic AMP or calcium ions to carry and enhance the signal within the cell, while intracellular receptors tend to have an effect on particular genes, which impacts transcriptional activity. The receptor-binding mechanism is significant in how hormones influence various tissues, as seen in the research of regulatory mechanisms of estrous behavior in dairy cattle, where estradiol (E2) has emerged as a major modulator of reproductive processes by its influence on neural networks and gene expression (Boer et al., 2010). The complexity of hormone signaling is also apparent from the part G protein-coupled receptors (GPCRs) play in mediating a response to multiple hormones, including corticotropin-releasing hormone (CRH). Upon binding by hormone, G proteins become activated and then activate downstream signals that influence various cellular activities , such as gene expression, cytoskeletal organization, and neurotransmitter release. Recent studies on CRH signaling, its action in the hypothalamic-pituitary-adrenal (HPA) axis, for example, suggest that this intricate signaling pathway plays a pivotal role in the modulation of physiological as well as behavioral responses to stress. Importantly, understanding the specificity of CRH interaction with its receptors, for example, recently discovered processes of cAMP generation, enhances the knowledge on neuroendocrine control and its translation to disorders of stress and mood (Inda et al., 2017). Moreover, the combination of genomic techniques and mathematical modeling with the study of hormone signaling offers special promise as a way to continue the illumination of endocrine physiology. By means of systems biology approaches, researchers can investigate the interactions between hormonal signaling cascades and gene expression, enabling improved understanding of how molecular changes produce larger-scale physiological responses. This multidisciplinary interface sheds light on the adaptive as well as maladaptive mechanisms of animal reproductive behavior, as well as the resulting maladaptive responses ensuing from metabolic stress in high-yielding dairy cows. These advancements not only decipher the fundamental principles of hormone action but also usher in novel possibilities for therapeutic modalities aimed at the restoration of reproductive impairment as well as other disorders related to hormonal malfunction (Boer et al., 2010) (Figure 4.12).

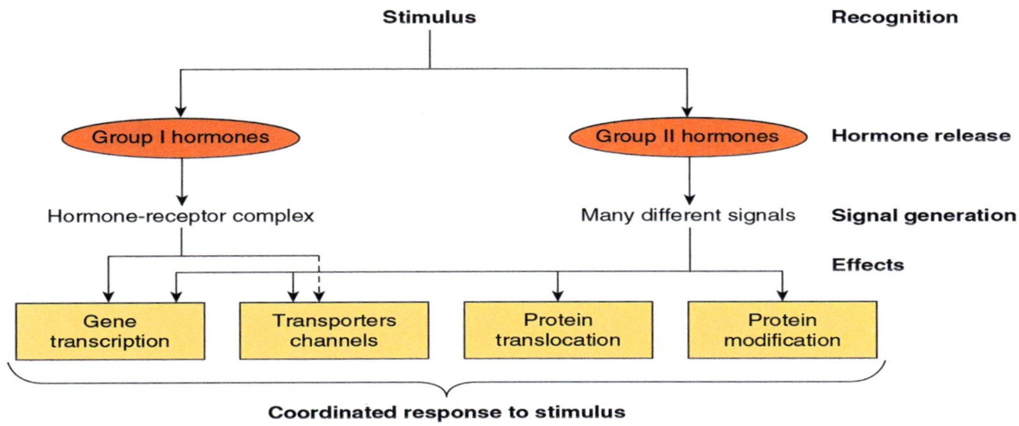

Figure 4.12. Hormone receptors and signal transduction.

Source: https://basicmedicalkey.com/wp-content/uploads/2017/02/image02222.gif.

4.4.1. Types of Hormone Receptors

In the complex setting of endocrine physiology, the hormone receptors are key effectors of hormonal action, classifying into two groups: membrane-bound and intracellular receptors. The membrane-bound receptors, which occur frequently with peptide and protein hormones, are part of the plasma membrane of target cells. These receptors are likely to operate through secondary messenger systems, e.g., cyclic ADP-ribose or inositol trisphosphate, to convey the hormone's signal within the cell. This process enables the rapid physiological response, a necessity for processes like glucose metabolism and ion transport, demonstrating the efficiency of membrane receptors in eliciting acute biological responses. Intracellular receptors, usually tasked with binding steroid and thyroid hormones, associate with signals by direct interaction with DNA and mediate changes in gene expression after prolonged periods. Hence, the knowledge of the distinction between the receptor types enhances our comprehension of hormonal signal pathways in various physiological conditions. Intracellular hormone receptors play a fundamental role in regulating gene expression as transcription factors that control the formation of specific proteins. Thyroid hormones like triiodothyronine (T3) and thyroxine (T4) are classic examples of this process, in which they bind with thyroid hormone receptors (TRs) in the nucleus and influence metabolic processes that extend up to sexual and reproductive function. Experiments have established the presence of TRs within the male and female reproductive systems, supporting the postulate of thyroid hormones having a significant role in fertility and reproductive health. The detection of TRs in the gonads was the initial clue to a shift in paradigm towards the understanding of an extended interaction between thyroid and reproductive physiology (Carosa et al., 2018). Studies defining this interaction suggest that thyroid disease can lead to adverse reproductive outcomes, uncovering the extended role of hormone receptor function in endocrine health and disease. Furthermore, hormone-receptor interaction goes beyond the traditional pathways, portraying a multifaceted system of hormonal control. For instance, thyroid hormones not only control their pathways but also communicate with other endocrine functions, including the sex steroid hormone axis. Evidence reveals that variation in thyroid hormone status can influence the secretion of other hormones , such as estrogen and testosterone, hence sexual function and behavior. Scientific studies, particularly in animal models, have revealed significant interactions between thyroid function and sexual behavior, with findings indicating that absence of TRs is to blame for disturbed sexual differentiation and behavior (Gross et al., 2001). These results lead to increased exploration of hormone receptor subtypes, a description for the intricate and often reciprocal system of hormone action underlying endocrine physiology and its medical relevance to human health (Figure 4.13).

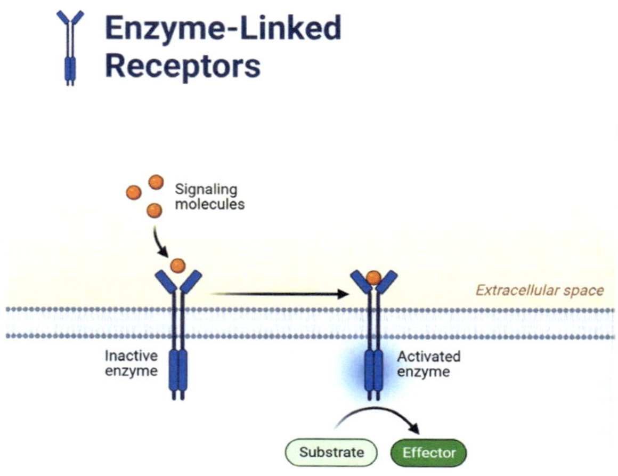

Figure 4.13. Types of hormone receptors.

Source: https://endoconsult.b-cdn.net/wp-content/uploads/enzyme-coupled-receptors.png.

4.4.2. Mechanisms of Signal Transduction

Signal transduction is an elementary process through which hormonal information is conveyed across cells, thereby initiating a chain of intracellular events that ultimately result in various biological responses required for homeostasis. This process is centered on hormone receptors, predominantly located on the cell membrane or the cytoplasm, which interact with specific hormones to generate a chain of intracellular phenomena. When it binds to its receptor, a hormone , such as estradiol would likely cause conformational changes that result in the activation of downstream signaling. For example, when considering estrous behavior in dairy cows, estradiol has been found to be a key regulator of many hormonal and behavioral events during the estrous cycle. This implies that the sensitivity and responsiveness of the endocrine system to hormonal changes are essential for reproductive fitness and overall health in such animals and is therefore important to value the intricate processes of signal transduction (Boer et al., 2010). The relationship between hormones and signal transduction pathways is complex and intricate, at times being in the form of G protein-coupled receptors (GPCRs) and other signaling molecules. Corticotropin-releasing hormone (CRH), for instance, is a component of the hypothalamic-pituitary-adrenal axis, and it contributes to adaptively responding to stress by influencing humoral as well as behavioral responses.

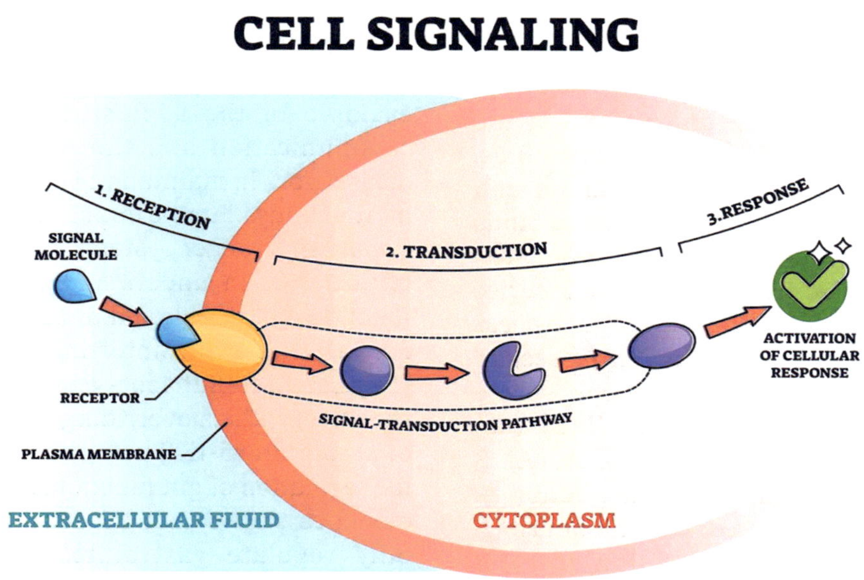

Figure 4.14. Signal-transduction.

Source: https://www.creativebiomart.net/incl/images/2-signal-transduction-1.jpg.

Signaling mechanisms for CRH include the activation of GPCRs, such as, CRHR1 and CRHR2, leading to the generation of second messengers , such as cyclic AMP (cAMP) and subsequent activation of extracellular signal-regulated kinases (ERK1/2). This cascade illustrates the way in which signal transduction leads to maximal physiological changes, highlighting the critical functions these pathways have in both regular and stress-related hormonal responses within the endocrine system (Inda et al., 2017). Moreover, the dynamic nature of systems biology provides a holistic view of how it is possible to comprehend the complex networks involved in hormone signaling and transduction. With the merging of physiological and genomic data with mathematical modeling, researchers anticipate that the complicated dance between various hormonal stimuli and their cell reactions will be unlocked. This is particularly informative in terms of explaining the mechanisms of gene expression governing the control of estrous behavior, as research has shown in recent studies that specific regions of the brain, such as, the hypothalamus, are influenced by estrogen-induced gene expressions. With the evolving genomic technologies, systems biology will be in a position to complement endocrine physiology intelligence by facilitating the study of interactions among components at different levels of biological organization toward enhancing understanding of fertility and related disorders (Boer et al., 2010) (Figure 4.14).

4.4.3. Role of Second Messengers

Second messengers play a crucial role in the signaling pathways activated by hormones, serving to integrate extracellular stimuli and intracellular responses. When a hormone binds to its receptor on a target cell membrane, the receptor becomes active and triggers a series of biochemical reactions. The activation process typically consists of the production of second messengers like cyclic adenosine monophosphate (cAMP) or inositol trisphosphate (IP3) that amplify the original signal. For instance, cAMP, which is produced from ATP by the action of adenylate cyclase, activates protein kinase A (PKA), causing the phosphorylation of many target proteins. The resulting changes produce various physiological effects, such as, controlling gene expression, altering enzyme activity, or changing cellular metabolism. This gain of effect makes the second messengers significant factors in endocrine physiology control and highlights their pivotal position in hormone action. Apart from cAMP, calcium ions (Ca^{2+}) are also crucial second messengers in most hormonal communications. Ca^{2+} entry in a cell can be induced by more than one stimulus, e.g., the activation of G-protein-coupled receptor (GPCR). For instance, the cellular response to hormones , such as oxytocin and vasopressin is caused by Ca^{2+}-dependent mechanisms that influence muscle contraction and secretory processes. The intricate role of Ca^{2+} as a second messenger extends even further into its involvement in the release of neurotransmitters from synapses, which speaks to its versatility in both endocrine and nervous system signaling. Ca^{2+} levels are also controlled with exquisite precision by numerous channels and pumps so that cells can properly respond to hormone signals. This fascinating regulation is a prime example of the sophistication of endocrine communication and the necessity of second messengers in maintaining homeostatic balance in the body. Furthermore, the physiology of second messenger systems also plays a growing critical role in understanding gastrointestinal function and its relation to neurological activity. For instance, gastrointestinal enterochromaffin (EC) cells are nutrient- and neurotransmitter-sensitive, with an overriding role in the secretion of serotonin (5-HT) as a secondary messenger for regulation of gut functions. The most current evidence shows that EC cells' signals will not only regulate gastrointestinal motility but also affect satiety and visceral perception by coordination with the central nervous system (Alcaino et al., 2025). This is a two-way traffic between the brain and intestine through second messengers, which emphasizes the interdependence of endocrine functions. These findings emphasize the importance of second messengers in elucidating the complexity of hormone action and their potential therapeutic site for gut disorders (Dsouki et al., 2024).

Test Your Knowledge

1. Differentiate between cell surface receptors and intracellular hormone receptors with examples.
2. Explain the role of G protein-coupled receptors (GPCRs) in hormone signal transduction.

4.5. Effects of Hormones on Target Tissues

Learning Outcome

1. Identify the hormonal regulation of metabolism;
2. Define the hormonal influence on growth and development;
3. Describe the hormonal effects on homeostasis.

Hormone action with target tissues is a fundamental aspect of endocrine physiology in which the hormones serve as messenger molecules that modulate a broad range of physiological processes. Secreted into the bloodstream, hormones travel to specific target tissues where they bind to specific receptors. Receptor-mediated action triggers a series of intracellular processes with resulting physiological consequences, including changes in gene expression, cellular metabolism, and tissue function. For instance, steroid hormones , such as testosterone and estrogen exert a significant influence on reproductive processes and metabolic functions, influencing fertility all the way to energy homeostasis. Intricate pathways of such signaling indicate that the role of hormones in maintaining homeostasis and organizing body functions is essential, indicative of their utility in health and illness.

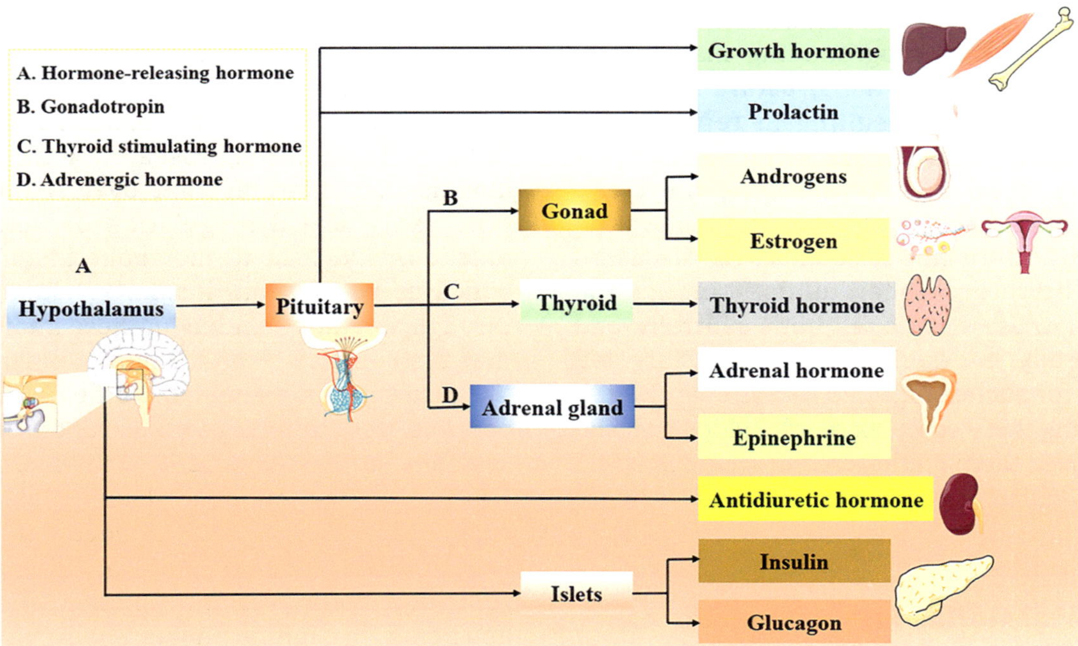

Figure 4.15. Target organs regulated by endocrine hormones.

Source: https://www.researchgate.net/publication/349226561/figure/fig1/AS:1022199515340809@1620722764287/Target-organs-regulated-by-endocrine-hormones.png.

The varied activities of hormones in target tissues also extend to the central nervous system, where hormones can affect psychological processes and behavior. The neuroendocrine interface shows that hormones like estrogen and progesterone, instead of being engaged merely with reproduction, are vital to brain function and neuroprotection. Evidence is present that these steroid hormones can influence neuronal plasticity and resilience, particularly with respect to neurodegenerative disease.

For example, the neuroprotection conferred by progesterone illustrates the far-reaching significance of hormonal regulation. Such findings not only identify the multifunctional roles of hormones but also open avenues for therapeutic interventions against hormonal processes in various neurological diseases, further solidifying the intricate interaction between neural function and endocrine signaling (Zubeldia-Brenner et al., 2016). Furthermore, the effect of hormones on target tissues can result in many pathological processes if it becomes dysregulated. Hormonal imbalances may contribute to the pathogenesis of disorders , such as polycystic ovary syndrome and metabolic syndrome, where harmony between hormonal signaling and tissue responsiveness becomes extremely crucial. Disruption in normal hormonal programming may induce significant changes in the structure as well as function of tissue, resulting in reproductive or metabolic disease. For instance, elevated androgen levels in conditions like polycystic ovary syndrome correlate with shifts in ovarian function and insulin resistance. As discussed in the literature today, understanding the effect of these hormones both centrally and peripherally is essential in shaping targeted therapy for such conditions (Gross et al., 2001). Unraveling these complex relationships can lead to improved therapeutic outcomes and improved understanding of endocrine physiology (Figure 4.15).

4.5.1. Hormonal Regulation of Metabolism

The hormonal regulation of metabolism functions by complex interaction of various endocrine messages that coordinate energy balance in the body. Focal to this regulation are hormones , such as insulin, glucagon, and epinephrine, each playing various but crossover roles in metabolic pathways. Insulin from the pancreas facilitates glucose uptake and glycogen storage, while glucagon does the opposite, stimulating glycogen breakdown and gluconeogenesis under fasting. In addition, epinephrine mobilizes energy substrates during exercise or stress, which initiates a quick metabolic response. The interaction of the hormones enables the body to maintain energy stores and respond accordingly to changing physiological demands, demonstrating the complexity of endocrine signaling and metabolic control. Apart from these classic metabolic hormones, other processes , such as the autonomic nervous system, significantly influence metabolic regulation. The sympathetic and parasympathetic branches control energy balance through their effects on hormone secretion and organ function. For instance, during overfeeding, shifts in sympathetic and parasympathetic outflow are evident that are associated with shifts in metabolism, like increased parasympathetic outflow, increasing insulin sensitivity and reduction of lipid storage. In addition, research with animal models demonstrates that overfeeding over time can cause dysregulation of autonomic functions and lead to metabolic disturbances , such as obesity and insulin resistance. It is through an understanding of these interactions that the complexity of hormonal regulation in the maintenance of metabolic health and the possible implications of disturbances in these systems become apparent (Scheurink et al., 1996). Examination of regulatory mechanisms for hormonal regulation of metabolism has expanded significantly, shedding light on gene expression and the function of specific hormones in significant metabolic pathways. As an example, recent literature suggests estrogen plays a central role in regulating estrous behavior in female mammals with broad implications for metabolic health. Estradiol (E2), an extremely effective estrogen, controls energy metabolism by controlling gene expression in a variety of tissues, with the hypothalamus playing a critical role in energy homeostasis. A combination with other hormones , such as progesterone and insulin-like growth factor-1, illustrates a multifaceted control of metabolic response. These findings underscore the value of exploring hormonal regulation by systems biology approaches in a bid to seize the complexity of fertility and metabolism, particularly in high-yielding dairy cows, where metabolic stress is known to influence reproductive function (Boer et al., 2010) (Figure 4.16).

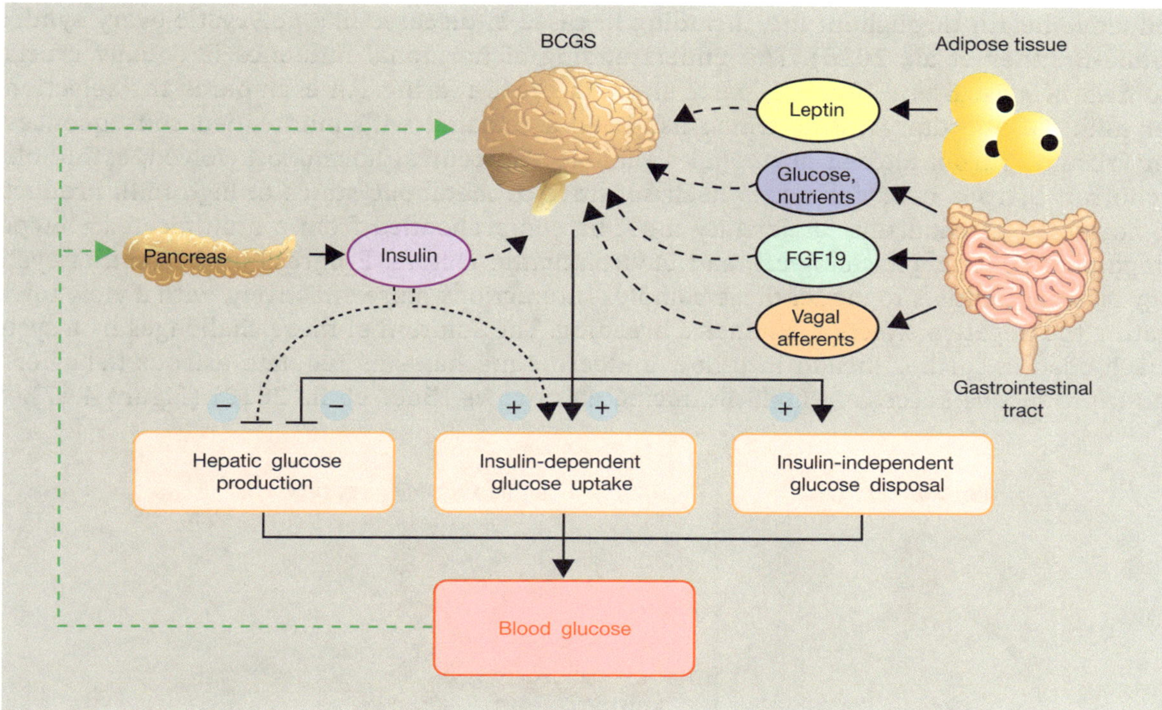

Figure 4.16. Hormonal regulation of metabolism.

Source: https://els-jbs-prod-cdn.jbs.elsevierhealth.com/cms/attachment/02215242-cb24-4dc2-9382-04e8a359a46f/gr2_lrg.jpg.

4.5.2. Hormonal Influence on Growth and Development

The intricate interaction of hormones deeply influences growth and development across various biological systems. Some of the major hormones include growth hormone (GH), insulin-like growth factors (IGFs), and sex steroids, which play key roles at all stages of life. Growth hormone, secreted from the anterior pituitary gland, initiates growth in almost every tissue by stimulating protein synthesis and cell division. This hormone synergizes with the IGFs that mediate the action of GH in growth during puberty. Sex steroids like testosterone and estrogen, in their turn, are the central molecules not only responsible for sexual development but also for bone development and growth. Understanding all these interactions informs us about how hormonal imbalance disturbs the growth pattern and the necessity of comprehensive research in the field of endocrine physiology to be utilized in the formulation of treatments for growth disorders. Besides, it is not possible to overlook the importance of steroid hormones in reproductive behavior and development. Estradiol and progesterone hormones are crucial in controlling the reproductive cycle. Their actions extend beyond the mere aspects of reproduction; they also influence secondary sexual characteristics and behavioral patterns. Estradiol, for instance, causes the onset of ovulation and sets up mating behaviors through neuroendocrine mechanisms. Existing research indicates that the steroid hormones have enduring effects upon brain structure and function, establishing connections that underpin metabolic and reproductive functions. Such mechanisms have the effect of highlighting the subtlety of hormonal regulation and the need for more studies into how these endocrine signals affect reproductive health throughout life, including in cases of diseases like polycystic ovary syndrome (Zubeldia-Brenner et al., 2016). The understanding of hormonal influence is equally crucial in the context of agricultural practice, particularly in cattle rearing. An example is the selection for higher milk yield in dairy cattle, which has been associated with unintended consequences for fertility resulting from altered hormonal signaling. The central hormone involved, estradiol, not only controls estrous behavior but is itself sensitive to metabolic states of high milk production. Thus, hormonal mechanisms for fertility must be comprehended from a multifaceted viewpoint, encompassing genetic, physiological, and environmental factors. Progress in the field of systems biology allows scientists to model these complex interactions more effectively, with a view towards mitigating the negative effects of intensive breeding. The solution of these challenges by a systems approach enables further insight into how endocrine mechanisms regulate estrous behavior and overall reproductive success in high-producing dairy cows (Boer et al., 2010) (Figure 4.17).

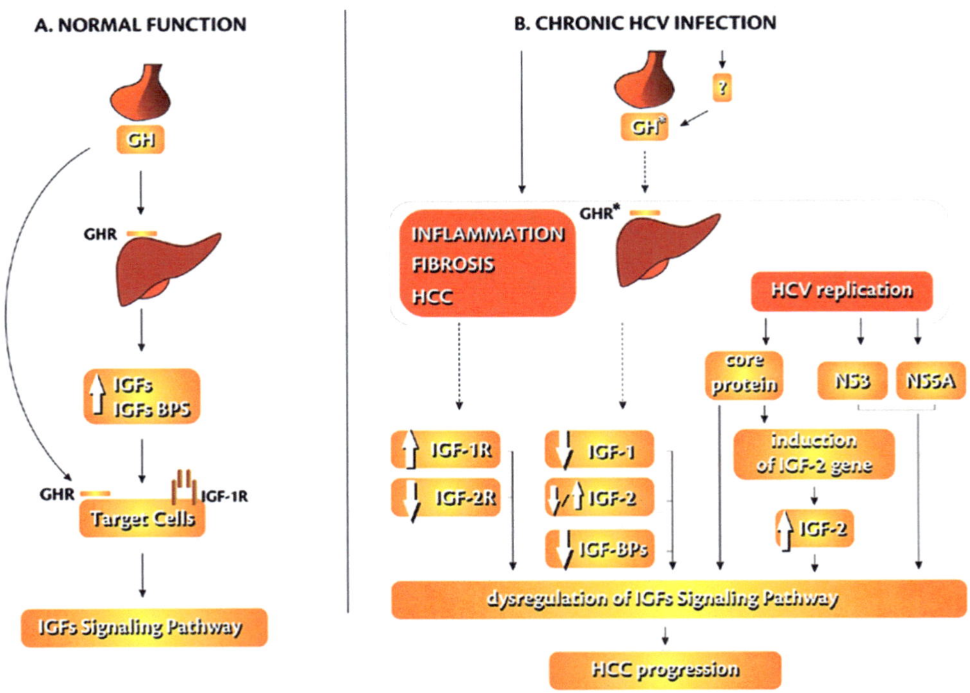

Figure 4.17. The insulin-like growth factor (IGF).

Source: https://www.spandidos-publications.com/article_images/ijo/41/6/IJO-41-06-1919-g02.jpg.

4.5.3. Hormonal Effects on Homeostasis

The relationship between homeostasis and hormones is a cornerstone of endocrine physiology, which demonstrates how the body maintains a constancy of the internal environment despite varying conditions in the external environment. The chemical messengers hormones transmit crucial information from tissues and organs to elicit responses that adjust physiological functions , such as metabolism, immune function, and fluid balance. A prime example is in the operation of the $Na+/K^+$ pump that not only generates electrochemical gradients but also underlies larger mechanisms in hormonal signaling required for cellular homeostasis. More recent discoveries have revealed that the endogenous ligand Ouabain plays a critical role in these mechanisms. Its involvement in many pathophysiological conditions illustrates how hormonal regulation extends far beyond mere ion transport into influencing cellular stress response and signaling cascades that are essential to maintaining homeostasis despite changing physiological demands (Elendu et al., 2025). Beyond the glucocorticoids and mineralocorticoids that directly regulate metabolic activity, other hormones greatly influence homeostasis indirectly by virtue of their secondary effects. As an example, insulin plays a central role in glucose and energy metabolism, stimulating cells to take up glucose in times of plenty of energy. In addition to providing immediate energy to cells, this action also sustains blood glucose levels constant and prevents hyperglycemia or hypoglycemia from occurring. Furthermore, the hormone leptin, secreted by fat cells, informs the brain regarding energy stores and regulates appetite and metabolism. They collectively create a web of feedback interactions that underscore the importance of hormonal interaction in homeostatic balance, particularly in nutritional and environmental stresses. Endocrine disruptors , such as phytoestrogens, demonstrate how exogenous substances may disrupt hormonal processes and affect homeostasis. From various plant sources, the phytoestrogens are structurally analogous to estrogens and capable of binding to estrogen receptors with pro-estrogenic and anti-estrogenic activities. The interaction can yield significant disruptions in hormonal regulation, potentially leading to developmental and reproductive abnormalities like endometriosis. As this disease reflects a breakdown in maintaining hormonal equilibrium, it is critical that studies on phytoestrogens be part of comprehending the implications of dietary factors on well-being. The absence of deficiency signs of phytoestrogenic activity also complicates the measurement of their total effects. Thus, it is important to distinguish between the positive and negative endocrine disturbances when formulating dietary recommendations for improving homeostasis, but not the adverse effects of endocrine-disrupting chemicals (Szukiewicz, 2023).

Test Your Knowledge

1. How do hormones exert specific effects on target tissues despite circulating throughout the body?
2. Describe the cellular and physiological effects of insulin on the liver, muscle, and adipose tissue.

4.6. Disorders of the Endocrine System

Learning Outcome

1. Describe the common endocrine disorders;
2. Define the impact of hormonal imbalances;
3. Discuss the treatment options for endocrine disorders.

Endocrine disorders comprise a range of conditions with hormonal imbalance that can result in significant interference with regular body functions. Endocrine disorders may be caused by a single or multiple etiologies, including genetic causes, environment, or lifestyle. An example includes anorexia nervosa, a psychiatric condition that entails excessive self-imposed food restriction, resulting in complete malnutrition and hormonal imbalance. This specific condition highlights the close association between psychological health and endocrine function as it results in functional amenorrhea and compromises reproductive ability through abnormalities in the hypothalamic-pituitary-ovarian axis. Such disruptions can be of a permanent nature, compromising fecundity and resulting in pregnancy comorbidities, highlighting the overriding importance of addressing both mental and endocrine health in individuals so affected (Poterasu et al., 2020).

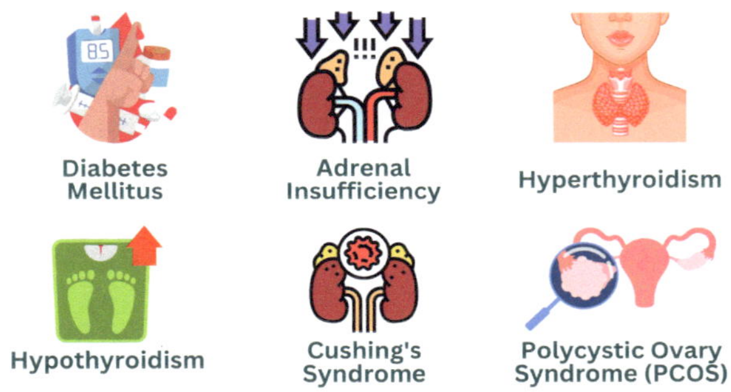

Figure 4.18. Common endocrine system disorders.

Source: https://cdn.shopify.com/s/files/1/0789/3781/7379/files/25.png?v=1720715274.

A better understanding of the molecular underpinnings of endocrine disease reveals the intricate roles receptors and signal transduction processes play in hormone action and regulation. Research has shown that steroid hormones, among numerous others, rely on specific receptors for their activities, which can be regulated by a variety of cofactors acting as co-activators or co-repressors. The receptor-mediated actions of these hormones, nonetheless, are not limited to genomic actions; there also exist non-genomic actions, meaning the sophistication of these hormones. More recently, the identification of endocrine disruptors—environmental pollutants that interfere with hormonal signaling—has introduced new challenges in public health. Disruptors can activate or inhibit natural hormones, leading to reproductive dysfunction and developmental disorders when acting on estrogen receptors or other critical pathways of signaling (Indarto & Izawa, 2017). The consequences of endocrine illness extend beyond individual health, with implications for broader societal and healthcare functions. The spread of illnesses , such as diabetes and thyroid diseases, for instance, demands a comprehensive response from public health systems. Advances in research have been central to the development of therapeutic practices and diagnostic methods aimed at minimizing the impact of such illnesses. Besides, the knowledge of the role of endocrine disruptors encourages regulatory action towards reducing exposure to these substances in the environment. As there is continuous advancement in endocrine physiology, interdisciplinarity with endocrinology, environmental science, and public health will be imperative in working on the complex problems related to endocrine disorders (Figure 4.18).

4.6.1. Common Endocrine Disorders

Familiarity with common endocrine disorders is required to appreciate the nuances of endocrine physiology and its strong impact on human health. Diabetic mellitus, hypothyroidism, and polycystic ovary syndrome illustrate the diverse consequences of hormonal dysregulation. In diabetes, for example, failure of the body to manage blood glucose levels due to insulin deficiency or resistance can lead to profound metabolic disturbances. Similarly, hypothyroidism results from improper synthesis of thyroid hormones that may result in symptoms as simple as fatigue or as complex as weight gain and depression. These conditions depict the importance of the regulation of hormones in homeostasis and reflect the need for proper interventions to correct hormonal deficiencies or resistance among patients. In addition, sex hormones play a pivotal role in the pathophysiology of most endocrine diseases, particularly in females. An example is the polycystic ovary syndrome (PCOS) that results in an imbalance of the two major sex hormones, testosterone and estrogen, causing ovarian dysfunction and infertility.

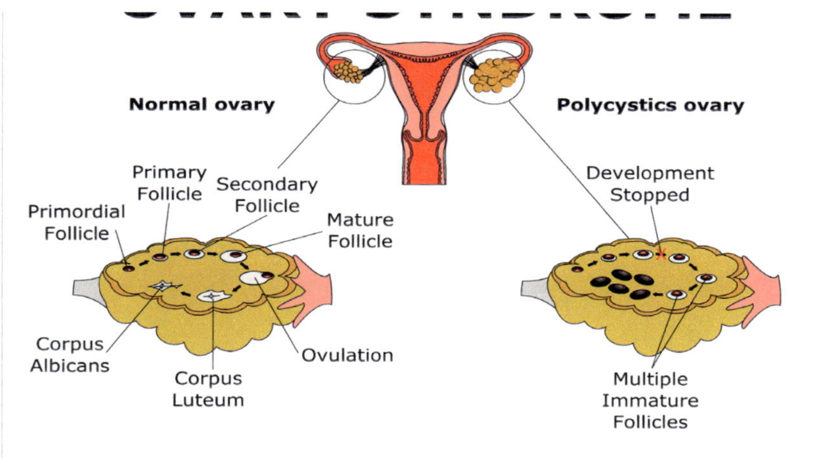

Figure 4.19. Polycystic ovary syndrome (PCOS).

Source: https://1.bp.blogspot.com/-0WzI8WQK4eM/ XvwSP4n5pWI/AAAAAAAAAgk/ VGPZlmeta RwfQauYt6jv 3PHKCi1k8fjM ACLcBGAsYHQ/s1600/polycystic-ovary- syndrome-pcos-explained.png.

The impact of such hormonal disruption is not limited to fertility but penetrates into metabolic health and predisposition to insulin resistance. Identifying the role of sex hormones in endocrine disorders is important for evolving patient care and creating gender-based treatment modalities. It is noted that the interaction of gender and hormonal regulation can have a significant impact on both disease progression and responsiveness to treatment, thus highlighting the need for more sensitized practice in endocrinology (Lauretta et al., 2018). Psychiatric disorders , such as anorexia nervosa (AN) also point to the sophisticated interplay between mental illness and endocrinology. AN patients typically manifest with extreme caloric deficiency, with significant disruption of endocrine function, including functional amenorrhea due to hypothalamic-pituitary-ovarian axis dysfunction. Endocrine changes can have lasting consequences on reproduction, affecting fertility as well as pregnancy complications. While some consequences can be reversed with recovery of the eating disorder, the potential for irreversible impact necessitates an understanding of the hormonal derangements involved in the pathophysiology. Consequently, the interconnection between endocrine function and mental health highlights the complexity of recurrent endocrine disorders and the need for interdisciplinarity in treatment approaches (Poterasu et al., 2020) (Figure 4.19).

4.6.2. Impact of Hormonal Imbalances

Hormonal imbalance can have serious implications for overall health, influencing a wide range of body processes. Imbalance is triggered by different factors like genetic constitutions, environmental exposures, and behavioral patterns. Hypothyroidism and hyperthyroidism are examples that show that alterations in thyroid hormone levels can lead to severe metabolic abnormalities. In hypothyroidism, the deficient production of thyroid hormone causes weight gain, lethargy, and depression, while hyperthyroidism induces symptoms , such as weight loss, agitation, and tachycardia. By having a complete appreciation of the biochemical mechanisms of these imbalances, researchers can better guide interventions aimed at reestablishing hormonal equilibrium, thus maximizing quality of life in those impacted.

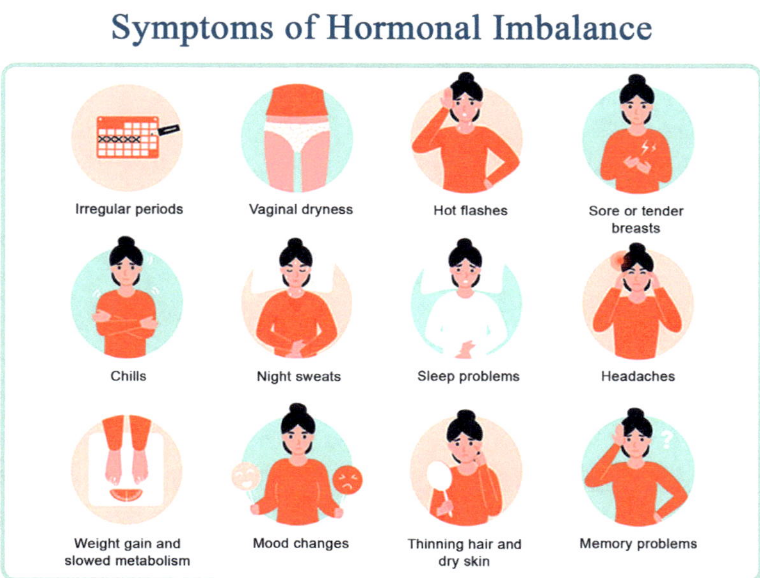

Figure 4.20. Symptoms-of-hormonal-imbalance.

Source: https://www.womenshealthnetwork.com/wp-content/uploads/2022/11/Symptoms-of-Hormonal-Imbalance-1.jpg.

These findings emphasize the necessity for continuous endocrinology research, especially in the case of the complex interaction between hormones and body functions. The complex interrelationship of hormonal imbalances with other conditions includes reproductive health as well in both males and females. In females, for instance, endocrine alterations that accompany the menstrual cycle can lead to premenstrual syndrome (PMS) or polycystic ovary syndrome (PCOS). They are characterized by irregular menstrual cycles, ovarian cysts, and elevated androgen levels, with signs including weight, acne, and excess hair growth. Men do not escape hormonal issues either, with testosterone imbalances leading to low desire, infertility, and muscle wasting. Research on how hormonal imbalance influences reproductive health offers a twofold opportunity for clinical and public health intervention. By treating and identifying these hormonal imbalances, clinicians are able to offer customized therapeutic treatments to improve reproductive function and health in the individual. Beyond their direct effect on health, hormonal imbalances also demonstrate more global systemic associations within the body that influence long-term diseases , such as obesity and diabetes. For example, insulin resistance resulting from chronic hyperinsulinemia leads to metabolic syndrome and type 2 diabetes. Pathophysiologic mechanisms involve complex interactions between insulin and hormonal processes, which ultimately regulate glucose metabolism and fat storage. Similarly, evidence suggests that other hormones, including cortisol, are also pivotal in regulating stress response and hunger, hence linking physical and emotional well-being. Understanding these complex hormonal pathways is essential to developing effective treatment paradigms. Furthermore, the influence of environmental factors , such as endocrine disruptors, on hormonal homeostasis must be addressed to mitigate long-term health effects. In doing so, such a synergy calls for the implementation of a multi-dimensional approach to addressing hormonal imbalance as well as the extensive influence on health and disease management (Aggarwala, 2024; Karim et al., 2025) (Figure 4.20).

4.6.3. Treatment Options for Endocrine Disorders

Endocrine disorders are best treated by several methods because they can possibly impact numerous physiological processes. Hormone replacement therapy is one of the commonly employed treatments, and it is utilized in numerous conditions, including hypothyroidism or adrenal insufficiency. This type of therapy alleviates symptoms and processes related to deficiency through the replacement of normal hormone levels. For instance, thyroid disease patients generally experience symptoms of fatigue and weight gain; hence, the application of synthetic thyroid hormone improves metabolic function and general health. Moreover, the need for differentiated patterns of treatment cannot be overstated, as patients respond differently based on their own levels of hormones, which illustrates the importance of individualized therapeutic interventions in the treatment of endocrine illnesses. Aside from hormone replacement therapy, pharmacologic management using targeted agents serves as an important second-line option for the treatment of many endocrine disorders. As an example, erectile dysfunction (ED) has phosphodiesterase type 5 (PDE5) inhibitors as the current therapeutic standard, which is effective through mechanisms of enhancing blood supply via nitric oxide signaling pathways. However, for patients who are refractory to PDE5 inhibitors, secondary treatments , such as intracorporeal injections or vacuum erection devices are also entertained (Benea et al., 2016). These therapies expand the array of available treatments with which clinicians are able to act using an effective method in managing the multifactorial pathophysiology of ED. Aside from this, current research looks for new pharmacological agents that may possess improved efficacy or fewer side effects, testimony to the dynamic evolution of endocrine treatment options. New treatments also point to the necessity for innovative thinking, particularly in managing disorders linked to hormonal imbalance, such as, Irritable Bowel Syndrome (IBS) and Inflammatory Bowel Disease (IBD). Research has indicated that hormones, especially those interacting with the gastrointestinal system, may play a crucial role in symptomatology, suggesting hormone-based therapies as potential treatments. Specifically, interventions targeting hormones like progesterone could ameliorate symptoms by restoring balance and addressing underlying mechanisms, rather than merely alleviating manifestations (Linson, 2013). It's a perspective that deflects attention to explaining the interactions of hormones and the regulatory mechanisms that result in endocrine disorders, giving an opening to novel therapeutic mechanisms to be employed in order to enhance patient outcomes in the long term.

Test Your Knowledge

1. Differentiate between primary, secondary, and tertiary endocrine disorders with suitable examples.
2. What are the causes and symptoms of hyperthyroidism and hypothyroidism?

SUMMARY

The study of endocrine physiology shows that hormones play central roles in regulating body processes and their workings are often mixed with the health implications. The relationship between prolonged sedentary behavior and cognitive function indicates the wide-ranging impact of hormones , such as brain-derived neurotrophic factor, dopamine, and serotonin. They are triggered by lifestyle modifiers that raise extreme health risks. The hypothesis assumes that interrupting extended sitting can enhance cognitive functions by modifying these hormonal levels and overall cognitive function. Thus, addressing such sedentary behaviors can have tangible and measurable effects on workplace effectiveness and mental well-being, justifying the activation of interventions geared toward addressing physiological well-being among office employees (Chandrasekaran et al., 2021). Furthermore, insulin is also a good illustration of how hormones not only modulate glucose homeostasis but also other anabolic and catabolic processes in the body. The ambivalence of insulin action, wherein low and high concentrations both can be harmful, exemplifies the complexity of endocrine communication. Hyperinsulinemia is a good representation of how imbalance in hormones can have severe health implications, such as, obesity, type 2 diabetes, and cardiovascular disease. Selective insulin responses reveal differential interference with signal pathways, the implications of which are pivotal to guide treatment intervention and life changes intended to regulate insulin levels optimally. This understanding promotes the relevance of ensuring hormonal homeostasis in managing overall well-being (Kolb et al., 2020). Lastly, the multifaceted mechanisms of hormone action present an avenue to understand action in endocrine physiology. From cognitive function via physical training to the metabolic action of insulin, the potential of hormonal interactions is vast. Emphasizing the function of attaining hormonal equilibrium through lifestyle alteration has the capacity to impact public health policy and clinical intervention alike. Future research will have to look into these mechanisms in greater detail, as well as their potential for disease treatment. By forming a holistic perspective of hormones and their effects, one can improve health outcomes, enhance thought processes, and negate the health effects of hormonal imbalance, thereby forming a holistic process of endocrine wellness and health.

The endocrine system entails a sophisticated interaction of glands that release hormones, which play a crucial role in the preservation of physiological homeostasis. Hormones are chemical messengers responsible for coordinating a diverse array of biological processes from metabolism to mood. An understanding of the subtle mechanisms by which these hormones function is the cornerstone of the field of endocrine physiology. Various hormones act by two major channels of signaling: the lipophilic hormones, which can diffuse through cell membranes and bind intracellular receptors, and hydrophilic hormones, which bind surface receptors to trigger cascades of intracellular activity. This duplicity exists because hormonal communication is diverse and relies upon receptor specificity and signal transduction processes in regulating physiological response. Studies have further implicated the role of the gut microbiota on the endocrine regulation, namely through the microbiota-gut-brain axis, which highlights the interwoven nature of body systems. The trillions of microorganisms of the gut microbiome produce metabolites , such as SCFAs that can modulate neuro-endocrine function, suggesting a two-way effect between hormonal and gut health. It has been demonstrated in research that microbiota compositional variations can affect the biosynthesis of hormones like cortisol and insulin. Further, stress can affect this axis at any point in life, opening up the likelihood of drastic modifications in endocrine function. Thus, the understanding of microbiota interactions offers new opportunities for therapy against hormonal pathology and emphasizes the significance of dietary influence on hormonal balance (Cryan et al., 2019; Silva et al., 2020). Ultimately, the research into endocrine physiology and mechanisms of hormones opens up a rich brocade of interdisciplinary paradigms within which numerous factors converge. From the complex causal pathways of classical hormonal mechanisms to recent findings regarding microbiota interactions, the adaptable control of bodily processes is increasingly understood as a sophisticated interwoven composite of both internal and external influences. Although there has been remarkable progress in elucidating these relationships, many of the mechanisms are poorly characterized and offer avenues for further study. The repercussions of these discoveries extend far beyond the scientific community, as they could translate into novel treatments for diseases associated with hormonal disturbances, like metabolic syndromes and neuropsychiatric illnesses. By continuing to analyze the complex interactions within the endocrine system, scientists can build on our knowledge of health and disease pathways, opening the door to sophisticated interventions that capture this complexity.

KEY TERMS FROM THIS CHAPTER

- Adrenal cortex
- Endocrine glands
- Glucagon
- Homeostasis
- Hypothalamus
- Intracellular signaling
- Parathyroid hormone (PTH)
- Cortisol
- G protein-coupled receptors (GPCRs)
- Growth hormone (GH)
- Hormones
- Insulin
- Negative feedback
- Peptide hormones

CRITICAL THINKING QUESTIONS

1. **Which of the following hormones acts through an intracellular (nuclear) receptor?**
   a. Insulin
   b. Cortisol
   c. Glucagon
   d. Epinephrine
2. **The second messenger most commonly associated with G protein-coupled receptors is:**
   a. Calcium
   b. ATP
   c. Cyclic AMP (cAMP)
   d. Phospholipase A
3. **Which hormone is secreted by the posterior pituitary gland?**
   a. Growth hormone
   b. Prolactin
   c. Oxytocin
   d. ACTH
4. **What is the primary mechanism of action of peptide hormones?**
   a. Direct activation of nuclear transcription
   b. Binding to cytoplasmic receptors
   c. Binding to cell surface receptors and activating second messengers
   d. Diffusing through the membrane and altering DNA transcription directly
5. **Which of the following best describes negative feedback in endocrine regulation?**
   a. Hormone stimulates another hormone to increase secretion
   b. Hormone levels remain constant despite physiological needs
   c. Increased hormone levels inhibit further secretion
   d. Hormones are only secreted during stress

Short Answer Questions

1. What is a hormone? Give two examples of endocrine glands.
2. Differentiate between endocrine, paracrine, and autocrine signaling.
3. Name the second messenger systems used by peptide hormones.
4. What are the primary differences between steroid and peptide hormones in terms of receptor location and mechanism of action?
5. Which hormones are secreted by the anterior pituitary gland?
6. How does negative feedback regulate hormone levels? Give one example.
7. Discuss the regulation of blood glucose by insulin and glucagon, including their mechanisms of action.
8. Explain the synthesis, transport, and physiological actions of thyroid hormones.
9. Describe the hormonal response to stress, focusing on the adrenal medulla and cortex.

Answers to Critical Thinking Questions

1. (b); 2. (c); 3. (c); 4. (c); 5. (c).

REFERENCES

1. Herrera M, Mancera JM and Costas B (2019) The Use of Dietary Additives in Fish Stress Mitigation: Comparative Endocrine and Physiological Responses. Front. Endocrinol. 10:447. doi: 10.3389/fendo.2019.00447 (accessed on 28th June 2025).
2. Aggarwala, K. (2024). Pathological eye growth in myopia: A limited review on endocrine physiology for future research. *Physiology*. https://www.semanticscholar.org/paper/f25c51eea773607065f96c2d241a75582bbf6f0d (accessed on 28th June 2025).
3. Alcaino, C., Guccio, N., Miedzybrodzka, E. L., Quale, J. R., Davison, A., Smith, C. A., Overington, E., et al. (2025). Mechanisms of activation and serotonin release from human enterochromaffin cells. *bioRxiv*. https://www.semanticscholar.org/paper/477dea010d8306f4fc70f0570165b75a6cb32b71 (accessed on 28th June 2025).
4. Scheurink, A. J., Balkan, B., Strubbe, J. H., van Dijk, G., & Steffens, A. B. (1996). Overfeeding, autonomic regulation and metabolic consequences. *Cardiovascular drugs and therapy, 10 Suppl 1*, 263–273. https://doi.org/10.1007/BF00120496 (accessed on 28th June 2025).
5. Lauretta, R., Sansone, M., Sansone, A., Romanelli, F., & Appetecchia, M. (2018). Gender in Endocrine Diseases: Role of Sex Gonadal Hormones. *International journal of endocrinology, 2018*, 4847376. https://doi.org/10.1155/2018/4847376(accessed on 28th June 2025).
6. Inda, C., Armando, N. G., Dos Santos Claro, P. A., & Silberstein, S. (2017). Endocrinology and the brain: corticotropin-releasing hormone signaling. *Endocrine connections*, *6*(6), R99–R120. https://doi.org/10.1530/EC-17-0111 (accessed on 28th June 2025).
7. Gross, Timothy S.,Arnold, Beverly S.,Spulveda, Maria S.,McDonald, Kelly (2021). Relations of environmental contaminants, algal toxins, and diet with the reproductive success of American alligators on Florida Lakes. http://hdl.handle.net/1834/18957 (accessed on 28th June 2025).
8. Boer, H. M., Veerkamp, R. F., Beerda, B., & Woelders, H. (2010). Estrous behavior in dairy cows: identification of underlying mechanisms and gene functions. *Animal : an international journal of animal bioscience*, *4*(3), 446–453. https://doi.org/10.1017/S1751731109991169(accessed on 28th June 2025).
9. Benea, V., Georgescu, S. R., Mitran, C. I., Mitran, M., et al. (2016). The current treatment of erectile dysfunction. https://core.ac.uk/download/144552982.pdf (accessed on 28th June 2025).
10. Carosa, E., Jannini, E. A., & Lenzi, A. (2018). Thyroid hormone receptors and ligand, tissue distribution and sexual behavior. https://core.ac.uk/download/160052696.pdf (accessed on 28th June 2025).
11. Goldsworthy, G., Mullen, L., Opoku-Ware, K. and Chandrakant, S. (2003), Interactions between the endocrine and immune systems in locusts. Physiological Entomology, 28: 54-61. https://doi.org/10.1046/j.1365-3032.2003.00314.x (accessed on 28th June 2025).
12. Mabilleau, G., Pereira, M., & Chenu, C. (2018). Novel skeletal effects of glucagon-like peptide-1 (GLP-1) receptor agonists. *The Journal of endocrinology*, *236*(1), R29–R42. https://doi.org/10.1530/JOE-17-0278accessed on 28th June 2025).
13. Poterasu, M., Rowland, D. L., Ciobanu, C., & Fica, S. (2020). Anorexia Nervosa and Reproduction: Connecting Brain to Gonads. Journal of Mind and Medical Sciences, 7(1), 1-8. https://doi.org/10.22543/7674.71.P18 (accessed on 28th June 2025).

14. Cryan, J. F., O'Riordan, K. J., Cowan, C. S. M., Sandhu, K. V., Bastiaanssen, T. F. S., Boehme, M., Codagnone, M. G., et al. (2019). The microbiota-gut-brain axis. *Physiological Reviews, 99*, 1877–2013. https://doi.org/10.1152/physrev.00018.2018 (accessed on 28th June 2025).

15. Di Pietro, G., Forcucci, F., & Chiarelli, F. (2023). Endocrine disruptor chemicals and children's health. *International Journal of Molecular Sciences, 24*. https://www.semanticscholar.org/paper/492db7e660f5ee6e846c7e397cd7b42b71330f5d (accessed on 28th June 2025).

16. Elendu, C., Amaechi, D. C., Elendu, T. C., Amaechi, E. C., Elendu, I. D., Ajakaye, A. A., Ubi, E. S., et al. (2025). The pump, the exchanger, and the holy spirit: Tracing the 40-year evolution of the ouabain-Na^+ pump endocrine system concept. *Annals of Medicine & Surgery*. https://www.semanticscholar.org/paper/12db3f18cf4ec93cb20755483514fced7d3eff5f (accessed on 28th June 2025).

17. Lisa DeLisle Judith Estrine (2006). Stress: Putting the brain back into medicine. An Interdisciplinary Workshop of the INTERNATIONAL LONGEVITY CENTER–USA https://core.ac.uk/download/71356692.pdf (accessed on 28th June 2025).

18. Frøbert, A. M., Toews, J., Nielsen, C., Brohus, M., Kindberg, J., Jessen, N., Frøbert, O., et al. (2022). Differential changes in circulating steroid hormones in hibernating brown bears: Preliminary conclusions and caveats. *Physiological and Biochemical Zoology, 95*, 365–378. https://www.semanticscholar.org/paper/8303dffcdee14d5af3a5b5c50ec4f3280aab14e9 (accessed on 28th June 2025).

19. Gasser, P. J., & Lowry, C. A. (2018). Organic cation transporter 3: A cellular mechanism underlying rapid, non-genomic glucocorticoid regulation of monoaminergic neurotransmission, physiology, and behavior. https://core.ac.uk/download/213087190.pdf (accessed on 28th June 2025).

20. Zubeldia-Brenner, L., Roselli, C. E., Recabarren, S. E., Gonzalez Deniselle, M. C., & Lara, H. E. (2016). Developmental and Functional Effects of Steroid Hormones on the Neuroendocrine Axis and Spinal Cord. *Journal of neuroendocrinology, 28*(7), 10.1111/jne.12401. https://doi.org/10.1111/jne.12401(accessed on 28th June 2025).

21. Indarto, D., & Izawa, M. (2017). Steroid hormones and endocrine disruptors: Recent advances in receptor–mediated actions. https://core.ac.uk/download/12345745.pdf (accessed on 28th June 2025).

22. Karim, M. A., Park, C., Cho, H. J., Sebastian, A. E., Ryu, C., Yoon, J., & Kim, Y. J. (2025). Leveraging AlphaFold models to predict androgenic effects of endocrine-disrupting chemicals through zebrafish androgen receptor analysis. *Toxicology Mechanisms and Methods*. https://www.semanticscholar.org/paper/9e1492b9ea9cd21d8c0daa23c007368125fae22a (accessed on 28th June 2025).

23. Kolb, H., Kempf, K., Röhling, M., & Martin, S. (2020). Insulin: Too much of a good thing is bad. *BMC Medicine, 18*. https://doi.org/10.1186/s12916-020-01688-6 (accessed on 28th June 2025).

24. Koyama, T., Saeed, U., Rewitz, K., & Halberg, K. V. (2025). The integrative physiology of hormone signaling: Insights from insect models. *Physiology*. https://www.semanticscholar.org/paper/11e06865d14f34d6e5ae56ae6ab1de65400b8790 (accessed on 28th June 2025).

25. Linson, E. A. (2013). The interplay between hormones and irritable bowel disease. https://open.bu.edu/bitstream/2144/12149/6/Linson_Elyse_2013_nosig_nocv.pdf (accessed on 28th June 2025).

26. Patwardhan, K. (2008). Concepts of human physiology in Ayurveda. https://core.ac.uk/download/pdf/87482.pdf (accessed on 28th June 2025).

27. Silva, Y. P., Bernardi, A., & Frozza, R. L. (2020). The role of short-chain fatty acids from gut microbiota in gut-brain communication. *Frontiers in Endocrinology, 11*. https://doi.org/10.3389/fendo.2020.00025 (accessed on 28th June 2025).

28. Szukiewicz, D. (2023). Insight into the potential mechanisms of endocrine disruption by dietary phytoestrogens in the context of the etiopathogenesis of endometriosis. *International Journal of Molecular Sciences, 24*. https://www.semanticscholar.org/paper/93b020a2c4279f1ea9c5f0d383a920cb3b87de9a (accessed on 28th June 2025).

29. Yaglova, N., Obernikhin, S., Nazimova, S., & Timokhina, E. (2024). Developmental exposure to endocrine disruptor DDT alters parameters of sex steroid production in male rats. *Russian Journal of Biological Physics and Chemistry*. https://www.semanticscholar.org/paper/37a51d08200170b8b49b3a73240c45dffa7b97b7 (accessed on 28th June 2025).

METABOLIC PHYSIOLOGY AND ENERGY BALANCE

5

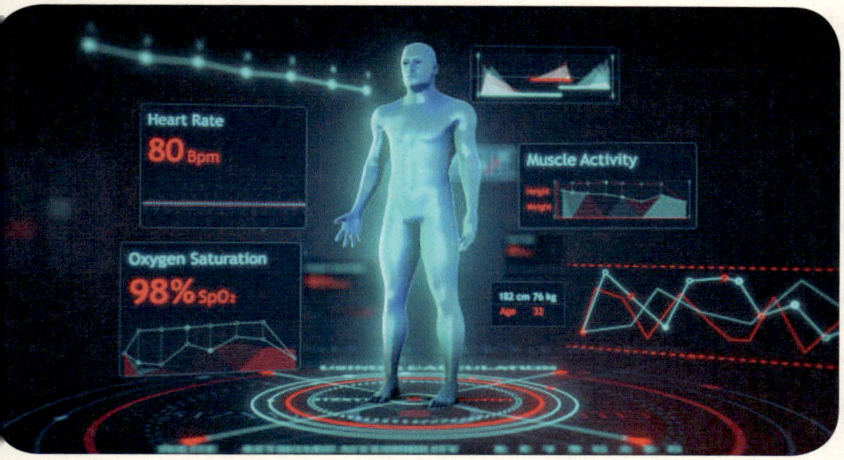

LEARNING OBJECTIVES

After studying this chapter, you will be able to:

1. Describe the basics of metabolism.
2. Explain the energy sources for metabolism.
3. Discuss the energy expenditure.
4. Define the hormonal regulation of metabolism.
5. Learn about factors affecting energy balance.
6. Understand the metabolic disorders.

Introduction

Metabolic physiology and energy balance knowledge are also critical for solving the intricate mechanisms determining how food is converted into energy by living things and for how homeostasis is controlled. Basically, metabolic physiology investigates the biochemical processes of substrate metabolism by carbohydrates, fats, and proteins to fulfill cellular energy requirements. The energy intake and expenditure balance is what determines energy balance, a state in which the number of calories ingested is equal to the number of calories spent during basal metabolism, activity, and thermogenesis. Energy balance is important to growth, reproduction, and health because positive and negative energy imbalances have undesirable outcomes like obesity or malnutrition. When learning metabolic physiology, one must consider external factors like environmental conditions and diet that influence energy balance. The literature highlights the role of photoperiod on metabolic rates and feeding behavior in general, and particularly in animals like the Japanese quail, where variation in light exposure significantly impacts weight gain and energy considerations. As an example, broilers grown under prolonged photoperiods exhibited greater weight gains, driven largely by changes in the supply of food and metabolic activity as a result of exposure duration. These findings illustrate the ways in which the ambient environment serves multifaceted roles in affecting metabolic functions and suggest that energy balance cannot be adequately understood unless one takes into consideration the multifaceted interactions between biology and environmental conditions (Boon et al., 2000). The exercise contribution to energy balance also warrants significant consideration, particularly concerning the way that exercise impacts metabolic responses and appetite regulation. Evidence has shown that post fasting exercise can result in a different physiological response than post-feeding exercise. More specifically, postprandial exercise has been shown to be more suppressive of appetite than fasted exercise but without generating significant differences in total energy intake between trials. This occurs as a result of the timing of exercise in relation to meal times, which influences energy balance, once more making it more complex to interpret metabolic physiology (Deighton et al., 2012). Thus, environmental factors and lifestyle, and exercise patterns are responsible for determining a person's energy balance and metabolic status (Figure 5.1).

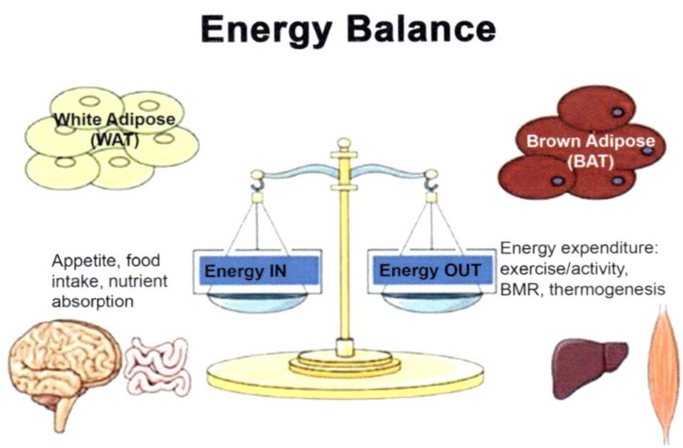

Figure 5.1. Energy balance.

Source: https://external-content.duckduckgo.com/iu/?u=https%3A%2F%2Fbing.com%2Fth%3Fid%3DOIP.z9ub7qapl3nx9ME7Q5PtewHaFj%26cb%3Dthvnextc2%26pid%3DApi&f=1&ipt=0c5521185dcf92eb5825480e432723fb832ac6fc661b489244910001feb0e157.

Definition of Metabolic Physiology

Metabolic physiology is an essential science regarding how living organisms obtain energy from diet and how, in the process, the overall health and functioning of an organism are influenced. It entails the study of biochemical processes that form life, including catabolism and anabolism, which play a vital role in maintaining homeostasis in the biological system. As living things engage with the world around them, the efficacy of these metabolic processes is crucial to energy equilibrium—the equilibrium between energy intake and energy output. The discipline highlights the importance of micro and macro-interactions, from cellular metabolism to body system function, and how energy production and consumption regulate biology. By exploring metabolic physiology in detail, researchers can uncover intricate relationships that define health, disease, and the evolutionary advantage of various metabolic modes and thus construct an integrative framework for the examination of energy dynamics in living organisms. Central to the exploration of metabolic physiology is the concept of carbon use efficiency (CUE), which is a measure of how effectively microbes use substrates to yield biomass under varying environmental conditions.

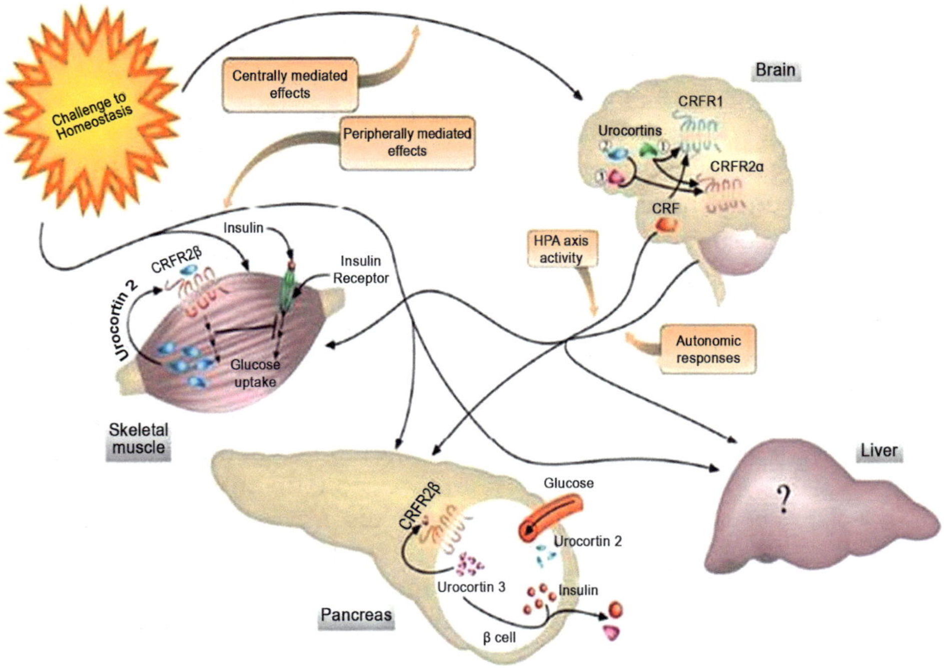

Figure 5.2. Physiology of metabolism and energy.

Source: https://cf.ppt-online.org/files1/slide/7/7SlrZPiWoDBz21av39H6yqh4wVe5mnKXcbLuMAYkj/slide-2.jpg.

This conceptual framework can be scaled up to larger metabolic processes by illustrating the dependency of energy loss and biomass formation at different ecological scales. CUE is separated into three definitions: population-scale, community-scale, and ecosystem-scale efficiency, each of which defines different yet complementary aspects of metabolic behavior. Population-scale CUE concerns how certain microbial taxa perform under specific metabolic and thermodynamic regimes. On the other hand, CUE at the community level examines gross biomass production versus substrate assimilation within brief periods of time, with a focus on current energy usage as opposed to recycling. Utilizing these definitions of CUE in the overall framework of metabolic physiology gives essential insights into terrestrial carbon flows and the ecological implications of energy balance, hence making it a crucial element of the field (Geyer et al., 2016). Secondarily, coupling metabolic physiology with energy balance yields a more general concept of homeostasis, the body's capacity to maintain constant internal conditions despite variable external conditions. This holistic consideration necessitates one's consideration of the interaction of various physiological processes and how they yield energy input and output. The theoretical concept of homeostasis is that energy intake must equal energy expenditure for physiological constancy. When disturbed, it is possible to make adjustments in any component of this equation to restore equilibrium, rather than looking at the initial disturbance alone. This speaks to the necessity of systems biology, breaking with reductionism, in order to make stronger connections between biochemical machinery and clinical utility. Understanding these principles is a step towards new medical techniques and improved health since it encompasses fundamental processes that define energy expenditure across life (Spasojevic, 2011) (Figure 5.2).

Importance of Energy Balance in Human Health

Energy balance is a fundamental principle behind comprehending human health, particularly in relation to weight regulation and metabolism. Energy balance is achieved when calories consumed from food equal calories lost through basal metabolic processes and physical exercise. This balance must be set in maintaining the body at a healthy weight; imbalance—whether through excessive caloric consumption or insufficient energy output—will lead to obesity or malnutrition. Obesity specifically is a major public health issue, requiring extensive knowledge of the countless factors impacting energy balance, such as, behavioral, environmental, and genetic factors. The modern-day obesity epidemic points towards the importance of tackling these factors collectively towards optimal weight control and overall well-being. This multi-dimensional approach is required for the formulation of interventions that solve the root causes of energy imbalance and induce improved lifestyles in varied populations (McMinn, 1984). Moreover, the interaction between sleep, circadian rhythms, and energy balance has emerged as a field of utmost significance within the discipline of metabolic physiology. Research shows that sleep disruptions significantly impact metabolic health, and affect insulin sensitivity and hunger regulation. These disturbances have the capacity to disturb energy balance by provoking weight gain and increasing the risk of developing diabetes. For instance, sleep loss over time can lead to alterations in hormonal regulation, which provokes increased hunger and the urge to eat high-calorie foods. Sleep-disordered breathing, an incredibly common disease in millions of people, has also been associated with metabolic dysregulation. To identify the long-term impact on energy balance and health, these sleep disturbances need to be restored. As we progress with these interactions, we realize that the integration of sleep science into research in metabolic health can potentially provide more holistic interventions for obesity and diabetes prevention (Arble et al., 2015). Second, interventions aimed at preserving healthy energy balance must take into consideration the multifactorial interaction between eating habits, activity, and lifestyle factors. Encouraging a diet that consists of a large proportion of whole foods, with active transport, can facilitate a more positive energy balance. Interventions should also, though, respond to individual differences, including genetic influence and metabolic differences. The studies emphasize that metabolism may be defined by thousands of variables, including the activity of specific enzymes and tissues in energy expenditure. Recognition of these nuances lies at the heart of devising personalized health plans that cater to distinctive metabolic signatures. Continued research into the mechanisms that control energy balance will improve our knowledge base for optimal promotion of ideal health and the prevention of obesity and metabolic disease and thereby build a healthier society (McMinn, 1984; Arble et al., 2015).

5.1. Basics of Metabolism

Learning Outcome

1. Describe the metabolism;
2. Focus on types of metabolism: catabolism and anabolism;
3. Learn about the role of enzymes in metabolic processes.

Metabolism is a biochemical process of reactions that convert food into energy to maintain the basic functions of the body. Understanding such processes is crucial for examining energy balance, caloric consumption versus expenditure. Metabolism is usually classified as catabolism or the breakdown of complex molecules for the release of energy and anabolism, or the building up of new compounds to form growth and repair. This dynamic interaction maintains homeostasis and enables the body to adjust to shifting energy requirements. Skeletal muscle, in particular, makes significant contributions to metabolic function. It is a focal point for glucose storage and uptake, thereby regulating overall energy balance. Creation of insulin signal transduction pathways, more so their coordination with metabolic substrates, is significant in effective determination of these mechanisms since disruption leads to metabolic diseases, thus the importance of further studies in metabolic pathways through studies like those presented in LaBarge et al., (2015). Increased metabolic disorder incidence, primarily in obesity and aging, stresses the importance of learning metabolic physiology. Type II Diabetes Mellitus, previously noted predominantly in adults, is now being diagnosed more commonly in children, indicating a disconcerting trend that is linked to environmental and lifestyle determinants. Heterogeneity of this condition arises from its involvement being modulated by combined genetic and environmental factors, making it a multifactorial disorder. Modifiable risk factors , such as diet, physical activity, and obesity, have primary roles in the etiology of Type II Diabetes, with a need for preventive intervention in young people. Focusing intervention strategies on environmental modification—e.g., improved diet, increased exercise—can significantly reduce the incidence of the condition. This proactive step would decrease the co-morbid load of Type II Diabetes, as discussed in Kapke (2015). These metabolic complications need serious attention to energy balance and how that relates to health outcomes. A clear comprehension of the metabolism and the regulation that takes place is needed for proper planning of treatment for metabolic disorders. Investigation of the acetylation of insulin signal transducing proteins, for instance, yields valuable insight into the dysfunctions underlying insulin resistance. The interface between such biochemical alterations and glucose metabolism reveals key pathways that could be targeted to offer therapeutic intervention. As metabolic disorders increasingly rise globally, especially amongst vulnerable populations, the need to counteract underlying metabolic dysfunctions becomes progressively urgent. This research not only contributes to scholarship but also informs practical strategies for improving long-term health implications of metabolic diseases, eventually helping public health initiatives towards improved well-being (Figure 5.3).

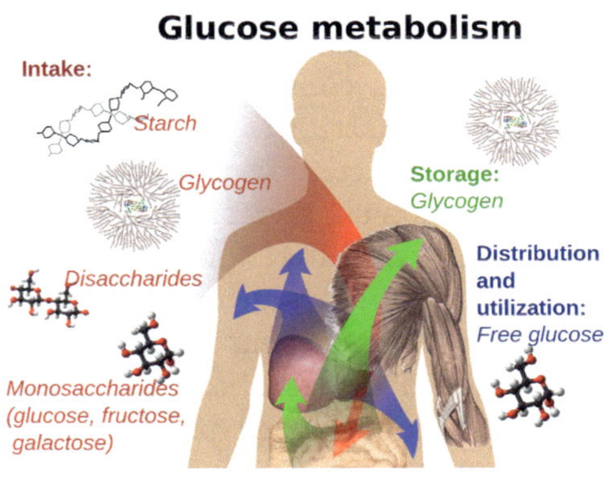

Figure 5.3. Glucose-metabolism.

Source: https://i1.wp.com/gettinghealthier.com/wp-content/uploads/2015/06/Glucose-metabolism.png?ssl=1.

5.1.1. Definition of Metabolism

Metabolism is a heterogeneous collection of biochemical processes by which living things maintain life, into two broad categories of which are catabolism and anabolism. Catabolism is the breakdown of molecules to provide energy, and anabolism is the construction of all the materials needed for the development and restoration of cells. The balance between the two processes ensures energy homeostasis, allowing organisms to adapt to variations in energy demand and nutrient availability. Such dependence not only highlights the effectiveness of metabolic pathways but also the activity of various enzymes and hormones regulating metabolic processes. For instance, insulin activates anabolic pathways to enable the uptake and storage of glucose, while glucagon and adrenaline trigger catabolic pathways to mobilize stores of energy under fasting or stress conditions. This interplay is complex and offers essential information regarding metabolic physiology and its applicability towards the general energy balance. Cellular-wise, the term "metabolism" is expanded to encompass a collection of environment-condition- and cell-requirement-dependent metabolic phenotypes. Overflow metabolism is one of them, in which cells , such as Escherichia coli develop under fermentative modes even in the presence of oxygen, yielding metabolic byproducts. The shift in metabolism is a compensatory mechanism to overcome constraints by high cellular macromolecular concentration and constraint of resource allocation characteristic of the protein allocation constraint in cellular physiology. By the creation of equilibrium between oxidative phosphorylation and fermentation, the organism is able to modulate metabolic strategies for the optimization of energy production under different environments. The flexibility not only emphasizes the metabolism's dynamism of pathways but also highlights the necessity for the appreciation of metabolic flexibility with respect to energy balance, particularly under fluctuating dietary conditions. Moreover, metabolism efficiency is also made complex by microbial carbon use efficiency (CUE), a key parameter governing greater ecological and biogeochemical processes. CUE is the percentage of carbon retained in microbial biomass against carbon substrate consumed, showing varying scales of efficiency: population, community, and ecosystem levels. These account for the complexities of relationships governing energy transfer in ecosystems, affecting soil organic matter processes and ecosystem productivity. Because CUE combines the internal limitations along with the external environmental factors, CUE is a critical step in determining the ecological impact of microbial metabolism in carbon cycling. By understanding the intricate definitions and roles of metabolism, researchers can better quantify and model energy balance across a variety of biological and ecological systems, expanding our understanding of metabolic physiology's role in regulating global carbon fluxes and ecosystem health (Geyer et al., 2016; Vazquez & Oltvai, 2016) (Figure 5.4).

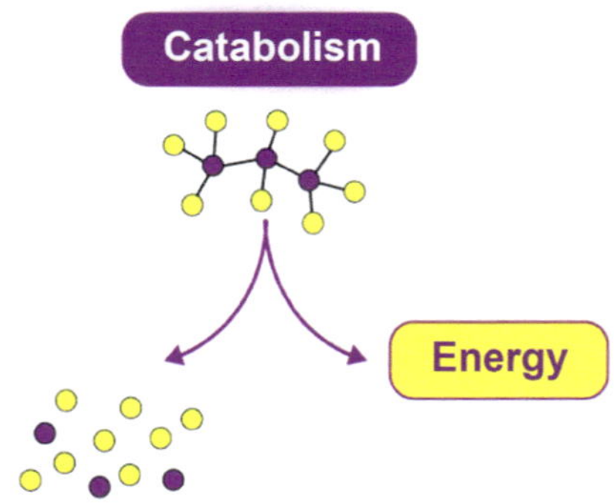

Figure 5.4. Catabolism.

Source: https://external-content.duckduckgo.com/iu/?u=https%3A%2F%2Fcdn1.byjus.com%2Fwp-content%2Fuploads%2F2017%2F08%2FCatabolism-1-700x351.png&f=1&nofb=1&ipt=414d0ec1d531a5c47ba3243e0cfce6130e9343b29865f20a60eb291271499e45.

5.1.2. Types of Metabolism: Catabolism and Anabolism

The intricate interaction between anabolism and catabolism forms the very foundation of metabolic physiology, which is paramount to the control of energy balance within the body. Catabolism, which involves the breakdown of complex molecules into simpler ones, is significant in order to supply the energy necessary to sustain cellular processes. This energy, primarily in the form of adenosine triphosphate (ATP), is produced during carbohydrate, fat, and protein catabolism. In fasting or periods of severe exercise, catabolic processes are particularly marked, as the body tries to break down stored energy in an effort to fulfill short-term needs. Anabolism, in contrast, is the biosynthetic reactions that construct larger, more complex molecules from simpler ones, employed particularly to facilitate growth, repair, and tissue maintenance.

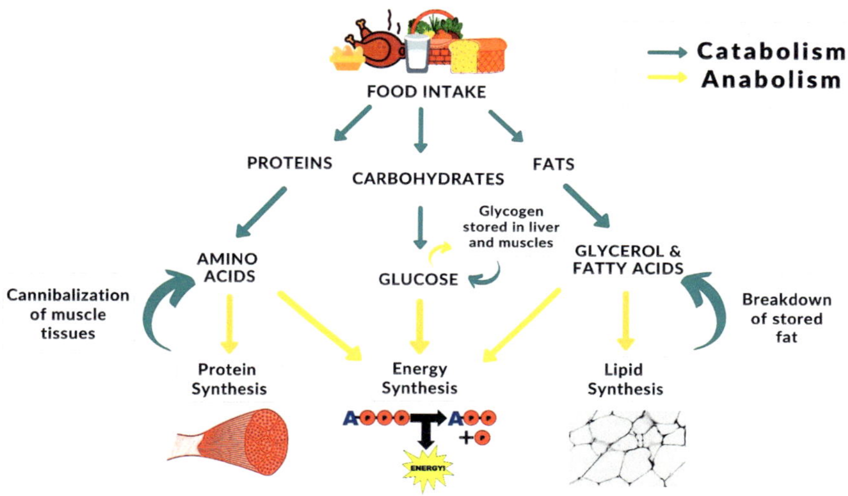

Figure 5.5. Catabolism and anabolism.

Source: https://external-content.duckduckgo.com/iu/?u=https%3A%2F%2Fwww.biologyonline.com%2Fwp-content%2Fuploads%2F2019%2F10%2FCatabolism-and-Anabolism-diagram.jpg&f=1&nofb=1&ipt=698a3c2a9aca1c499e883ed753b89f42c92f95cf9d70b724f0d9475ecb97c306.

Thus, these two metabolic processes need to be learned so that one learns how energy is extracted from food and utilized for body processes. Anabolism vs catabolism is not related to metabolism alone but has significant repercussions on both the health and well-being of an individual. During growth or recuperative states, e.g., adolescent existence or following exercise muscle repair, anabolic functioning is preferred in order to construct new proteins and repair tissues. Hyper catabolism, on the other hand, can lead to a deleterious state of cachexia, frequently observed in chronic disease, in which muscle wasting occurs at a shocking pace. This group is particularly susceptible to such imbalances, which result in conditions like sarcopenia, characterized by progressive loss of skeletal muscle mass. These effects can be mitigated by interventions resulting in an anabolic state, i.e., resistance training and maximal protein intake. Thus, interventions to optimize metabolic balance are of utmost importance for healthy aging and improving the quality of life, supporting the validation that metabolic health is a prime determinant in world well-being (Hayes

& Cribb, 2008). In Chinese medicine, paradigms parallel to those of modern metabolic thinking do exist, wherein dualities—catabolic and anabolic processes—are considered relative to constitutional medicine. This perspective focuses on the need for individual metabolic responses to food intake and activities and illustrates how unique constitutions determine the effectiveness of metabolism. For example, the intake and storage of Qi and body fluids are indicative of metabolic processes like catabolism and anabolism, suggesting a wholistic process in attaining health. The personalized application of this philosophy assures that dietary and exercise regimens need to consider individual differences to optimize metabolic function. Research on these integrative strategies may also provide more insight into how to improve metabolic function in other populations, emphasizing the potential benefits of employing individualized strategies for maintaining optimal health and even preventing metabolically linked diseases (Kim & Pham., 2009) (Figure 5.5).

5.1.3. Role of Enzymes in Metabolic Processes

Enzymes play a fundamental role in energizing metabolic reactions required to sustain energy homeostasis in the body. Such biochemical catalysts significantly accelerate chemical reactions, allowing metabolic pathways to operate with high efficiency and respond to varying demands for energy. Each enzyme is specific to certain substrates, catalyzing distinct biochemical reactions that constitute higher-order metabolic networks. For instance, during hypoxia, the organism requires a subtle balance between oxygen demand and supply to maintain cellular function. The enzyme nitric oxide synthase (NOS), which catalyzes the synthesis of nitric oxide, is one such example in that it causes vasodilation and enhanced blood flow to counteract tissue oxygen levels. Therefore, the intricate relationship between enzymes and metabolic reactions speaks for their critical function in maintaining physiological homeostasis, particularly when exposed to conditions of stress on energy homeostasis (Dyson et al., 2013). Secondly, exercise adaptations are closely related to enzymatic activity in skeletal muscle, demonstrating the considerable impact of enzymes on metabolic efficiency. Physical exercise causes an increase in the expression of metabolic enzymes, and this is primarily regulated at the transcription level. This regulation is done through the action of histone deacetylases (HDACs), and HDAC5 is focused on, which binds to transcription factors necessary for the expression of metabolic genes. Inhibition and nuclear exportation of HDAC5 by exercise, mediated by kinases , such as AMP-activated protein kinase, increases the transcription of energy metabolic genes. These enzymatic changes point to the plasticity of skeletal muscle in response to exercise, resulting in better energy homeostasis and overall metabolic well-being (McGee, 2007). So, not just do enzymes catalyze fundamental processes of metabolism, they also manifest the body's ability to adjust to changed energy needs in molecular terms. In addition to their role in traditional metabolic processes, enzymes also control how cells respond to stress in the environment, such as, fluctuations in the oxygen level. An excellent example of this kind of response is nitric oxide synthase, whose activity has a critical role in the control of blood flow during hypoxia. Through induction of vasodilation, nitric oxide promotes increased oxygen delivery to the tissues, augmenting the body's attempt to compensate for energy deficiency due to decreased oxygen. Furthermore, metabolic modulation induced by nitric oxide involves cellular energy expenditure adjustments to ensure optimal consumption of substrates that are available. This dual role of enzymes, and most importantly in the generation of nitric oxide, illustrates their key function in metabolic and physiological adaptation. Understanding the mechanisms helps enhance our comprehensibility as to how enzymatic functions are precisely entangled with maintaining metabolic physiology and energy homeostasis, especially under periods of physiological stress (Dyson et al., 2013).

Test Your Knowledge

1. What is the difference between anabolic and catabolic pathways in metabolism?
2. Describe the role of ATP in metabolic reactions.

5.2. Energy Sources for Metabolism

Learning Outcome

1. Explain the macronutrients: carbohydrates, proteins, and fats;
2. Define the micronutrients and their role in energy production;
3. Learn about the role of water in metabolic processes.

Understanding of substrates for energy metabolism constitutes the foundation for the science of metabolic physiology and energy homeostasis. Metabolism employs an array of substrates, primarily carbohydrates, lipids, and proteins, as energy sources for various physiological activities. Carbohydrates, being the first choice for energy, are readily mobilized through glycolysis to provide an immediate release of energy for utilization as and when needed. On the other hand, fats are employed in prolonged low-intensity activities and yield more ATP per gram of substance than carbohydrates, further solidifying their value in energy production. Proteins are generally a resort of last resort for energy, being catabolized only after other sources of energy are exhausted. The interaction and hierarchy of these sources of energy not only influence the energy balance of an organism but also potentially act as a proxy for the metabolic status of an organism, highlighting the importance of understanding metabolic pathways and their regulation. Lipid metabolism, a significant source of energy in physiological situations, is a key function regulated by nuclear receptors. Research with model organisms, e.g., C. elegans, has illuminated the means by which nuclear receptors, including NHR-49, control gene expression involved in various metabolic processes. These receptors control energy balance by virtue of their capacity to manage lipid binding, degradation, and remodeling. Most notably, studies have revealed that NHR-49 also influences mitochondrial biogenesis, a critical process for energy production within cells. NHR-49 co-factors identification has revealed insights into the regulatory mechanisms of NHR-49, demonstrating how various signals from various tissues intersect to govern appropriate transcriptional responses for the maintenance of metabolic homeostasis (Pathare, 2011). All this precise information can be utilized to guide metabolically directed therapeutics. In addition to the intrinsic regulation of metabolism, environmental stressors outside of the organism have also been found to affect energy metabolism. For instance, heat stress can lead to increased metabolic demand and energy imbalance in poultry that would need adaptive adjustments to mitigate negative effects. Alteration of feeding habits, altering nutrient intake timing or composition, has been shown to reduce the heat load under hot conditions (Syafwan et al., 2011). By enabling maximum nutrient utilization and minimal energy costs for thermoregulation and digestion, such responses can serve to optimize the overall health and effectiveness of affected species. This convergence of environmental stress with metabolic response reveals the multidimensional dynamics that govern energy intake in biological systems and emphasizes the ongoing relevance of inquiry into adaptive response across contexts of metabolic physiology (Figure 5.6).

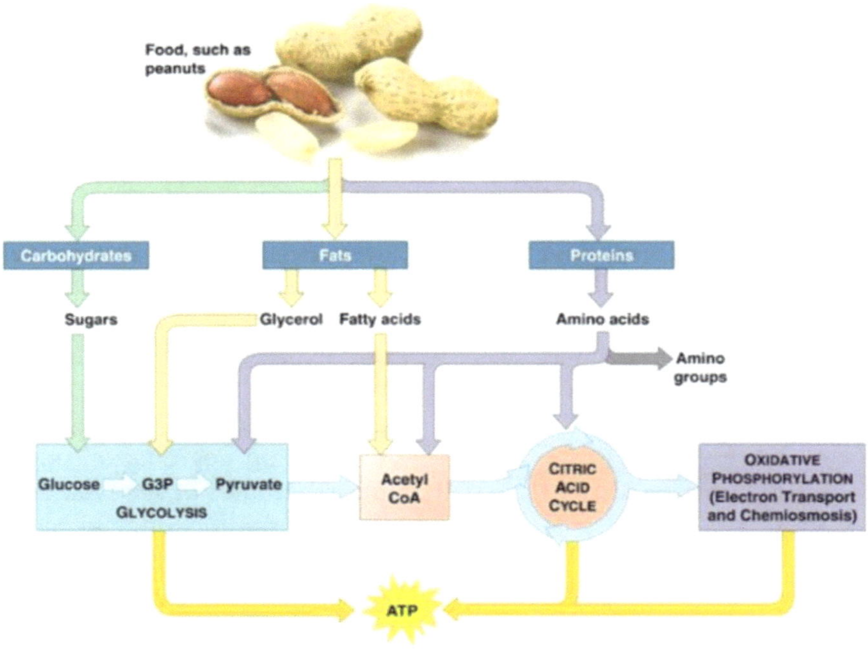

Figure 5.6. The metabolism of energy sources.

Source: https://image1.slideserve.com/2594015/v-the-metabolism-of-energy-sources-l.jpg.

5.2.1. Macronutrients: Carbohydrates, Proteins, and Fats

The energy balance in the human body relies greatly on three major macronutrients, namely carbohydrates, proteins, and fats, and all of them play important roles in metabolic physiology. Carbohydrates are especially essential as they serve as a key source of energy, mainly during high-level exercise. According to the International Olympic Committee, athletes should consume sufficient carbohydrate-rich foods that enhance recovery and performance, noting on balanced diet (Price, 2021). However, studies have indicated that the majority of athletes, particularly those competing in some college sports, do not meet these carbohydrate consumption guidelines, which will lower their energy reserves and overall performance. Therefore, adequate carbohydrate consumption is important for athletes and reflects a broader need for nutritional sensitivity across various populations that are active. Proteins are of great importance among macronutrients, particularly due to their roles in muscle repair and synthesis. They are made up of amino acids, the constituent building blocks required for various physiological functions, e.g., hormone secretion and immune function. During energy balance, protein can also serve as an alternative source of energy during long-term exercises or poor caloric intake. Most recent research has shown that collegiate athletes have a propensity to exceed protein recommendations, without necessarily being directly associated with increased performance or recovery (Price, 2021). This result points to a common misconception that the higher protein intake proportionally increases one's sports ability. Instead, a more balanced approach prioritizing total macronutrient distribution could promote better metabolic function and energy balance. Fats are generally misunderstood whenever they are brought up, when referring to macronutrients, since they are associated with negative health conditions. However, they are critical constituents of the body, maintaining hormonal balance and providing a compact source of energy that suits low to moderate-level exercise. The recommended intake of fat among exercising populations is typically 15-20% of total energy intake, but many athletes may be above this amount, with potential implications for performance and metabolic health (Price, 2021). Also, incorrect facts concerning fats, largely based on media coverage, can hinder individuals from understanding their complex role in energy metabolism. A better balanced understanding of fats is thus needed in the promotion of a balanced diet that addresses both energy needs and general health, and accordingly, education must address these myths assertively (Figure 5.7).

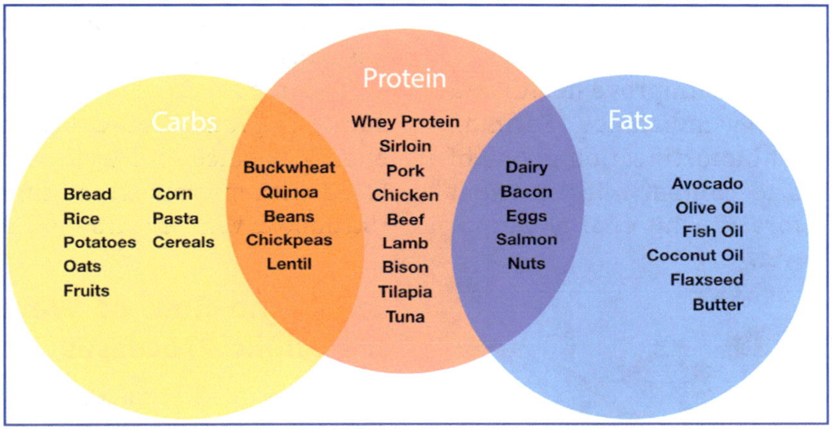

Figure 5.7. The macronutrients: carbohydrates, proteins, and fats.

Source: https://external-content.duckduckgo.com/iu/?u=https%3A%2F%2F1.bp.blogspot.com%2F-BriN8OW3i74%2FV5ggHkcVSZI%2FAAAAAAAAAiQY%2FNKKBbZQNNRQ2RwT5DIu75-vmPBMZZHDcACLcB%2Fs1600%2F Macronutrients%252BProtein%25252C%252BFat%252 Band%252BCarbohydrates.n.2.jpg&f=1&nofb= 1&ipt=7ee2df5f1ed8bd4fe7990371f82427d4c3fd5d3fe8cf29610da37040346f20ec.

5.2.2. Micronutrients and Their Role in Energy Production

Micronutrients play a central role in energy production within the context of metabolic physiology and energy balance. Essential vitamins and minerals serve as cofactors for an array of biochemical reactions, particularly those involved in cellular respiration and energy metabolism. For instance, B-vitamins B1, B6, and B9 are pivotal for carbohydrate, protein, and fat metabolism to be able to transform macronutrients into ATP, the cells' universal currency of energy. With below-requisite levels of these micronutrients, metabolic activities are hampered, leading to lowered energy output and general metabolic function. With the situation of concealed hunger, which encompasses over two billion individuals globally, highlighting the overriding importance of adequacy in micronutrients, it is understood that addressing micronutrient deficiency is required to guarantee energy homeostasis and optimal physiological functions among individuals globally (Strobbe & Van Der Straeten, 2018). In addition, the mechanism of action for micronutrients does not solely lie in energy production but also regulates and controls overall metabolism and homeostasis. Micronutrients are key to ensuring enzymatic activity balance as well as assisting processes within the cell that influence energy equilibrium. B-vitamins, for instance, are part of coenzyme formation that is indispensable in the Krebs cycle and oxidative phosphorylation, where energy is produced by the efficient conversion of substrates. Insufficient intake of these vitamins leads to metabolic disorders with symptoms of fatigue and reduced physical performance. Hence, understanding the intricacies of micronutrient functions and interactions with metabolic pathways can inform nutritional interventions to improve health and avert diseases of energy imbalance (Sarmidi, 2012). The concept of biofortification is one of the promising ways to combat micronutrient malnutrition, therefore raising energy output at the population level.

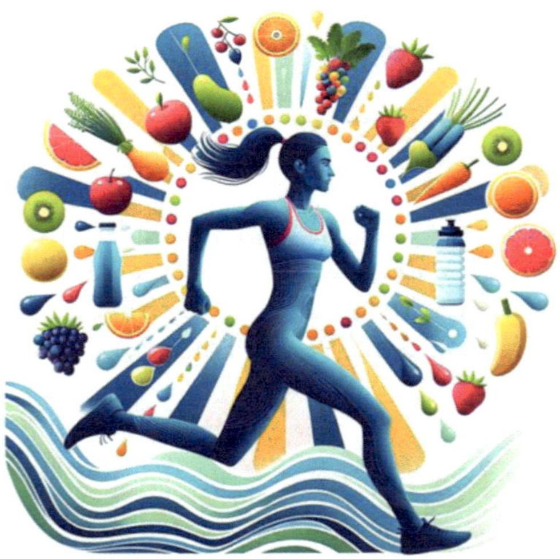

Figure 5.8. The role of micronutrients and hydration in physical performance.

Source: https://external-content.duckduckgo.com/iu/?u=https%3A%2F%2Ftse3.mm.bing.net%2Fth%3Fid%3DOIP.5H7K2jX2wv-bxPZlHp71DAHaHa%26pid%3DApi&f=1&ipt=a44e6ff6b28cbe5f22ed6b6313f8c18a2d4932e9e5bbbf37cad83b3a21a7f7f3.

Enhancing the content of micronutrients in staple food through breeding or genetic modification can enable public health programs to focus on nutritional enhancement and diet quality enhancement for the vulnerable populations. For example, efforts at biofortifying crop quantities with B-vitamins have been encouraging at lowering malnutrition and its consequent impacts—particularly in low-income areas where B diversification of food supplies may be limited. Biofortification that works not only helps fight hidden hunger but also facilitates increased metabolic ability by ensuring the individual has the micronutrients needed for maximal cellular functioning. Lastly, such programs could significantly increase energy balance and well-being in populations faced with micronutrient deficiency challenges (Strobbe & Van Der Straeten, 2018) (Figure 5.8).

5.2.3. The Role of Water in Metabolic Processes

Water is an integral component of metabolic reactions, and it plays a crucial function in sustaining homeostasis and contributing to biochemical processes within the body. Its polarity and capacity to function as a solvent make it capable of dissolving various essential substances , such as nutrients, ions, and metabolic wastes. This characteristic is significant in biological functions since it facilitates transportation across cell membranes and in fluid bodies so that cellular metabolism occurs effectively. Furthermore, water has an intricate function in hydrolysis, the process by which large molecules are broken down into smaller components, easing the digestion and absorption of nutrients. Without adequate intake of fluids, such metabolic processes would be less effective, greatly affecting overall energy balance and body function, and thus making water an integral part of the intricate metabolism association of metabolic physiology. Furthermore, thermoregulation's role in water strengthens water's importance in metabolic function. Regulation of body temperature is crucial for optimal enzymatic activity because most biochemical reactions are temperature-sensitive. The high specific heat of water allows it to accumulate and retain heat and therefore keep the body at the appropriate temperature, irrespective of changes in the environment. Such a feature is particularly vital during physical exercise when metabolic requirement is increased and body temperature increases. It requires a good cooling system to prevent overheating and promote metabolic efficiency, particularly for sportsmen or individuals performing intense activities. Thus, it can be noted that hydration is directly involved in thermoregulation and accordingly influences energy expenditure, as considered in some studies that compare total energy expenditure (TEE) with metabolic rates while undertaking different activities of the body. Apart from its functions in structure and regulation, water is also involved in the metabolic processes associated with energy production. Cellular respiration bioenergetics, for instance, relies on water as a substrate and product of redox reactions in the mitochondria. Some of these are the reactions necessary for the production of ATP, cellular energy currency. Water functions extends beyond mere participation in chemical reactions; it also affects the effectiveness of energy storage and transfer by interacting with the mitochondrial membranes. Moreover, inadequate hydration can interfere with metabolic adaptation to energy deficits, leading to energy balance distortion and causing deleterious health effects. Thus, the understanding of the intricate functions water plays within metabolism is crucial for ensuring effective guidelines and interventions are accessible to address hydration needs (Nowak et al., 2007).

Test Your Knowledge

1. How does the body utilize carbohydrates, fats, and proteins for energy under different physiological conditions?
2. Compare aerobic and anaerobic pathways for ATP generation in terms of efficiency and by-products.

5.3. Energy Expenditure

Learning Outcome

1. Explain the basal metabolic rate (BMR);
2. Define the physical activity and its impact on energy expenditure;
3. Describe the thermic effect of food (TEF).

Understanding energy expenditure is paramount to the exploration of metabolic physiology, i.e., in terms of energy balance. Energy expenditure can be defined as the absolute quantity of energy that an individual expends over an interval, which encompasses basal metabolic rate (BMR), physical activity, and thermogenesis. The BMR refers to the quantity of energy required to maintain essential physiological processes during resting conditions, while physical activity refers to any energy spent on movement. Thermogenesis is energy dissipated during processes , such as digestion and temperature control. These parameters all together explain total energy balance, which plays an essential role in weight and overall health maintenance. An imbalance between consumption and expenditure of energy can lead to malnutrition or obesity and hence the need to understand the energy expenditure patterns within various populations in terms of both environmental factors and lifestyle. The relationship between environmental factors and energy expenditure cannot be over-stressed. Various species have varying adaptive mechanisms in response to different environmental factors, such as, temperature and humidity. For instance, research in the Malagasy bat species *Triaenops menamena* has illustrated how energy expenditure and metabolic rate can be influenced by thermoregulatory mechanisms. These bats are extremely flexible in physiological reaction to the occurrence of large thermal fluctuations, varying the rates of metabolism between normothermia and torpor for optimal energy conservation. This ability is essential, especially during the age of climate change, when organisms need to adapt to increasingly challenging ecological environments. As highlighted in these findings, the capacity for controlling energy expenditure in a way that responds to environmental stressors is important for survival and also underscores the importance of energy control as part of metabolic physiology (Remmers, 2024). With respect to human physiology, an understanding of energy expenditure gives insight into lifestyle disorder management, particularly obesity. The philosophy developed by Acharya Charaka in the Charaka Samhita revolves around the interaction between energy intake and energy expenditure through the practice of Santarpana. The system in this ancient era recognizes the fact that an imbalance between energy intake and energy expenditure can lead to various disorders. Specifically, hormones , such as leptin and ghrelin regulate appetite and energy homeostasis and dictate how the body utilizes absorbed energy. Harmony of diet (Santarpana Ahara) and living (Vihara) is the key to facilitating healthy metabolic processes. Against the backdrop of modern lifestyles, we can integrate these age-old axioms with physiology so that our approaches to wellness and health become more efficient, as emphasizing energy expenditure would ensure a constant metabolic state and prevent lifestyle disease (Roji et al., 2021) (Figure 5.9).

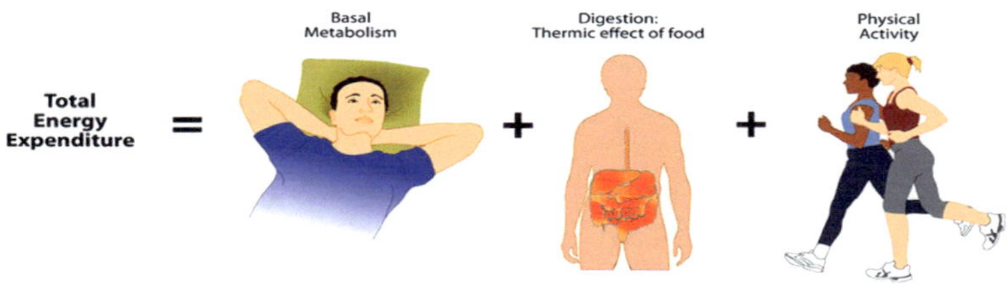

Figure 5.9. Components of energy expenditure.

Source: https://external-content.duckduckgo.com/iu/?u=https%3A%2F%2Fbodybuilding-wizard.com%2Fwp-content%2Fuploads%2F2020%2F12%2Fcomponents-of-energy-expenditure.jpg&f=1&nofb=1&ipt=e0a04961fe33dedcd246c3fe637648a6285b8266a805338c401d6fda3bd43b9e.

5.3.1. Basal Metabolic Rate (BMR)

Basal Metabolic Rate (BMR) is the cornerstone of understanding big concepts in metabolic physiology and energy balance. BMR refers to the amount of calories one consumes when the body is resting completely, with no energy burned from exercise and digestion. These factors of age, sex, body composition, and genetic predisposition influence BMR. For instance, individuals with greater lean body mass will have greater BMR owing to increased expenditure of energy by muscle tissue compared to fat tissue. This heterogeneity has strong implications for energy control since increased BMR translates to increased energy expenditure overall, which affects obesity and weight maintenance. Lastly, accurate knowledge of individual BMR is indispensable in individualizing diet and exercise protocols to maximize the best energy balance and well-being. In the context of overall energy expenditure (TEE), the interaction of BMR and physical activity level (PAL) then becomes the pivotal area of interest. The TEE to BMR ratio, otherwise known as PAL, indicates the level of lifestyle of individuals by categorizing them as either active or sedentary.

The PAL value of about 1.2 suggests very low levels of physical activity, while values approaching 4.5 signify high energy expenditure levels commonly associated with severe exercise or hard work. Experiments verify the relevance of BMR as a useful indicator for TEE, indicating that the lifestyle change-induced variation in BMR can have significant impacts on energy requirements over time. This context is of very high utility for planning effective interventions for weight management or the improvement of physical fitness, since the achievement and manipulation of BMR estimates make possible more efficient and effective solutions to energy balance and metabolic regulation. Also, application of BMR is relevant in clinical practice, as accurate assessments of energy requirements are essential in the management of patients. Data on an individual's BMR can inform treatment for various conditions, including obesity, malnutrition, and metabolic disorders. Furthermore, stability of BMR over a period of time, as borne out by large amounts of research evidence, makes it a valid marker of energy requirements across different populations. For example, the relationship between BMR and overall health status emphasizes the value of individualized dietary guidance according to metabolically driven principles. Knowing how endogenous and exogenous factors dictate BMR, health practitioners can better facilitate gains in health in specific populations, particularly under weight loss or energy-restricted diets (Chen et al., 2017). With ongoing research and tailored procedures, the correct application of BMR as a key indicator can vastly enhance metabolic physiology and energy balance measures (Figure 5.10).

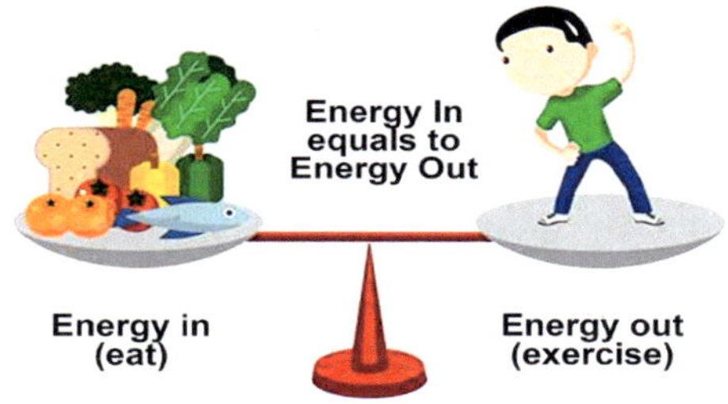

Figure 5.10. Basal metabolic rate calculator.

Source: https://external-content.duckduckgo.com/iu/?u=https%3A%2F%2Fcalculator-online.net%2Fimages%2FWhat%2520is%2520BMR.jpg&f=1&nofb=1&ipt=b4bcc99902042045036a7ce7171a050eae8bbc5aeca484e7e7cbfa4e081fcc14.

5.3.2. Physical Activity and Its Impact on Energy Expenditure

Physical activity and energy expenditure is also one of the simplest yet most essential metabolic physiology concepts that have an immediate effect on the net energy balance. Physical activity refers to the generic term encompassing all active movements , such as sports, exercise, and everyday activities, all of which are contributors to the overall energy expenditure (TEE). Energy utilized in physical activities may be considerably different based on a number of variables , such as the type of activity, intensity, and length.

For instance, intense aerobic exercise like cycling not only demands higher energy expenditure during activity but also can elevate post-exercise oxygen consumption, thereby enhancing overall energy expenditure in the recovery phase. Understanding these dynamics is critical for the development of effective interventions for weight control and metabolic health. Physical activity-related health outcomes are significantly influenced by patterns of energy expenditure. Evidence indicates that habitual physical activity may modulate appetite and energy intake, influencing the body's overall energy balance. For instance, a study that investigated the acute effects of cycling on energy intake reported an hour of exercise resulted in a significant reduction in relative energy intake during the next meal in active people. This indicates that exercise may exert a beneficial effect on appetite regulation and satiety in order to promote a more harmonized energy intake relative to expenditure. The research also highlighted the observation that individuals with more active living experienced a heightened sensitivity in their physiological response to hunger and satiety cues, supporting the linked association between physical activity, energy expenditure, and metabolic regulation (Broom et al., 2018).

In addition, physical activity's effects on energy expenditure are not only restricted to short-term adaptations but extend to long-term health outcomes. Continued execution of physical activity is associated with an exercise-induced increase in resting metabolic rate (RMR), which is the energy expended during rest. The rise in RMR can be accounted for by a progression of adjustments in the muscle mass and in the metabolic processing of nutrients as exercise is performed relentlessly. Consequently, individuals who integrate physical activity into their regimen of everyday tasks exhibit more favorable energy balance, thus reducing obesity as well as consequent disease risks. Systemic effects of long-term physical activity also highlight its necessity in maintaining metabolic health, supporting the importance of developing a physically active lifestyle. As research continues to study this association, it reveals not only exercise's acute effects but also its long-term contribution to energy balance and overall well-being (Chen et al., 2017) (Figure 5.11).

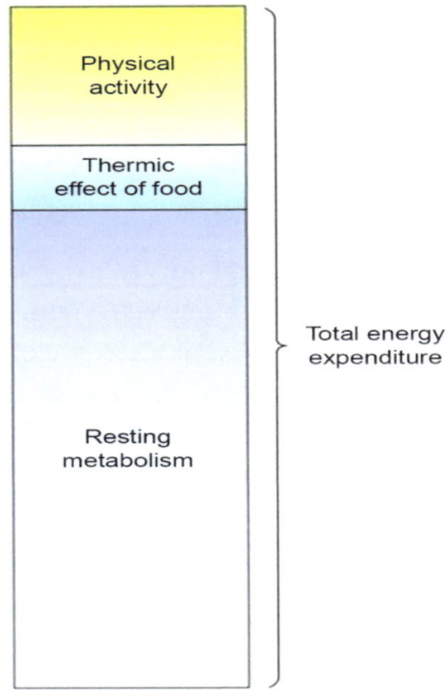

Figure 5.11. Total energy expenditure.

Source: https://external-content.duckduckgo.com/iu/?u=https%3A%2F%2Fimage3.slideserve.com%2F6356164%2Fcomponents-of-total-energy-expenditure-tee-l.jpg&f=1&nofb=1&ipt=645b4a8746b51be873b0035a6dccd692a5f386238c3698eb7481b722a69b00fd.

5.3.3. Thermic Effect of Food (TEF)

The thermic effect of food (TEF) is a significant component of metabolic physiology, which is a quantitative measure of the increase in the metabolic rate following food ingestion. Metabolic response is primarily caused by the cost of energy for the digestion, absorption, and assimilation of nutrients. The composition of the food determines the quantity of TEF, as macronutrient composition varies in its thermogenic activity. In particular, protein carries a higher TEF than fats and carbohydrates, and this can have implications for weight control, diet composition and overall energy balance. Therefore, an understanding of TEF's contribution to daily energy expenditure can aid in better nutritional strategies to optimize metabolic health and body weight management. Research has explored the influence of individual diets on the thermic effect, particularly in patients with special metabolic disorders. For instance, one study was used to highlight that TEF in patients receiving a phenylketonuria (PKU) diet generated significantly less postprandial energy expenditure when compared to a control diet, while expressing concerns regarding adverse effects on energy balance in subjects receiving very restrictive diets. Interestingly, the PKU group had a TEF of 10.2% on their special meal versus 13.2% in the control diet, suggesting that some dietary restrictions inadvertently have an impact on metabolic rate in vulnerable groups (Alfheeaid et al., 2018). These findings underscore the relevance of incorporating TEF into formulations for dietary plans, particularly for individuals who require specific nutritional accommodations. In addition, the relationship between TEF and energy consumption is an indication of the complexity of hunger control. Nutritional high-energy supplements (HENSDs) have recorded a multifaceted impact on energy consumption, manifesting a short-term inhibiting impact on appetite but inducing an overall net increase in energy intake. In a clinical trial of healthy women, energy intake was shown to decrease substantially following the consumption of HENSDs, illustrating how the outside food ingredients can affect TEF as well as appetite modulators , such as CCK and PYY (Arvanitidou et al., 2015). This exchange reveals the importance of understanding TEF in the broader context of energy balance, since it can influence weight management approaches as well as knowledge on metabolic disorders, towards a holistic solution of nutritional science.

Test Your Knowledge

1. What are the main components of total daily energy expenditure (TDEE)?
2. How is basal metabolic rate (BMR) measured and what factors influence it?

5.4. Hormonal Regulation of Metabolism

Learning Outcome

1. Identify the role of insulin in energy storage;
2. Define the effects of glucagon on energy release;
3. Describe the influence of thyroid hormones on metabolic rate.

The intricate interaction of the hormones in regulating metabolism is very important in maintaining the balance of energy in the body. Hormones , such as insulin, glucagon, thyroid hormone, and other sex hormones regulate metabolic processes, influencing how the body utilizes and stores energy. Insulin, for instance, promotes the entry of glucose into cells, consequently lowering the blood glucose concentration and facilitating the storage of excess nutrients as glycogen in the liver and muscle or adipose tissue fat. This activity is counteracted by glucagon, which increases glycogenolysis and gluconeogenesis, particularly during fasting states. The balance of these hormonal messages allows for the presence of energy when needed as well as for storage of surplus energy, thus ensuring homeostasis vital to overall physiological well-being. Circadian rhythms also profoundly influence metabolic regulation through hormonal means. The suprachiasmatic nucleus (SCN) of the hypothalamus plays a role in synchronizing daily cycles of metabolism with environmental light-dark cycles.

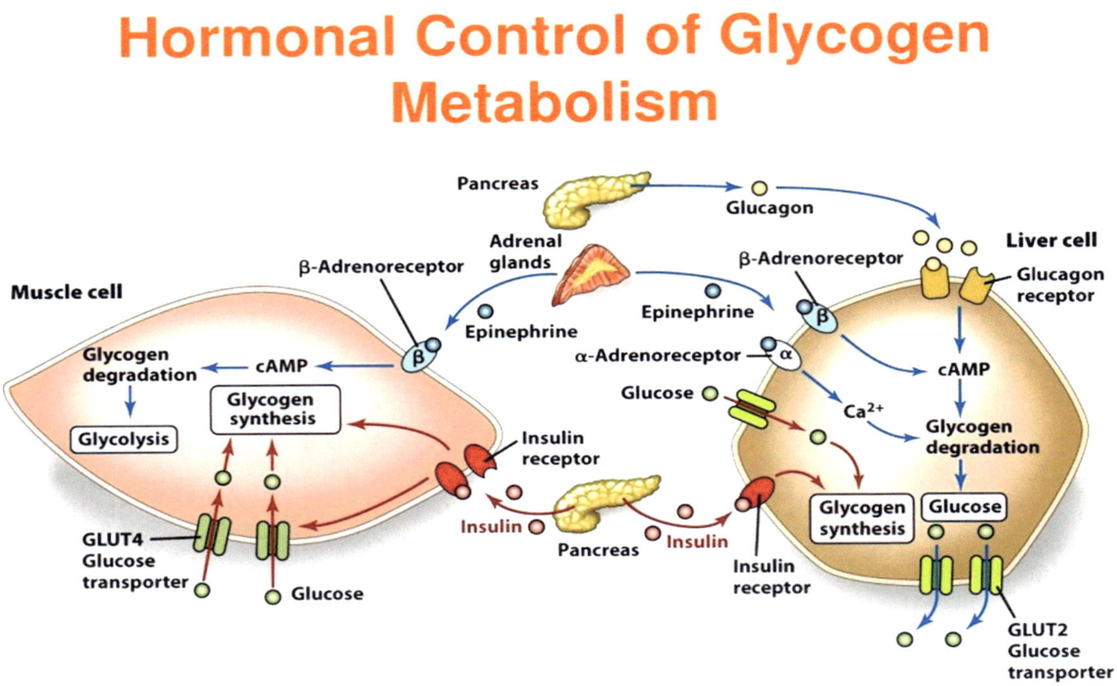

Figure 5.12. Hormonal-control-of-glycogen-metabolism.

Source: https://image4.slideserve.com/9181759/hormonal-control-of-glycogen-metabolism-l.jpg.

This regulation, according to studies, is the coordination of energy expenditure and feeding behavior, emphasizing the importance of timing of hormones in metabolism. Achieving or disruption of the SCN and its entrainment to peripheral oscillators by factors , such as shift work or chronic jet lag can lead to misalignments that are detrimental to metabolic health. Specifically, these disruptions have been linked to increased risks for metabolic disorder, diabetes, and obesity as hormonal regulation of metabolism becomes deregulated, leading to inefficient energy use and storage (Plano et al., 2017). The interaction of the reproductive hormones with metabolism even better illustrates the complexity of hormonal control. In cows, high milk production has been associated with reduced fertility in a relationship reinforcing the metabolic demand of high milk yield on endocrine homeostasis. Estradiol is an important hormone to regulate estrous activity and is hypothesized to be in interaction with other hormones like progesterone and insulin-like growth factor-1 in regulating reproductive cycles. The metabolic stress generated by overproduction of milk reprograms estrous behavior-related gene expression, demonstrating the ways in which physiological need can disrupt hormonal pathways (Boer et al., 2010). Understanding these interactions is significant since it demonstrates the mechanisms involved in not just metabolic health but also reproductive function, and how vital an integrative approach to the study of hormonal regulation of metabolism is (Figure 5.12).

5.4.1. Role of Insulin in Energy Storage

Insulin's role in energy storage is at the core of metabolic physiology since it integrates the regulation of glucose and lipid metabolism. When one eats, particularly carbohydrates, blood glucose levels rise, triggering pancreatic beta cells to secrete insulin. The hormone facilitates the entry of glucose into muscle and adipose cells so these cells can metabolize glucose to form glycogen and fat in their respective cells. The insulin-mediated enzymic activities , such as glycogenesis and lipogenesis, are significant in the establishment of energy storage. Besides promoting storage of energy, insulin also inhibits gluconeogenesis and lipolysis and therefore maintains homeostasis during periods of nutrient abundance. This regulatory function illustrates the very significant balance insulin establishes between excess and deficiency energy so that the body is able to store energy efficiently for subsequent metabolic needs, a key element both of the preservation of metabolic balance and of well-being. In overfeeding and obesity, though, insulin's function is less straightforward.

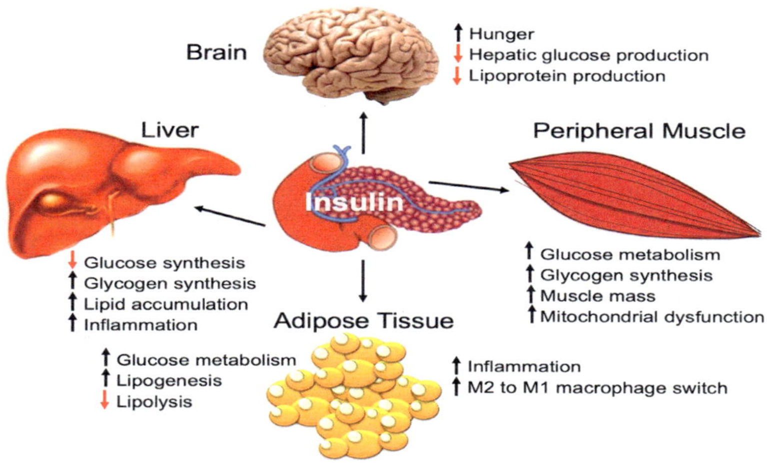

Figure 5.13. Insulin is a major regulator of metabolism and organ function.

Source: https://www.researchgate.net/publication/339383295/figure/fig1/AS:860640382038023@1582204065716/Insulin-is-a-major-regulator-of-metabolism-and-organ-function.png.

Excess caloric intake triggers hyperinsulinemia, an insulin value that is elevated and reflects the body's reaction to surplus energy. This pathophysiological state generates excess fat gain and altered energy substrate metabolism as insulin compels the storage of surplus nutrients. The intrinsic feedback mechanism governing energy homeostasis is derailed in such a scenario and resulting in increased adiposity and the accompanying metabolic illness. It has been discovered in research that obesity does have major changes in autonomic nervous system control. For instance, there is raised parasympathetic output with the intake of food associated with heightened insulin response, demonstrating a complicated interaction between autonomic control and insulin-stimulated energy storage pathways (Scheurink et al., 1996). Understanding insulin's regulatory mechanisms extends beyond glucose and lipid metabolism because it suggests broader implications for energy homeostasis in metabolic disease. Feedback mechanisms and organizational closure in the endocrine system offer the complexity of insulin's influence on energy homeostasis. Rather than acting through simple feedback mechanisms, insulin operates in a web of functional constraints such that its actions are connected to other metabolic effects. This perspective suggests that insulin's ability to provide energy storage support is less a result of its secretion and more the dynamic interaction between varied metabolic routes and hormonal signals (Bich et al., 2020). Thus, disruptions of insulin signaling have severe metabolic implications, emphasizing its prime position in maintaining energetic homeostasis as well as preventing pathologies of metabolic dysfunction (Figure 5.13).

5.4.2. Effects of Glucagon on Energy Release

The hormone glucagon is central to the management of energy release in the body through its effects on glucose metabolism. Glucagon is produced by the alpha cells of the pancreas and is indispensable in the management of blood glucose when the body is fasting or avoiding food for extended periods. When the glucose level goes down, glucagon stimulates glycogenolysis, the hydrolysis of glycogen, the form of glucose stored in the liver, into glucose and release into the bloodstream.

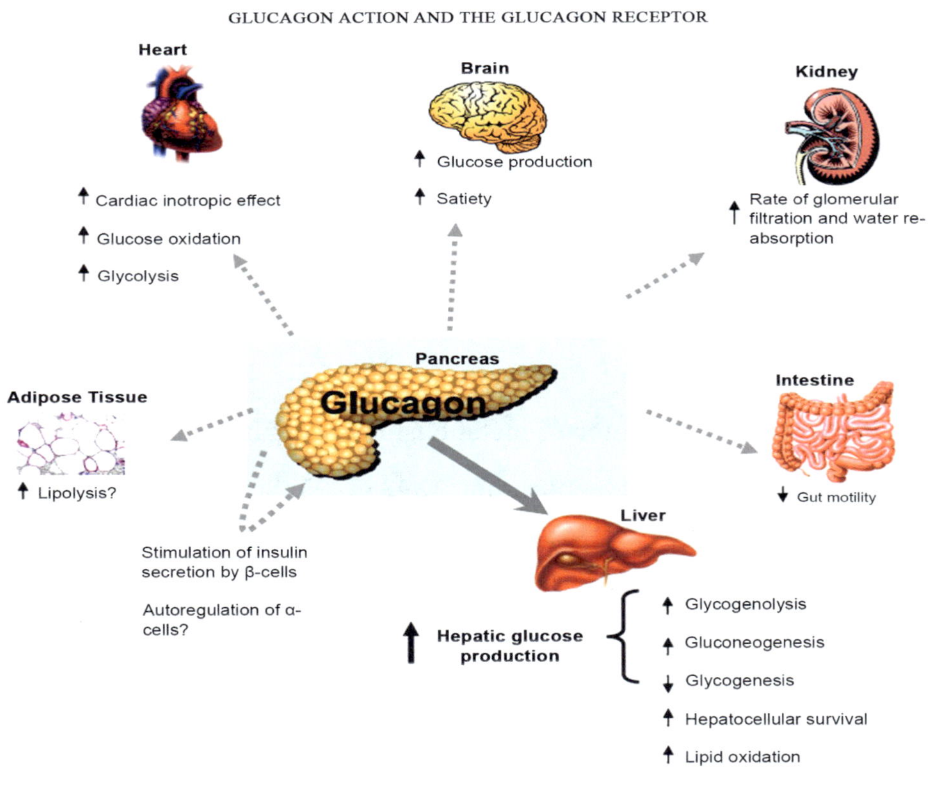

Figure 5.14. The effects of glucagon on various organs.

Source: https://collab.its.virginia.edu/access/content/group/61ef6ea0-869d-476a-990a-9738e3899823/1/32_YahandaA_GlucagonReceptorGPCR-Homo%20sapiens_4L6R/32_YahandaA_GlucagonReceptorGPCR-Homo%20sapiens_4L6R_images/img_2_1.png.

Besides supplying the brain and other vital organs with sufficient energy, it stimulates gluconeogenesis, wherein the non-carbohydrate precursors are converted into glucose. These metabolic changes point to the function of glucagon in energy balance, particularly in cases where external sources of energy are limited, highlighting its indispensable function to maintain homeostasis (Bich et al., 2020). In addition, glucagon's role in energy metabolism transcends the control of glucose release as it also encompasses the control of fat metabolism. Upon depletion of energy stores, glucagon triggers lipolysis, the breakdown of triglycerides in fat cells to free fatty acids and glycerol. The free fatty acids may then be utilized by other tissues as an energy source. Besides, glucagon also prompts the liver to absorb these fatty acids, where they are either oxidized for energy or utilized to synthesize ketones, a fuel for the brain and muscles in the case of prolonged fasting or a very-low-carbohydrate diet. This mobilizing activity of fat not only increases an optimal supply of energy but also reflects glucagon's critical role in adjusting the body's metabolic pathways to energy balance under different physiological states (Plano et al., 2017). In metabolic physiology, glucagon's action on energy release indicates its basic part in a complex feedback mechanism composed of various hormones and metabolic pathways. For instance, the glucagon-insulin interaction is a regulatory mechanism to control energy metabolism. While glucagon facilitates the mobilization of the stored energy, insulin, conversely, promotes the storage of energy after food is consumed. Metabolic conditions like diabetes with insulin resistance and inappropriately high levels of glucagon can be the consequence of the imbalance between these hormones. Appreciation of the role in energy release provides a clue to more universal principles of metabolic physiology, in which the intricate interaction between hormones decides energy homeostasis and overall health outcome. The kinetic nature of glucagon's responses not only signifies the energy needs of the body but also reflects the significance of retaining balance of metabolism (Bich et al., 2020) (Figure 5. 14).

5.4.3. Influence of Thyroid Hormones on Metabolic Rate

The function of thyroid hormones in metabolic rate is a significant area of research in metabolic physiology and energy balance. Thyroid hormones, thyroxine (T4) and triiodothyronine (T3), are crucial to regulating the metabolic activities of nearly all tissues in the body. Thyroid hormones elevate basal metabolic rate (BMR) by accelerating oxygen consumption and heat production, which is important to maintain physiological homeostasis. Additionally, they control carbohydrate, fat, and protein metabolism, thus assigning priority to energy expenditure. Lower levels of thyroid hormones may lead to a remarkable decline in metabolism, which leads to additional impacts on energy balance as well as overall health. Hyperthyroidism, however, leads to an increase in metabolic rates, with weight loss, among other issues, as a consequence. Understanding the balance of these hormones is important in the development of therapeutic treatment for metabolic disorders. Thyroid hormones also significantly influence energy metabolism at the cellular level by their control over mitochondrial function. Mitochondria, which are the powerhouse of the cell, are important in generating ATP and energy control. T3, in particular, has actions on activating mitochondrial biogenesis as well as enhancing the rate of ATP generation and thereby increasing the net energy yield of muscle and other tissues. The influence of thyroid hormones transcends the control of metabolic rate; their action on cellular respiration can have implications for the overall energy homeostasis and weight regulation. Apart from that, thyroid hormones also have intricate interactions with other endocrine systems within the body, i.e., insulin and glucagon, which go on to add to the difficulty of regulating energy metabolism. These interactions point towards the need for comprehensive knowledge of metabolic physiology in the context of thyroid function, especially to design targeted therapeutic strategies for metabolic dysfunction (Brinkmann et al., 2016). Research on the gender role and sex differences in thyroid hormone function has opened new horizons in metabolic physiology understanding. What is proven is that sex hormone fluctuation can affect thyroid metabolism and function, leading to differential metabolic responses in either sex. For instance, thyroid hormone interactions with estrogen will regulate metabolic rates, particularly during menstrual periods and menopause. This association emphasizes the necessity of taking both biological and gender aspects into account when researching thyroid function and metabolic well-being. In-depth studies suggest that these endocrine interactions are able to guide personalized treatment strategies, particularly in the management of metabolic disorders (Lauretta et al., 2018). The identification of the additional effects of thyroid hormones on metabolic rate can therefore promote successful interventions and facilitate the progress of patient-oriented medicine.

Test Your Knowledge

1. How does insulin regulate glucose, fat, and protein metabolism in the fed state?
2. Describe the role of glucagon during fasting and its effect on liver metabolism.

5.5. Factors Affecting Energy Balance

Learning Outcome

1. Identify the genetic influences on metabolism;
2. Define the environmental factors and lifestyle choices;
3. Describe the psychological aspects of eating behavior.

The intricate energy balance dynamics are highly dependent on various interacting variables within a person's lifestyle and physiological state. Physical activity is one of such prime determinants that not only influences energy expenditure but also influences appetite and energy intake. For instance, one study examining the effect of fasted compared with postprandial exercise found that individuals exercising postprandial reported greater suppression of appetite compared to subjects exercising in fasted states. Of note, while both exercise modes induced a negative energy balance with respect to sedentary conditions, total intake of energy was not varied between trials, demonstrating the complexity of appetite regulation and energy expenditure during active conditions. This timing-exercise interaction on control of appetite underscores the need for unique approaches to management of energy balance by physical activity across various groups (Deighton et al., 2012). In addition to exercise, sleep cycles and circadian rhythms have a great impact on metabolism and energy balance.

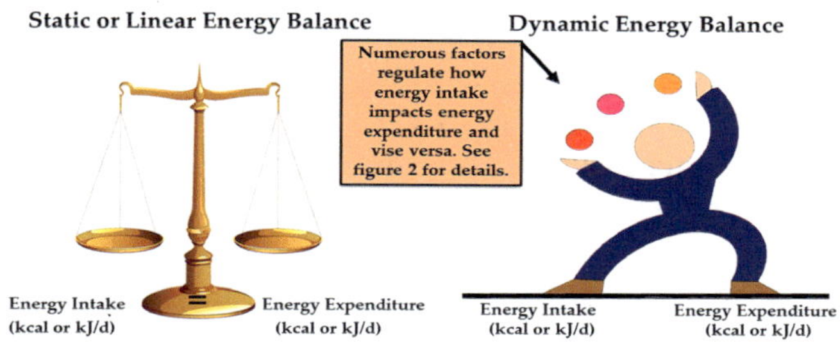

Figure 5.15. Dynamic energy balance.

Source: https://pub.mdpi-res.com/nutrients/nutrients-09-00905/article_deploy/html/images/nutrients-09-00905-g001.png?1569504612.

The SCN plays an essential role in synchronizing the body's internal clock with the external environment by regulating daily fluctuations in physiological processes, including metabolism. Disruptions of these circadian rhythms, often the consequence of modern lifestyle habits , such as shift work or irregular sleep patterns, could lead to metabolic dysregulation. Indications exist that the likelihood of mismatched circadian rhythms being one of the explanations for the imbalance between expenditure and intake of energy and thereby increasing the risk of obesity and other metabolic disorders. Therefore, circadian alignment importance should be understood in order to enhance perfect energy balance and avoid chronic diseases, underscoring the urgency for incorporating sleep health into the consideration of metabolic physiology (Plano et al., 2017). In addition, food composition and timing of nutrition are also vitally important in influencing energy balance. The macronutrient composition of meals, or the ratio of carbohydrate, protein, and fat, may impact metabolic and satiety-signaling responses. The most recent studies have suggested that specific timing of nutrients, for example, carbohydrate intake after exercise, may aid in recovery and have differential effects on subsequent energy intake and expenditure. In addition, meal timing relative to one's internal clock also has an important role to play; consuming meals at times that align with circadian rhythms can potentially maximize metabolic efficiency and overall energy expenditure. Thus, taking both quality and timing of nutrition into account could be a strategic approach in maintaining effective energy balance and maximizing metabolic health outcomes (Deighton et al., 2012; Plano et al., 2017) (Figure 5.15).

5.5.1. Genetic Influences on Metabolism

The relationship between genetics and metabolism is complex but significant to the energy balance of the human body. Differences in genes have significant impacts on metabolic processes, from substrate usage to energy dissipation. Such genetic differences have the potential to cause variations in how individuals respond to alterations in diet or exercise. For instance, gene polymorphisms that affect adiposity and insulin sensitivity can make individuals susceptible to obesity or metabolic disorders, even with large impacts on their energy balance. Also, recent research indicates the role of specific genes in the regulation of metabolic pathways and the manner in which genetic susceptibilities manifest as distinct metabolic patterns. This is the genetic underpinning of metabolism that is potentially opening the field of personalized nutrition and targeted treatments with emphasis on the need to consider genetics in developing obesity prevention and metabolic health improvement plans. Some of the metabolic pathways have been found to be tightly regulated by genes, which can alter the metabolic response to the environment and diet of an individual. Overfeeding, for example, is often accompanied by dramatic changes in autonomic nervous activity, reflecting the situation that genetic predisposition can increase or alter the effects of caloric excess. Investigations using genetically modified animal models, such as, hyperphagic rats, are illuminating the relationship between imbalance of the metabolism and genetic causes. Enhanced sympathetic tone and increased parasympathetic outflow observed in such models reflect how genetic elements can facilitate or hinder metabolic adaptations during phases of overconsumption. The finding is central to the creation of complete strategies towards metabolic disorders with consideration of genetic contributions towards energy homeostasis and appetite regulation, thereby opening a window of view into more effective clinical therapies. Furthermore, genetic influences contribute to the effects of microbiomes on metabolism, introducing another aspect of energy balance complexity. Interactions between host genomes and microbial populations can affect metabolic outcomes, suggesting genetic makeup as an aspect that possibly governs the structure and function of gut microbiota. This microbe-mediated influence can also affect nutrient absorption and energy harvest from diets, regulating metabolic outcomes. Recent research has highlighted the use of model organisms, e.g., Sphagnum species, as models for peatland ecosystems, to aid in unscrambling these intricate interactions among genetics and microbial function in carbon cycling, as cited in Gu et al. (2014). Similarly, evidence regarding the autonomic nervous system indicates that genetic predispositions are able to mirror changes in metabolic control following overfeeding, confirming the hypothesis that genetics plays an important part in establishing the individualized metabolic patterns, confirming the interdependence of genetic, diet, and environmental determinants of metabolic physiology and energy homeostasis as underscored in Scheurink et al. (1996) (Figure 5.16).

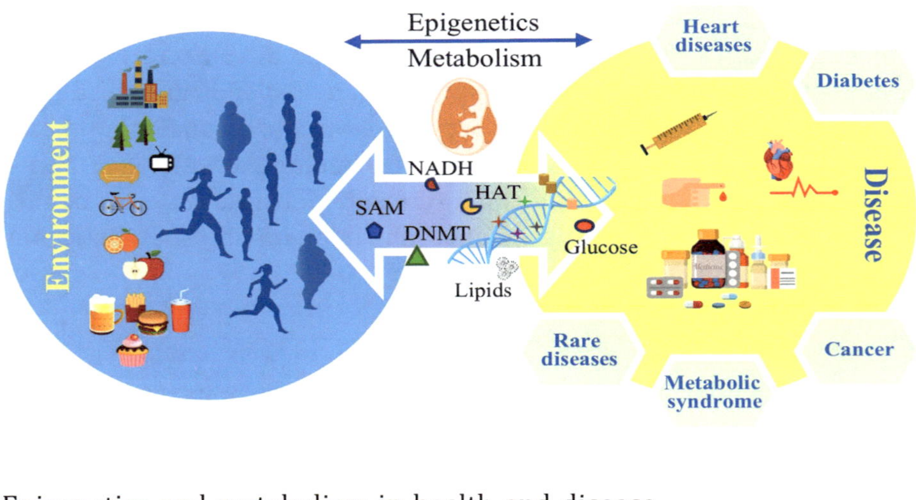

Figure 5.16. Epigenetics and metabolism in health and disease.

Source: https://www.frontiersin.org/files/Articles/410886/fgene-09-00361-HTML-r2/image_m/fgene-09-00361-g001.jpg.

5.5.2. Environmental Factors and Lifestyle Choices

The relationship between lifestyle and environment is a critical determinant of metabolic physiology and energy balance. The conditions that facilitate easy access to high-calorie foods and physical inactivity enable lifestyles leading to weight gain and metabolic derangement. As individuals navigate through their everyday lives, they are at times dominated by structural and social characteristics of their surroundings, and these will determine dietary options as well as activity opportunities. Basal metabolic rate (BMR) is a cornerstone in comprehending the variation of body composition and energy expenditure according to these external factors. Thus, for instance, variability in BMR must be accounted for in the determination of total energy expenditure (TEE), particularly in cases where lifestyles and dietary habits vary. An eco-friendly design with a preference for healthy foods, along with incentives for promoting physical activity, is capable of effectively modifying individual behavior towards a direction more favorable to better metabolic processes.

Revealing the role of acculturation in lifestyle change further supports environmental pressures on metabolic health. The acculturation hypothesis postulates that immigrant groups slowly come to adopt unhealthy behavioral habits prevalent in the host setting as they are integrated into new environments. This process can promote increased risk for obesity by altering eating habits and physical activity levels. Obesity disparities between immigrant groups, such as, Hispanics and East/Southeast Asians, indicate the diversity of lifestyle integration. While Hispanics exhibited elevated body mass index levels, East/Southeast Asians maintained healthier dietary patterns, indicating that there are strong cultural determinants of lifestyle following migration (Plano et al., 2017). Comprehension of these dynamics is critical to developing specialized interventions for promoting enhanced behaviors among various populations and combating the rising obesity epidemic linked to rising environments. Ultimately, the convergence of environmental dynamics and lifestyle patterns highlights the importance of customized public health interventions geared towards maximizing enhanced metabolic health. Urban physical activity, availability of recreational space, and dietary education can empower communities to make informed lifestyle choices. Furthermore, interventions must consider migration-related stressors that are known to heighten the challenges of adopting healthy habits. Through consideration of the intricate dynamics between environmental contexts, psychological well-being, and lifestyles, stakeholders can establish enabling frameworks that promote healthier lifestyles. These combined approaches are essential in optimizing energy equilibrium among vulnerable population groups at risk of metabolic disease and in designing an environment that will sustain sustained health benefits (Plano et al., 2017).

5.5.3. Psychological Aspects of Eating Behavior

The psychosocial factors of food consumption are inextricably linked to metabolic physiology and energy homeostasis, which mirror the complex mind-body interaction. Psychological factors like mood, emotions, and mental health are significant regulators of eating behavior and food selection. For instance, individuals utilize food to deal with stress and anxiety, which could be one of the reasons for emotional eating and, consequently, could disrupt energy balance. The macronutrient contribution to the effect of these behaviors does not need to be exaggerated. Carbohydrate-rich food can trigger serotonin production, affect mood and hunger, whereas proteins may stimulate satiation and satisfaction. The connection underscores the importance of understanding the psychological and affective factors in the act of consumption as a mechanism for promoting better eating habits and achieving metabolic equilibrium, as highlighted in current behavioral studies (Bellisle et al., 2017).

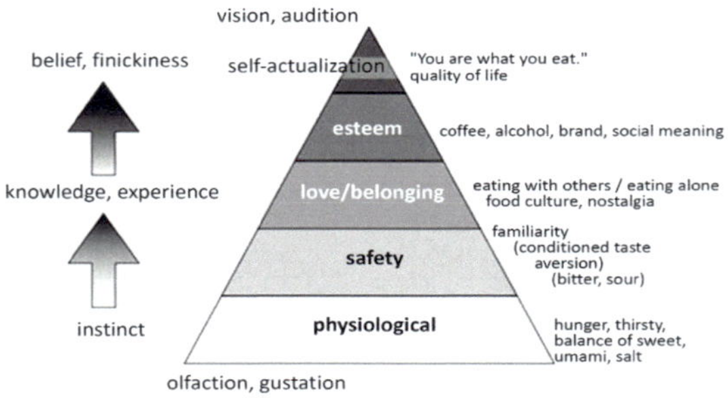

Figure 5.17. Psychological aspects of eating behavior.

Source: https://psychologyinrussia.com/images/volumes/psych_1_2014_2_2.jpg.

Adding to the interaction between psychology and eating is the complication of genetic influences mediating responses to dietary interventions. New evidence shows that polymorphisms of genes, notably those involved in neurotransmitter systems, could predict how a person will respond to vitamin and mineral supplementation, with effects on both mood and eating. For example, certain alleles of dopamine and serotonin pathways have been linked to the improvement of mood by micronutrient supplementation. This suggests that tailored nutrition can be an effective approach in managing eating behavior and enhancing mental welfare. Being aware of these genetic influences is significant for developing effective eating plans that not only address metabolic physiology but also individual psychological needs. Thus, exploring these genetic influences in association with psychological factors can offer more effective interventions in maintaining energy balance (Benton & Young, 2017). Furthermore, the influence of ingredients from food on psychological states signifies the importance of diet on overall mental health. Various studies have demonstrated that various foods and nutrients possess the ability to exacerbate or modulate psychiatric symptoms, which is important in the understanding of disordered eating behaviors. Some food additives and high-intensity sweeteners have been suggested to be contributing factors to behavioral alterations and affective states, like increased anxiety or dysphoria. This interaction highlights the two roles of food as both a nutriment and an energizer of mental health. Addressing these psychological dimensions is central to advancing nutritional care for energy homeostasis. In doing so, clinicians and healthcare professionals can better craft dietary recommendations that strike a balance between metabolic needs and mental health, toward more integrative health promotion (Bellisle et al., 2017) (Figure 5.17).

Test Your Knowledge

1. What is energy balance and how is it maintained in the human body?
2. List and explain physiological factors that influence energy intake and expenditure.

5.6. Metabolic Disorders

Learning Outcome

1. Identify the overview of common metabolic disorders;
2. Define the impact of metabolic disorders on energy balance;
3. Describe the treatment and management strategies.

Metabolic diseases are critical to learn about in the context of metabolic physiology and energy balance due to the fact that they have a direct effect on how the body acquires and utilizes energy. Metabolic diseases, comprised of several serious illness conditions , such as obesity, diabetes, and metabolic syndrome, are likely to occur due to imbalances between energy intake and expenditure. Because individuals consume more calories than the body is able to metabolize, they may experience a cascade of changes at a physiological level that can lead to insulin resistance and impaired glucose metabolism. Such imbalances require comprehensive strategies that not only address dietary changes but also deal with the overall importance of lifestyle elements , such as exercise and sleep cycles, in metabolic health. Research has increasingly demonstrated the interplay of sleep, circadian rhythm, and metabolic function, and has shed new light on how disruption in these areas results in metabolic disorders. Workshop presentations at the National Institute for Diabetes and Digestive and Kidney Diseases have illustrated the potential for synergy in studies to further elucidate these relationships. It is becoming more appreciated that disruption in sleep can enhance insulin resistance and result in weight gain. As mentioned, intervention on such factors as obstructive sleep apnea through interventions like CPAP may help decrease the risk of diabetes in the target group. Such findings could lead to improved prevention and treatment strategies, showing evidence of a more holistic model of metabolic health management that integrates both behavior and physiology (Arble et al., 2015).

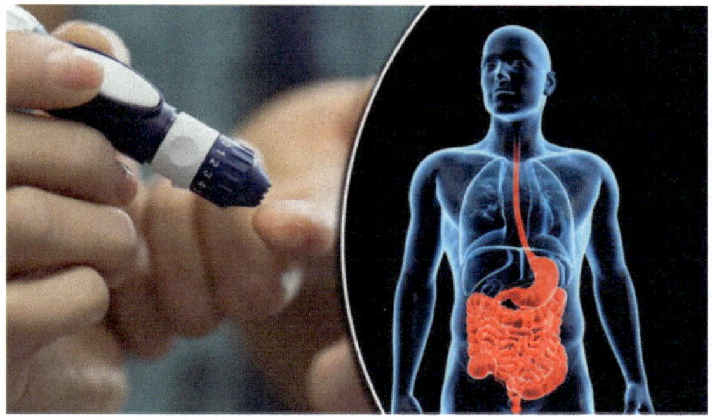

Figure 5.18. Connection between diabetes and digestive health.

Source: https://www.fitpaa.com/wp-content/uploads/2024/01/Untitled-design-37-jpg.webp.

The relationship between diet and metabolic disease also warrants closer examination, with more focus placed on how patterns of eating help to preserve health and homeostasis. Nutritional biochemistry, process engineering, and human physiology are backgrounds for understanding the impact of diet components on metabolic and overall health. For instance, excessive intake of trans fats and refined carbohydrates promotes inflammation and metabolic disorders leading to type 2 diabetes. Alternatively, whole-foods-based diets that are rich in fiber and healthy fats may be beneficial to metabolic health by enhancing cellular homeostasis and reducing the risk of metabolic pathology. Appreciation of these nutritional balances in their role of designing response-directed food strategies to avoid or reverse metabolic impairment and obtain energy homeostasis is crucial (Sarmidi, 2012) (Figure 5.18).

5.6.1. Overview of Common Metabolic Disorders (e.g., Diabetes, Obesity)

Understanding such prevalent metabolic diseases as diabetes and obesity is relevant to appreciating the broader implications of metabolic physiology and energy homeostasis. Diabetes, particularly Type 2, is characterized by insulin resistance and impaired glucose metabolism, generally aggravated by lifestyle factors , such as improper diet and absence of physical activities. This disease has far-reaching health implications in the form of cardiovascular illness, renal failure, and neuropathy. Obesity, defined by excessive fat accumulation, is a similar potent risk factor because not only does it induce derangement of metabolic homeostasis, but it is also a potent predictor for the development of insulin resistance and, consequently, diabetes. A critical review of the conditions demonstrates the duality of metabolic health and lifestyle measures, emphasizing the need for lifestyle-differentiated public health intervention. The complicated interaction between sleep patterns, circadian rhythms, and metabolic disease compounds the landscape of diabetes and obesity even further. Recent findings point towards the mechanisms by which sleep disturbance can have adverse effects on energy balance and lead to metabolic dysregulation. Studies have shown that sleep disturbances can be the cause of altered appetite-regulating hormones, ultimately leading to overeating and increased weight. Furthermore, identification of sleep factors as potentially causing metabolic disease opens up new avenues for intervention. For instance, examining the merit of CPAP therapy in obstructive sleep apnea patients would help avoid the risk of diabetic complications in at-risk groups, thereby exemplifying interdisciplinary characteristics of these diseases (Arble et al., 2015). The intersection of sleep science and metabolic science points toward the need for an integrative health approach. Last but not least, diet is essential for the regulation of metabolic disease. Understanding biochemistry and the interaction between food and metabolism can facilitate strategies for the achievement of metabolic homeostasis. A balanced diet of whole foods will help regulate energy intake and utilization, critical in preventing and reversing obesity and diabetes. Furthermore, new approaches , such as timed nutrition or temporal restricted feeding have shown promise for improving metabolic health. These methods focus not just on what one consumes, but when, to capitalize on the body's internal rhythm (Sarmidi, 2012). With ongoing advances in research, it is necessary to translate these findings to beneficial dietary recommendations, promising improved health for individuals afflicted with metabolic disorders (Figure 5.19).

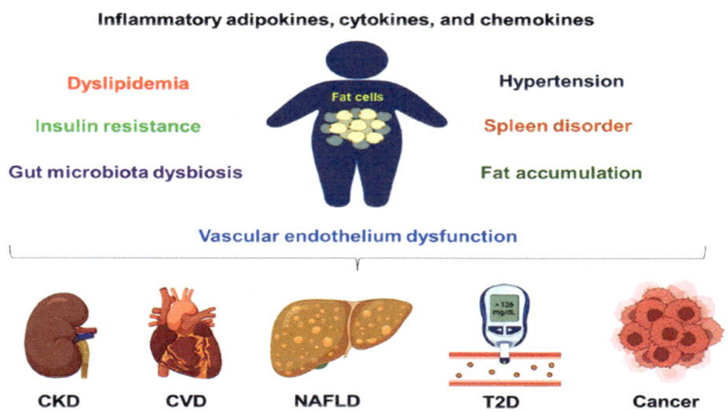

Figure 5.19. The related metabolic diseases and treatments of obesity.

Source: https://pub.mdpi-res.com/healthcare/healthcare-10-01616/article_deploy/html/images/healthcare-10-01616-g001-550.jpg?1661417514.

5.6.2. Impact of Metabolic Disorders on Energy Balance

Metabolic disturbances significantly affect energy balance because metabolic disease has the potential to alter both energy expenditure and intake. Obesity and diabetes, for instance, demonstrate how dysregulation affects body functions in the context of energy maintenance. Obesity, for instance, is often generated by an imbalance in which energy input exceeds that of output, leading to excess body fat accumulation. This may create a vicious cycle; increased fat storage can further impair metabolic functions, exacerbating the disorder. Moreover, as indicated by recent studies, the relationship between metabolic health and regulation of energy is not merely caloric intake, but rather an emphasis on the need to establish the underlying biological mechanisms (Arble et al., 2015). Overcoming these challenges is essential in determining effective interventions to restore energy balance and improve overall metabolic health. Comorbid conditions, such as, obstructive sleep apnea (OSA), also complicate the energy balance profile. It is reported that OSA individuals exhibit disturbed sleep patterns, which drive insulin resistance and hunger. This interaction describes the function of sleep and circadian cycles in energy metabolism. In this context, metabolic diseases interact with sleep disease to produce synergistic effects on energy homeostasis. According to research, effective management of sleep disorders may be critical to improving metabolic outcomes among affected patients. Through the analysis of combined models that address sleep quality and metabolic function at the same time, researchers are capable of uncovering new fronts for preventive health interventions to be pursued (Murphy & Mercer, 2013).

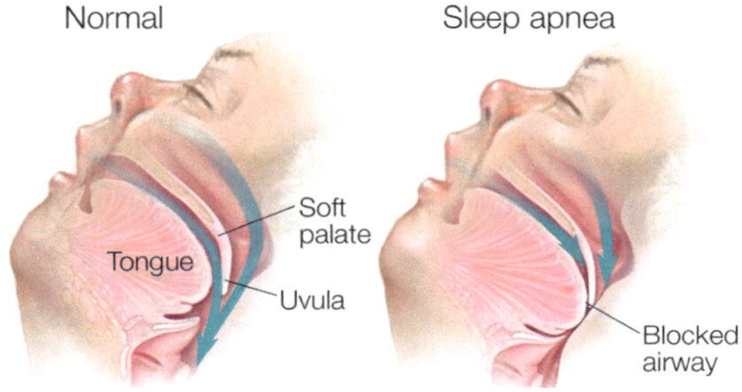

Figure 5.20. Obstructive Sleep Apnea (OSA)

Source: https://thumbayuniversityhospital.com/wp-content/uploads/2022/05/sleep-apnea.jpg.

Such an integrated perspective is necessary in advancing knowledge of energy balance and the impacts of metabolic disease. Moreover, interdisciplinary studies are most important in explaining the complex interaction between energy balance and metabolic disease. Integration of data from sleep science and metabolic studies has the ability to produce a rich picture of how variables interact to lead to energy dysregulation. Recent advances have suggested that coordination among researchers within these research areas could be valuable in providing information about the mechanisms affecting energy imbalances within specific populations. For example, examining treatments like continuous positive airway pressure (CPAP) in pre-diabetic patients with OSA may uncover whether or not solving sleep problems prevents continued metabolic decline. Investigating such relationships will not only add to current literature but may also open up new therapeutic options to promote metabolic health and reach energy balance (Arble et al., 2015) (Figure 5.20).

5.6.3. Treatment and Management Strategies

Optimal metabolic physiology and energy equilibrium among various organisms, particularly under stressor-induced environments , such as temperature or salinity fluctuations, are critical for proper treatment and management. In poultry, for instance, heat stress induces severe physiological deviations, among which include hyperthermia. To act against the foregoing implications, some feeding strategies have been employed; among them is restricted feeding. Through feeding for long enough before large heat exposure, the negative impacts of heat can be reduced. In addition, through choice feeding with diets of varying make-up in terms of nutrients—e.g., protein and energy density—self-regulation of nutrients by the birds is made possible to suit their metabolic needs, hence stabilizing their energy balance during heat stress (Syafwan et al., 2011). In marine environments, the regulation of alterations in salinity is yet another issue that needs special intervention measures. Such species as the delta smelt are subjected to fluctuating salinity regimes caused by anthropogenic influences, which can significantly impact their osmoregulation. Research determines that the fish are able to rapidly adjust physiological adaptations in order to resist alterations in salinity, but such activities are energetically costly. As such, optimal physiological performance is a result of constant monitoring and control of their habitat to reduce these stressors. By merging physiological response with habitat control, scientists validate predictions of how these species will be affected by continuing environmental changes, ensuring that efforts are catered to their survival and energy balance demands (Komoroske et al., 2016). As these examples illustrate, treatment and management responses must be tailored to specific environmental and species-specific needs, utilizing combinations of nutrition and habitat treatments to optimize metabolic health. In chickens, feeding regimes must be modified as a component of avoiding heat stress and optimizing energy utilization. Similarly, in marine ecosystems, the upkeep of stable salinity concentrations through effective management practices can enhance the viability and reproductive success of such sensitive organisms as the delta smelt. Both approaches highlight the importance of research-driven management measures that consider the intricate interactions between environmental factors and metabolic physiology. Through such holistic management practices, we can accomplish healthier stocks and sustainable strategies in progressively challenging ecosystems (Syafwan et al., 2011; Komoroske et al., 2016).

Test Your Knowledge

1. What are inborn errors of metabolism, and how do they affect biochemical pathways?
2. Describe the pathophysiology and symptoms of diabetes mellitus as a metabolic disorder.

SUMMARY

The research of metabolic physiology and energy balance is worth noting the interconnectedness of energy expenditure, consumption, and the physiological mechanisms by which they are controlled. Energy balance regulation is not a matter of calories in, calories out; it is the interaction between metabolic processes, hormonal controllers, and behavioral factors. In addition, recent research highlights the role of lifestyle components , such as sleep and circadian rhythms, with evidence that disruptions in these categories have a major impact on metabolic health. As identified through recent research, collaboration between sleep science and metabolic health is a high priority in translating laboratory findings into real-world applications that can promote public health (Arble et al., 2015). Such interdisciplinarity will not only expand our understanding of energy balance but also inform interventions designed to reverse obesity and diabetes. Additionally, the emergence of high-intensity interval training (HIIT) protocols underscores the necessity for individualized approaches to exercise in the control of energy balance and maximal metabolic health. Individual differences in thresholds of tolerance to exercise imply that one size will not fit all. By applying tailored HIIT protocols based on each subject's physiological responses, as illustrated in recent research (Ferguson et al., 2013), coaches can optimize training intensity and duration, leading to improved results in energy expenditure and general metabolic function. Such an individualized approach leads to better adherence to exercise programs, ultimately leading to healthy lifestyle choices. The potential of HIIT to transform the exercise science domain is a reflection of the worth of integrating state-of-the-art research with working models for improving metabolic health. Lastly, understanding the nuances of metabolic physiology and energy balance plays a crucial role in the resolution of the rising rate of metabolic diseases in contemporary society. As science develops, more research must bridge the gap between foundational findings and the translation of these findings into real-world applications across different populations. Emphasis on the role of whole-system approaches—e.g., dietary modification, exercise, and mental health interventions—can ultimately result in more effective control of health disorders associated with energy imbalance. Interdisciplinary collaboration between scientists, health practitioners, and public health professionals will be critical in spearheading a multifaceted understanding of the complex interplay. Ultimately, the guarantee that scientific advancement leads to tangible improvements in real-world health for society remains a significant objective within the framework of metabolic physiology (Arble et al., 2015).

In metabolic physiology, an integrated understanding of energy balance is necessary to explain how organisms regulate their metabolic process. Among the key subjects emphasized are the intricate relationships between calorie consumption, energy expenditure, and the role of macronutrients in driving metabolic processes. The body's energetic requirement changes with different parameters , such as exercise, environmental supply, and hormonal regulation and hence constitutes a dynamic framework for energy regulation. This dynamic character underscores the capacity of metabolic systems to adapt to fluctuating physiological states, attesting to the importance of an active area of research into metabolic rates and their health relevance, as well as in disease. These adaptations are crucial not just for efficient performance of day-to-day tasks but also for long-term energy homeostasis during the development of metabolic disorders, thereby motivating additional studies into the modulatory mechanisms governing such processes. Furthermore, the metabolic pathways of substrate metabolism to produce energy are complex and highly regulated by endogenous and exogenous factors. Metabolic flux variation has been recently discovered to have profound impacts on energy balance with differential physiological outcomes. By integrating steady-state and dynamic labeling approaches in experiments, researchers can gain insight into metabolic control in organisms. Interestingly, how external influences affect metabolic networks delivers critical details in interpreting energy use and distribution in different tissues. Metabolic flux is a significant concept as it showcases how cells can modify their metabolic reactions to accommodate environmental transitions, with a view to maintaining viability and function. This knowledge can prove to be vital for therapeutic treatments in the management of metabolic disease since we gain a better insight into cellular energy metabolism (Fernie & Morgan, 2013). Lastly, as metabolic physiology and energy balance continue to be studied, these new challenges and future directions strengthen the discussion. One of the fundamental issues of contention is the intricate compartmentation of cell metabolism, rendering the investigation of metabolic fluxes challenging. Facts are at hand that understanding these compartmentalized processes is the master key to an understanding of the way metabolic networks operate under varying conditions. In addition, kinetic modeling developments have significant potential for dissecting these intricate metabolic pathways. Enhanced methods to label distribution analyses are supporting significant advances in exploring cellular responses to metabolic change. Thus, responding to theoretical issues as well as experimental challenges is nonetheless at the forefront for understanding plant metabolism and its subsequent impact on metabolic health (Bake et al., 2014).

KEY TERMS FROM THIS CHAPTER

- Adipose tissue
- Anabolism
- Basal metabolic rate (BMR)
- Catabolism
- Ghrelin
- Glycolysis
- Krebs cycle (Citric acid cycle)
- AMPK (AMP-activated protein kinase)
- ATP (adenosine triphosphate)
- Caloric balance
- Energy expenditure
- Glucose homeostasis
- Insulin resistance
- Leptin

CRITICAL THINKING QUESTIONS

1. **Which hormone plays the most significant role in lowering blood glucose levels?**
   a. Glucagon
   b. Epinephrine
   c. Cortisol
   d. Insulin
2. **Which of the following processes is responsible for generating glucose from non-carbohydrate sources?**
   a. Glycogenesis
   b. Glycolysis
   c. Gluconeogenesis
   d. Lipogenesis
3. **What is the primary energy currency of the cell?**
   a. NADH
   b. $FADH_2$
   c. ATP
   d. Glucose
4. **Which hormone is released during fasting to maintain blood glucose levels?**
   a. Insulin
   b. Leptin
   c. Glucagon
   d. Thyroxine
5. **Leptin, a hormone secreted by adipose tissue, primarily functions to:**
   a. Increase hunger
   b. Stimulate insulin secretion
   c. Promote fat storage
   d. Suppress appetite and increase energy expenditure

Short Answer Questions

1. Define basal metabolic rate (BMR) and list two factors that affect it.
2. What is the difference between catabolism and anabolism?
3. Name the major metabolic hormones and their primary effects on metabolism.
4. What is gluconeogenesis, and when does it occur?
5. Which hormone promotes lipolysis during fasting?
6. Explain the process of energy production from glucose, including glycolysis, the Krebs cycle, and oxidative phosphorylation.
7. Discuss the role of insulin and glucagon in maintaining blood glucose homeostasis.
8. Describe the metabolic changes that occur during prolonged fasting or starvation.
9. Explain how the body balances energy intake and expenditure, and the role of hypothalamic regulation.
10. Discuss the role of brown adipose tissue in thermogenesis and energy balance.

Answers to Critical Thinking Questions

1. (b); 2. (c); 3. (a); 4. (b); 5. (c).

REFERENCES

1. Akhtar Roji, A. Y., & Paliwal, M. (2021). Concept of *Santarpana*: A scientific analysis. https://core.ac.uk/download/478522086.pdf (accessed on 28th June 2025).
2. Alfheeaid, H., Cochrane, B., Elhauge, M., Gerasimidis, K., et al. (2018). Impact of phenylketonuria-type meal on appetite, thermic effect of feeding and postprandial fat oxidation. https://core.ac.uk/download/80696977.pdf (accessed on 28th June 2025).
3. Scheurink, A. J., Balkan, B., Strubbe, J. H., van Dijk, G., & Steffens, A. B. (1996). Overfeeding, autonomic regulation and metabolic consequences. *Cardiovascular drugs and therapy, 10 Suppl 1*, 263–273. https://doi.org/10.1007/BF00120496(accessed on 28th June 2025).
4. Kim, J. Y., & Pham, D. D. (2009). Sasang constitutional medicine as a holistic tailored medicine. *Evidence-based complementary and alternative medicine : eCAM, 6 Suppl 1*(Suppl 1), 11–19. https://doi.org/10.1093/ecam/nep100(accessed on 28th June 2025).
5. Lauretta, R., Sansone, M., Sansone, A., Romanelli, F., & Appetecchia, M. (2018). Gender in Endocrine Diseases: Role of Sex Gonadal Hormones. *International journal of endocrinology, 2018*, 4847376. https://doi.org/10.1155/2018/4847376accessed on 28th June 2025).
6. Arble, D. M., Bass, J., Behn, C. D., Butler, M. P., et al. (2015). Impact of sleep and circadian disruption on energy balance and diabetes: A summary of workshop discussions. https://core.ac.uk/download/213087763.pdf (accessed on 28th June 2025).
7. Arvanitidou, E. I., Fatima, S., Gerasimidis, K., Malkova, D., et al. (2015). Response of appetite and potential appetite regulators following intake of high energy nutritional supplements. https://core.ac.uk/download/42363118.pdf (accessed on 28th June 2025).
8. Bake, T., Morgan, D. G., & Mercer, J. G. (2014). Feeding and metabolic consequences of scheduled consumption of large, binge-type meals of high fat diet in the Sprague-Dawley rat. *Physiology & behavior*, *128*(100), 70–79. https://doi.org/10.1016/j.physbeh.2014.01.018 (accessed on 28th June 2025).
9. Benton, D., & Young, H. A. (2017). Reducing Calorie Intake May Not Help You Lose Body Weight. *Perspectives on psychological science : a journal of the Association for Psychological Science*, *12*(5), 703–714. https://doi.org/10.1177/1745691617690878(accessed on 28th June 2025).
10. Boer, H. M., Veerkamp, R. F., Beerda, B., & Woelders, H. (2010). Estrous behavior in dairy cows: identification of underlying mechanisms and gene functions. *Animal : an international journal of animal bioscience*, *4*(3), 446–453. https://doi.org/10.1017/S1751731109991169(accessed on 28th June 2025).
11. Bellisle, F., Blundell, J. E., Dye, L., Fantino, M., et al. (2017). Functional food science and behaviour and psychological functions. https://core.ac.uk/download/85217796.pdf (accessed on 28th June 2025).
12. Bich, L., Mossio, M., & Soto, A. M. (2020). Glycemia regulation: From feedback loops to organizational closure. https://core.ac.uk/download/287611700.pdf (accessed on 28th June 2025).
13. Boon, P., Daan, S., & Visser, G. H. (2000). Effect of photoperiod on body weight gain, and daily energy intake and energy expenditure in Japanese quail (*Coturnix c. japonica*). https://core.ac.uk/download/pdf/12941316.pdf (accessed on 28th June 2025).

14. Brinkmann, L., Gerken, M., Hambly, C., Riek, A., et al. (2016). Thyroid hormones correlate with field metabolic rate in ponies, *Equus ferus caballus*. https://core.ac.uk/download/131024388.pdf (accessed on 28th June 2025).

15. Broom, D. R., Dalton, C. F., Hopkins, M., Paxman, J. R., et al. (2018). An acute bout of cycling does not induce compensatory responses in pre-menopausal women not using hormonal contraceptives. https://core.ac.uk/download/228178402.pdf (accessed on 28th June 2025).

16. Chen, L., Delville, C., Derous, D., Douglas, A., et al. (2017). The effects of graded levels of calorie restriction: VIII. Impact of short-term calorie and protein restriction on basal metabolic rate in the C57BL/6 mouse. https://core.ac.uk/download/80685984.pdf (accessed on 28th June 2025).

17. Colthorpe, K. (2004). Action learning project: Using an inquiry-based practical class to enhance student understanding. https://core.ac.uk/download/14981959.pdf (accessed on 28th June 2025).

18. Komoroske, L. M., Jeffries, K. M., Connon, R. E., Dexter, J., Hasenbein, M., Verhille, C., & Fangue, N. A. (2016). Sublethal salinity stress contributes to habitat limitation in an endangered estuarine fish. *Evolutionary applications*, *9*(8), 963–981. https://doi.org/10.1111/eva.12385(accessed on 28th June 2025).

19. Hayes, A., & Cribb, P. J. (2008). Effect of whey protein isolate on strength, body composition and muscle hypertrophy during resistance training. *Current opinion in clinical nutrition and metabolic care*, *11*(1), 40–44. https://doi.org/10.1097/MCO.0b013e3282f2a57d(accessed on 28th June 2025).

20. Deighton, K., Stensel, D. J., & Zahra, J. C. (2012). Appetite, energy intake and resting metabolic responses to 60 min treadmill running performed in a fasted versus a postprandial state. https://core.ac.uk/download/29018536.pdf (accessed on 28th June 2025).

21. Dyson, A., Audibert, G., Berne, R. M., Blitzer, M. L., Boutilier, R. G., Brown, I. P., Devlin, C., et al. (2013). The key role of nitric oxide in hypoxia: Hypoxic vasodilation and energy supply-demand matching.

22. Fernie, A., & Morgan, J. (2013). Analysis of metabolic flux using dynamic labeling and metabolic modeling. https://core.ac.uk/download/210620021.pdf (accessed on 28th June 2025).

23. Geyer, K.M., Kyker-Snowman, E., Grandy, A.S. *et al.* Microbial carbon use efficiency: accounting for population, community, and ecosystem-scale controls over the fate of metabolized organic matter. *Biogeochemistry* **127**, 173–188 (2016). https://doi.org/10.1007/s10533-016-0191-y(accessed on 28th June 2025).

24. Plano, S. A., Casiraghi, L. P., García Moro, P., Paladino, N., Golombek, D. A., & Chiesa, J. J. (2017). Circadian and Metabolic Effects of Light: Implications in Weight Homeostasis and Health. *Frontiers in neurology*, *8*, 558. https://doi.org/10.3389/fneur.2017.00558(accessed on 28th June 2025).

25. Gu, L., Muchero, W., Schmutz, J., Shaw, J., et al. (2014). *Sphagnum* physiology in the context of changing climate: Emergent influences of genomics, modelling and host-microbiome interactions on understanding ecosystem function. https://core.ac.uk/download/305124687.pdf (accessed on 28th June 2025).

26. Kapke, D. R. (2015). Childhood type II diabetes: The risks and complications. https://core.ac.uk/download/58826199.pdf (accessed on 28th June 2025).

27. Syafwan, S., Kwakkel, R. P., & Verstegen, M. W. A. (2011). Heat stress and feeding strategies in meat-type chickens. *World's Poultry Science Journal*, *67*(4), 653–674. https://doi.org/10.1017/S0043933911000742(accessed on 28th June 2025).

28. LaBarge, S., Migdal, C., & Schenk, S. (2015). Is acetylation a metabolic rheostat that regulates skeletal muscle insulin action? https://core.ac.uk/download/323065531.pdf (accessed on 28th June 2025).

29. McGee, S. L. (2007). Exercise and MEF2–HDAC interactions. http://hdl.handle.net/10536/DRO/DU:30025017 (accessed on 28th June 2025).

30. McMinn, M. R. (1984). Mechanisms of energy balance in obesity. https://digitalcommons.georgefox.edu/cgi/viewcontent.cgi?article=1276&context=gscp_fac (accessed on 28th June 2025).

31. Murphy, M., & Mercer, J. G. (2013). Diet-regulated anxiety. *International journal of endocrinology*, *2013*, 701967. https://doi.org/10.1155/2013/701967(accessed on 28th June 2025).

32. Nowak, A. J., Bach, V., Bell, E., Bolton, C., Brück, K., Cengel, Y., Elabbassi, H., et al. (2007). A combined study of heat and mass transfer in an infant incubator with an overhead screen. https://core.ac.uk/download/334376.pdf (accessed on 28th June 2025).

33. Vazquez, A., & Oltvai, Z. N. (2016). Macromolecular crowding explains overflow metabolism in cells. *Scientific reports*, *6*, 31007. https://doi.org/10.1038/srep31007 (accessed on 28th June 2025).

34. Pathare, P. (2011). The role of *C. elegans* NHR-49 in regulating global lipid homeostasis. https://core.ac.uk/download/299066887.pdf (accessed on 28th June 2025).

35. Price, F. (2021). Macronutrient intake: A multi-sport study of female Division I collegiate athletes. https://core.ac.uk/download/487620584.pdf (accessed on 28th June 2025).

36. Remmers, S. (2024). Ready for climate change? The importance of adaptive thermoregulatory flexibility for the Malagasy bat species *Triaenops menamena*. http://arxiv.org/abs/2401.13012 (accessed on 28th June 2025).

37. Sarmidi, M. R. (2012). Food is our medicine. https://core.ac.uk/download/11801185.pdf (accessed on 28th June 2025).

38. Spasojevic, I. (2011). Integrative concept of homeostasis: Translating physiology into medicine. https://core.ac.uk/download/pdf/290549.pdf (accessed on 28th June 2025).

39. Strobbe, S., & Van Der Straeten, D. (2018). Toward eradication of B-vitamin deficiencies: Considerations for crop biofortification. https://core.ac.uk/download/158346323.pdf (accessed on 28th June 2025).

40. Ferguson C, Wilson J, Birch KM, Kemi OJ (2013) Application of the Speed-Duration Relationship to Normalize the Intensity of High-Intensity Interval Training. PLoS ONE 8(11): e76420. https://doi.org/10.1371/journal.pone.0076420(accessed on 28th June 2025).

REPRODUCTIVE PHYSIOLOGY

6

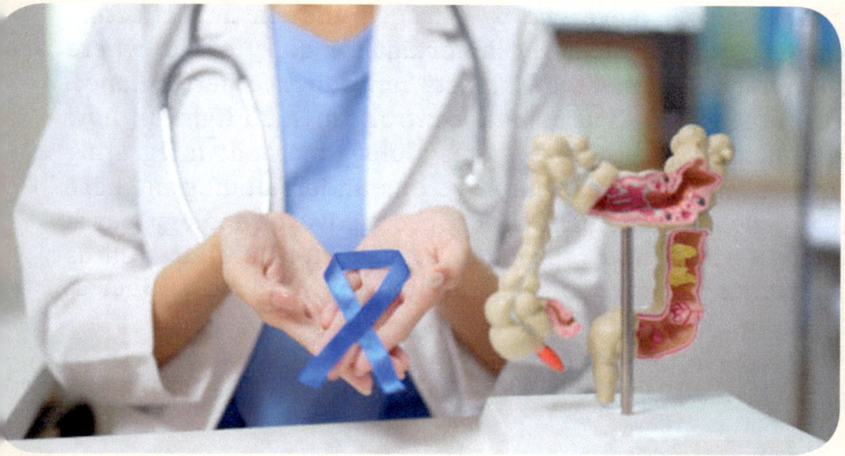

LEARNING OBJECTIVES

After studying this chapter, you will be able to:

1. Discuss the anatomy of the male reproductive system.
2. Explain the anatomy of the female reproductive system.
3. Discuss the hormonal regulation of reproduction.
4. Define gametogenesis.
5. Describe the fertilization and early development.
6. Evaluate the reproductive health and disorders.

Introduction

Reproductive physiology is the science of those intricate biological mechanisms that manage the reproductive processes in various organisms. It is central to the field to possess some understanding of endocrine processes directing the cycle of reproduction, which are significant in determining fertility and reproductive success. Estradiol is a critical hormone that plays a key role in the coordination of endocrine events and behavioral expressions, particularly in mammals. For instance, in cows, altered hormone levels can cause lower expressions of estrous behavior, thus affecting fertility rates. This low reproductive success is often linked to increased milk production, pointing towards a correlated set of physiological demands and reproductive capacity. By examining such interactions, researchers can gain insights about the biological processes that control reproduction, leading to better management practices in agricultural and conservation efforts. Reproductive physiology is not only about hormonal regulation but also about variation in individuals' responses to physiological stressors, as suggested by studies on grey seals. Such studies showed substantial inter-individual variation in baseline heart rate variability or HRV, which relates to coping styles—a highly pertinent factor in understanding reproductive health. Such coping styles, which include proactive and reactive processes, influence mothering behavior as well as reproductive success. In female grey seals, the individuals with higher baseline HRV were related to alternative maternal investment strategies. Contrarily, females with lower HRV were related to higher maternal transfer efficiency, reflecting the physiological mechanisms that underpin reproductive success. This correlation supports the inclusion of behavioral and physiological models in reproductive physiology to correctly express the complexity of reproduction in different species. Further clarifying the mechanisms that govern reproductive physiology, there has been new evidence directed toward the role of gene expression in governing estrous behavior. Various animal models have indicated that expression of genes within the brain area, the hypothalamus, is governed by estrogen, thus in turn affecting reproduction-related behavior. Such knowledge is particularly important for dairy cattle, where greater milk yields are associated with metabolic stress that impacts reproductive performance. Knowledge of the interactions of endocrine signaling and genetic control can shed light on how metabolic conditions affect reproductive function. Moreover, systems biology methods integrating physiological information with mathematical modeling can improve our understanding of these complex biological pathways. The convergence of genomics with reproductive physiology paves the way for novel strategies for enhancing fertility and reproductive health for rural as well as wildlife populations, broadening the horizon of investigations currently being conducted (Boer et al., 2010; Brannan & Bobbie, 2017) (Figure 6.1).

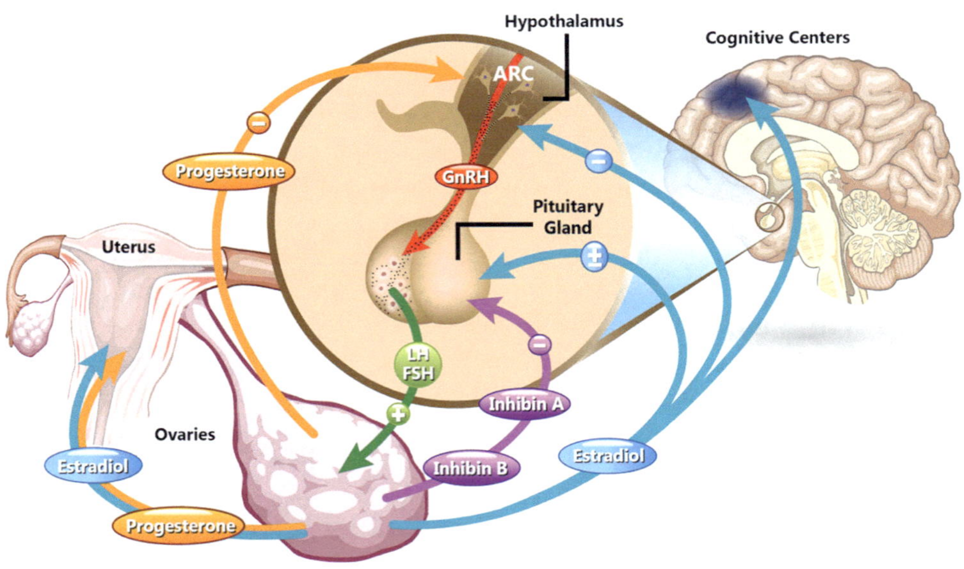

Figure 6.1. Reproductive physiology.

Source: https://www.niehs.nih.gov/sites/default/files/research/atniehs/labs/assets/images/q_r/rpp_graphic.jpg.

Definition and Importance of Reproductive Physiology

Reproductive physiology is the scientific discipline concerned with the biological processes and systems through which reproduction occurs, encompassing a very broad range of functions from gametogenesis to the intricate hormonal control in cycles of reproduction. Reproductive physiology has a crucial role to play in explaining how organisms reproduce, develop, and establish species continuity. Reproductive physiology, at the cellular level, is the study of the nature of gametes, processes of fertilization, and embryonic development. In addition, it describes the interaction among various physiological systems, noting the interdependence and complexity of the biological processes that enable reproduction. Such knowledge can still point out how reproductive health is maintained and how disruptions in these processes can lead to infertility, congenital abnormalities, or other reproductive health issues, demonstrating its significant role in individual health and species reproduction. The implications of reproductive physiology extend beyond mere survival and reproduction; they carry profound meaning for evolutionary and environmental biology, and for human health. Outcomes of the study of reproductive systems inform conservation of endangered species and farming practices by enhancing the reproductive potential of farm animals. In medical contexts, information obtained from reproductive physiology is critical in the formulation of treatments for reproductive disease, assisting in vitro fertilization methods, and enhancing prenatal treatment. Furthermore, knowing the regulation of reproduction by hormones helps solve problems associated with hormonal diseases, menopause, and androgen diseases. Reproductive physiology, thus, stands at the interface of fundamental science and practical health, providing the background constructs required for a number of interdisciplinary sciences like medicine, ecology, and genetics. Moreover, the advances in reproductive physiology put into perspective the value of understanding the interaction between cellular arrangement and reproductive outcome. Organizational arrangement of multicellular systems is most critical, since differences in cellular interaction and spatial arrangement can have a gigantic effect on reproductive efficiency and success.

For instance, the extracellular matrix plays a significant role in the regulation of cell behavior and fate across reproductive systems and modulates processes that cover spermatozoa maturation to embryonic implantation. With the understanding of the functional structure of intercellular space, researchers can have an even better-informed vision of reproductive processes. Interestingly, these revelations can make valuable contributions to solving problems in reproductive medicine, such as, those concerning cancer and aging, which interfere with normal reproductive function. Thus, the physiology of reproduction is not merely necessary to study reproductive well-being but also crucial in the growth of medical and biological sciences generally (Farinelli et al., 2016; Bich et al., 2019) (Figure 6.2).

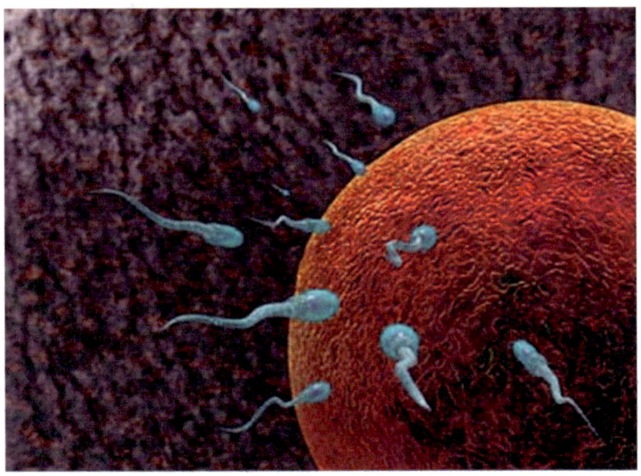

Figure 6.2.

Source: https://www.smarteach.com/wp-content/uploads/2014/11/1_60Reproductive-Physiology.jpg.

Overview of Reproductive Systems in Different Species

The difference in reproductive systems across species illustrates the complicated modifications organisms have undergone to ensure successful reproduction. In mammals, for instance, reproductive strategies can differ from the human placental viviparity to the oviparous adaptations of animals , such as monotremes, the platypus, which lays eggs. This divergence illustrates how environmental pressures and evolutionary paths shape reproductive anatomy and physiology. Reptiles, however, can express any level of oviparity and viviparity, and some, such as, certain snakes, provide live birth while others lay eggs in nests. It is essential to the research of reproductive physiology that these be understood because they provide a way of understanding how different mechanisms operate and the evolutionary benefits they hold, which further influence survival and reproductive success. Aquaculture has had a significant influence on research into reproductive systems, particularly in aquatic animals , such as fish and shrimp. Aquaculture, as a developing industry, has progressed without an adequate appreciation of the physiological mechanisms involved in reproductive success in these creatures. In particular, aquaculture for shrimp, there is a critical necessity to possess a deeper understanding in reproductive physiology because when one understands the biological process, it can improve breeding programs and aquaculture management. A study indicates that maximizing physiological characteristics will enhance productivity and resilience in aquaculture systems. The ability to select for desirable reproductive traits in breeding schemes holds potential advantages, eventually contributing towards increased sustainability and productivity in food production (Balasubramanian, 2009). Reproductive physiology has a direct link with the efficiency of production in livestock, particularly dairy cows. Selection for greater milk production has, unfortunately, been accompanied by reduced fertility levels, associated with diminished expression of estrous behavior. The endocrinological regulation of the estrous cycle in dairy cows has been well studied, revealing that hormones , such as estradiol play significant roles in influencing both reproductive hormones and behavioral activities of estrus. Interactions of the hormones regulate elements , such as gene expression and metabolic stress, which are fundamental to managing fertility problems in high-yielding dairy cows. The recent studies on gene expression in various animals, including rodents, reveal that determining the neural mechanisms affected by estradiol could bring new advancements in raising fertility in dairy cattle (Boer et al., 2010). Utilization of these physiological insights into animal breeding is paramount for guaranteeing productive and sustainable agricultural systems.

6.1. Anatomy of the Male Reproductive System

Learning Outcome

1. Describe the structure and function of testes;
2. Focus on the role of accessory glands;
3. Learn about the pathway of sperm production and transport.

The anatomy of the male reproductive system is a well-coordinated assemblage of structures that each play distinctive roles essential to reproduction. Exclusively located in the pelvic cavity, the system consists of the testes, seminal vesicles, prostate gland, and penis, which collectively function to produce and convey sperm. The testes, which represent the primary reproductive organs, are located within the scrotum to maintain the temperature control that is essential to successful spermatogenesis. This development starts in the embryonic phase, where mesonephric ducts are the precursor to the male reproductive organs, underlining the subtle inter-relationship of embryonic anatomy and organ differentiation (Satchi & Muneer, 2021). Each anatomical element from the spermatic cord to the urethra plays a crucial part in the whole functionality of the system, showing the evolutionary compensations that optimize male fertility. Parallel to its anatomy, the male reproductive system is under complex physiological mechanisms that regulate fertility and reproductive health. System development is regulated strictly by the hypothalamic–pituitary–gonadal (HPG) axis, which orchestrates hormone release necessary for the onset of spermatogenesis (Scribner & Tadros, 2021). Hormones such as the luteinizing hormone (LH) and the follicle-stimulating hormone (FSH) are key modulators of both testosterone production and sperm development within the seminiferous tubules. This endocrine relationship is central to reproductive success because testosterone influences not only secondary sexual characteristics but also prepares the spermatozoa for subsequent maturation. This sophisticated orchestration of endocrine signals underscores the significance of the endocrine system in providing for the health of male reproductive organs. The process of sperm transport from the testes through the male reproductive system once more demonstrates the complexity of the system's design. During transport through the epididymis, the sperm undergo important maturation processes, which enhance motility and fertility, from immotile to functional spermatozoa (Scribner & Tadros, 2021). Maturation is important because it guarantees that viable sperm are ejaculated. The journey from the epididymis to the urethra is facilitated by muscle spasms and the input of seminal fluid from accessory glands, creating a better condition for sperm viability. The higher-order anatomical structure of the male reproductive system, its regulating hormones, and nourishing fluids show the intricate nature of the system, built for reproduction success and continuation of the genetic line (Figure 6.3).

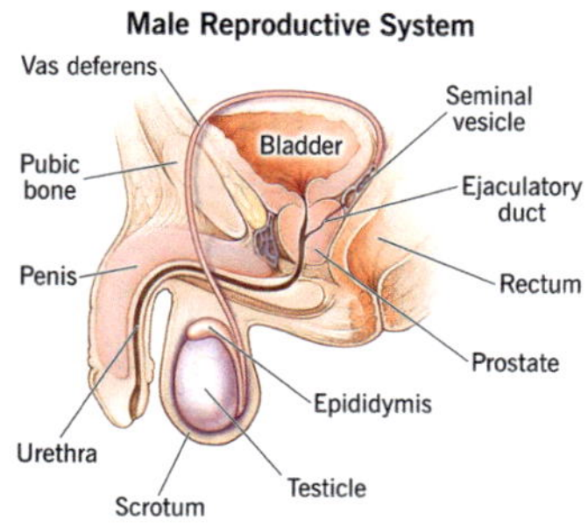

Figure 6.3. Male-reproductive-system.

Source: https://my.clevelandclinic.org/-/scassets/images/org/health/articles/9117-male-reproductive-system.

6.1.1. Structure and Function of Testes

The testicular structure is particularly functional to facilitate the main functions of the testes: spermatogenesis and hormone secretion. Located in the scrotum, the testes consist of seminiferous tubules where sperm cells are produced. There are hundreds of these tubules in each testis that are covered in Sertoli cells, which give the growing sperm cells the necessary support and nutrition. The intratubular spaces are filled by Leydig cells, which play a role in testosterone production, a hormone with crucial functions in male reproductive physiology, like the establishment of secondary sexual characteristics and regulation of spermatogenesis. The structural organization of the testes provides ideal temperature regulation for optimal spermatogenesis, an essential process for male fertility. Spermatogenesis comprises a variety of different stages: mitosis, meiosis, and spermiogenesis. These begin by dividing by mitosis into primary spermatocytes, which then go through meiosis to become haploid spermatids. This complicated process is concluded by spermiogenesis, during which the spermatids are converted by morphological alteration to mature spermatozoa. During this period of transformation, structures like the acrosome and flagellum are formed to enable the motility of the sperm and the fertilization of an egg. Interestingly, the testes are implicated as well in seminal fluid production in terms of sperm secretions from accessory glands. The fluid consists of proteins serving diverse functions in reproduction, as reports on male seminal fluid proteins (SFPs) among different species, including tsetse flies, have shown and detail the complexities of ejaculate composition (Scolari et al., 2016). The function of the testes can be significantly determined by the environment, leading to a disruption in reproductive health. For instance, exposure to estrogenic chemicals can impact reproductive development and function, such as, in domestic poultry exposed to EE2 and o,p-DDT chemicals. Exposure may lead to diminished male reproductive functions by way of testicular morphological changes and changes in hormone levels, as well as diminished sperm production and quality (Hermansson, 2007). Thus, the delicate balance of the hormonal and structural components of the testes is not just vital to individual reproductive success but also to species perpetuation. An understanding of the effects of environmental factors on testicular function is important for future conservation and reproductive management plans for a variety of species (Figure 6.4).

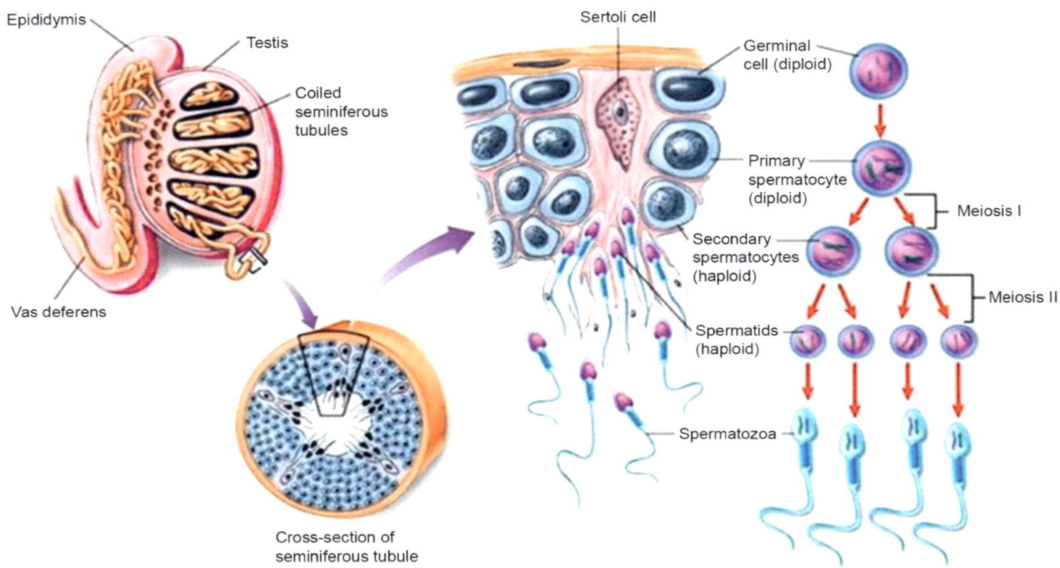

Figure 6.4. Testis function.

Source: https://ars.els-cdn.com/content/image/3-s2.0-B9780123864567051029-f05102-05-9780123864567.jpg.

6.1.2. Role of Accessory Glands

Accessory glands play a vital role in reproductive physiology, notably through seminal fluid protein (SFP) synthesis and secretion, which are essential for successful fertilization and resulting reproductive processes. In the majority of species, as in insects , such as *Aedes aegypti*, accessory glands have a significant impact not only on sperm viability, but also on female reproductive biology and behavior. Accessory glands discharge proteins that are known to initiate sperm motility, modify female receptivity, and even transfer essential nutrients to the sperm for successful fertilization (Degner et al., 2018). Importantly, the engagement of these proteins with the physiology of the female can induce behavioral changes, such as, refractoriness to further mating, indicating the intricate dynamics of reproductive strategy and selection pressures in mating systems across species. The evolutionary significance of accessory glands is emphasized by their convergent evolution, which indicates an ongoing interaction between male reproductive tactics and female reproductive tactics. Evidence indicates that SFPs, particularly in polyandrous mating systems of species, are subject to rapid evolution under the pressures of sexual selection, including sperm competition and female choice (Sepil et al., 2018). This evolution has repercussions for the reproductive success of individual males, as well as for population dynamics and general species adaptability. By controlling female physiology via such SFPs, males thus maximize their chances of paternity in situations where multiple mating is common, and so confirm the accessory glands' pivotal role in reproductive success determination and influencing evolutionary processes. Besides, the accessory glands are involved in complex biochemical communication processes that go beyond mere reproduction. Through the release of SFPs, the accessory glands not only cater to the short-term reproductive needs but also contribute to the general health and lifespan of offspring. The seminal fluid can impact offspring development and postnatal health, and studies confirm this, highlighting the vast influences of accessory gland secretions on more than fertilization itself (Degner et al., 2018). As scientists learn more about the function and structure of these proteins, their findings offer new approaches to pest control and regulation of reproductive health. Discovering the molecular details of accessory glands offers potential areas of intervention, especially in such vectors as Aedes aegypti that are powerful agents of public health because they serve as disease vectors (Figure 6.5).

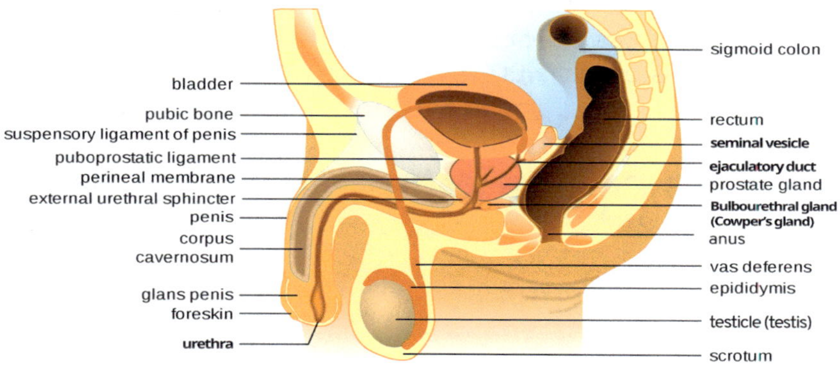

Figure 6.5. Accessory glands.

Source: https://iastate.pressbooks.pub/app/uploads/sites/43/2022/02/male-reproductive-system.png.

6.1.3. Pathway of Sperm Production and Transport

The sperm generation and transport process is a multicellular physiological process that commences in the seminiferous tubules of the testis, wherein spermatogenesis occurs. Spermatogenesis is the process of division and maturation of spermatogonia stem cells into mature sperm cells and entails several stages involving mitosis, meiosis, and spermiogenesis. Spermatozoa are transported to the epididymis once they are produced, where they mature and gain motility. The epididymal setting is crucial since it allows for sperm membrane reorganization and storage of essential proteins. Under the setting, sperm experience dramatic biochemical changes that enhance their function. Study of these processes of development is a cornerstone since they directly affect fertility and any impairment has the capacity to lead to male infertility, thus making reproductive physiology essential to understand in detail. Transport of sperm from the epididymis to the female reproductive tract involves a coordinated series of motions and biochemical events. Sperm are transported into the vas deferens during ejaculation and they are mixed with seminal fluid from accessory glands to form semen. The highly developed mixture is not only a nutrient-rich environment to support sperm motility but also contains molecules that protect sperm against oxidative damage. Capacitation—a key process of maturation—occurs in the oviduct or female reproductive tract, wherein sperm are rendered fertile to fertilize an oocyte. Of specific importance at this stage is the activity of bicarbonate ions (HCO_3^-), stimulating adenylate cyclase and producing cyclic AMP (cAMP). The mechanisms of how bicarbonate is transported in sperm cells remain a subject of current research, and therefore, the intricacies of sperm transport are within cellular signaling pathways to regulate capacitation and, eventually, fertilization (Austin et al., 2017). Compounding the intricacies of the sperm transport pathway is the metabolic regulation that influences sperm behavior and viability. Current studies show that sperm metabolic activity not only facilitates ATP production but also plays a part in cellular signaling, regulating motility and the acrosome reaction, an important step in sperm penetration of the egg protective capsules. Sperm metabolism interaction with cell fate decisions highlights the importance of the microenvironment in the immediate vicinity of the sperm as it moves through the female reproductive tract. Studies of these metabolic processes can also give clues to how outside forces, i.e., culture conditions, impact embryonic growth and reproductive health overall. As we learn more about the metabolic needs of sperm at various points, such as, capacitation, its significance for fertility therapy increases (Lewis & Sturmey, 2015).

Test Your Knowledge

1. List the primary and accessory organs of the male reproductive system and describe their functions.
2. Describe the structure and function of the testes, including the seminiferous tubules.

6.2. Anatomy of the Female Reproductive System

Learning Outcome

1. Explain the structure and function of ovaries;
2. Define the role of the uterus and fallopian tubes;
3. Learn about the menstrual cycle and its phases.

The female reproductive anatomy constitutes a system of organs that cooperate to ensure reproduction. The key organs within this system are the ovaries, whose functions include the production of ova and the secretion of hormones like estrogen and progesterone. The ovaries, placed one on each side of the uterus, discharge eggs through the process of ovulation. These eggs are subsequently swept up by the fallopian tube fimbriae, where they can be fertilized if there are sperm present. The muscular uterus, or womb, is crucial in holding the developing fetus while pregnant, and the lining of this organ, referred to as the endometrium, becomes thickened to prepare for potential implantation of an egg. An understanding of these organs is necessary to realize how hormonal fluctuations impact female reproductive health and physiology. Aside from the organs listed above, the female reproductive system includes the vagina and the cervix, both of which have crucial functions in reproduction and menstrual processes. The cervix is a canal linking the vagina and the uterus, regulating the flow of sperm during sexual intercourse and providing a barrier to protect the uterine environment from infections. Further, during labor, the cervix also opens up to allow the passage of the infant. The vagina is both the receptacle for the sperm and the birth canal, emphasizing its dual role in reproduction.

The system is regulated by hormones with difficulty, and the interaction between the ovaries and the pituitary gland controls a cyclical phenomenon that is central to fertile health, emphasizing the importance of an integrated understanding of female reproductive anatomy in reproductive physiology. Despite the crucial role played by the female reproductive system in general health, findings identify a wide gap in knowledge regarding reproductive anatomy among students. For instance, studies have proven that first-year non-medical health care students perform badly on tests of their knowledge regarding reproductive systems, indicating the need for improved learning systems in such a setting (Albeitawi et al., 2024). This difference underlines the importance of more reproductive education to foster educated attitudes and behavior towards sexual health. Sexual reproductive health training programs, particularly in non-clinical settings, can enable people with the necessary information to make educated choices regarding their reproductive well-being. These interventions can enhance deeper knowledge of anatomy, physiology, and the importance of regular gynecological check-ups, thereby improving community health outcomes (Figure 6.6).

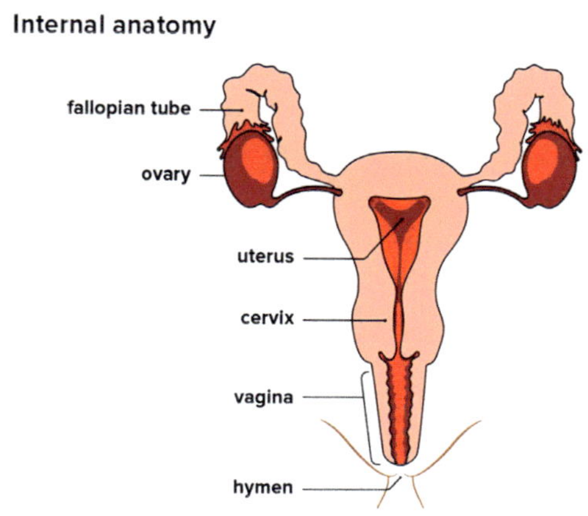

Figure 6.6. Female reproductive organ anatomy.

Source: https://i0.wp.com/post.medicalnewstoday.com/wp-content/uploads/sites/3/2021/08/158819-female-anatomy-uterus-1296x728-body-1024x692.jpg?w=1155&h=1839.

6.2.1. Structure and Function of Ovaries

Ovaries, which are organs of the female reproductive system, have several crucial functions, primarily the production of oocytes and hormone production. Ovaries are almond-shaped organs situated bilaterally in the pelvic cavity, each being covered with a fibrous tunica albuginea. Internally, the ovaries have two distinct regions: the outer cortex, with the ovarian follicles, and the inner medulla, with blood vessels and connective tissue. Ovarian follicles, at various stages of development, are where oocyte maturation occurs and are responsible for hormone secretion, particularly estrogen and progesterone. Understanding the structural intricacies of the ovaries is useful in comprehending their capacity and function in female reproductive processes. Ovarian function is greatly regulated by hormonal stimulation, in this instance, through the mechanism of action of gonadotropins like follicle-stimulating hormone (FSH) and luteinizing hormone (LH). The anterior pituitary gland releases these hormones and plays a critical role in being regulators of ovarian function as well as being pivotal in the menstrual cycle. The FSH-ovarian follicle interaction is implicated in the promotion of follicular growth and estrogen release, which are essential for the preparation of the endometrium for potential implantation. RFRP3, a neuropeptide of the hypothalamus, also plays an interesting role as it can inhibit gonadotropin release and consequently affect ovarian function. This feedback regulatory process emphasizes the complexity of ovarian physiology, in which intricate hormone interaction controls both follicular development and overall reproductive readiness (Wilsterman et al., 2019). aside from these hormonal feedback processes, the ovaries also involve local factors that influence follicle development and steroidogenesis. It was discovered through research that RFRP3 is expressed in the ovaries and has the ability to influence follicle viability and function. Experiments on the effects of RFRP3 on ovarian follicles, particularly in domestic cats, show its inhibitory action on steroidogenesis and follicle integrity at certain concentrations. This is a significant observation for understanding how local influences affect ovarian physiology, with emphasis on the necessity of careful evaluation of both systemic and local effects on the ovaries. These results are not only within the general knowledge body of reproductive physiology but also have implications for captive breeding and fertility management of wildlife and also understanding ovarian dysfunction-related pathologies (Yom-Din et al., 2016) (Figure 6.7).

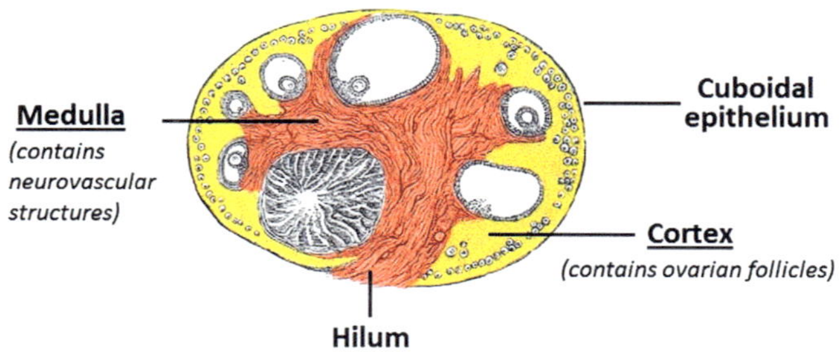

Figure 6.7. Structure and function of ovaries.

Source: https://teachmeanatomy.info/wp-content/uploads/Cross-Section-of-an-Ovary-Medulla-Cortex-Epithelium.jpg.

6.2.2. Role of the Uterus and Fallopian Tubes

The uterus and the fallopian tubes play a key role in reproductive physiology and are essential organs for fertilization and gestation. The muscular uterus is designed to accept and nourish a fertilized ovum. Its endometrial lining cyclically changes under hormonal control to become receptive for implantation. When fertilization occurs in the fallopian tubes, the fertilized egg, or zygote, is transported to the uterus to be implanted in the receptive endometrium. This movement from the tube into the uterus gives prominence to the interaction of these organs, with spatial and functional coordination being crucial for successful reproduction. Besides, the uterine microenvironment is finely regulated to support embryo development through various biochemical signals, demonstrating its active role in fertility and pregnancy success. Apart from physical structures, the uterine and fallopian tubes also host a complex microbiota that can influence reproductive well-being. Current studies show that despite the fact that vaginal microbiota has been adequately characterized, the upper genital tract, including the uterus and tubes, comes into being slowly and having distinctive microbial communities (Peric et al., 2019).

The microbial communities are likely to have positive and negative impacts on the reproductive process, and thus, our theory of female fertility is further insoluble. For instance, some strains of bacteria may help maintain the health of the reproductive environment and may have a commensal role, while others may be involved in inflammation or reproductive disease. The emerging field of reproductive microbiome sciences demands reexamination of the sterile environment paradigm, thus revealing new dimensions of human reproduction and fertility issues. Lastly, besides the aforementioned causes of infertility, oxidative stress (OS) has emerged as a critical factor in determining the uterine and fallopian tube function. Reproductive homeostasis is reliant on the balance between ROS and antioxidants; disruption leads to negative impacts on reproductive fertility in females (Lu et al., 2018). Studies indicate that elevated levels of ROS can potentially disrupt normal signaling processes in reproductive tissues, resulting in conditions like polycystic ovary syndrome (PCOS) and endometriosis. Interestingly, the fallopian tubes, which are frequently exposed to varying oxidative milieus, may suffer oxidative damage, compromising their fertilizing capacity and gamete-transport properties. Understanding the oxidative processes affecting these reproductive tissues offers new targets for treatment intervention to enhance female fertility and address reproductive health disorders (Figure 6.8).

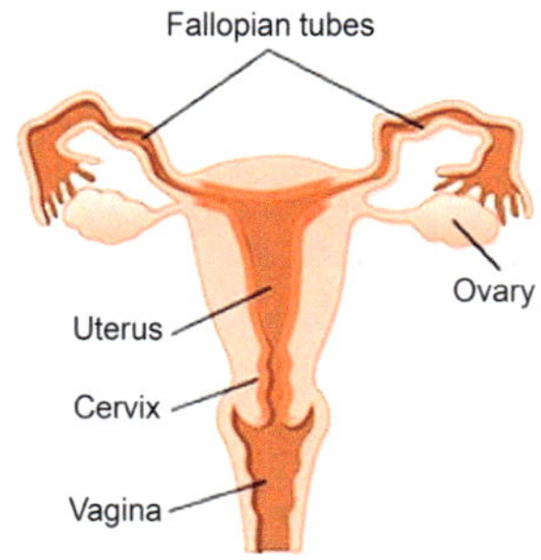

Figure 6.8. Fallopian tube recanalization.

Source: https://stanfordhealthcare.org/medical-treatments/f/fallopian-tube-recanalization/_jcr_content/tab-nav-component/tab-nav-parsys/imagewithcaption_0/image.img.full.high.jpg/1474756072516.jpg.

6.2.3. Menstrual Cycle and Its Phases

The menstrual cycle is a diverse physiological process governed by intricate interactions of hormones that prepare the body of a female for potential pregnancy. The cycle, which takes approximately 28 days on average, is divided into four mutually exclusive phases: menstrual phase, follicular phase, ovulation, and luteal phase. During the menstrual phase, the uterine lining is shed if there is no conception, resulting in menstruation. This is followed by the follicular phase, in which hormones , such as follicle-stimulating hormone (FSH) trigger the growth of ovarian follicles. Both phases play significant roles in reproductive physiology, with the follicular phase contributing significantly to cycle variability. Studies indicate that in regularly cycling women, the variation in cycle length can be greatly variable, often greater than seven days in nearly half of the cases being studied (Fehring et al., 2006). This physical variability addresses the dynamic nature of the menstrual cycle and the importance of the menstrual cycle within reproductive health. Ovulation marks the beginning of the second most important stage of the menstrual cycle. With a surge of

LH, ovulation typically occurs mid-month in the menstrual cycle. It does this to encourage fertility, as it releases a mature egg from the ovaries, making it available for fertilization. The timing of ovulation is not fixed, influencing the fertile window—a very critical period when intercourse can lead to pregnancy. The highest reading of fertility, as observed in clinical trials, will usually mirror this point of ovulation and is the peak of reproductive capacity. Curiously, the luteal phase follows ovulation when the corpus luteum forms, producing progesterone to prepare the uterine lining for potential implantation of the embryo. Understanding the alteration in hormone levels during these phases facilitates effective control over reproductive health, like the use of contraceptive measures and fertility treatments. The luteal phase also reiterates the function of uterine action on the backdrop of reproductive physiology. During the luteal phase, the hormonal environment not only influences the endometrium lining but also uterine contractility, which latter plays a role in ensuring overall success of reproduction. Studies with transabdominal electro hysterography have begun to clarify uterine patterns of contraction during the menstrual cycle, and significant differences between phases have been identified, particularly between the menstrual and luteal phases (Sammali et al., 2018). The findings potentially provide insight into conditions , such as dysmenorrhea and endometriosis, where abnormal uterine contractility is prevalent. By means of sophisticated evaluation methods like electro hysterography, researchers anticipate gaining greater insight into the role of the uterus in the nonpregnant female and, thereby, improving the management of reproductive diseases associated with uterine dysfunction.

Test Your Knowledge

1. Describe the structure and functional zones of the uterus.
2. What are the roles of the ovaries in reproduction and hormone production?

6.3. Hormonal Regulation of Reproduction

Learning Outcome

1. Explain the key hormones involved in male reproduction;
2. Define the key hormones involved in female reproduction;
3. Describe the feedback mechanisms in hormonal regulation.

Hormonal regulation takes a pivotal role in the intricate mechanisms of reproduction, which influence anything from gametogenesis to metabolic functions associated with reproductive well-being. At the root of hormonal regulation are steroid hormones, including estrogens and testosterone, that have been described by their uber activity at both the peripheral and central components of the neuroendocrine axis. This regulatory network activity is evident not only in reproductive potential and sexual differentiation but also in overall metabolic programming and neurological health. For example, hormonal programming of reproductive function can impact diseases such as polycystic ovary syndrome, suggesting the importance of realizing the interaction and balance of the hormones involved. The multifaceted functions of steroid hormones cut across various physiological scenarios, highlighting their pivotal role in reproductive health and disease prevention (Zubeldia-Brenner et al., 2016). For the male reproductive system, it is crucial to understand the physiological underpinnings of hormone control in a bid to deliver meaningful medical responses. Testosterone, the key male sex hormone, is pivotal in male reproductive organ growth and maintenance, sperm production, and libido regulation. The intricate feedback mechanisms involving the hypothalamus, pituitary gland, and gonads depict the inherent interrelation of regulators and hormones. Furthermore, a thorough understanding of these hormonal processes benefits clinicians in managing male reproductive disorders, including infertility and sexual dysfunction.

There remain huge lacunae in our comprehension of the entire field of male reproductive endocrinology. Closing such gaps can enhance the efficacy of hormonal therapies, and more research in this critical field of reproductive physiology is called for (Clavijo & Hsiao, 2018). The hormonal regulation of reproduction is further complicated by the influence of environmental and health-related factors that have the potential to interfere with the proper functioning of hormones. Endocrine disrupting chemicals, for instance, can manipulate the routes of hormonal signaling and lead to reproductive pathology. Understanding how these external influences on hormonal balance are important in order to develop preventive measures within reproductive health. Additionally, investigation into the behavioral components that are shaped by hormonal alteration, such as, sexual orientation and strategy of reproduction, can give insight into reproductive physiology evolution. By investigating both the internal physiological hormonal processes and external influences that control reproduction, researchers can gain a better understanding of the workings of reproductive physiology. This integrative strategy is essential for addressing problems of today in reproductive health and for creating effective prevention and treatment strategies (Zubeldia-Brenner et al., 2016) (Figure 6.9).

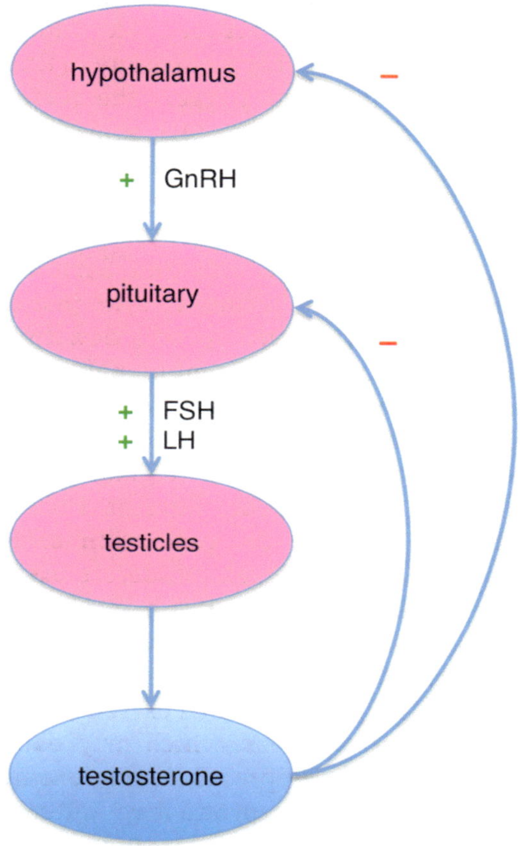

Figure 6.9. Hormonal regulation of the reproductive system.

Source: https://bio.libretexts.org/@api/deki/files/78931/s-pituitary-testicles-axis.png?revision=1.

6.3.1. Key Hormones Involved in Male Reproduction

Among the intricate physiology of male reproductive functions, certain primary hormones have a pivotal role to play in regulating many diverse facets of spermatogenesis and overall reproductive well-being. Testosterone, secreted predominantly in the testes, is essential to the development of male secondary sexual characteristics and for inducing spermatogenesis. It affects Sertoli cells, which nourish and support young spermatozoa cells that develop within seminiferous tubules. In addition, gonadotropin-releasing hormone (GnRH) from the hypothalamus triggers the secretion of luteinizing hormone (LH) and follicle-stimulating hormone (FSH) from the anterior pituitary. LH stimulates testosterone secretion by Leydig cells, whereas FSH is essential in regulating spermatogenesis and Sertoli cell function. Thus, these hormones synergistically facilitate effective sperm production that is viable, an essential component of male fertility. Additionally, outside factors , such as health status and exercise also influence the balance of reproductive hormones. Regular exercise has been found to enhance hormonal balance, particularly through the regulation of FSH, testosterone, and LH levels. Moderate exercise is favorable to the quality of sperm by increasing motility and morphology, while overexercise can lead to hormonal imbalances that impair fertility. A pertinent study indicates that exercise not only reduces oxidative stress, which may damage sperm DNA, but also improves insulin sensitivity, resulting in better reproductive outcomes. Significantly, this interaction suggests that male reproductive hormones are significantly determined by lifestyle choices, highlighting the relevance of comprehensive interventions in reproductive health. These results are critical to understanding the interactions among various factors and their influence on male fertility. Genetic and molecular technologies have paved the way for new contraceptive modalities, expanding deliberation of male reproductive hormones. Although the evolution of non-hormonal contraceptives for selective genes and proteins in spermatogenesis is on the horizon, the understanding of the action of the major hormones remains vital. For instance, recent studies with long-read sequencing technologies have identified the crucial genomic areas involved in sperm motility and sperm production. These findings provide targets for the development of targeted inhibitors that do not disrupt global hormone control. Progress in small molecule inhibitors affecting such pathways as those regulated by STK33 and CDK2 points towards a promising future for male contraception. With the coming together of genetic information and hormonal biology, the field is moving towards an integrated understanding of male reproductive physiology that promises to make reproductive health care safer and more effective (Adelowo et al., 2024; Garcia & Matzuk, 2024) (Figure 6.10).

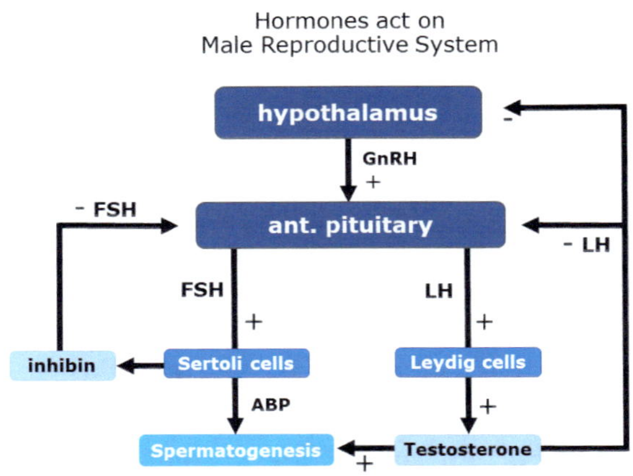

Figure 6.10. Hormones Involved in Male Reproduction.

Source: https://iastate.pressbooks.pub/app/uploads/sites/43/2023/02/Slide1-e1701380214733.png.

6.3.2. Key Hormones Involved in Female Reproduction

The intricate female reproduction mechanisms are mostly controlled by diverse primary hormones, and the central regulating point is the hypothalamic-pituitary-gonadal (HPG) axis. Gonadotropin-releasing hormone (GnRH) produced in the hypothalamus has a primary regulatory function of stimulating the release of luteinizing hormone (LH) and follicle-stimulating hormone (FSH) produced in the anterior pituitary gland. These gonadotropins are instrumental in ovarian function, stimulating the growth of follicles and causing the secretion of estrogen and progesterone by the ovaries. The balance and interaction between these hormones are vital not only for menstrual cycle regulation but also for fertility. Deviation from normal levels can initiate reproductive disorders, thereby underlining the importance of understanding these hormonal interactions in the overall picture of reproductive physiology and health. Yet another hormone that is important in female reproduction is leptin, which has traditionally been associated with energy balance but is now known to have a role to play in reproductive processes. Leptin influences oocyte growth, embryonic development, and puberty onset and is a metabolic signal that connects energy status to reproductive competence. It is mainly secreted by adipocytes in mammals and plays a role in ovarian follicle and steroid hormone regulation via the HPG axis. Notably, recent findings have indicated that leptin also enhances ovarian function at some point in life, e.g., energy deficit periods, suggesting that it may modulate reproductive adaptation to various metabolic conditions (Ahmadi & Ohkubo, 2025). This is thus the type of function leptin illustrates in terms of the complex interaction between nutritional status and reproductive physiology. Further, circadian control of reproductive hormones has increasingly been reported, particularly through the agency of the Bmal1 gene in the HPG axis. This gene is essential for orchestrating the intricate hormonal cues needed for female fertility, as evidenced by studies in Bmal1-knockout mice with abrogated estrous cycles and impaired ovarian function (Zhang et al., 2024). Removal of Bmal1 causes alterations in chief reproductive hormones , such as prolactin and progesterone, which signal a chain of changes that ultimately reduce fertility. These findings accentuate the manner in which endogenous circadian rhythms can significantly impact reproductive well-being and shed light on potential therapeutic strategies for the treatment of female infertility. Cumulatively, these hormones illustrate the intricate bidirectional interconnection of female reproduction between metabolic, neuroendocrine, and circadian regulation required for reproductive success (Figure 6.11).

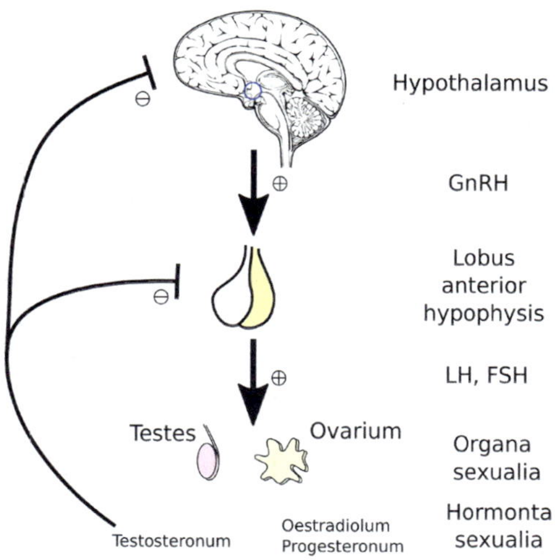

Figure 6.11. Hypothalamic pituitary gonadal axis.

Source: https://upload.wikimedia.org/wikipedia/commons/5/57/Hypothalamic%E2%80%93pituitary%E2%80%93gonadal_axis.svg.

6.3.3. Feedback Mechanisms in Hormonal Regulation

The intricate interaction of the hormones in the reproductive system is the hallmark of the importance of feedback mechanisms in hormonal regulation. Feedback loops in male and female physiology offer an equilibrium coordination of the hormones, which is essential in reproductive functions. For instance, in the female menstrual cycle, shifts in levels of estrogen and progesterone have regulatory effects on the secretion of luteinizing hormone (LH) and follicle-stimulating hormone (FSH). A rise of estrogen during the follicular phase induces positive feedback and results in an LH surge, leading to ovulation. Post-ovulation, levels of progesterone rise and induce negative feedback on FSH and LH so that repeat ovulation during the same cycle is prevented. This delicate equilibrium is of extreme importance since any disruption in hormones could yield issues in reproductive well-being, thereby necessitating the understanding of such mechanisms of feedback to tackle disorders , such as amenorrhea or infertility (Temirova & Asadova, 2025). Male reproductive physiology is also regulated to a large degree by feedback mechanisms that exhibit the complexity of endocrine control. Testosterone, the hormone of male sex, acts primarily through a negative feedback system between the pituitary gland and the hypothalamus. Upon increasing to a certain threshold, testosterone triggers the hypothalamus to reduce the release of gonadotropin-releasing hormone (GnRH) and inhibit the secretion of LH and FSH by the pituitary gland. The feedback system helps regulate appropriate levels of testosterone, which are needed for spermatogenesis as well as overall male reproductive health. Furthermore, the disruption of this feedback mechanism can result in hypogonadism disorders to infertility, and therefore male reproductive and sexual medicine specialists must possess a proper understanding of these physiological mechanisms (Clavijo & Hsiao, 2018). Overall, feedback mechanisms in hormone regulation offer a foundation on which the physiology of reproduction depends and ensure an appropriate environment for peak reproductive function. As science continues to advance, individual feedback loops are increasingly accurately interpreted, providing a more realistic reproduction of health representations. As a case in point, the discovery of inhibin and activin function as regulators of FSH levels adds further complexity to the male and female reproductive system feedback mechanisms. Moreover, therapeutic maneuvers directed toward these feedback mechanisms, such as, hormonal treatments, illustrate the practical significance of this insight in the clinical setting. Hormonal imbalance treatment via targeted intervention requires comprehension of these dynamics of hormonal control, teaching us something about both reproductive health and endocrine function in general. Thus, the study of feedback mechanisms remains essential to both scientific research and clinical application in reproductive physiology (Temirova & Asadova, 2025).

Test Your Knowledge

1. Describe the role of the hypothalamus and pituitary gland in regulating reproductive hormones.
2. How do FSH and LH influence ovarian and testicular function?

6.4. Gametogenesis

Learning Outcome

1. Identify the process of spermatogenesis;
2. Define the process of oogenesis;
3. Describe the comparison of gametogenesis in males and females.

Gametogenesis is a fundamental reproductive physiology process, encompassing gamete production—sperm in the male, oocytes in the female. It is a multistep, intricate process with mitosis, meiosis, and differentiation, regulated strictly by a combination of hormones and genetics. The pivotal factor in gametogenesis is the interaction of the brain-pituitary-gonad axis, regulating the hormonal environment necessary for gamete production. The onset of this process can be induced by a number of different external influences , such as nutrition, environmental influences, and social interaction, thus making it a dynamic aspect of reproductive biology. These regulatory processes need to be understood to enable scientists as well as practitioners to regulate breeding programs effectively and attain successful reproduction in both wild as well as domestic animals. The mechanism of gametogenesis depicts a remarkable interaction between intrinsic as well as extrinsic processes.

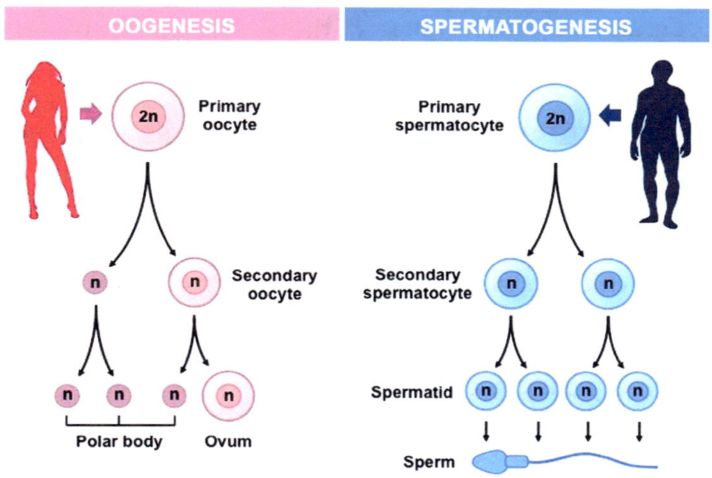

Figure 6.12. Gametogenesis.

Source: https://old-ib.bioninja.com.au/_Media/gametogenesis_med.jpeg.

For instance, nutritional condition, temperature, and photoperiod can significantly affect the timing and efficiency of gamete production. It has been shown that in fish, puberty onset at the earliest would be connected with the highest growth rates, which is necessary for gametogenesis. Environmental stress can also lead to variation in age and size at sexual maturity in organisms. These contrasts illustrate the plasticity of reproductive strategies in different species and have bearing on both wild population viability and aquaculture businesses. Such attention thus becomes important to the fine-tuning of such environmental pressures, not only for the conservation of species but also for enhancing the efficiency of production in farming systems. It has been demonstrated that genetically controlled responses to environmental conditions are important in regulating gametogenesis.

For example, the discovery of clock genes in aquatic bivalves reflects the complex regulation that manages reproduction cycles that can be modulated by environmental variations , such as day-night cycles and seasonal fluctuations. The research implies that endogenous clock processes can further synchronize gametogenesis to allow species to prepare and respond to fluctuating environmental cues. Moreover, sexually dimorphic expression of such genes indicates the intricacy of regulatory networks involved in gamete development. With advancing knowledge, particularly concerning the interaction of genetic and environmental factors, it has the potential to improve breeding practice, raise aquaculture production, and overcome challenges faced in wildlife conservation programs (Carrillo et al., 2010; Chapman, 2019) (Figure 6.12).

6.4.1. Process of Spermatogenesis

The process of spermatogenesis is an orderly and intricate physiological process central to the fertility of the male. It occurs in the seminiferous tubules of the testes, during which germ cells go through a series of changes to become mature spermatozoa. It is a multi-step process that can be sub-divided into three principal stages: mitosis, meiosis, and spermiogenesis. Initially, spermatogonia, being diploid cells, undergo mitosis to produce a large number of cells that will form the sperm. Afterwards, during the meiotic phase, spermatocytes undergo two divisions to give haploid spermatids. This reduction of chromosome numbers is crucial since it ensures that when fertilization occurs, the resulting zygote will have the correct diploid number of chromosomes—a process of utmost significance in maintaining genetic stability from generation to generation. Proceeding from meiotic divisions to spermiogenesis, round spermatids develop dramatically into long spermatozoa. This involves extensive morphological transformation, including the development of the acrosome, the formation of the flagellum, and the condensation of the nucleus. All this is vital in bringing mobility to the sperm as well as fitness for fertilization of the oocyte. Moreover, the role of the microenvironment in the seminiferous tubules cannot be overstated, as Sertoli cells provide structural support and required nutrients throughout spermatogenesis. Specifically, germ cell-Sertoli cell communication is very important in regulating the efficacy of spermatogenesis.

The coordination of these cellular communications ensures maximum sperm production and indicates the intricate biological network employed in the male reproductive physiology. Research on the endocrine regulation of spermatogenesis has enlighteningly analyzed the mechanisms of testosterone and other endocrine regulators to modulate this complex process. Testosterone, produced predominantly by Leydig cells, is crucial for sperm maturation as well as for Sertoli cell function. Research has indicated that variations in the level of testosterone significantly influence histological testicular structures as well as the rates of sperm production. In particular, evidence has shown that positive correlations exist between testosterone levels and the most significant testicular morphometric parameters, pointing to the key role of the hormone in the regulation of spermatogenesis (Abdul-Rahman et al., 2017). In addition, recent evidence reports the impact of environmental pollutants and endocrine disruptors on spermatogenic activity in various species, thereby suggesting that the understanding of spermatogenesis has implications for wildlife conservation and reproductive medicine (Caneppele et al., 2016). In general, the complex interplay among hormonal signals, cellular dynamics, and environmental influences points to the necessity for further investigation of reproductive physiology (Figure 6.13).

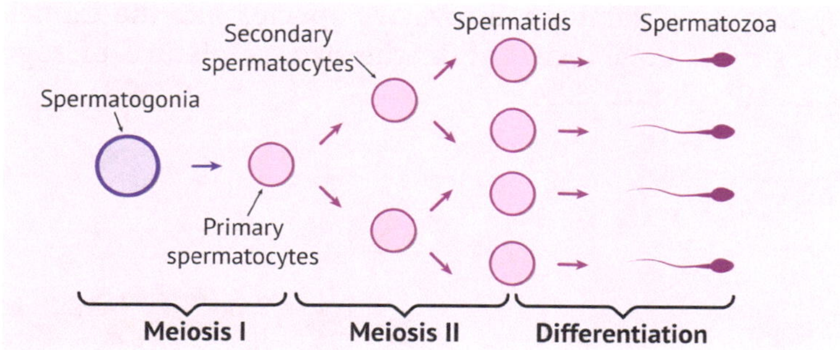

Figure 6.13. Spermatogenesis-phase-meiotic.

Source: https://www.invitra.com/en/wp-content/uploads/2014/07/spermatogenesis-phase-meiotic.png.

6.4.2. Process of Oogenesis

Oogenesis is a fundamental part of the reproductive physiology in which the development of the female gamete is ensured. It is a sophisticated biological process commencing with the early stages of embryonic development when primordial germ cells migrate to the developing ovaries and become oogonia. The oogonia go through a number of mitotic divisions, producing a group of primary oocytes which initiate the first meiotic division. There is extensive cell investment in this phase, as the oocytes accumulate organelles and nutrients. The primordial follicles surround the main oocytes, which are preserved in an inactive condition until puberty, emphasizing the lengthy developmental span of oogenesis. Understanding of this initial phase accentuates the significance of oocyte viability and environmental influences that may impact reproductive success, as in studies of aquatic animals like the Chinese pond mussel, with varying reproductive specializations depending on their habitats (Labecka & Domagała, 2018). With puberty approaching, hormonal activation of maturation of oocytes leads to reactivation of growth of oocytes to mature the primary oocytes into secondary oocytes by the completion of the first meiotic division. This is marked by the release from meiotic arrest so that secondary oocytes will continue to the second meiotic division, which is usually left incomplete until the time of fertilization. Here, oocytes undergo key biochemical alteration, e.g., vitellogenesis, in which yolk proteins are synthesized and stored within the oocyte, thereby enhancing its nutritional content. This growth forms the basis of the later embryonic process, as it provides the necessary finances for the early cleavage divisions. Regulation of such processes is derived from a complex interaction of hormonal cueing and local follicular dynamics, guiding reproductive potential of the organism and supporting strategies observed throughout different species, such as, brooding habits described in the Chinese pond mussel (Gross et al., 2001). Lastly, the climax of oogenesis is the discharge of the mature ovum at ovulation, a process closely linked with the female reproductive cycle. This is the climax of meiosis, producing a haploid ovum and a polar body, a residual of the meiotic division. The regulation of hormonal signals, particularly by the hypothalamus and pituitary gland, at this time is very important in guiding the ovarian follicles to prepare for ovulation and subsequent fertilization. In addition, oocyte maturation is aided by support cells of the follicle that further contribute through paracrine signaling. This orderly physiological process underscores the importance of oogenesis not just for individual reproductive success but also for population dynamics and evolutionary adaptation in the long term. The different reproductive strategies that are observed in other species, like the steady output of gametes in invasive species like the Chinese pond mussel, also demonstrate the complexity of oogenesis within the overall picture of reproductive physiology (Labecka & Domagała, 2018) (Figure 6.14).

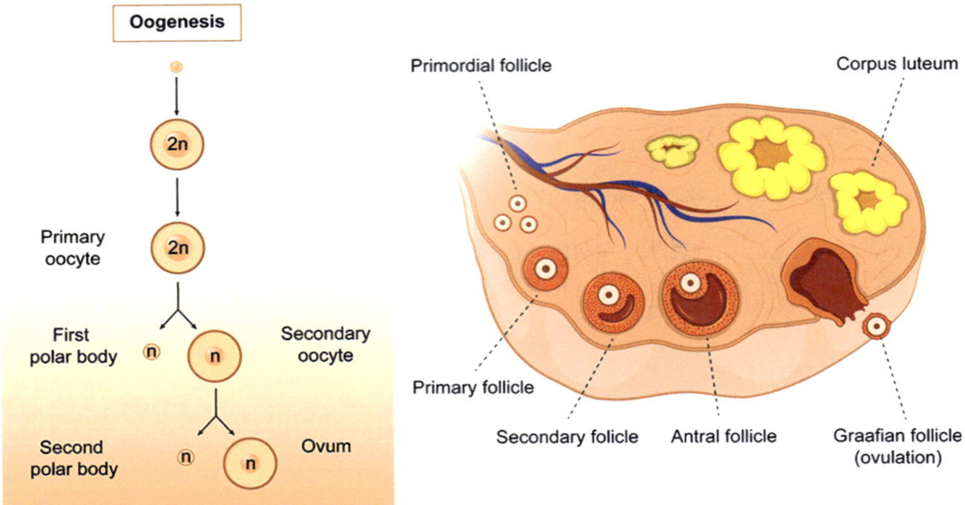

Figure 6.14. The process of oogenesis.

Source: https://www.researchgate.net/publication/372929799/figure/fig3/AS:11431281258620735@1720122333887/The-process-of-oogenesis-Oogenesis-starts-with-a-transformation-of-the-oogonia-into-the.tif.

6.4.3. Comparison of Gametogenesis in Males and Females

Gametogenesis or the production of gametes is quite different in male and female. Spermatogenesis occurs in the testes of a male, where a diploid germ cell undergoes mitosis to give rise to spermatogonia, which develop into spermatozoa by going through meiosis. Spermatogenesis is a relatively continuous process and millions of sperm are produced daily throughout the reproductive life of a male. By contrast, oogenesis in women occurs in the ovaries and is characterized by an evident cyclical nature. Women are born with a few immature oocytes that are arrested in prophase I until puberty, when hormonal changes induce them to mature. This fundamental difference produces an imbalance of gametes in terms of numbers, males producing in great numbers small, motile sperm and females producing in few numbers large, immotile ova required for the embryonic stage. The duration and regulation of gametogenesis differ greatly between the sexes as well. Male spermatogenesis can take several weeks and is an ongoing process due to hormonal signals like testosterone, which result in the proliferation and maturation of sperm. It is regulated primarily by the hypothalamic-pituitary-gonadal axis so that the reproductive potential is comparatively elastic and responds to males' environmental as well as physiological conditions. Oogenesis, however, is a more cyclical process with regulation by the hormonal cycles occurring during the menstrual cycle. Each cycle develops one main follicle into a secondary oocyte, with the remaining follicles degenerating through atresia. The cycle not just impacts fertility but also reflects the evolutionary pressures on female reproductive tactics, where gamete quality rather than quantity is ideally prioritized. In addition, the physiological process of gametogenesis further illustrates sexual dimorphism in reproductive physiology. In males, seminal fluid protein synthesis (SFPs) during the process of sperm development is vital as these proteins aid post-mating function in females, for example, increased egg production and lowered receptivity to successive attempts at mating. Such a relationship bears evidence of the sophisticated gamete interaction and corresponding biochemical environments that influence reproductive success. In women, the cyclical hormonal alterations that accompany oocyte maturation also prepare the body for future pregnancy, affecting not only the quality of the gamete but also the uterine environment. These differences are mirrored in the evolutionary situation, where each sex's gametogenesis has developed to optimize their reproductive success within various environmental paradigms, and thus their relevance to learning about these processes in the broader disciplinary context of reproductive physiology (Avila et al., 2010; Bowman et al., 2017).

Test Your Knowledge

1. Describe the key stages of spermatogenesis and indicate where each stage occurs.
2. Outline the process of oogenesis and explain how it is regulated hormonally.

6.5. Fertilization and Early Development

Learning Outcome

1. Identify the mechanisms of sperm-egg interaction;
2. Define the stages of fertilization;
3. Describe the early embryonic development and implantation.

In reproductive physiology, fertilization is a critical juncture in the life cycle of many species and is the first event to initiate development. Once the gametes have fused, there is a sensitive chain of cellular and molecular events that ultimately guide the zygote through a series of stages of embryonic development. The process is subject to external forces, including environmental factors and hormonal regulation. As an example, in laboratory experiments with bluemouth Helicolenus dactylopterus, there is evidence of robust seasonality in reproductive cycles, with specific time-periods for fertilization linked to hormonal changes in association with spawning behavior. Investigation of gametic interactions and early developmental stages emphasizes the need to be at the right time because optimum conditions for fertilization directly impact viability of early embryonic development and, by extension, survival rates. With progression from zygote to embryo, species-specific adaptations play a critical role in determining early stages of success. In the yellowfin tuna species, spawning behavior has been studied meticulously to reveal some of the intricacies involved in this phase of reproductive physiology. Organized courtship and spawning rituals are documented and demonstrate remarkable consistency, suggesting that body and biological processes largely control reproductive success. Most interestingly, the temperature of water becomes an important environmental variable that controls egg development and spawning time. Yellowfin tuna, for instance, have a predictable spawning cycle that is closely related to optimal water temperatures, illustrating how environmental variables can enhance reproduction success and enhance the viability of the species' larvae, thereby ensuring continuity of the species. Also evidenced is the relationship between physiological processes and early development by the hormonal oscillations governing the reproductive events. In bluemouth Helicolenus dactylopterus, rapid fluctuations in sex steroid levels have been reported, in particular the pre-mating surge of 17,20-dihydroxypregn-4-en-3-one. This suggests an exquisitely controlled hormonal environment that not only influences behavior but also plays a role in the timing of fertilization and embryogenesis. Thus, the intricate interaction between physiological response and hormonal control during fertilization is the key to understanding reproductive strategy in various species. Scientists opine that information gleaned from such studies is vital to guiding conservation efforts and maximizing aquaculture, as it is the key to unlocking fundamental traits of early development vital to the survival and adaptability of species in a dynamically changing environment (Figure 6.15).

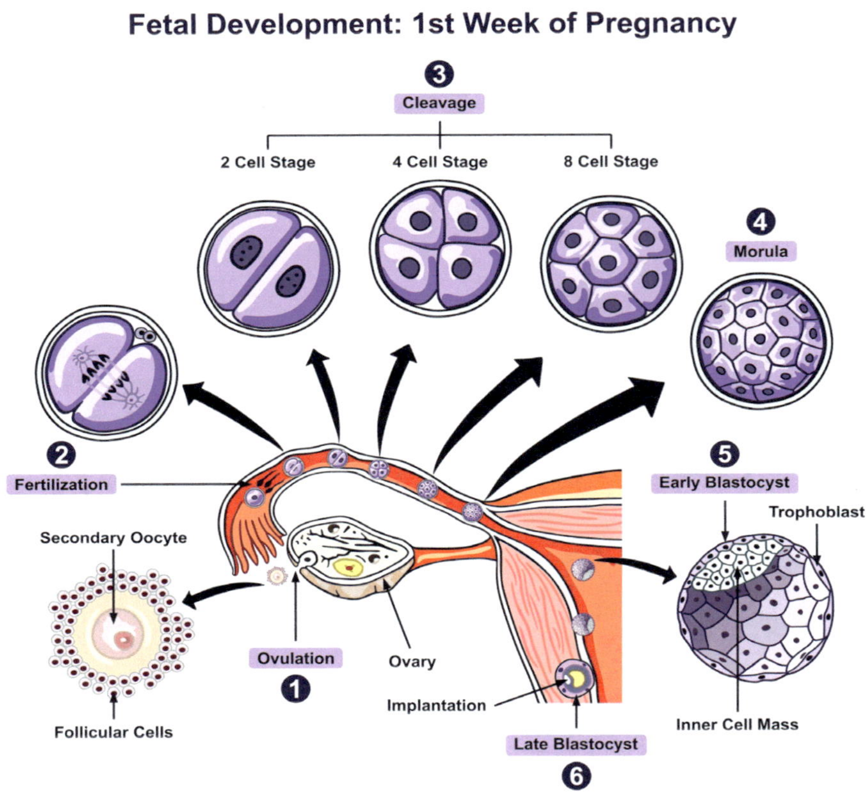

Figure 6.15. Fertilization and Early Development.

Source: https://iastate.pressbooks.pub/app/uploads/sites/43/2021/03/AdobeStock_505384740-scaled.jpeg.

6.5.1. Mechanisms of Sperm-Egg Interaction

Understanding mechanisms of sperm-egg interaction is at the center of reproductive physiology knowledge. Initial stages of fertilization depend on complex biochemical interactions that facilitate sperm to reach and penetrate the egg. A key element is the role played by the zona pellucida, the egg's glycoprotein covering that not only shields oocytes but also serves as a critical recognition barrier. Sperm must bind to specific receptors on the zona pellucida to fertilize, showing a highly sophisticated system of compatibility necessary for the successful sperm-egg union. This intricate process forms the foundation of mammalian fertilization, as it ensures only sperm possessing compatible qualities are able to initiate the fusion effectively. Furthermore, recent studies have highlighted the contribution of environmental elements to impacting the functionality and viability of sperm. Per- and polyfluoroalkyl substances (PFASs), widespread environmental pollutants in human tissues, disrupt critical reproductive mechanisms. Findings indicate that PFAS exposure can impair sperm motility, quality, and viability, adversely affecting the sperm's ability to swim to and fertilize the egg (Maxwell et al., 2025).

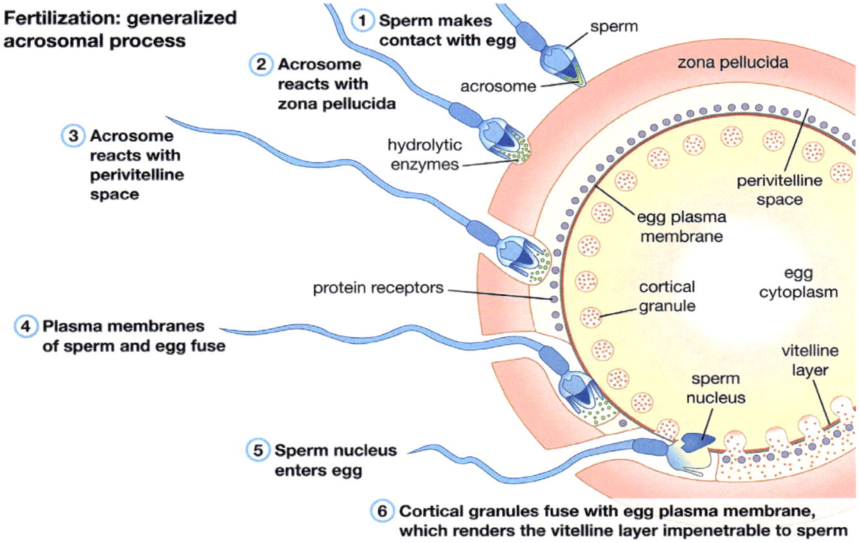

Figure 6.16. Mechanisms of sperm-egg interaction.

Source: https://cdn.britannica.com/22/194822-050-336EB737/sperm-cell-changes-layers-contact-prominence-spermatozoa.jpg.

The chemicals also disrupt endocrine mechanisms by altering critical reproductive hormones, which have indirect impacts on the sperm-egg interaction process. The implications of such interference are complex, in addition to questioning the short-term impact on fertility, also raising concerns regarding long-term reproductive health effects, necessitating more research on how toxins in the environment affect reproductive processes. Another subject of interest for study in the sperm-egg interaction is the phenomenon of sperm competition, pointing to the evolutionary mechanisms involved in fertilization success. Scientific studies indicate that sperm exhibit competitive behavior, and fertilization success is a function of competition among sperm of various males. Such competition could influence sperm motility as well as sperm selection activities in the female reproductive tract. Surprisingly, studies in Cd9-null female mice have revealed that the absence of specific proteins can result in disparity in the sperm to egg ratio, suggesting normal sperm-egg interactions are highly reliant upon specific molecular signals that control attraction and fusion mechanisms (Stickler & Avella, 2024). Such awareness not only outlines the intricacy of fertilization but also focuses on the evolutionary pressures that shape reproductive strategies across species (Figure 6.16).

6.5.2. Stages of Fertilization

Fertilization steps are important processes that determine significant reproductive success as well as subsequent embryonic development. Sperm capacitation forms the beginning of the process, which conditions spermatozoa to successfully penetrate the zona pellucida protective layers surrounding the oocyte. The biological readiness is necessary because only capacitated sperm will acutely respond to the biochemical cues generated by the oocyte in causing the acrosome reaction. During this phase, enzymes are released that lyse the zona pellucida and allow penetration by the sperm into the oocyte.

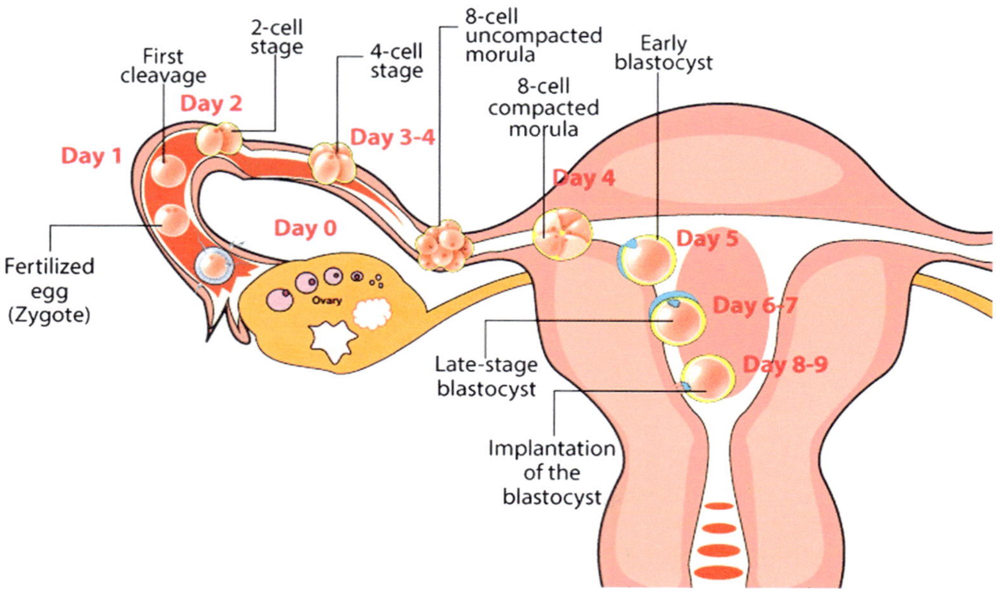

Figure 6.17. Fertilization-and-implantation.

Source: https://cdn1.byjus.com/wp-content/uploads/2017/11/fertilization-and-implantation.png.

Such intricate interaction highlights the importance of cellular communication and the physiological changes in both gametes, as well as the intricacy of the reproductive physiology. Once a sperm enters the oocyte, fertilization leads to the attainment of the meiotic maturation of the ovum with its characteristic entry into metaphase II. This process actually triggers the resumption of meiotic division of the oocyte, leading to the formation of a healthy zygote. Upon fertilization, the combination of both sperm and oocyte genetic material not only initiates the zygotic genome but also marks the beginning of embryonic development. The resulting zygote, then a unicellular organism, continues to later cleavage divisions that progressively increase its cell number without significant growth in size. These early events of fertilization form the groundwork for ongoing differentiation and subsequent tissue development, sustaining the intricacies of reproductive physiology. However, extrinsic factors , such as hormonal regulation may also have a considerable influence on the success of fertilization and embryonic development. For instance, excessive concentrations of cortisol, often the result of stress, have been shown to have an adverse effect on oocyte development and viability. Research has also indicated that increased cortisol levels can significantly suppress meiotic maturation of the cattle's oocytes and negatively impact embryonic development following fertilization, evident in decreased cleavage rates and lower percentages of blastocyst formation (Mahdy, 2018). Such findings are attributed to the interaction between reproduction mechanisms and environment, necessitating better knowledge of how reproductive physiology may be tuned towards improved fertility in human and livestock settings (Farinelli et al., 2016) (Figure 6.17).

6.5.3. Early Embryonic Development and Implantation

The intricate process of early embryonic development is a pivotal time of reproductive physiology characterized by a series of carefully regulated events leading to successful implantation and continued gestation. After fertilization, the zygote undergoes rapid cleavage divisions to form a multi-cellular structure known as the morula. This transition is crucial, as it sets the stage for what is to come in differentiation to the blastocyst, a stage where cells begin to specialize into trophoblasts and the inner cell mass. This specialization is particularly significant in implantation, as the trophoblasts are responsible for plugging into the uterine wall so the embryo may be secured tightly to the mother's environment. This intricate dance of cellular processes is regulated in synchrony with the mother's physiology, emphasizing the need for precise timing and efficient communication between maternal and embryonic systems to facilitate successful implantation and early embryonic growth (Boden et al., 2013). As the embryo develops to the stage of a blastocyst, ensuing developmental milestones are initiated, including culmination in implantation within the uterine wall. Implantation is not a mechanical process per se; it involves a highly advanced biochemical dialogue between the developing embryo and the endometrium. It is orchestrated by a set of signaling factors and growth factors that impact the embryo as well as the maternal tissues, such that conditions for implantation are maximized.

Research demonstrates that the control of genes that are engaged in progesterone generation and implantation of the embryo, such as, TIMP1 and TCTP, is central to this process, enhancing the potential of embryos to anchor in the uterine tissue (Pokharel et al., 2020). Thus, any disruption to this balance can lead to unsuccessful implantation, demonstrating how important it is that genetic and endocrine interaction takes place in early embryonic development in reproductive physiology. The preimplantation phase is particularly crucial as it's the time when most pregnancies can fail or struggle to survive. Indeed, studies reveal that most pregnancy losses in ruminants occur during this period of initial development, and thus, it is critical to reproductive success. Maternal well-being, hormone levels, and environmental influences can significantly alter the course of early development. Of particular interest are differences in gene expression between species, as revealed in comparative analyses between breeds like Finn sheep and Texel, elucidating the complex biological processes involved in implantation and early pregnancy maintenance (Pokharel et al., 2020). The identification of differentially expressed genes, particularly regarding embryo viability and capacity for implantation, lays the groundwork for optimizing reproductive outcomes and is also indicative of possible therapeutic interventions in reproductive medicine. Hence, understanding the nuances of early embryonic development and implantation is essential to inform advancing basic reproductive biology and clinical application in reproductive health.

Test Your Knowledge

1. Describe the sequence of events that occur during fertilization of the ovum by a sperm cell.
2. What mechanisms ensure species-specific and monospermic fertilization?

6.6. Reproductive Health and Disorders

Learning Outcome

1. Describe the common male reproductive disorders;
2. Define the common female reproductive disorders;
3. Discuss the impact of lifestyle and environment on reproductive health.

Reproductive health forms a vital component of overall well-being and specifically understanding various disorders that can undermine reproduction and outcomes. In women, disorders of reproduction , such as polycystic ovary syndrome (PCOS) and endometriosis, are prevalent, and they lead to problems , such as infertility, abnormal menses, and increased risk of metabolic disorders. They lead to dysfunction in the normal physiology of reproduction by altering hormone levels and ovarian function. For instance, PCOS is characterized by hyperandrogenism, ovulatory dysfunction, and polycystic ovaries, which have a profound effect on fertility. The pathophysiologic mechanisms of the disorder—ranging from insulin resistance to chronic inflammation—highlight the need for an interdisciplinary diagnostic and treatment approach that aims to tackle both the somatic and psychological aspects of the disorder. Moreover, certain psychiatric disorders, and anorexia nervosa in particular, can have a tremendous effect on reproductive health. Anorexia patients tend to have substantial hormonal profile changes with restricted caloric intake, leading to disruption of the hypothalamic-pituitary-ovarian axis. This impacts the function of amenorrhea, in which menstruation is lost, essentially affecting fertility. Besides the direct reproductive effect, the long-term consequence of anorexia complicates future pregnancy, and thus the pregnancy may have implications for maternal and fetal development. The clinical presentation of reproductive disorders in anorexia is careful observation of the relationship between psychiatric illness and reproductive physiology because careful observation is required to avoid risks associated with fertility and pregnancy outcomes (Poterasu et al., 2020). Funding research and efforts have contributed significantly to the body of knowledge concerning reproductive health disorders and consequences. Landmark studies funded by various organizations have explored the biological and behavioral mechanisms of such diseases and illuminated pathways most likely to provide new treatment strategies. Continuing commitment to investigation is crucial since it facilitates the development of evidence-based treatments specifically tailored to individuals affected by reproductive disorders. Such studies not only contribute to our knowledge of the complications associated with reproductive health but also create an awareness of the need for holistic approaches to healthcare that address both psychological and physiological needs. A broad understanding of reproductive disorders, enabled by vast research efforts, is essential for improving health outcomes and fertility prospects among sufferers (Stevenson et al., 2018) (Figure 6.18).

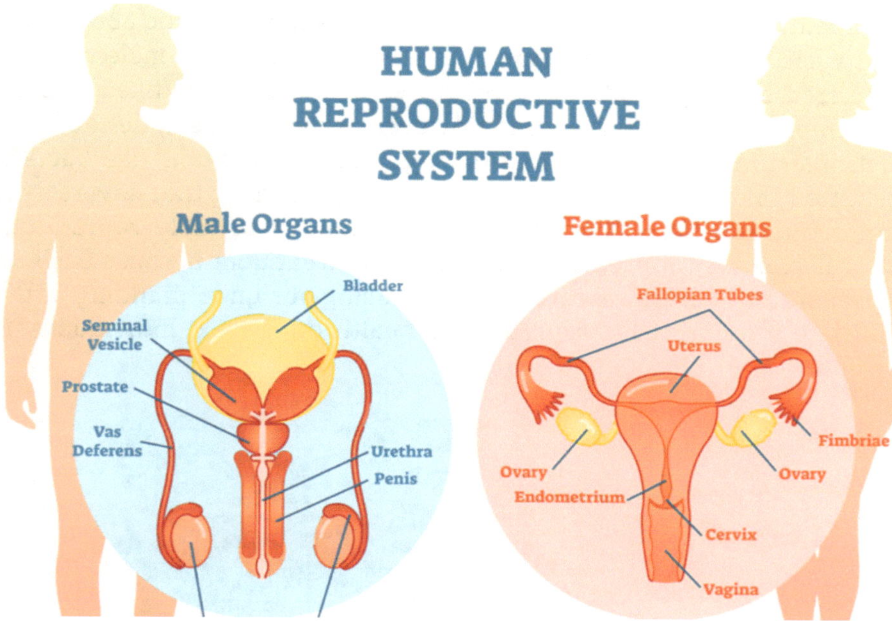

Figure 6.18. Reproductive Health and Disorders.

Source: https://www.niehs.nih.gov/sites/default/files/health/assets/images/reproductive_health_og.jpg.

6.6.1. Common Male Reproductive Disorders

The male reproductive system is susceptible to a variety of disorders, which can have a serious impact on fertility. Of all the conditions, one of the most frequent is male infertility, with approximately 50% of couples experiencing difficulty conceiving being impacted. There are several underlying factors for infertility, including endocrine disorders, testicular abnormalities, and environmental influences. Of particular significance is the fact that mitochondrial function plays an important role in sperm health because spermatozoa depend on mitochondrial oxidative metabolism for fertilization and motility. Of special significance on the outer mitochondrial membrane are voltage-dependent anion channels (VDACs) because they facilitate important energy generation and metabolite exchange processes. Recent studies have begun to uncover the unique roles of VDAC isoforms, particularly VDAC2 and VDAC3, in the male reproductive tract and suggest a critical relationship between mitochondrial physiology and infertility disorders that must be investigated (Nibali et al., 2024). Subclinical hypothyroidism (SCH) is another widespread disorder affecting male reproductive function and can induce significant derangement in sperm quality. The many symptoms of this endocrine disorder often remain undiagnosed, further mandating exhaustive examinations in the assessment of infertility. Current meta-analyses have reported the adverse effect of SCH on various parameters of sperm, with declines seen in the volume of seminal fluid, total number of sperm, and motility. These findings help to affirm the importance of thyroid function in fertility, specifically, evidence that even minimal dysregulation of hormones can significantly affect fertility. Moreover, the study also found that while SCH was associated with decreased sperm morphology, it was associated with a higher concentration of sperms of moderate order. Revealing such complex associations among endocrine disorders and male fertility can lead to more effective diagnostic and therapeutic measures (Bahreiny et al., 2024). Apart from the above conditions, other conditions , such as varicocele, cryptorchidism, and infection, also affect male reproductive health. Varicocele, characterized by the dilatation of scrotal veins, is generally linked with reduced levels of testosterone and impaired spermatogenesis. However, cryptorchidism, defined as undescended testes, can result in infertility if left untreated during infancy. Infections like bacterial prostatitis and sexually transmitted infections lead to inflammation and scarring that adversely impact sperm quality and reproductive function. The multifactorial etiology of male reproductive disorders necessitates an interdisciplinary approach to diagnosis and treatment because each disorder might have to be treated separately. Future research and enhancing our understanding of these disorders will ultimately translate into improved reproductive health in affected individuals (Figure 6.19).

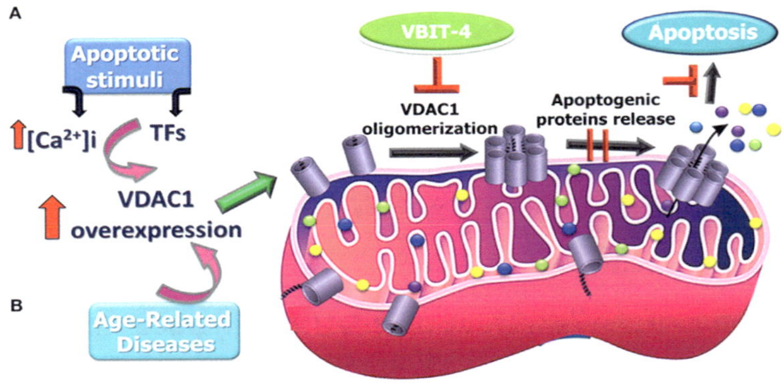

Figure 6.19. Significance of voltage-dependent anion channels (VDACs).

Source: https://www.frontiersin.org/files/Articles/249194/fonc-07-00060-HTML/image_m/fonc-07-00060-g002.jpg.

6.6.2. Common Female Reproductive Disorders

The female reproductive system is susceptible to a variety of disorders that can significantly influence physical status and quality of life. The most commonly met among the disorders are polycystic ovary syndrome (PCOS) and endometriosis, both of which possess intricate pathophysiologic mechanisms. PCOS usually presents in the form of oligomenorrhea or amenorrhea, hyperandrogenism, and infertility, occasionally with concomitant metabolic disturbances like insulin resistance. Recent studies highlight the high genetic correlation between reproductive disorders and body mass index (BMI), wherein the high BMI is specifically highlighted as a causative factor in several conditions, like gestational diabetes mellitus and endometrial carcinoma. Analysis of the genetic basis of such disorders will help researchers identify common pathways and therapeutic targets, unearthing the intricate relationship between obesity and reproductive health (Shao et al., 2025). Endometriosis, a prevalent illness in most women of reproductive age, is the proliferation of endometrial-type tissue outside the uterus and leads to chronic inflammation and discomfort. Research indicates that inflammatory markers may be playing a role in the causation of this condition. For instance, elevated levels of monocyte chemoattractant protein-1 have shown a positive causal correlation with PCOS, and raised levels of interleukin-9 with risk of endometriosis (Alesi et al., 2024). They suggest that inflammation can disrupt the normal immunoendocrine interactions that are necessary for reproductive function, although clear causal links remain to be demonstrated. Clarification of these correlations not only better elucidates the pathophysiology of such disorders but also identifies putative pathways for specific treatments aimed at modulating inflammation in affected subjects. Furthermore, considerations of these female reproductive disorders extend beyond their direct physiological effect; they are often entangled with psychosocial aspects and quality of life concerns. Women with conditions , such as PCOS and endometriosis also often report high levels of emotional distress, which can worsen the physical symptoms themselves. This bidirectional relationship highlights the necessity of a holistic diagnosis and management strategy involving both medical therapy and counseling. As increasing research uncovers the shared genetic and inflammatory pathways that underlie these disorders, clinicians are better able to individualize interventions to address both the biological and psychosocial determinants of reproductive health. It is therefore crucial to address these factors in order to maximize patient outcomes and enhance overall well-being in women presenting with reproductive disorders (Figure 6.20).

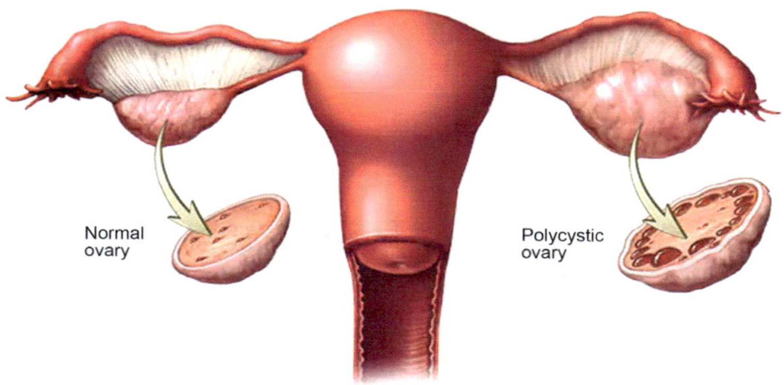

Figure 6.20. Polycystic ovary syndrome (PCOS).

Source: https://www.mayoclinic.org/-/media/kcms/gbs/patient-consumer/images/2013/08/26/10/42/ds00423_im04151_mcdc7_polycystic_ovarythu_jpg.jpg.

6.6.3. Impact of Lifestyle and Environment on Reproductive Health

The intricate relationship among lifestyle components and environmental conditions heavily influences reproductive well-being, defining problems related to fertility, pregnancy, and general reproductive physiology. Poor dietary habits, characterized by high consumption of processed foods and low use of required nutrients, lead to reproductive malfunction. For instance, micronutrient-deficient diets , such as those in folic acid, omega-3 fatty acids, and antioxidants, have been linked to conditions , such as polycystic ovary syndrome (PCOS) and irregular menstrual cycles in females. Further, lifestyles that include smoking, excessive alcohol consumption, and physical inactivity have also been linked to adverse reproductive health outcomes, hence agreeing with the necessity of adopting a holistic model that includes nutrition and lifestyle modification for optimal reproductive potential. The environment also plays a major role in reproductive health, as exposure to toxins and environmental pollutants has been discovered to compromise reproductive function. Endocrine pathways are disrupted by chemicals , such as heavy metals and pesticides, causing fertility concerns among women and men. For example, studies have established that industrial pollutants can impact spermatogenesis in males, reducing sperm quality and increasing the risk of infertility. At a macro-level, heightened urbanization and industrialization have placed reproductive health results in correlation with the biological effects of the surrounding environment, pointing toward the way industrial processes act as intermediaries between lifestyle patterns and reproductive physiology (Comacchio et al., 1998). Knowledge of these environmental impacts, therefore, becomes imperative for ensuring the safety of reproductive health in contemporary society. Moreover, socio-economic conditions are crucial in determining reproductive health, subject to access to healthcare facilities, education, and health-practice awareness. Groups and individuals who have limited access to quality healthcare report more augmented reproductive health issues. Ignorance about the involvement of lifestyle and environmental determinants in reproductive outcomes further exacerbates such inequality, necessitating intervention with comprehensive education and outreach activities. Public health initiatives are therefore challenged to advocate for greater awareness about how lifestyle choices and the wider environment might affect reproductive well-being, fostering a preventative approach to reproductive health. These initiatives are essential to advocating for lifestyle modification and to addressing environmental substrates for reproductive physiology, in order that risk related to the alignment of these determinants can be minimized (Fehring et al., 2009).

Test Your Knowledge

1. How do sexually transmitted infections (STIs) affect reproductive health, and what are some preventive measures?
2. Explain the role of education, contraception, and public health policies in promoting reproductive well-being.

SUMMARY

The intricacies of reproductive physiology reflect the wide-ranging impact of environmental determinants on physiological processes, particularly light-hormone interaction. The action of artificial light-at-night on urbanized animals , such as blackbirds, highlights the adaptive adjustment of wildlife to new surroundings. This is not solely a matter of behavior; it suggests enormous change in the control of hormones, particularly melatonin release. As observed in the research, the evolution of daily rhythms in these birds is associated with decreased nocturnal melatonin secretion, reflecting a transition in circadian processes. Knowledge of how these mechanisms function is vital in crafting useful conservation measures and controlling the ecological impacts of urbanization. A closer inspection shows that the effects of changed reproductive physiology go beyond single species and affect larger-scale ecological as well as behavioral tendencies. Changes in hormonal profiles can lead to mismatches in reproductive timing vis-à-vis environmental signals, and therefore potentially disrupt breeding cycles and population dynamics. This is particularly concerning in urban environments where light pollution exaggerates these mismatches. The dissimilar responses between urban and countryside populations of birds highlight organism plasticity but also indicate likely sensitivities (Dominoni et al., 2013). Researchers have an obligation to conduct investigations of these dynamics to inform policies that mitigate artificial light effects on wildlife and maintain ecological stability in increasingly urbanized landscapes. Ultimately, research into the effects of light-at-night provides important insight into species' reproductive biology and survival. The interrelatedness of environmental forces and biological processes necessitates that a holistic study be conducted that examines the long-term effect of human-altered conditions on wildlife. The attempts to counteract light pollution can regulate endocrine and hormonal fluctuations and preserve natural patterns of breeding in species, which are crucial for preserving resilience. It is clear that as the growing urbanization continues, growing awareness of reproductive physiology with these adjustments in view will be imperative towards the preservation of biodiversity and inducing sustainability of ecosystems amidst anthropogenic pressures (Stevenson et al., 2018).

The intricate reproductive physiology underscores the functions of various biological parameters and environmental stimuli. Of particular significance, the aryl hydrocarbon receptor (AhR) emerged as a significant factor in male reproductive physiology, given its influence over spermatogenesis and endocrine regulation. The receptor is immediately affected by both endogenous ligands , such as food-derived metabolites and exogenous toxicants , such as dioxins, which introduce oxidative stress and endocrine disturbance. Interference with AhR signaling can lead to alterations in sperm quality and fertility, revealing the critical relationship between environmental exposure and reproductive function. Such interactions must be elucidated if male infertility issues are to be overcome, particularly where environmental toxins are prevalent, hence paving the way for potential therapeutic modalities in reversing reproductive dysfunctions related to AhR activity (Bustani et al., 2025). Moreover, the recent advances achieved in reproductive physiology exceed classical species, as witnessed with proteomic investigations of shark semen. The establishment of an extensive proteome database for small-spotted catsharks is a pioneering effort at deciphering reproductive success in this remarkable taxon. This research has identified significant variation in protein composition of seminal plasma and spermatozoa between wild and aquarium individuals, revealing the reproductive function adaptations in different environments. The differential abundance proteins would prove a valuable tool to identify fertility-related biomarkers, which are crucial for conservation measures for chondrichthyans. These findings underscore the need for interdisciplinary approaches to reproductive physiology, integrating molecular biology and ecological conservation to facilitate effective breeding schemes (Mñoz-Baquero et al., 2024). Lastly, cross-talk among environmental pollutants, biological pathways, and fertility indicates the nature of complexity of reproductive physiology. Environmental xenobiotics, through receptor-mediated pathways like AhR, significantly influence endocrine regulation and sperm function. As evident from the shark experiments, an understanding of the proteomic changes underlying them can enhance our knowledge of reproductive mechanisms and inform the development of fertility-promoting interventions in other species. Integrating proteomic information with environmental information allows for a comprehensive view of the determinants of reproductive health. Future research must explore these correlations further, especially in light of increasing anthropogenic pressures on wildlife and the potential consequences for species persistence and biodiversity. Combined, these results contribute to a broad understanding of reproductive physiology, linking ecological health with reproductive success in diverse organisms.

KEY TERMS FROM THIS CHAPTER

- Androgens
- Estrogen
- Follicle-stimulating hormone (FSH)
- Human chorionic gonadotropin (hCG)
- Implantation
- Menopause
- Oogenesis
- Corpus luteum
- Fertilization
- Gonads
- Hypothalamic-pituitary-gonadal (HPG)
- Luteinizing hormone (LH)
- Menstrual cycle
- Ovulation

CRITICAL THINKING QUESTIONS

1. **Which hormone is primarily responsible for triggering ovulation?**
   a. Estrogen
   b. Progesterone
   c. Follicle-stimulating hormone (FSH)
   d. Luteinizing hormone (LH)
2. **Where does fertilization of the ovum typically occur?**
   a. Uterus
   b. Cervix
   c. Fallopian tube
   d. Ovary
3. **Which structure produces progesterone after ovulation?**
   a. Graafian follicle
   b. Corpus luteum
   c. Endometrium
   d. Pituitary gland
4. **In males, which cells are responsible for the production of testosterone?**
   a. Sertoli cells
   b. Leydig cells
   c. Germ cells
   d. Epididymal cells
5. **Which hormone stimulates the development of ovarian follicles in females?**
   a. LH
   b. Progesterone
   c. FSH
   d. Oxytocin

Short Answer Questions

1. What is the role of luteinizing hormone (LH) in males and females?
2. Define the menstrual cycle and name its main phases.
3. What is spermatogenesis and where does it occur?
4. Name two functions of testosterone.
5. What hormone triggers ovulation, and when does it typically occur?
6. Describe the hormonal regulation of the female menstrual cycle, including feedback mechanisms.
7. Explain the process of spermatogenesis and the hormonal control involved.
8. Discuss the physiological changes that occur during pregnancy and the role of placental hormones.
9. Describe the mechanisms of hormonal contraception and how they interfere with normal reproductive physiology.
10. Explain the regulation of male reproductive function, including the roles of the hypothalamus, pituitary gland, and testes.

Answers to Critical Thinking Questions

1. (d); 2. (c); 3. (b); 4. (b); 5. (c).

REFERENCES

1. Scolari, F., Benoit, J., Michalkova, V. *et al.* The Spermatophore in *Glossina morsitans morsitans*: Insights into Male Contributions to Reproduction. *Sci Rep* **6**, 20334 (2016). https://doi.org/10.1038/srep20334 (accessed on 28th June 2025).
2. Abdul-Rahman, I. I., Jeffcoate, I. A., & Obese, F. Y. (2017). Developmental changes in the histological structure of the testes, and testosterone profiles in male guinea fowls (*Numida meleagris*). https://core.ac.uk/download/84591459.pdf (accessed on 28th June 2025).
3. Adelowo, O. E., Akindele, B. M., Adegbola, C. A., Oyedokun, P., Akhigbe, T. M., & Akhigbe, R. (2024). Unraveling the complexity of the impact of physical exercise on male reproductive functions: A review of both sides of a coin. Frontiers in Physiology, 15. https://www.semanticscholar.org/paper/33660bfb9750286b7cb745fc5f64f63b6cdf46b5 (accessed on 28th June 2025).
4. Ahmadi, S., & Ohkubo, T. (2025). A bird's-eye overview of leptin and female reproduction–With mammalian comparisons. The Journal of Poultry Science, 62. https://www.semanticscholar.org/paper/4a6bf833b5af9165bf9147d59ee4ebf19ce847e8 (accessed on 28th June 2025).
5. Yom-Din, S., Hollander-Cohen, L., Aizen, J., Boehm, B., Shpilman, M., Golan, M., Hurvitz, A., Degani, G., & Levavi-Sivan, B. (2016). Gonadotropins in the Russian Sturgeon: Their Role in Steroid Secretion and the Effect of Hormonal Treatment on Their Secretion. *PloS one, 11*(9), e0162344. https://doi.org/10.1371/journal.pone.0162344(accessed on 28th June 2025).
6. Albeitawi, S. N., Al-Alami, Z. M., Hattab, D., Jarrar, W., Alrbeiqi, A., Jabata, D., & Elisabetta, G. (2024). Do school students' study enough about the reproductive system? Data from Jordan. BMC Medical Education, 24. https://www.semanticscholar.org/paper/10b0e0ccf302ed8fc86675f1884200c91f841654 (accessed on 28th June 2025).
7. Alesi, S., Teede, H., Moran, L., Enticott, J., De Silva, K., & Mousa, A. (2024). Exploring causal associations between serum inflammatory markers and female reproductive disorders: A Mendelian randomization study. Biomolecules, 14. https://www.semanticscholar.org/paper/3908b182e1edc275c22d4e721d806225ecbf05f1 (accessed on 28th June 2025).
8. Fernanda Farinelli a, b, c, 1, Mauricio B. Almeida a,d , Peter L. Elkinb,d and Barry Smithb,c,d (2016). OntONeo: The obstetric and neonatal ontology. Conference: International Conference on Biomedical Ontology 2016At: Corvallis, Oregon, USA https://core.ac.uk/download/131214730.pdf (accessed on 28th June 2025).
9. Stevenson, T. J., Alward, B. A., Ebling, F. J. P., Fernald, R. D., Kelly, A., & Ophir, A. G. (2018). The Value of Comparative Animal Research: Krogh's Principle Facilitates Scientific Discoveries. *Policy insights from the behavioral and brain sciences, 5*(1), 118–125. https://doi.org/10.1177/2372732217745097(accessed on 28th June 2025).
10. Gross, Timothy S.,Arnold, Beverly S.,Spulveda, Maria S.,McDonald, Kelly (2021). Relations of environmental contaminants, algal toxins, and diet with the reproductive success of American alligators on Florida Lakes. http://hdl.handle.net/1834/18957(accessed on 28th June 2025).
11. Temirova Niginabonu & Asadova Feruza Djumaevna(2025). The mechanism of hormonal regulation of the sexual cycle. The Mechanism of Hormonal Regulation of the Sexual Cycle. (2025). *American Journal of Pediatric Medicine and Health Sciences (2993-2149), 3*(1), 249-

252. https://grnjournal.us/index.php/AJPMHS/article/view/6770 (accessed on 28th June 2025).

12. Austin, C., Berger, T., Bobadilla, M., Buffone, M., et al. (2017). Essential role of CFTR in PKA-dependent phosphorylation, alkalinization, and hyperpolarization during human sperm capacitation. https://core.ac.uk/download/159287934.pdf (accessed on 28th June 2025).
13. Avila, F. W., Sirot, L. K., LaFlamme, B., Rubinstein, C. D., & Wolfner, M. F. (2010). Insect seminal fluid proteins: Identification and function. Annual Review of Entomology, 56, 21–40. https://doi.org/10.1146/annurev-ento-120709-144823 (accessed on 28th June 2025).
14. Bahreiny, S. S., Ahangarpour, A., & Aghaei, M. (2024). Assessment of the effects of subclinical hypothyroidism on male reproductive parameters: A meta-analysis approach. Reproductive and Developmental Medicine, 9, 57–65. https://www.semanticscholar.org/paper/9090bb719b0f608d337819238f4d40d726da1dd0 (accessed on 28th June 2025).
15. Balasubramanian, C. P. (2009). Physiology in aquaculture with special reference to penaeid shrimp aquaculture—Winter school on recent advances in breeding and larviculture of marine finfish and shellfish. https://core.ac.uk/download/33015486.pdf (accessed on 28th June 2025).
16. Sequeira, V., Couto, E., Neves, A., Vieira, A. R., Paiva, R. B., Canario, A. V. M., & Gordo, L. S. (2017). Zygoparity and sex steroid hormone profiles in bluemouth Helicolenus dactylopterus. *Journal of fish biology*, *90*(5), 2157–2169. https://doi.org/10.1111/jfb.13299(accessed on 28th June 2025).
17. Boer, H. M., Veerkamp, R. F., Beerda, B., & Woelders, H. (2010). Estrous behavior in dairy cows: identification of underlying mechanisms and gene functions. *Animal : an international journal of animal bioscience*, *4*(3), 446–453. https://doi.org/10.1017/S1751731109991169(accessed on 28th June 2025).
18. Wilsterman, K., Bentley, G. E., & Comizzoli, P. (2019). RFRP3 influences basal lamina degradation, cellular death, and progesterone secretion in cultured preantral ovarian follicles from the domestic cat. *PeerJ*, *7*, e7540. https://doi.org/10.7717/peerj.7540(accessed on 28th June 2025).
19. Bich, L., Moreau, J. F., & Pradeu, T. (2019). Understanding multicellularity: The functional organization of the intercellular space. https://core.ac.uk/download/228134961.pdf (accessed on 28th June 2025).
20. Boden, M., Kennaway, D., & Varcoe, T. (2013). Circadian regulation of reproduction: From gamete to offspring. https://core.ac.uk/download/19445268.pdf (accessed on 28th June 2025).
21. Bowman, J. L., Kohchi, T., Yamato, K. T., Jenkins, J., Shu, S., Ishizaki, K., Yamaoka, S., et al. (2017). Insights into land plant evolution garnered from the Marchantia polymorpha genome. Cell, 171, 287–304.e15. https://doi.org/10.1016/j.cell.2017.09.030 (accessed on 28th June 2025).
22. Brannan, N., & Bobbie, L. (2017). Investigating the physiological underpinnings of proactive and reactive behavioral types in grey seals (*Halichoerus grypus*): Trial deployment of a minimally invasive data logger for recording heart rate and heart rate variability in a wild free-ranging breeding pinniped species. https://core.ac.uk/download/76946367.pdf (accessed on 28th June 2025).

23. Bustani, G. S., Alghetaa, H., Mohammed, A., Nagarkatti, M., & Nagarkatti, P. (2025). The aryl hydrocarbon receptor: A new frontier in male reproductive system. Reproductive Biology and Endocrinology: RB&E, 23. https://www.semanticscholar.org/paper/a40cd2ef8aaf862d400785152210f0b9858de96f (accessed on 28th June 2025).

24. Caneppele, D., Honji, R. M., Lo Nostro, F. L., Moreira, R. G., et al. (2016). A case of intersex occurrence in *Steindachneridion parahybae* (Steindachner, 1877) (Siluriformes: Pimelodidae) under captivity condition: A cytogenetic and morphological study. https://core.ac.uk/download/161784355.pdf (accessed on 28th June 2025).

25. Carrillo, M., Felip, A., Taranger, G. L., Zanuy, S., et al. (2010). Control of puberty in farmed fish. https://core.ac.uk/download/36054675.pdf (accessed on 28th June 2025).

26. Chapman, E. C. (2019). The molecular basis of circadian and seasonal rhythms in the blue mussel *Mytilus edulis*. https://core.ac.uk/download/556180898.pdf (accessed on 28th June 2025).

27. Poterasu, M., Rowland, D. L., Ciobanu, C., & Fica, S. (2020). Anorexia Nervosa and Reproduction: Connecting Brain to Gonads. Journal of Mind and Medical Sciences, 7(1), 1-8. https://doi.org/10.22543/7674.71.P18(accessed on 28th June 2025).

28. Clavijo, R., & Hsiao, W. (2018). Update on male reproductive endocrinology. https://core.ac.uk/download/323070097.pdf (accessed on 28th June 2025).

29. Comacchio, C. (1998). Metamorphosis: Science, management, and "human machinery" in industrial Canada, 1900–45. https://core.ac.uk/download/143679868.pdf (accessed on 28th June 2025).

30. Degner, E. C., Ahmed-Braimah, Y. H., Borziak, K., Wolfner, M. F., Harrington, L. C., & Dorus, S. (2018). Proteins, transcripts, and genetic architecture of seminal fluid and sperm in the mosquito Aedes aegypti. Molecular & Cellular Proteomics, 18, S6–S22. https://doi.org/10.1074/mcp.ra118.001067 (accessed on 28th June 2025).

31. Labecka, A.M., Domagala, J. Continuous reproduction of *Sinanodonta woodiana* (Lea, 1824) females: an invasive mussel species in a female-biased population. *Hydrobiologia* **810**, 57–76 (2018). https://doi.org/10.1007/s10750-016-2835-2(accessed on 28th June 2025).

32. Dominoni, D. M., Goymann, W., Helm, B., Partecke, J., et al. (2013). Urban-like night illumination reduces melatonin release in European blackbirds (*Turdus merula*): Implications of city life for biological time-keeping of songbirds. https://core.ac.uk/download/16458859.pdf (accessed on 28th June 2025).

33. Fehring, R. (2009). Current medical research Winter 2008–Spring 2009. https://core.ac.uk/download/213086359.pdf (accessed on 28th June 2025).

34. Fehring, R., Raviele, K., & Schneider, M. (2006). Variability in the phases of the menstrual cycle. https://core.ac.uk/download/213077040.pdf (accessed on 28th June 2025).

35. Garcia, T. X., & Matzuk, M. M. (2024). Novel genes of the male reproductive system: Potential roles in male reproduction and as non-hormonal male contraceptive targets. Molecular Reproduction and Development, 91. https://www.semanticscholar.org/paper/b70727db8267a8ea09a371f711eeb50430e24a9f (accessed on 28th June 2025).

36. Goetz, A. T., Pound, N., & Shackelford, T. K. (2005). Psychological and physiological adaptations to sperm competition in humans. https://core.ac.uk/download/333188.pdf (accessed on 28th June 2025).

37. Zubeldia-Brenner, L., Roselli, C. E., Recabarren, S. E., Gonzalez Deniselle, M. C., & Lara, H. E. (2016). Developmental and Functional Effects of Steroid Hormones on the Neuroendocrine Axis and Spinal Cord. *Journal of neuroendocrinology*, *28*(7), 10.1111/jne.12401. https://doi.org/10.1111/jne.12401(accessed on 28th June 2025).

38. Hermansson, A. (2007). Effects on the reproductive system in domestic fowl (Gallus domesticus) after embryonic exposure to estrogenic substances. https://core.ac.uk/download/11695140.pdf (accessed on 28th June 2025).

39. Pokharel, K., Peippo, J., Weldenegodguad, M., Honkatukia, M., Li, M. H., & Kantanen, J. (2020). Gene Expression Profiling of *Corpus luteum* Reveals Important Insights about Early Pregnancy in Domestic Sheep. *Genes*, *11*(4), 415. https://doi.org/10.3390/genes11040415(accessed on 28th June 2025).

40. Hunt, S. L., Margulies, D., Nakazawa, A., Olson, R. J., et al. (2007). Spawning and early development of captive yellowfin tuna (Thunnus albacares). https://core.ac.uk/download/11023447.pdf (accessed on 28th June 2025).

41. Imam, J., Barnabas, M. K., Amshi, A. K., Julius, S., Abdullahi, S. A., & Ali, M. N. (2024). Anatomy and physiology of reproductive system of bovine species: A review. Journal of Veterinary and Biomedical Sciences. https://www.semanticscholar.org/paper/75dd385f2fce5fa0612abe845740d22c668c14f0 (accessed on 28th June 2025).

42. Kageyama, J. (2025). On the intertemporal allocation of consumption, mortality and life-history strategies. https://core.ac.uk/download/pdf/7127417.pdf (accessed on 28th June 2025).

43. Sammali, F., Kuijsters, N. P. M., Schoot, B. C., Mischi, M., & Rabotti, C. (2018). Feasibility of Transabdominal Electrohysterography for Analysis of Uterine Activity in Nonpregnant Women. *Reproductive sciences (Thousand Oaks, Calif.)*, *25*(7), 1124–1133. https://doi.org/10.1177/1933719118768700(accessed on 28th June 2025).

44. Lewis, N., & Sturmey, R. (2015). Embryo metabolism: What does it really mean? https://core.ac.uk/download/151161377.pdf (accessed on 28th June 2025).

45. Lu, J., Wang, Z., Cao, J., Chen, Y., & Dong, Y. (2018). A novel and compact review on the role of oxidative stress in female reproduction. Reproductive Biology and Endocrinology, 16. https://doi.org/10.1186/s12958-018-0391-5 (accessed on 28th June 2025).

46. Mahdy, A. K. H. (2018). Effect of cortisol on bovine oocytes maturation and further embryonic development after *in vitro* fertilization. https://core.ac.uk/download/225139900.pdf (accessed on 28th June 2025).

47. Maxwell, D. L. B. S., Petriello, M. C., Pilsner, R. P. M. J., Gaskins, A. J., & Minguez-Alarcon, L. (2025). PFAS exposure and male reproductive health: Implications for sperm epigenetics. *Seminars in Reproductive Medicine*. https://www.semanticscholar.org/paper/c1a8db64d44b1e24258ccc8307d7746b54b9e60c (accessed on 28th June 2025).

48. Muñoz-Baquero, M., Lorenzo-Rebenaque, L., García-Domínguez, X., Valdés-Hernández, J., García-Párraga, D., Marín, C., García-Vázquez, F. A., et al. (2024). Proteomic insights into seminal plasma and spermatozoa proteins of small-spotted catsharks, Scyliorhinus canicula: Implications for reproductive conservation in aquariums. Animals: An Open Access Journal from MDPI, 14. https://www.semanticscholar.org/paper/476ee5978de6b101516cf18fd22d3cb144687ff6 (accessed on 28th June 2025).

49. Nibali, S. C., Battiato, G., Pappalardo, X., & De Pinto, V. (2024). Voltage-dependent anion channels in male reproductive cells: Players in healthy fertility? Biomolecules, 14. https://www.semanticscholar.org/paper/6b8cbe4f0cf6db22975fc4b8062294fdd5ed1ba9 (accessed on 28th June 2025).

50. Peric, A., Weiß, J., Vulliemoz, N., Baud, D., & Stojanov, M. (2019). Bacterial colonization of the female upper genital tract. *International Journal of Molecular Sciences, 20*, 3405. https://doi.org/10.3390/ijms20143405 (accessed on 28th June 2025).

51. Satchi, M., & Muneer, A. (2021). Embryology, anatomy, and physiology of the male reproductive system. In CRC Press eBooks. https://doi.org/10.1201/9780429285813-12 (accessed on 28th June 2025).

52. Scribner, R. T., & Tadros, N. N. (2021). Anatomy and Physiology of the Male Reproductive System. Cambridge University Press eBooks. https://doi.org/10.1017/9781108867245.002 (accessed on 28th June 2025).

53. Sepil, I., Hopkins, B. R., Dean, R., Thézénas, M. L., Charles, P. D., Konietzny, R., Fischer, R., et al. (2018). Quantitative proteomics identification of seminal fluid proteins in male Drosophila melanogaster. Molecular & Cellular Proteomics, 18, S46–S58. https://doi.org/10.1074/mcp.ra118.000831 (accessed on 28th June 2025).

54. Shao, H., Xu, C., Wang, H., Lu, N., Gu, H., Zhang, C., Li, L., et al. (2025). Dissecting the genetic determinants and biological associations between body mass index and female reproductive disorders based on genome-wide association study. Reproductive Biology and Endocrinology: RB&E, 23. https://www.semanticscholar.org/paper/cde91d0c80fc2a4c06640e0b40091f2876d0c120 (accessed on 28th June 2025).

55. Stickler, E., & Avella, M. (2024). Disruption of gamete fusion alters the sperm-egg ratio at gamete interaction. Journal of Translational Medicine, 22. https://www.semanticscholar.org/paper/747a1cd33bd7e1de7f777eb093399771bc63a337 (accessed on 28th June 2025).

56. Zhang, A., Li, S., Huang, L., Jiang, Y., Chen, Y., Zhu, S., Xiong, F., et al. (2024). *Bmal1* regulates female reproduction in mice via the hypothalamic–pituitary–ovarian axis. *The FASEB Journal, 38*. https://www.semanticscholar.org/paper/de818692df35894b6b726d6618b9d13d24f6b007 (accessed on 28th June 2025).

IMMUNOPHYSIOLOGY AND INFLAMMATION

7

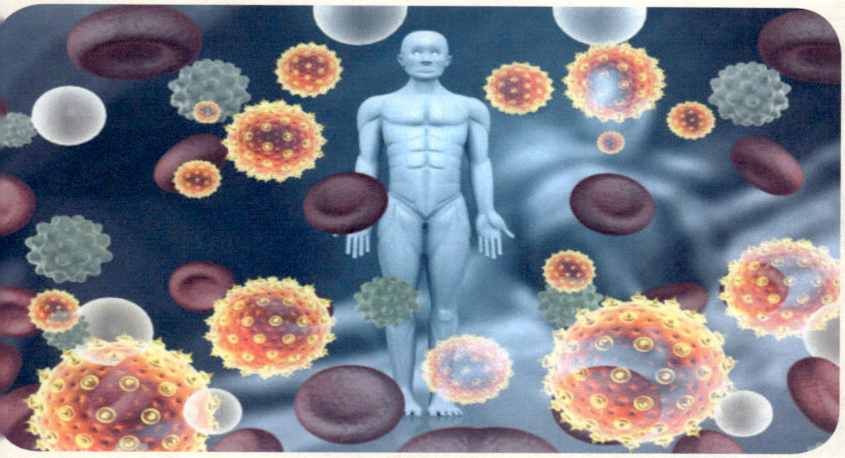

LEARNING OBJECTIVES

After studying this chapter, you will be able to:

1. Discuss the immune system.
2. Explain the mechanisms of inflammation.
3. Identify the role of cytokines in inflammation.
4. Determine the chronic inflammation and disease.
5. Learn about the relationship between immunophysiology and inflammation.
6. Evaluate the therapeutic approaches to modulate inflammation.

Introduction

The complex interaction between inflammation and immunophysiology is a key area of research, particularly in the context of how immune functions are controlled in sickness and health. Immunophysiology is the science of the physiological mechanisms and processes engaged in the functioning of the immune system, which is a key defense against pathogens. Inflammatory reactions—traditionally considered a double-edged sword—play a protective role in preventing the body from infection but potentially contribute to tissue injury and chronic disease under circumstances of dysregulation. An understanding of these mechanisms is essential for the development of targeted therapeutic approaches, particularly in those disorders in which inflammation is inappropriate or excessive, such as, autoimmune illnesses, allergies, and chronic inflammatory diseases. Recent research has highlighted some of the molecular mechanisms involved in these complex interactions, particularly the role of receptors , such as Toll-like receptor 4 (TLR4) in enabling immune responses. For instance, research has demonstrated that the expression of TLR4 varies strongly across different physiological states, such as, hibernation, and suggests its potential role in reproduction and immune adaptation (Kelley, 1992). This dynamic modulation highlights the significance of investigating how these immune receptors operate under different physiological conditions. In addition, TLR4's role in mediating inflammation and controlling cellular responses offers significant information on how immune systems can be both protective and pathological depending on the context of the inflammatory response. Furthermore, delving into the effects of immunophysiology is not just a matter of understanding but also of preparation for designing novel treatments to modulate inflammatory processes. For example, the realization of immune signaling pathways' complex nature can guide approaches to designing drugs that would specifically and selectively target overactive immunity without wasting resources on causing damage to tissues and instead facilitating healing. The significance of this work is illustrated by research funded by large institutions, such as, grants from the National Institutes of Health and the USDA, which aim to unravel these intricate biological processes (Kelley, 1992). Ultimately, our advances in the understanding of immunophysiology and inflammation will revolutionize treatment modalities for chronic inflammatory conditions and related health problems (Figure 7.1).

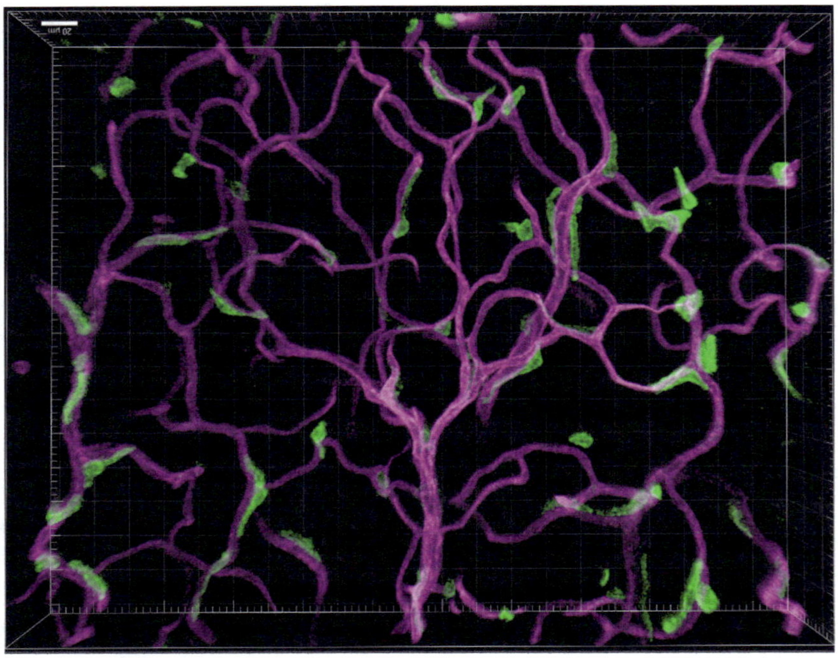

Figure 7.1. Immunophysiology.

Source: https://images.squarespace-cdn.com/content/v1/61e1f174 05c31f76db00b5ae/1642258008871-0T0NBUGXTBBN0NSPS5R1/ Macrophages+in+gren+wraping+blood+vessels+in+the+fat+in+magenta.png.

Definition of Immunophysiology

Immunophysiology, an interdisciplinary science incorporating immunology and physiology, seeks to explain the sophisticated mechanisms of how the immune system intersects with a broad variety of physiological processes across the body. The focus of this interdisciplinarity is on the critical role of immune responses in maintaining homeostasis and health. Examining how immune function acts in response to physiological states enables one to tackle fundamental questions regarding disease susceptibility, protection against pathogens, and tissue injury healing. This subfield is particularly relevant to conditions , such as inflammation, in which it not only analyzes the responses to pathogenic agents but also the physiological effects of such responses on the host. Immunophysiology is crucial to know in order to distinguish between successful immunity and pathogenesis of disease, and as such is a vital pursuit in therapeutic development and medical investigation.

Besides examining immune response, immunophysiology also examines how other systemic conditions, such as, metabolic stress and the environment, might affect immune function. This is especially important in disease tolerance research, where disease tolerance is referred to as an organism's ability to survive infection without presenting significant declines in health. By application of various methodologies, including performance monitoring and welfare evaluation, scholars aim to create a framework that differentiates successful disease tolerance from mere pathogen resistance. Such a nuanced understanding of disease tolerance allows for more thorough control of health in farm and medical settings, especially in the case of animals, where environmental stress may modulate immune responses (Nakov et al., 2019). Through this integrated strategy, the field offers practical information that fills gaps between traditional immunology and health practice applications. The use of biomarkers in immunophysiological studies has emerged as a revolutionary tool to uncover disease mechanisms and therapeutic effectiveness. Identifying particular markers of biological activity relevant to immune responses allows researchers to better track disease development and therapeutic effectiveness. This is particularly relevant in multifactorial complex disorders, where immune reactions may be regulated by an interaction of genetic, environmental, and lifestyle determinants (Kersten et al., 2017).

The poised analysis of a compound linked to inflammation and immune regulation presents pathways to design therapies with a targeted approach that have the potential to advance patient outcomes. With the progression of the field of immunophysiology, so will the emphasis be placed on biomarkers and, therefore, on their function in promoting the translation of lab results into clinical applications, ultimately toward more efficient therapeutic interventions in treating inflammatory illnesses and toward improved understanding of immune interaction.

Importance of Studying Inflammation

Inflammation has become a major subject of concern in the field of immunophysiology, as it is a simple biological response that is necessary in the maintenance of homeostasis and the battle against disease. Inflammation is a complex physiological reaction involving various immune cells, cytokines, and signaling molecules that work in perfect concert to seal off and kill the pathogens or irritating stimuli. Knowledge of the cellular and molecular processes of inflammatory reactions can provide fruitful information on acute as well as chronic conditions, such as, autoimmune diseases, infections, and inflammatory diseases.

For instance, bile duct epithelial cells, the cholangiocytes, have been found to be involved in liver tissue inflammation and repair and reflect why inflammation should be investigated in relation to organ-specific disease and therapy. This knowledge not only further our knowledge on the disease process but also helps in the development of new therapeutic avenues to prevent inflammation and improve outcomes.

Moreover, the complexity of the regulatory aspects of the immune system demands an extensive exploration of inflammation and its impact on autoimmune diseases. The role of regulatory T cells (Tregs) is to maintain immunological tolerance by preventing inflammatory reactions that cause tissue damage. A hyperactive immune response through an overabundance of effector T cells and insufficient Tregs can induce the production of autoimmune disease, leading to poor morbidity (Aker, 2016). Inflammation is thus not simply a cellular response; it entails an understanding of what dysregulation in various clinical presentations means. Conclusions derived from examining inflammatory pathways have the potential to direct the development of targeted therapies that restore balance to the immune system, thus reducing the occurrence of autoimmune diseases and enhancing patient quality of life. Furthermore, inflammation holds far-reaching implications for the pathogenesis of chronic disease, and additional research in this area is advisable. Chronic inflammatory diseases have been implicated in a wide range of diseases, including cardiovascular disease and diabetes, and even certain types of cancer, suggesting that inflammation is not only a local reaction but an overall phenomenon that can lead to the spread of disease. By understanding the interplay between inflammation, cellular signaling, and tissue damage, scientists can identify potential biomarkers and targets for early treatment. In addition, having an understanding of how chronic inflammation reshapes cell behavior can lead to new treatments that can cut down on the long-term consequences of continuous inflammatory reactions. Lastly, the importance of studying inflammation not only consists in understanding its pathologic functions but also in using such information to stimulate innovation in medical science and therapeutics (Figure 7.2).

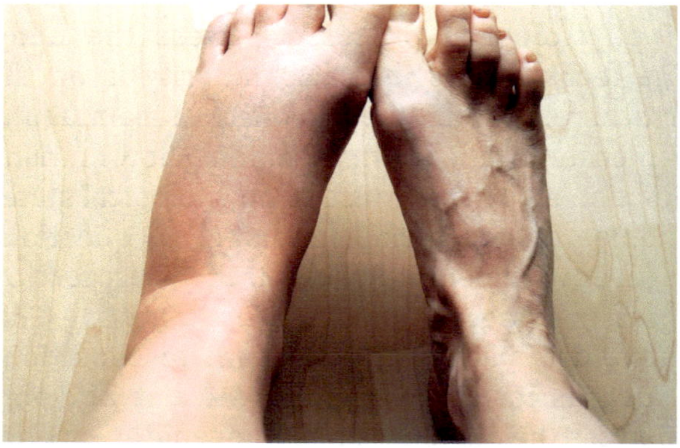

Figure 7.2.

Source: https://cdn.britannica.com/12/198812-050-1E607680/leg-Human-Foot-inflammation.jpg.

7.1. The Immune System: An Overview

Learning Outcome

1. Describe the components of the immune system;
2. Focus on types of immunity: innate and adaptive;
3. Learn about the role of immune cells in defense.

The immune system is a complex network that plays a vital role in the body's defense against infection and in the attainment of homeostasis. It is composed of innate and adaptive immunity, both of which have distinct roles. The innate immunity provides the first line of defense through physical barriers , such as skin and mucous membranes and cellular responses , such as phagocytes and natural killer cells. This system is able to have a rapid, albeit not specific, response to infection. The adaptive immune system, however, possesses traits of specificity and memory and contains lymphocytes like B cells and T cells that recognize distinct antigens. How these two branches of immunity work together is crucial; when the innate system recognizes an invader, it calls upon the adaptive system to permit a more efficient and accurate response, which permits long-term immunity. Understanding this synergy is important in developing therapeutic strategies that intervene in the immune response in inflammatory disease and infection. The complexity of the immune system is also seen in immune disorders in individuals, which illustrate its complex functionality. Interferonopathies, characterized by overexpression or underexpression of interferons, are one such disorder, typically leading to autoimmune conditions , such as systemic lupus erythematosus (SLE) and chronic viral infections. For instance, an excessive amount of type I interferon can be pathological and cause inflammation and tissue damage. Conversely, deficiency in IFNα/IFNβ or IFNγ causes profound susceptibility to infections, primarily viral and mycobacterial pathogens. Treatment with the use of recombinant human IFN therapies aims at correcting these imbalances, illustrating the delicate balance required for optimal immune function. Besides, growing knowledge of these disturbances allows scientists to explore new avenues of treatment with considerable clinical value to immune dysregulation. Further research on these diseases is under the fundamental relevance of the immune system to disease and health. Apart from its role in systemic immunity, the immune system is also involved in oral health, with implications poorly understood despite clinical relevance. The unique anatomy of the oral cavity, as a state of ongoing microbial exposure, creates difficult immune responses, requiring specialized mechanisms to balance tolerance and inflammation.

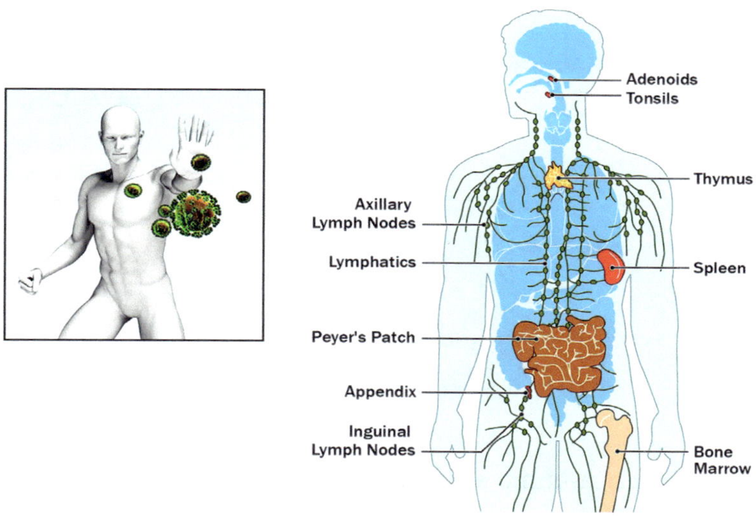

Figure 7.3. Immune System: Your Body's Defense.

Source: https://img.lb.wbmdstatic.com/vim/live/webmd/consumer_assets/site_images/article_thumbnails/BigBead/what-is-your-immune-system-bigbead/1800x1200-what-is-your-immune-system-bigbead.jpg?resize=750px:*&output-quality=75.

Diseases , such as periodontal diseases demonstrate the consequences of immune dysregulation within the oral cavity, causing inflammation with adverse effects on overall health. Current therapeutic approaches within dentistry often do not succeed because they do not prioritize such specific immune dynamics. By building our understanding of oral immunology, researchers can simplify treatment paradigms to treat oral pathology more effectively and promote quality of life. With the advancement of translational immunology research, there is hope of revolutionary transformation in dental practice that can significantly enhance oral health outcomes, thereby bridging the gap between systemic immunity and localized response in the oral cavity (Bozec et al., 2023) (Figure 7.3).

7.1.1. Components of the Immune System

The immune system consists of a complex array of cells, tissues, and organs that collectively defend the body from pathogens and other foreign invaders. At its core are leukocytes, or white blood cells, which consist of various types of such cells , such as neutrophils, lymphocytes, and monocytes. Leukocytes play significant roles in innate and adaptive immunity. Neutrophils are quick to respond to infection, often the first cells to reach sites of inflammation, while lymphocytes, like T cells and B cells, are integral to the identification of specific antigens and the generation of a targeted immune response.

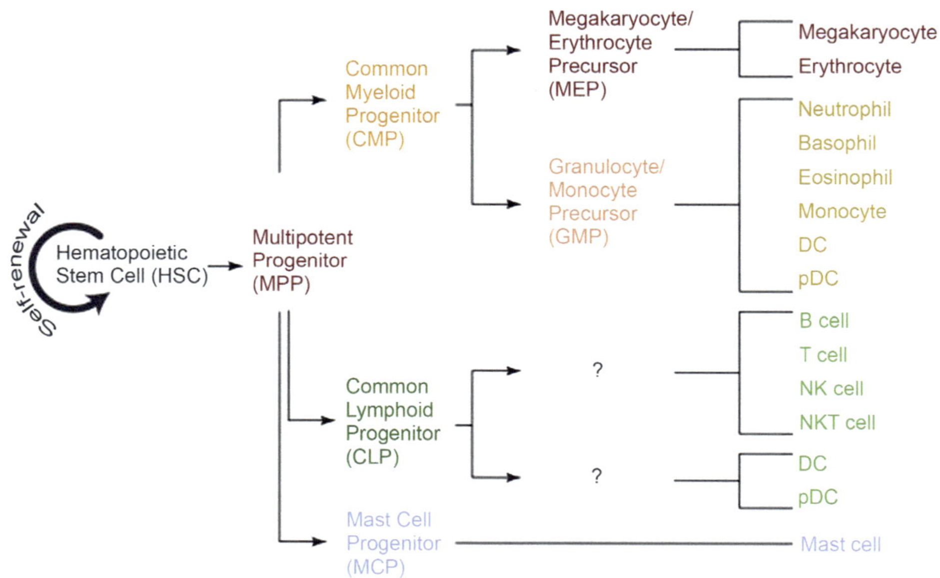

Figure 7.4. Components of the immune system.

Source: https://ars.els-cdn.com/content/image/3-s2.0-B9780123852458000029-f02-04-9780123852458.jpg.

These cells together are not only involved in the elimination of disease but also in the organization of the immune response, and emphasize the necessity for cell-to-cell communication and cooperation in the maintenance of homeostasis in the body. Another essential component of the immune system consists of many biological molecules , such as antibodies and cytokines. Antibodies are proteins secreted by B cells that bind specifically to antigens, marking them for destruction or inactivation by other immune cells. Signaling molecules known as cytokines enable cells to talk to one another in an immune response and thus modulate the extent and duration of these reactions. These molecules work together to maximize the effectiveness of the immune system and to ensure that the immune reactions are in proportion to the dangers posed. For instance, inflammation can be an example where pro-inflammatory cytokines can induce fever and recruit additional immune cells to the infected tissues, thus showing the fine balance in the immune system (Kelley, 1992). Lastly, the structural components of the body that facilitate immune function are the lymphatic system, thymus, and spleen. The lymphatic system is a system of drainage that supports the flow of lymph, an immune cell-rich fluid, through the body. The thymus is involved in the maturation of T cells so that they are well-suited to recognize and respond to foreign antigens. The spleen is also a filter of the blood, removing old or damaged cells and serving as a site for activation of the immune system. Collectively, these sites of anatomy serve to provide a means whereby the immune system can work effectively by providing regions of immune cell development, enlargement, and communication, again pointing out the fundamental nature of each one to both immunophysiology and the inflammatory process as a whole (Kelley, 1992) (Figure 7.4).

7.1.2. Types of Immunity: Innate and Adaptive

The immune system operates using two primary types of immunity: innate and adaptive. Innate immunity is the initial type of defense against pathogens, involving a rapid but nonspecific response. Innate immunity comprises many physical barriers , such as skin and mucosal surfaces, as well as immune cells , such as macrophages and neutrophils, that respond instantly to infections. The presence of pattern recognition receptors (PRRs), such as, Toll-like receptors (TLRs), on these immune cells facilitates detection of common pathogen-associated molecular patterns (PAMPs). For example, TLR4 has tissue-dependent expression variability, representing a dynamic immune response to environmental changes, as identified by research with animal models , such as Anatolian ground squirrels. This inherent immune component versatility is the basis of their critical function in initiating defense against attacking pathogens while concurrently initiating inflammation, which is critical to adequate healing and recovery (Kelley, 1992). In contrast to the innate immune system, adaptive immunity is characterized by specificity and remembrance. This type of immunity is slower to initiate but initiates a more specific response aimed at individualized pathogens. Adaptive immunity is mostly mediated by lymphocytes, including B cells and T cells, that mature and increase upon exposure to an antigen. The B cells produce antibodies, while the T cells assist with cytotoxic killing and organizing the immune response. The highly specialized approach allows for the recognition of pathogenically experienced pathogens and for long-term immunity. Of particular interest, the ability of lymphocytes to generate memory cells is an aspect of adaptive immunity, which is more often exploited in vaccination. It is important to comprehend the function of innate and adaptive immunity to be able to design effective treatment regimens for many infections and inflammatory diseases (Nesterova et al., 2019). Innate and adaptive immune systems do not operate in isolation; rather, they interact and communicate with each other to develop an integrated immune response. For instance, cytokines produced by innate immune cells can modulate the growth and activation of adaptive immune cells, thereby affecting the two systems. Moreover, the specific subpopulations of neutrophilic granulocytes , such as CD16+CD11b+NG, are excellent examples of this interaction since their expression patterns are significantly different in distinct states of disease. The literature indicates that the pattern of distribution of such subpopulations can serve as a biomarker for the differentiation between acute viral and bacterial infections. Detection of this interaction will enhance diagnostic accuracy and treatment regimens through the ability to target particular immune mechanisms that are relevant to the character of infection. This information regarding immunophysiology underscores the importance of a complete comprehension of inflammation and immunity (Nesterova et al., 2019) (Figure 7.5).

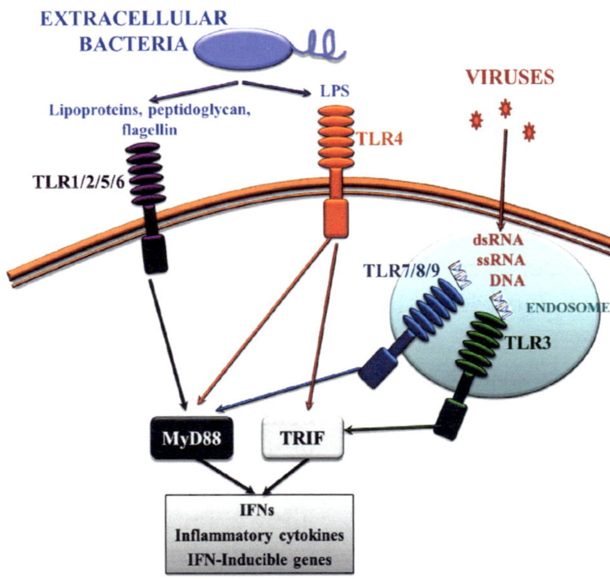

Figure 7.5. Pathogen-associated molecular patterns (PAMPs).

Source: https://www.researchgate.net/profile/Marta-Tejera-Alhambra/publication/307510943/figure/fig1/AS:405487402143745@1473687138427/Fig-1-Ligation-of-pathogen-associated-molecular-patterns-PAMPs-to-their-cognate.png.

7.1.3. Role of Immune Cells in Defense

The role of immune cells in defense is the fundamental element of immunophysiology, which allows the body to combat infection and maintain homeostasis. Immune cells like lymphocytes, macrophages, and dendritic cells are the front-line soldiers, detecting and responding to pathogens. Lymphocytes, particularly T and B cells, are significant in mediating adaptive immunity, in which they help recognize and eliminate specific invaders. Macrophages phagocytose and destroy pathogens and also partake in antigen presentation, which activates other immune cells. Such interaction between the cells is dynamic and is the most important factor in orchestrating an effective immune response. Moreover, their ability to be versatile and remember previous experience with pathogens makes the body more efficient in counteracting such pathogens in the future, pointing to the significance of activation and mitosis of immune cells in withstanding disease. Recent studies have discovered some immune receptors that are involved in such defensive processes. For instance, modulation of Toll-like receptor 4 (TLR4) has been demonstrated to adapt to adaptive environmental changes, such as, those during hibernation in certain animals, which suggests that immune cells can dynamically modify their function based on bodily conditions. Particularly, TLR4 was seen to be expressed more highly on spermatogonia and primary spermatocytes during hibernation, implying its role in reproductive as well as immune adaptation during periods of stress (Kelley, 1992). This adaptability is not merely restricted to reproductive cells; it implies a broader principle by which immune cell processes may be regulated based on environmental stresses and biological demand, once more drawing to the forefront the central significance of these cells in homeostasis. Furthermore, the intimate relationship between epithelial cells and immune cells, especially that of the intestinal environment, is a clear illustration of how immunity is fought on multiple fronts. Intestinal epithelium is both a barrier and home to a diverse group of immune cells and, therefore, is essential for immunity. Epithelial-to-immune cell interaction via cytokines and chemokines integrates responses necessary to maintain barrier integrity and combat pathogens (Andrews et al., 2018). In addition, this interaction also identifies how the immune response is not an independent action but a multifaceted network of signals that trigger both local as well as systemic immunity. Thus, the role of immune cells in defense is more than just mere pathogen fighting; it is a multifaceted interaction that regulates overall health and reduces inflammation, thus proving their role in immunophysiology as well as inflammation.

Test Your Knowledge

1. What are the main components of the innate and adaptive immune systems, and how do they differ in function?
2. Describe the roles of T lymphocytes and B lymphocytes in adaptive immunity.

7.2. Mechanisms of Inflammation

Learning Outcome

1. Explain the stages of the inflammatory response;
2. Define the chemical mediators involved in inflammation;
3. Determine the effects of inflammation on tissues.

Inflammation processes are intricate and pivotal to the response of body's response to injury, infection, and other stimuli. The core of this process is the neutrophils, which are some of the first immune cells to be mobilized to the inflammation site. These cells execute an extensive array of roles, including the production of reactive oxygen species (ROS) and the formation of neutrophil extracellular traps (NETs). These functions not only contribute to microbial clearance but also control the inflammatory environment, potentially leading to resolution or chronic inflammation. Further clarification of these processes is likely to generate new treatment strategies for inflammatory disease, highlighting the importance of neutrophils as more than mere sentinels against infection. The interaction between their protective roles and their ability to support inflammation highlights the complexity of the immune response in inflammatory disease (Marichal et al., 2020). Toll-like receptor 4 (TLR4) is a critical component in the recognition of inflammatory stimuli, particularly in innate immunity. Activation of TLR4 is responsible for intracellular signaling mechanisms that activate immune cells and induce the release of pro-inflammatory cytokines. This receptor's expression is dynamically altered across different tissues, which mirrors its adaptive role in adjusting inflammation based on various physiological and disease conditions. For instance, research on Anatolian ground squirrels reveals that TLR4 is highly localized at the hibernation phase, indicating its immunoadaptive role. These findings emphasize the role of TLR4 in the control of inflammatory processes, not just in acute but also chronic immune control, regulating adaptive mechanisms to physiological demand. Neutrophil and TLR4 involvement is complemented by the contribution of mediators , such as cytokines and alarmins in the orchestration of the inflammatory process. These molecules, which are produced by heterogeneous immune and non-immune cells, guide the recruitment and activation of additional immune cells to tissue damage or infection sites. Pro-inflammatory cytokines , such as interleukins and tumor necrosis factor-alpha (TNF-α), enhance local vascular permeability and facilitate the immigration of immune cells. Alarmins secreted from damaged or stressed cells serve as warning signals that can enhance the immune response. The creation of such a signal network demonstrates the complex interaction among diverse cellular and molecular actors in determining the inflammatory terrain, which in turn influences the trajectory of the inflammatory process. Such mechanisms are very important for the development of targeted therapies for many inflammatory diseases (Marichal et al., 2020) (Figure 7.6).

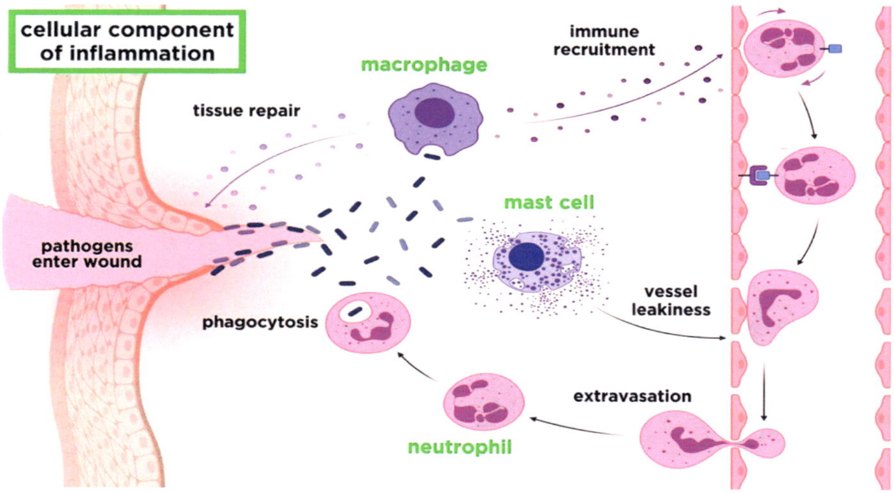

Figure 7.6. The inflammatory response.

Source: https://i.ytimg.com/vi/yIMz9pkT9xQ/maxresdefault.jpg.

7.2.1. Stages of the Inflammatory Response

The inflammatory reaction is a complex biological process that is initiated by infection or injury to the tissues, consisting of distinct stages that all work together to restore homeostasis. The initial stage begins with the recognition of pathogens or tissue injury by border immune cells, such as, macrophages and mast cells. These cells release pro-inflammatory cytokines, primarily interleukins and TNF-α, which are signaling molecules to trigger surrounding immune cells and attract them to the site of injury. This sequence of events sets the stage for the subsequent vascular and cellular responses that characterize acute inflammation. By inducing the dilation of blood vessels and increasing vascular permeability, these messages facilitate leukocyte and plasma protein migration from the bloodstream into the affected tissue, hence being a critical component of triggering an effective immune response against impending threats. As the inflammatory process continues, the second stage is characterized by infiltration of various leukocytes, primarily neutrophils, in the inflamed tissue. Neutrophils are some of the first to react to injury or infection and are the most important in terms of pathogen containment and clearance. Population heterogeneity of neutrophils, as shown by research on $CD16^{+}CD11b^{+}$ subpopulations, indicates that distinct phenotypes of the cells are associated with distinct immune challenges. The CD16brightCD11bbright population of neutrophils, for instance, is the dominant population in acute viral infections, while CD16dimCD11bbright is dominant in bacterial infections (Nesterova et al., 2019). This segregation allows the immune response to scale appropriately, resulting in rapid and efficient elimination of causative pathogens. Thus, it is important to elucidate such subpopulation dynamics for developing diagnostic modalities and therapeutic interventions involved in modulating inflammation towards a productive resolution. The resolution of the inflammatory response would lapse into healing, wherein tissue repair mechanisms are the overriding ones. This includes clearance of the dead cells and resolution of inflammation, which is significant in preventing chronic inflammation. Macrophages at this stage coordinate the repair process by clearing debris and the secretion of factors inducing tissue regeneration. Markers , such as serum cytokeratin-18 fragments (K18) have been found to be markers of cell apoptosis and are pertinent in the determination of disease severity, for instance, primary sclerosing cholangitis (Masuoka et al., 2015). The correlation of serum K18 with disease severity means that such markers should be tracked to determine the effectiveness of resolution of inflammation and repair of tissues. Finally, the inflammatory response process emphasizes the body's fine line between the defense mechanisms and healing processes, which are accountable for shaping the experience of various inflammatory diseases and treatment (Figure 7.7).

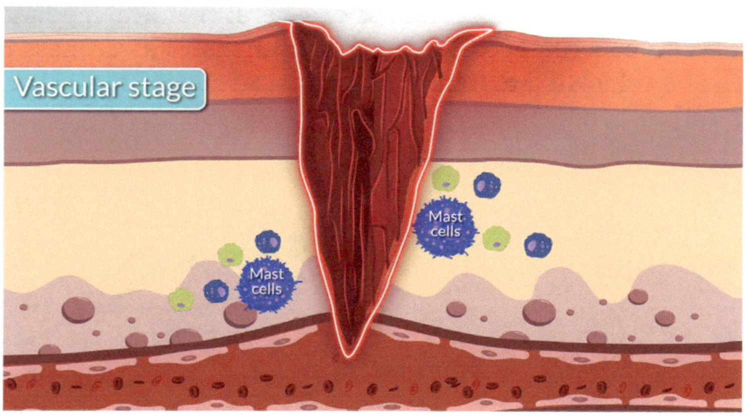

Figure 7.7. Inflammatory response.

Source: https://www.jove.com/files/media/science-education/science-education-thumbs/13233.jpg.

7.2.2. Chemical Mediators Involved in Inflammation

Inflammation is subtly regulated by a wide variety of chemical mediators, which play an integral role in orchestrating the body's response to injury or infection. The pro-inflammatory cytokines , such as interleukins (ILs), TNF-α, and interferons, are among the most important among these mediators. These cytokines are secreted by most of the immune cells, such as, the macrophages and T cells, and act to recruit additional immune cells into the inflamed tissues. Through the enhancement of vascular permeability and induction of acute phase responses, these mediators amplify the inflammatory reaction. Also, the balance between pro-inflammatory and anti-inflammatory cytokines largely dictates the duration and intensity of an inflammation, demonstrating the complex interaction between different mediators in immune reactions. Understanding the roles of these mediators can aid in the development of specific therapies for inflammatory disorders, thereby enhancing patients' well-being. Apart from cytokines, gas signaling molecules like nitric oxide (NO), carbon monoxide (CO), and hydrogen sulfide (H2S) are significant in the inflammatory response. The gaseous molecules endogenously produced possess unique characteristics and regulate various physiological responses, like vasodilation and oxidative stress regulation. In particular, NO has been identified to enhance blood perfusion and permit the transmission of messages among immune cells, hence playing a pivotal part in maintaining gastrointestinal mucosal integrity. Experiments have shown the synergistic effects of these gases, suggesting that they work conjointly to inhibit injury responses and activate healing in tissues. The study of such gases gives new avenues in the creation of anti-inflammatory agents that utilize their protective action to treat several gastrointestinal and systemic inflammatory disorders (Wallace et al., 2017). Further, the process of hormesis, which is believed to involve small doses of potentially harmful agents stimulating adaptive protective reactions, has gained attention as a mechanism to describe inflammation. Balneotherapy, through the use of medicinal waters' heat and therapeutic minerals, is a perfect example of this principle by tempering low-grade inflammation and conditions related to stress. The effectiveness of this measure can be attributed to neuroendocrine and immunological effects, which control the inflammatory response of the body (Gálvez et al., 2018). Prominent research into the mechanism of balneotherapy demonstrates that it triggers the induction of heat shock protein synthesis and influences the release of therapeutic mediators like H2S, thus reaffirming its therapeutic potential. Thus, the interconnectedness of several chemical mediators, either gaseous or cytokine-dependent, accentuates the necessity for comprehensive awareness of these mechanisms. Such a configuration can be translated to improved clinical strategies towards effectively modulating inflammation (Figure 7.8).

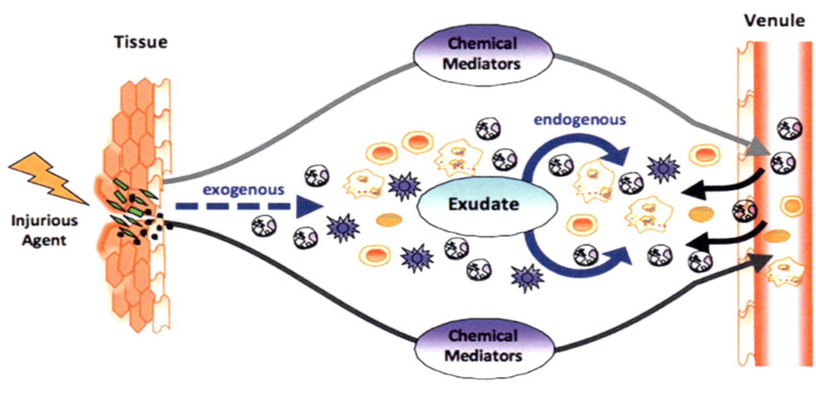

Figure 7.8. The role of chemical mediators in the acute inflammatory response.

Source: https://www.researchgate.net/publication/224919350/figure/fig1/AS:11431281239278250@1714292372249/The-role-of-chemical-mediators-in-the-acute-inflammatory-response-At-the-site-of-tissue.tif.

7.2.3. Effects of Inflammation on Tissues

Inflammation is a severe response to infection or trauma of the tissues and provokes a sophisticated cascade that profoundly impacts cellular structure and function. Under normal circumstances, it involves activation of the immune cells, release of inflammatory mediators, and subsequent repair. Once inflammation becomes chronic and ongoing, the tissue effects of inflammation are negative. For instance, persistent inflammation can lead to tissue remodeling with fibrosis, which replaces functional tissue with scar tissue and impairs organ function. This cytokine dysregulation shows the paradox that the initial protective process degrades into one that escalates tissue damage and dysfunction, particularly in organs , such as the lungs and liver. Therefore, understanding the balance between inflammatory and anti-inflammatory signals becomes critical for developing therapeutic interventions that reverse such harmful actions on tissues (Kelley, 1992). The role of the immune system in inflammation of tissues falls into sharp focus within the gastrointestinal tract, where the interaction of the immune cells with the epithelial tissues becomes crucial to maintaining homeostasis. The intestine is the largest barrier to environmental pathogens, requiring a balanced ratio to prevent over-inflammation while simultaneously defending against dangerous invaders. Inflammation in the intestine can modify the epithelial barrier, generating increased permeability and the potential for passing pathogens and toxins into systemic circulation. This breach not only enhances inflammatory responses but also has the potential to create chronic diseases like inflammatory bowel disease. Second, the production of cytokines and chemokines by both immune and epithelial cells controls such interactions, shaping the entire inflammatory environment. The understanding of these events highlights the role of regulatory mechanisms in regulating inflammatory responses in the intestine and their effects on tissue integrity (Andrews et al., 2018). Besides, the consequences of inflammation extend beyond localized tissue injury; it may have systemic implications. Activation of systemic inflammation produces downstream effects that alter metabolic pathways and result in the development of comorbidities. For instance, chronic inflammation has been associated with metabolic syndrome, cardiovascular disease, and autoimmune diseases. Elevation of inflammatory cytokines can induce insulin resistance, thus impairing glucose metabolism and rendering an individual susceptible to diabetes. Therefore, identification of the potential for tissue damage as a mediating process not only in tissue inflammation but in global physiological responses is necessary. The best management strategies that include not only signs of tissue inflammation but also the immune dysregulation underneath are essential in preventing a transition from the acute to chronic phases of inflammatory conditions (Kelley, 1992).

Test Your Knowledge

1. How do leukocytes migrate from the bloodstream to the site of tissue injury (i.e., the process of leukocyte extravasation)?
2. Compare acute and chronic inflammation in terms of causes, cellular involvement, and outcomes.

7.3. The Role of Cytokines in Inflammation

Learning Outcome

1. Explain the function of cytokines;
2. Define the types of cytokines involved in inflammation;
3. Describe the cytokine signaling pathways.

Cytokines are key signaling molecules that govern the inflammatory process as pro-inflammatory and anti-inflammatory mediators. Immune cells , such as macrophages and neutrophils, release pro-inflammatory cytokines , such as TNF-α and IL-1, in response to tissue injury or microbial infection. These cytokines facilitate immune cell recruitment and activation, which is essential to initiate the inflammatory cascade. At the cellular level, they alter vascular permeability to provide plasma proteins and leukocytes access to the injured area. The cytokine role in orchestrating these events testifies to their potential as therapeutic targets in most inflammatory disorders, wherein dysregulation of cytokine signaling is likely to lead to chronic inflammation and tissue injury, implying the necessity of careful modulation in the clinic (Marichal et al., 2020).

In addition to their pro-inflammatory roles, certain cytokines have anti-inflammatory effects that inhibit excessive inflammation and promote healing of the tissues. Interleukin-10 (IL-10), for instance, has been shown to inhibit the release of pro-inflammatory cytokines and enhance apoptosis of activated immune cells, hence curbing the inflammatory response. This balance between pro- and anti-inflammatory cytokines plays a crucial role in maintaining homeostasis in the immune system. Dysregulation may result in a variety of inflammatory illnesses, ranging from autoimmune disease to chronic inflammation. An understanding of this balance and the signaling pathways involved with cytokine release and action will give researchers and clinicians the potential to explore new types of treatment aimed at restoring balance in the hyper-inflammatory condition (Kelley, 1992). Moreover, the role of cytokines is not only in the initiation of inflammation; they are also pivotal in the adaptive immune response. For instance, cytokines , such as IL-6 and IL-12 are also involved in T cell differentiation and the production of memory cells. This aspect pinpoints the role of cytokines in not just transient immune responses but also persistent immunity and memory development. In chronic inflammation, cytokine patterns are prognostic of disease course and outcome and thus valuable biomarkers for diagnosis and monitoring. With continued investigation of the intricate cytokine network and its impact on immune response, it is increasingly clear that the manipulation of some cytokine pathways may hold promising therapies for a vast array of inflammatory and autoimmune diseases (Marichal et al., 2020) (Figure 7.9).

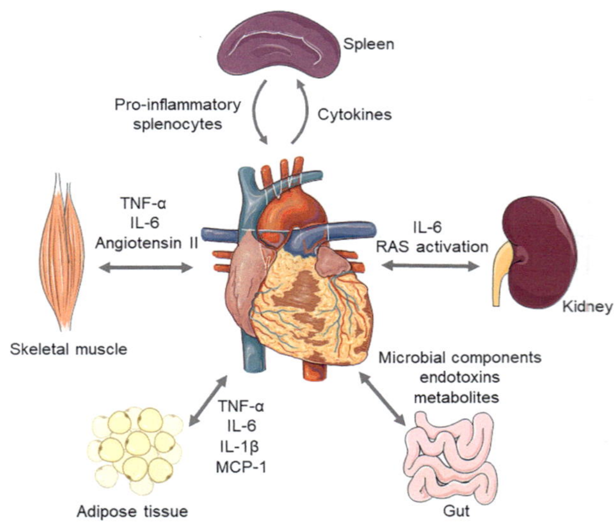

Figure 7.9. Inflammatory cytokines.

Source: https://www.frontiersin.org/files/Articles/695047/fphys-12-695047-HTML/image_m/fphys-12-695047-g001.jpg.

7.3.1. Definition and Function of Cytokines

Cytokines also play a key role in the regulation of immune responses as master signal molecules of the immunophysiology. Cytokines are secreted by various cells, including immune cells, and function to regulate the activity and behavior of other cells. By facilitating communication between immune cells, cytokines allow for the coordination of responses to pathogens, inflammation, and tissue repair. The complex family of cytokines includes interleukins, interferons, and tumor necrosis factors, each having specific roles that are able to initiate pro-inflammatory or anti-inflammatory effects, respectively, depending on the physiological context. The precise interplay between these signals can determine the collective immune response, thus attesting to their crucial function in normal physiology as well as pathology. One of the more stunning aspects of cytokines is that they are capable not only of influencing the immune system but also the neuroendocrine system, which involves a very complex interaction between the two. The neuroendocrine-immune regulation can be particularly observed in states of inflammation, where cytokines become involved in systemic processes involving other organ systems. For instance, cytokine release under stress or inflammation can modulate mood and behavior by influencing neurobiological processes. This adds evidence to the significance of cytokines as being more than immune phenomena because they have a vital role in maintaining homeostasis and regulating vital functions like growth, differentiation, and apoptosis. Thus, their dysregulation can lead to a wide range of disorders, from autoimmune disease to chronic inflammatory diseases, and they are important therapeutic targets. Additionally, cytokine function is not confined to chronic inflammation, in the sense that cytokines can sustain tissue damage and disease. In such situations, pro-inflammatory cytokines may become overexpressed, establishing a cycle of inflammation that can be detrimental to host tissue. This can be viewed particularly in diseases , such as rheumatoid arthritis and inflammatory bowel disease, in which ongoing cytokine activity alters normal healing to create pathological expression. Conversely, anti-inflammatory cytokines function to defend by acting against these pro-inflammatory signals, a reflection of the delicate balance needed for effective immunological function. Learning about these complex dynamics is central to developing targeted therapies that improve balance and counteract the detrimental effects of chronic inflammation, as suggested by recent studies that explore holistic approaches like balneotherapy, which can possibly regulate immune function via cytokine regulation (Ciraci et al., 2017; Gálvez et al., 2018) (Figure 7.10).

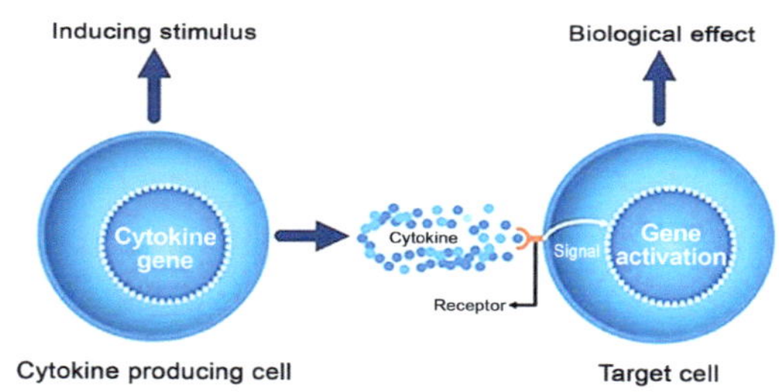

Figure 7.10. The function of cytokines.

Source: https://www.cusabio.com/statics/images/cytokine&receptor-interaction.jpg.

7.3.2. Types of Cytokines Involved in Inflammation

Cytokines are pivotal in regulating and sustaining inflammation as signaling molecules that facilitate interactions between immune cells. Various cytokines can be categorized based on their functions as well as the immune pathways they initiate. Pro-inflammatory cytokines , such as TNF-α, IL-1, and IL-6, are typically released in response to inflammatory stimuli and have a central role in the initiation and maintenance of the inflammatory response. They provoke leukocyte recruitment to the site of infection or injury, enhance the production of other inflammatory mediators, and influence systemic signs , such as fever. The relative balance between such pro-inflammatory cytokines and their regulatory counterparts is essential to the maintenance of homeostasis because dysregulation could lead to chronic inflammation and a range of associated diseases. Anti-inflammatory cytokines, conversely, serve to suppress and halt inflammation, thus restoring tissue integrity and homeostasis. Two of the key participants in this group are IL-10 and transforming growth factor-beta (TGF-β). These cytokines function primarily by inhibiting the action of pro-inflammatory cells and promoting an environment conducive to tissue repair. By downregulating immune cell activation and proliferation, they serve as a fundamental mechanism for preventing over-damage of host tissues during inflammation. In chronic illnesses, such as, autoimmune conditions, the ability of anti-inflammatory cytokines to contain inflammation can be deranged, which is indicative of the necessity for a delicate balance between these opposing forces so as not to have pathological consequences. The intricacy in cytokine interactions during inflammation has also been elucidated by new evidence, particularly within localized environments , such as the intestinal mucosa. The gut is inhabited by a diverse population of immune cells, and the epithelial layer is a key barrier to pathogens while simultaneously facilitating immune responses. Cytokines and chemokines produced by epithelial cells, such as, IL-22, play important roles in modulating epithelial cell proliferation, apoptosis, and permeability, and consequently immune cell behavior and tissue integrity. Epithelial cell and resident immune cell interaction through such soluble mediators plays an important role in coordinating effective immune responses to infection with avoidance of non-specific inflammation (Andrews et al., 2018). In addition, systemic modulators, including immune system stresses, may also control such cytokine responses, revealing the intricate network of interaction governing health and disease conditions (Gálvezet al., 2018) (Figure 7.11).

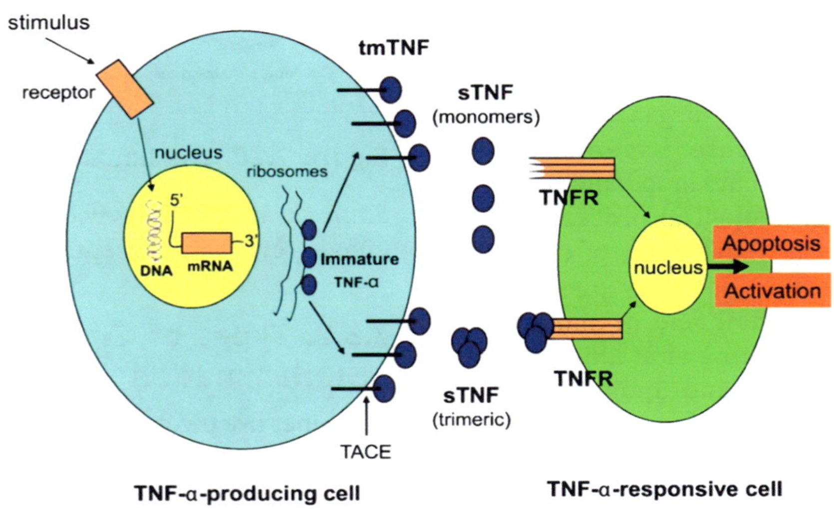

Figure 7.11. Tumor necrosis factor-alpha (TNF-α)

Source: https://ars.els-cdn.com/content/image/1-s2.0-S016557281100066X-gr1.jpg.

7.3.3. Cytokine Signaling Pathways

Cytokine signaling pathways are the core of the immune response and play a crucial role in homeostasis in the body. The pathways are based on the binding of cytokines, which are small signaling proteins secreted by numerous different cells, to receptors specifically found on target cells. Communication directs principal cellular responses, including proliferation, differentiation, and apoptosis. Of particular note is the fact that the intestinal epithelium, being the initial defense against environmental insults, is critically dependent on cytokine signaling to manage interactions with resident immune cells. This dynamic intercellular communication maintains a balanced immune response, averts overinflammation, and is also essential for the integrity of the intestinal barrier, which not only aids digestion but also protects against microbial invasion and sustains a healthy immune environment (Andrews et al., 2018). The significance of cytokine signaling extends beyond simple mediation of immune response; it is actually closely linked with several pathological conditions. Dysregulation of such pathways is responsible for extreme inflammatory diseases, including autoimmune diseases. For instance, faulty signaling of type I interferons , such as IFNα, has been implicated in certain diseases of chronic inflammation, among which systemic lupus erythematosus (SLE) and other interferonopathies are prominent examples. These states highlight the dualistic character of cytokines: although they are vital for a successful immune response, an excess or dysregulation thereof leads to detrimental host effects (Nesterova et al., 2020). As such, understanding these signaling pathways is not only at the core of immunophysiology but also at the core of creating targeted therapeutic strategies. More profound exploration of cytokine signaling pathways also illustrates their complexity and the many determinants influencing them, including diet, microbial contact, and cell-cell interactions within the immune microenvironment. As a case in point, some cytokines possess the ability to regulate the functional repertoire of the intestinal epithelium, influencing cellular functions like proliferation and barrier permeability. Dysfunctions in these signaling networks can magnify susceptibility to infection, produce inflammatory disease, and reconfigure the immune landscape. Therefore, cytokine signaling research uncovers not only immune regulation processes but also discloses avenues to novel types of interventions aimed at fixing homeostasis in varied inflammatory diseases. With growing knowledge, the potential for targeted treatments that could rectify cytokine imbalance grows, promising great potential for the treatment of chronic inflammatory diseases (Andrews et al., 2018).

Test Your Knowledge

1. Differentiate between pro-inflammatory and anti-inflammatory cytokines with examples.
2. How do interleukins, tumor necrosis factor (TNF), and interferons influence immune cell behavior during inflammation?

7.4. Chronic Inflammation and Disease

Learning Outcome

1. Identify the causes of chronic inflammation;
2. Define the diseases associated with chronic inflammation;
3. Describe the impact of chronic inflammation on health.

Chronic inflammation has been recognized as a major component of the pathophysiology of most diseases, negatively influencing overall health. The chronic inflammatory condition may be provoked by various stimuli, including infections, autoimmune disorders, and toxins. The continuous stimulation of the immune system results in tissue damage and potential formation of chronic diseases , such as cardiovascular disease, diabetes, and cancer. For instance, in autoimmune diseases like systemic lupus erythematosus (SLE), overproduction of type I interferon, particularly IFNα, has been linked with worsening and severity of the disease, emphasizing the importance of immunological dysregulation in chronic inflammation (Nesterova et al., 2020). Therefore, understanding the mechanisms of chronic inflammation is of paramount importance to uncover targeted therapeutic strategies that can effectively counteract its associated risks to health. Neutrophils, as a type of white blood cell, are key in acute and chronic inflammation, being not only protectors against infection but also key regulators of the inflammatory process. Neutrophils can mediate inflammatory responses through the generation of reactive oxygen species (ROS) and the formation of neutrophil extracellular traps (NETs), which in turn can perpetuate the inflammatory cycle (Marichal et al., 2020). Chronic diseases , such as psoriasis are an optimal example of this bivalency role, as activated neutrophils have been found in great numbers in skin lesions, contributing to the pathogenesis of the disease via ROS production and NETosis. Both processes explain how neutrophils can sustain chronic inflammation, and thus, due to that, are candidates for the development of therapeutic treatments against inflammatory diseases. Clarifying the functional neutrophil response is thus a requirement for the development of effective interventions in inflammatory disease.

The disease pathogenesis is complex and involves chronic inflammation, making prevention and treatment difficult. New therapeutic approaches, including the use of biologics directed against single pathways of inflammation, have shown effectiveness in the management of chronic inflammatory conditions. Certain therapies inhibiting the excessive production of IFNα have also been shown to decrease autoimmune disease symptoms with interferonopathies (Nesterova et al., 2020). Additionally, application of drugs that modify neutrophil function could be used to reduce tissue injury and inflammation in a wide variety of diseases (Marichal et al., 2020).

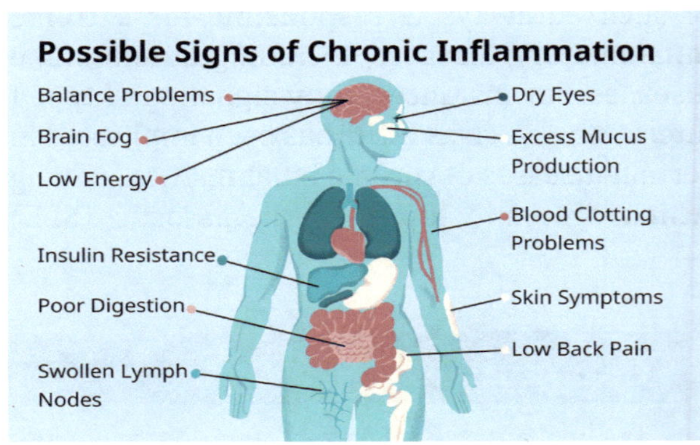

Figure 7.12. Chronic inflammation: symptoms, causes, treatment, and prevention.

Source: https://www.verywellhealth.com/thmb/MVxYxUTAweuooe8z7k0-7wF55JI=/1500x0/filters:no_upscale():max_bytes(150000):strip_icc()/11-atypical-signs-of-chronic-inflammation-5075765-FINAL-4-f5725e25e0764536876de79bceb3bb71.png.

With additional research unearthing the intricate interaction between inflammation and disease processes, it is essential to translate this knowledge into clinical practice. This will ensure that therapies in the future not only cure the symptoms of chronic inflammation but also its causes, ultimately translating into improved patient outcomes for many diseases (Figure 7.12).

7.4.1. Causes of Chronic Inflammation

Chronic inflammation is most often brought about by a range of factors that disrupt the homeostasis of the body, leading to ongoing stimulation of the immune system. One of the primary causes is repeated exposure to pathogens , such as viruses and bacteria, which induce chronic inflammation as the immune system continues to attempt elimination. For instance, diseases , such as tuberculosis illustrate how certain pathogens can evade the full immune destruction, resulting in chronic inflammatory pathways being activated for prolonged time periods. In addition, autoimmune diseases, including systemic lupus erythematosus (SLE), are characterized by a hyperactive immune response against self-antigens, and this also results in chronic inflammation. Abnormally high levels of interferon-alpha, an immune system-regulating cytokine, have been associated with such disorders, and this exhibits the complicated interplay between microbes, immunodeficiency, and conditions of chronic inflammation (Nesterova et al., 2020).

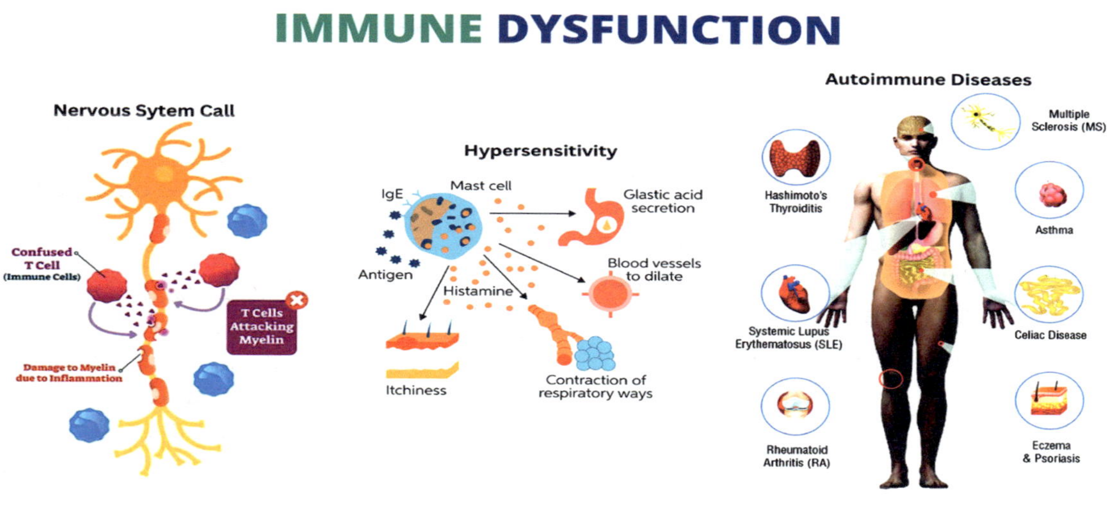

Figure 7.13. Thumbnail-immune-dysfunction.

Source: https://www.biocode.org.uk/wp-content/uploads/2021/10/Blog-Thumbnail-Immune-Dysfunction.png.

Environmental factors also contribute significantly to pathogenesis in chronic inflammation. Prolonged exposure to irritants , such as pollution, tobacco smoke, and certain chemicals can lead to repetitive injury to the tissues and inflammation. For example, particulate matter inhalation from air pollution has been recognized to instigate inflammation within the lungs, and in doing so, potentially be causal of chronic respiratory disease. Moreover, lifestyle components like inappropriate diet, obesity, and physical inactivity are also being recognized for their ability to modulate inflammatory responses. High consumption of processed meals and sugars will instigate the production of pro-inflammatory cytokines, which will worsen over time. Evidence has shown that chronic low-grade inflammation is highly prevalent in obese individuals, indicating that metabolic conditions and lifestyle are entangled well with the causality of persistent inflammatory responses (Suzaki et al., 1999). Chronic inflammation is also a result of dysregulation of the innate immune system, which can lead to an aberrant response to injury or stress. Situations , such as chronic stress and aging create an environment with activated inflammatory mediators at all times. The body releases a number of hormones during stress that can potentially modulate the immune response, creating an enhanced inflammatory profile. This can also be augmented by the age-related dysfunction of the efficacy of the immune system. In aging populations, greater levels of pro-inflammatory cytokines have been observed, which correlate with increased rates of chronic inflammatory disorders. Understanding the diversity of underlying causes of chronic inflammation is crucial in designing targeted treatments to reverse its long-term effects on health across different age groups (Chudilova et al., 2020) (Figure 7.13).

7.4.2. Diseases Associated with Chronic Inflammation

The link between chronic inflammation and most diseases is now established, and it is having a significant impact on public health worldwide. Chronic inflammatory conditions can lead to serious complications like autoimmune diseases, cardiovascular disease, and certain cancers. For instance, chronic inflammation of the body is a major underlying factor in systemic lupus erythematosus (SLE), a condition where the immune system of the body mistakenly identifies and attacks normal tissues, leading to serious complications. The chronic inflammation can result in an excess of pro-inflammatory cytokines that promote tissue dysfunction and injury. Additionally, chronic inflammation is typically accompanied by atherosclerosis, in which inflammatory lesions induce vascular injury resulting in heart attacks or strokes. The interaction between chronic inflammation and such cardiovascular diseases emphasizes the necessity for ongoing studies and development of targeted therapy designed to halt these detrimental effects. Among the airway disorders causally related to chronic inflammation, asthma and COPD have been of particular importance due to their high prevalence and morbidity. Small airway changes have emerged from studies as a key contributor to disease pathogenesis in asthma and COPD, where chronic inflammation is central to airway obstruction and hyperreactivity. The lung plumbing, that of the small airways (internal diameter <2 mm), is responsible for the successful management of such diseases. More recent initiatives by the Global Asthma Association and others emphasize the importance of an assessment of small airway involvement to better tailor treatment. With increasing evidence regarding the role of small airways in chronic disease, innovation , such as small-particle inhaled formulations is emerging as a valuable therapeutic modality, highlighting the intricate relationship between inflammation and respiratory disease (Braido et al., 2016). Moreover, the role of interferon (IFN) dysregulation in chronic inflammatory disease cannot be ruled out, particularly in the context of understanding the therapeutic modalities available to manage the diseases. Interferonopathies, caused by overproduction or type I interferon deficiency, are implicated in a variety of autoimmune diseases. For instance, in systemic lupus erythematosus, the inflammatory milieu is driven by an upregulation of IFNα, amplifying signs and disease activity. Conversely, an interferon defect makes an individual susceptible to recurrent infections or worsens chronic ongoing inflammatory conditions. Targeted therapies that modulate the IFN pathway, either by sequestering surplus IFNα with biologics or replacement therapy in case of deficiency, illustrate the need for a discriminative treatment approach. Improved knowledge of these correlations allows improved management approaches to stem chronic inflammation and its diseases, offering a tool for beneficial results in the implicated patients (Chudilova et al., 2020) (Figure 7.14).

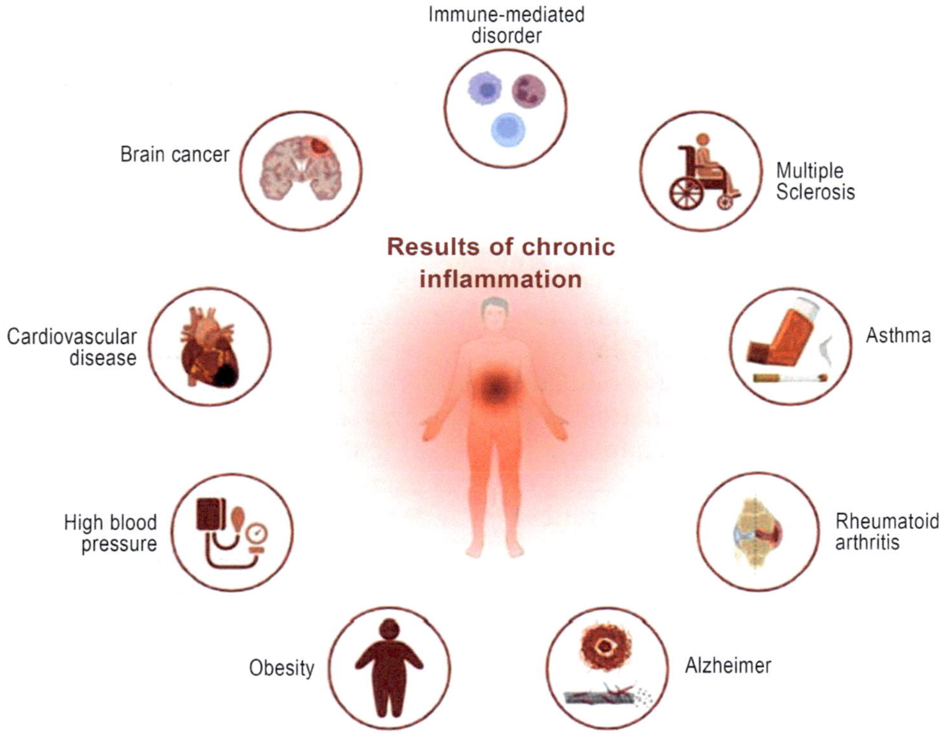

Figure 7.14. Chronic inflammation contributes to several diseases.

Source: https://www.researchgate.net/publication/375582874/figure/fig1/AS:11431281209554703@1701798995892/Chronic-inflammation-contributes-to-several-diseases.png.

7.4.3. Impact of Chronic Inflammation on Health

Chronic inflammation is a primary cause of a wide range of health conditions, like autoimmune, cardiovascular, and metabolic diseases. Chronic inflammation is characterized by the repeated activation of immune cells, leading to tissue damage and dysfunction. The involvement of small airways in respiratory diseases like asthma and chronic obstructive pulmonary disease (COPD) is the best example of the consequences of chronic inflammation. Research indicates that small airway dysfunction is the key to these diseases, given that a main factor determining airflow limitation and impaired lung function. Therefore, addressing small airway involvement using specialized treatment protocols will optimize disease management and patient outcomes, as a clear indication of direct correspondences between long-term inflammation and accompanying health complications (Braido et al., 2016). The acknowledgment of these complex interactions allows healthcare professionals to create targeted interventions that can mitigate the negative impacts of chronic inflammation. The role of neutrophilic granulocytes in chronic inflammation throws further light on its impacts on health. These natural defense cells are crucial in responding swiftly to infections and tissue damage. But repeated activation and recruitment of neutrophils may lead to tissue damage rather than repair, propagating multifaceted inflammatory diseases. Recent findings on CD16+CD11b+ neutrophil subsets indicate their magnitude could be decidedly altered among healthy and acute viral or bacterial infection patients. More specifically, alterations in these subsets reflect an imbalance in immune function that may promote chronic inflammation and the associated health risk. For example, the prevalence of specific neutrophil subpopulations during chronic inflammatory disease can reflect sustained immune dysregulation, and elucidation of such cellular dynamics is therefore key to successful therapeutic interventions (Chudilova et al., 2018). Thus, investigation of neutrophil function in inflammation emphasizes the sophistication of chronic inflammatory disorders. In comprehending the worldwide effects of chronic inflammation on health, lifestyle is found to play a significant role in its development. Lack of proper diet, inactivity, and high levels of stress typically lead to chronic inflammation, collectively producing pro-inflammatory states in the body. For example, diets rich in high-processed foods and sugars have the potential to enhance inflammation within the body, leading to obesity and type 2 diabetes, among other diseases. Lifestyle interventions , such as taking an anti-inflammatory diet or regular exercise, also have the potential to lower chronic inflammation and its resulting health impact. The implication that lifestyle measures have an effect on inflammation underscores the potential of preventive interventions to enhance public health. By addressing diet, exercise, and stress management, healthcare practitioners can help individuals avert the chronic inflammatory state that underpins numerous diseases, ultimately promoting healthier lives.

Test Your Knowledge

1. Describe the role of macrophages, lymphocytes, and fibroblasts in chronic inflammation.
2. How does chronic inflammation contribute to the pathogenesis of diseases like atherosclerosis, diabetes, or cancer?

7.5. The Relationship between Immunophysiology and Inflammation

Learning Outcome

1. Describe how to immune system regulates inflammation;
2. Define the feedback mechanisms in immune responses;
3. Understand the balance between pro-inflammatory and anti-inflammatory signals.

Inflammation is a central immunophysiological process that is the body's first line of defense against offending stimuli, including pathogens and injury. It is an active process with subtle interactions between immune cells, signaling molecules, and vascular remodeling that eventually lead to cure and reestablishment. Immune system activation causes the movement of leukocytes to sites of damage or infection, where they have protective and reparative functions. Yet when the inflammation reaction is uncontrolled or abnormally prolonged, it can lead to chronic inflammatory diseases, for instance, asthma or chronic obstructive lung disease (COPD) (Braido et al., 2016). One needs to understand this delicate equilibrium since it will guide therapeutic maneuvers meant to suppress inflammation and maximize disease status and global immunologic well-being. Immune response and inflammatory elements play pivotal roles in the pathogenesis of virtually all disease processes. For instance, recurrent inflammation may lead to cell damage, which can cause apoptosis or necrosis, such as, with primary sclerosing cholangitis (PSC) (Masuoka et al., 2015). Apoptosis markers of hepatocytes , such as cytokeratin-18 fragments, are great predictors of liver injury and severity of inflammation. Measurement of these markers in patients informs us about the severity of the underlying pathology and emphasizes the significance of inflammation in immunophysiology. With the quantification of levels of apoptotic markers, physicians can better individualize treatment for the regulation of inflammatory response, as well as its consequent effect on hepatocyte viability and function and illustrate the critical association of inflammation and immune health. Furthermore, with the understanding of lung physiology and the role of small airways in pathological conditions , such as asthma and COPD, the importance of understanding inflammation in immunophysiology is brought into focus. Their treatment involves a complete assessment of airway involvement, particularly in the patient with suboptimal disease control (Braido et al., 2016). That assessment includes the use of sophisticated diagnostic modalities in evaluating the function of small airways and determining the treatment modalities appropriate to the profile of the patient. In terms of functional and biological markers of inflammation, the clinician can advance therapy and, ultimately, enhance patient outcomes. The intricate interplay between inflammation and immunophysiology lies at the heart of comprehending the subtleties of disease mechanisms and effective management planning (Figure 7.15).

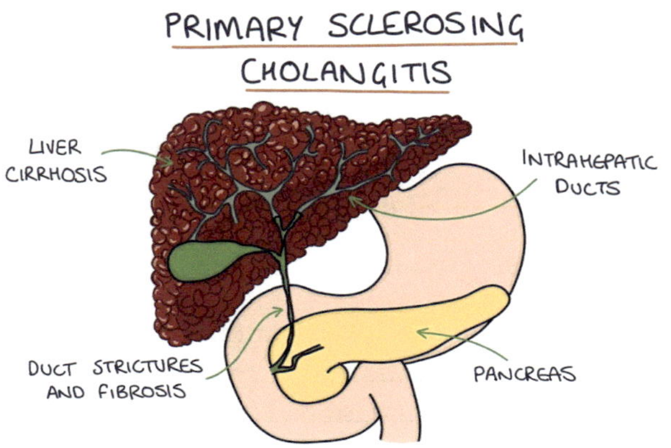

Figure 7.15. Primary sclerosing cholangitis.

Source: https://i.ytimg.com/vi/ZXs6FkjnBIs/maxresdefault.jpg.

7.5.1. How the Immune System Regulates Inflammation

The immune system also has the crucial role of regulating inflammation, balancing the need for a successful response with the risk of tissue damage. As soon as inflammation is initiated, innate immune cells , such as macrophages and neutrophils are rapidly summoned to the infection or injury site. They produce pro-inflammatory cytokines, which induce vasodilation and increased vascular permeability, allowing greater numbers of immune cells to enter. This cascade is very important in pathogen elimination and in the initiation of tissue repair. But if uncontrolled, the inflammatory process turns chronic and leads to a pathological condition in which tissues become subject to oxidative stress and injury. The immune system must thus utilize mechanisms that downregulate this response to ensure that inflammation is resolved effectively and does not progress to chronic disease, highlighting the importance of regulatory pathways in ensuring tissue integrity. As the inflammation continues, regulatory T cells and other anti-inflammatory mediators are instrumental in the re-establishment of homeostasis.

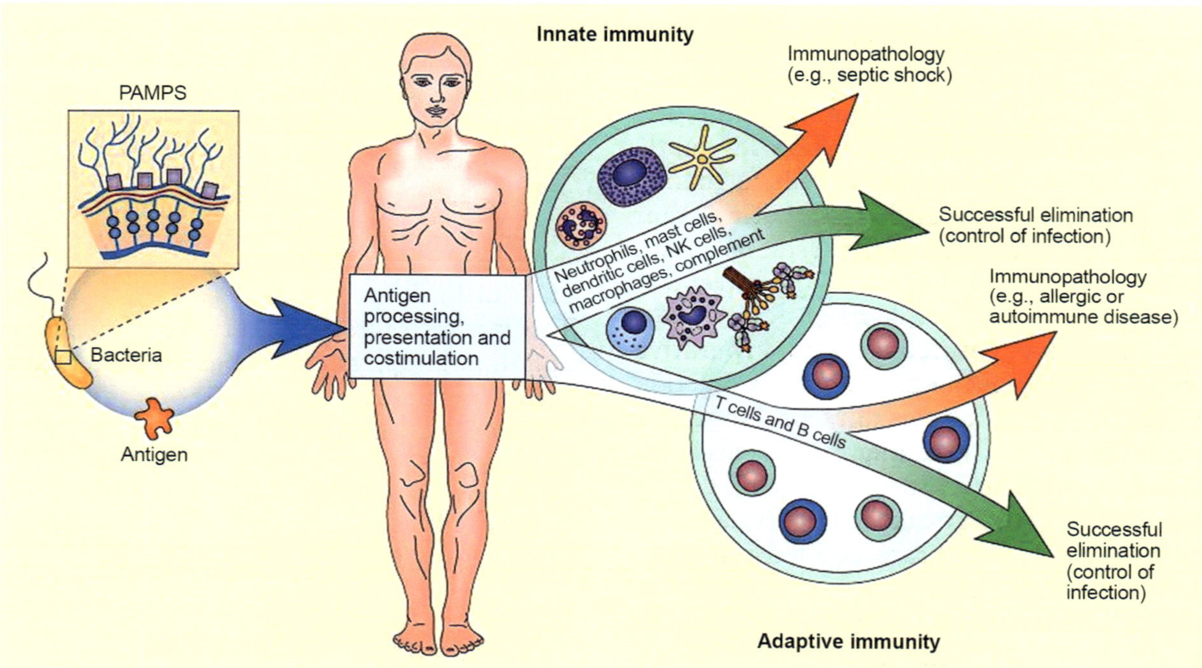

Figure 7.16. Inflammation and autoinflammation.

Source: https://www.immunopaedia.org.za/wp-content/uploads/2016/01/Figure-11.jpg.

They release anti-inflammatory cytokines, such as, IL-10 and TGF-β, that inhibit further activation of pro-inflammatory cells and cause apoptosis of overactive immune cells. In addition, resolution of inflammation is also achieved through the removal of apoptotic cells and the resolution of inflammatory mediators. Research has established that termination of inflammation is an active process involving specialized pro-resolving mediators (SPMs), which are synthesized from omega-3 fatty acids and actively promote the return to normal tissue function. Dysregulation of these processes leads to multiple inflammatory diseases, such as, autoimmune and chronic inflammatory diseases, and underscores the need for precise immune regulation during the inflammation response to enable efficient healing without collateral damage. Therefore, crosstalk between inflammation and the immune system is a highly developed equilibrium of signaling networks that need to be finely regulated. Pathology arises due to dysregulated inflammation in cardiovascular, diabetes, and neurodegenerative diseases. In recent research, pattern recognition receptors (PRRs), including Toll-like receptors (TLRs), were found to be crucial for recognizing tissue damage and guiding inflammation. For example, (Kelley, 1992) highlights the dynamic regulation of TLR4 in hibernation, consistent with alterations in immune adaptation determining reproductive processes and potentially associated with mechanisms responsible for inflammation regulation. In addition, (Kelley, 1992) reaffirms that there is a need to have a regulatory system to avoid chronic inflammation, further highlighting that this balance is crucial for health. Clarification of these complex interactions will facilitate the development of targeted therapies that are capable of immunomodulation to optimize outcomes for inflammatory disorders (Figure 7.16).

7.5.2. Feedback Mechanisms in Immune Responses

The interplay of feedback mechanisms in immune responses is necessary for homeostasis and effective defense against infection. Feedback control is achieved through complex signaling mechanisms that manage the activity of the immune response and modulate responses so that overinflammation and potential tissue damage do not result. For instance, pro-inflammatory cytokines and other signal molecules generated in the process of an immune response are able to induce the release of anti-inflammatory mediators. These mediators do prevent the continued activation of immune cells but instead allow resolution. There are such feedback systems not only that are significant for local immune responses but also for the regulation of the systemic responses. Such integral systems are known to show how the body balances the requirement for potent immune protection against the requirement to avoid detrimental overreactions that could lead to autoimmune disease or inflammatory chronicity. Modulation and expression of Toll-like receptors (TLRs) are typical of feedback in immune response, particularly in inflammation. TLRs are critical sensor molecules that detect pathogen-associated molecular patterns and trigger inflammatory responses to initiate defense against infection. The reported observations in recent studies have revealed the dynamic expression of TLR4, specifically in organs , such as the testis and epididymis under various physiological states, like hibernation and pre-hibernation. Notably, enhanced expression of TLR4 in the testis under hibernation suggests an adaptive process under altered physiological conditions, suggesting immune regulation sensitivity to environmental cues. This allows for an individualized immune response that not only encourages reproductive wellness but also a general immune adaptation process to maintain homeostasis in the dynamic environments (Kelley, 1992). Feedback mechanisms are also very critical in initiating and, at the same time, downregulating inflammatory processes, which is well-apparent in inflammatory diseases. Dysregulation of these feedback processes may lead to chronic inflammation, emphasizing the requirement for a balanced immune response. The interaction between pro-inflammatory and anti-inflammatory signaling demonstrates this balance. For instance, in chronic inflammatory disorders, pro-inflammatory cytokines' persistent activation could incapacitate regulatory feedback mechanisms, and an inflammatory vicious cycle is followed by tissue damage. This dysregulation highlights an important area of research in immunophysiology and raises the possibility that certain therapeutic approaches may attempt to reconstitute these feedback controls in an effort to achieve resolution of inflammation. Elucidation of these processes is central to the development of interventions that will effectively suppress chronic inflammatory disease and promote overall immune competence (Kelley, 1992) (Figure 7.17).

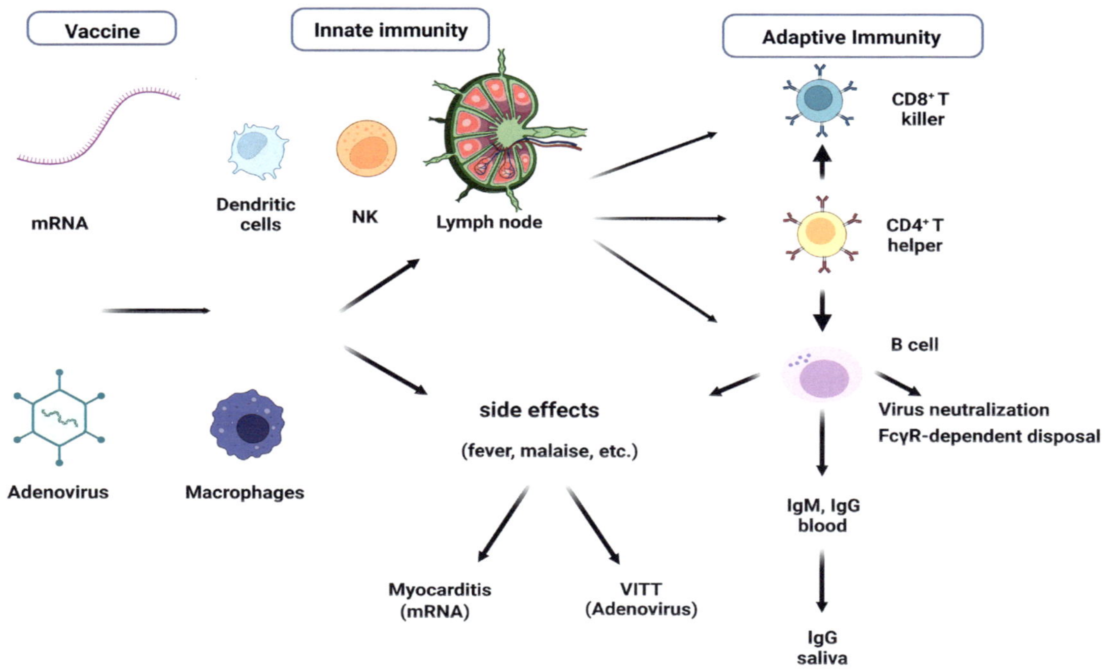

Figure 7.17. Activation of the immune response.

Source: https://ars.els-cdn.com/content/image/1-s2.0-S1471490623000054-gr1.jpg.

7.5.3. The Balance Between Pro-Inflammatory and Anti-Inflammatory Signals

The immune response operates through a complex interplay of pro-inflammatory and anti-inflammatory stimuli that create homeostasis and protect the organism from injury and pathogenic challenge. Pro-inflammatory stimuli, primarily mediated by cytokines , such as TNF-α and IL-6, are essential for initiating the inflammatory reaction. The stimuli evoke immune cell activation and recruitment into damaged or infected tissues, which results in the elimination of injurious agents. However, uncontrolled pro-inflammatory signaling is well known to induce tissue damage and chronic inflammation, leading to the development of several diseases, such as, autoimmune diseases. The delicate balance of these pro-inflammatory signals versus their counterparts is not only needed to respond to acute insults but also to the restoration of tissue homeostasis after injury, which emphasizes the dynamic role of the immune response and its contribution to health and disease. Conversely, anti-inflammatory signals are of paramount significance for the resolution and suppression of inflammation, thus acting as counterbalancing to pro-inflammatory signals. Suppressive mediators , such as IL-10 and transforming growth factor-beta (TGF-β) are accountable for suppression of inflammatory responses, promoting healing and tissue repair. This function of suppression is vital in preventing overactive immune responses that would otherwise lead to pathological processes. The intestinal epithelium itself, for instance, is a wonderful example of this balance; it is a key regulator in immune homeostasis within the gut and in modulating interactions between commensal microbiota and pathogens. Existing literature assures that proper communication among intestinal epithelial cells and resident immune cells via cytokines and chemokines is paramount to orchestrating appropriate immune responses (Andrews et al., 2018). This interactive equilibrium emphasizes the necessity for immune regulation to avoid potential dysregulation and subsequent disease. Inadequate regulation of the inflammatory response can lead to severe tissue damage and sustain chronic inflammation. The delicate equilibrium between anti-inflammatory and pro-inflammatory signals is particularly characterized in the testis, where immune privilege is crucial to protect germ cells against immune-mediated damage. Here, understanding of the testicular immune cells and their role with the germinal epithelium explains how an imbalance may lead to destructive outcomes. Inflammatory disease can disrupt this immune tolerance such that germinal epithelial destruction is caused by pro-inflammatory mediators (Kelley, 1992). This highlights the necessity for each to be in balance by the counteracting forces to avoid tissue damage and highlights the broader implications of immune control throughout physiology and disease, ultimately resulting in therapeutic targets for inflammatory disorders.

Test Your Knowledge

1. What roles do adaptive immune cells (T and B lymphocytes) play in sustaining or resolving inflammation?
2. How can dysregulation of immune responses lead to chronic inflammation and autoimmune diseases?

7.6. Therapeutic Approaches to Modulate Inflammation

Learning Outcome

1. Describe the anti-inflammatory medications;
2. Define the lifestyle changes to reduce inflammation;
3. Discuss the emerging therapies in immunophysiology.

Therapeutic approaches to modulate inflammation are of great clinical relevance in the management of various immunological disorders, thus bringing forth the necessity for targeted therapy. One prevailing approach is by making use of biologics, specifically in disease states with abnormal immune hyperactivation, such as, autoimmune disorders. Notably, type I interferonopathies, characterized by an overexpression of IFNα, are types of conditions that are treatable by such therapies. By employing bound treatments to IFNα, such therapies aim to rectify abnormal levels and restore immune balance. Recent developments over the last few years in interferon-corrective treatment have proven to be beneficial in the therapy for such disorders and represent a significant advancement over our ability to condition treatment for specific immune dysfunctions (Chudilova et al., 2020). In addition to biologics, the role of cytokines and chemokines in the regulation of inflammation cannot be overstressed, particularly within the intestinal microenvironment. The intestinal epithelial barrier is a critical interface between the external world and the immune system, fine-tuning immune responses by the secretion of these soluble mediators. This exquisite communication establishes homeostasis while defending against pathogens and regulating the immune response against commensals. Recent research is aimed at innovations in treatment regimens that modulate these signaling pathways for the enhancement of epithelial wellness, dampening excessive inflammatory reactions, and even curing inflammatory bowel disorders (Andrews et al., 2018). These approaches may yield new mechanisms to regulate immune functions and reduce inflammation, and it is an emerging area of focus for further study. Finally, the intersection of multi-dimensional treatment strategies underscores the multi-aspectual complexity of managing inflammation in various diseases. The interaction among diet, microbial exposure, and immune responses introduces another dimension to the concept of therapeutic modulation. New treatments are now beginning to investigate the influence of dietary components on cytokine production and immune modulation generally, showing potential for precision medicine in inflammatory disease. As researchers further refine our understanding of the complexity of these interactions, the use of patient-specific therapy becomes ever more possible. As proven by advances in the modulation of mediators from the epithelium and their interaction with immune cells, the therapeutic frontier is shifting, enabling clinicians to treat inflammation more holistically and individually (Andrews et al., 2018) (Figure 7.18).

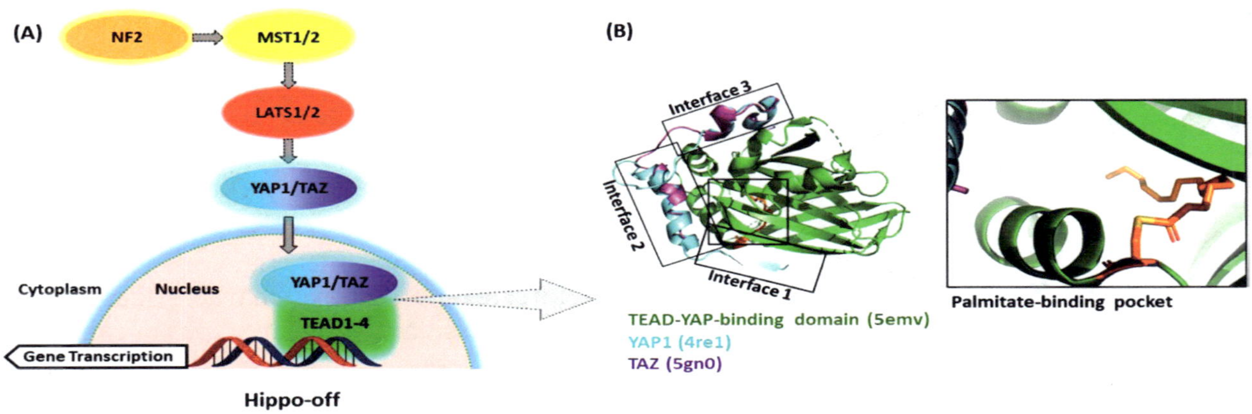

Figure 7.18. Recent therapeutic approaches to modulate the Hippo pathway in oncology.

Source: https://pub.mdpi-res.com/cells/cells-10-02715/article_deploy/html/images/cells-10-02715-g001.png?1633938471.

7.6.1. Anti-Inflammatory Medications

The use of anti-inflammatory medications has emerged as one of the key pillars in the management of both acute and chronic inflammatory conditions. They consist of nonsteroidal anti-inflammatory drugs (NSAIDs), corticosteroids, as well as other biologic agents and work by modulating the body's inflammatory process. NSAIDs , such as ibuprofen and aspirin work by inhibiting cyclooxygenase enzymes with the effect of reducing the synthesis of pro-inflammatory prostaglandins. This reduction is critical in alleviating symptoms , such as pain, inflammation, and fever, and for this reason, NSAIDs are frequently used in treating conditions such as arthritis and recent trauma. Corticosteroids , such as prednisone, however, exert more systemic action by influencing other immune processes, and are effective in suppressing a broad spectrum of inflammatory reactions. While effective, prolonged use of these drugs may be risky owing to gastrointestinal side effects and increased vulnerability to infections, raising questions about their safety profile in chronic therapy. Apart from traditional anti-inflammatory drugs, newer therapies have turned to biologic drugs that target inflammatory cytokines specifically. Such drugs as TNF-α inhibitors and interleukin antagonists have revolutionized the therapeutic landscape for autoimmune diseases , such as rheumatoid arthritis and inflammatory bowel disease. Through selective inhibition of mechanisms maintaining inflammation, these drugs have offered targeted therapy options with enhanced outcomes and reduced side effects compared to conventional treatments. As our understanding of immunophysiology advances, so too has the recognition of specific molecular targets for therapy, opening the door to targeted therapies. Such a movement toward biologics is a significant step forward in therapeutic strategy, particularly for those with inflammatory diseases that are not responsive to standard treatment regimens. Yet cost and access to these therapies are still significant obstacles to clinical practice, and additional research and effort must be applied to make them more widely available. The efficacy of anti-inflammatory medications also takes individual patient factors into consideration, including genetic vulnerabilities, co-morbidities, and extrinsic factors that influence inflammation. Personalized medicine, in which treatment options are tailored to a patient's unique characteristics, is progressively relevant in the treatment of inflammation. For instance, empirical studies are increasingly suggesting that the gut microbiota plays a significant role in modulating the inflammatory response and may impact the effectiveness of anti-inflammatory treatment protocols. Disruptions in the intestinal barrier, e.g., those encountered during conditions that are exacerbated by altitude or gastrointestinal impairment, lead to systemic inflammation that complicates management protocols (Bakshi et al., 2024). Similarly, oral and systemic inflammatory diseases should be taken into account since oral immunology has a significant effect on global immune response (Bozec et al., 2023). As the field of immunophysiology advances further, the integration of these personalized approaches into treatment strategies can potentially enhance patient outcomes for inflammation management (Figure 7.19).

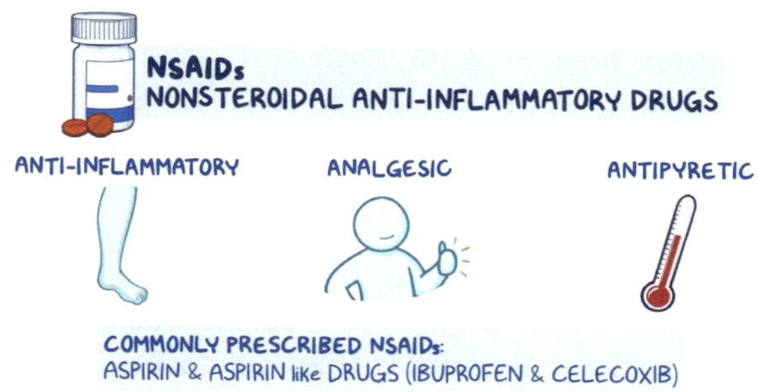

Figure 7.19. Nonsteroidal Anti-inflammatory Drugs (NSAIDs).

Source: https://external-content.duckduckgo.com/iu/?u=https%3A%2F%2Fosmose-it.s3.amazonaws.com%2FiYLvKJHST8GSLtxF3ToTeGQ8Rnm76IJG%2F_.jpg&f=1&nofb=1&ipt=138d9dff4a22520170eb81f51b3b62c015b3843852f23c9e71550ee723de55a7.

7.6.2. Lifestyle Changes to Reduce Inflammation

Dietary modifications are key to avoiding inflammation, a common underlying cause of chronic illnesses. A good diet with an emphasis on anti-inflammatory foods forms the foundation of this approach. Anti-inflammatory foods dense in such nutrients as fruits, vegetables, whole grains, legumes, and fatty fish are rich in antioxidants and omega-3 fatty acids that help combat oxidative stress and uphold immune function. Studies have shown that a Mediterranean diet, with an emphasis on those types of foods, can dramatically reduce inflammatory markers in the body. In addition, cutting down on processed foods containing high sugars and saturated fats can help prevent further inflammation from erupting. By eating whole, nutrient-rich foods first, individuals can establish an internal environment conducive to overall health and inflammation reduction, improving their body's capacity to maintain homeostasis and prevent chronic disease formation based on the concepts of immunophysiology and inflammation. Physical activity is another lifestyle modification that has immense control over inflammation. Exercise not only improves physical condition but also immune system regulation, thus lowering the levels of systemic inflammation. Engaging in moderate aerobic exercises , such as walking, cycling, or swimming has been shown to elicit the release of anti-inflammatory cytokines, with this resulting in an overall decrease in inflammatory biomarkers like C-reactive protein (CRP). Exercise also plays a core role in weight maintenance, with obesity being one of the main factors triggering chronic inflammation. By maintaining a healthy weight through ongoing exercise, individuals can reduce their risk for inflammatory diseases. Incorporating variety in the exercises one does via one's way of life gives rise to a blend of physical as well as mental health benefits, which overall give rise to overall reduction in inflammation and increased immunological welfare within the body. Stress-reducing techniques make up a significant aspect of lifestyle changes for reducing inflammation. Chronic stress can lead to ongoing cortisol levels, a hormone that, in excess, has the potential to initiate inflammatory responses throughout the body. Therefore, incorporating methods such as mindfulness meditation, yoga, and diaphragmatic breathing could significantly control the body's stress response as well as inflammation. Studies have indicated that these techniques can reduce markers of inflammation as well as improve psychological well-being. Furthermore, restful sleep plays a critical part in maintaining a well-balanced immune system; lack of sleep has been linked with increased inflammation. By ensuring stress management and restful sleep, individuals can establish a conducive environment for immune function and regulation of inflammation, as is the case with the overall topic of immunophysiology and inflammation under lifestyle influences (Figure 7.20).

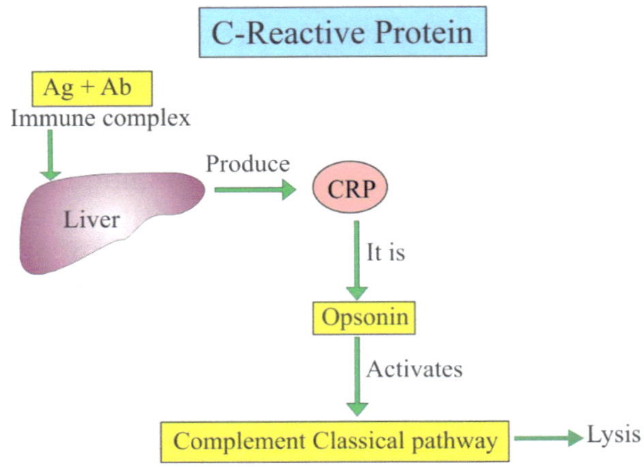

Figure 7.20. C-reactive protein (CRP).

Source: https://www.labpedia.net/wp-content/uploads/-c-reactive-protein-crp-high-sensitivity-crp-hs-crp-/CRP-6.JPG.

7.6.3. Emerging Therapies in Immunophysiology

Immunophysiology is going through revolutionary breakthroughs that hold the promise of enhancing inflammatory disease treatment modalities. New therapies are specifically targeting the intricate interaction in the immune system, utilizing cutting-edge molecular biology techniques and bioinformatics to analyze complicated inflammation pathways. Elucidation of these pathways has enabled researchers to identify new targets for immunomodulation that hold the promise for enhanced treatments. Traditional therapies can lack specificity in immune targets; therefore, such new strategies can even fill the gaps in present-day medical interventions. Such a shift towards personalized medicine can potentially offer strategies tailored to the immune status of each individual patient, enhancing efficacy and reducing side effects. One of the brightest areas of new therapies is the very robust growth of translational immunology, particularly with regard to oral health. Recent evidence indicates that a higher understanding of oral immunology may considerably improve the practice of therapeutic interventions for many oral diseases. The interplay of separate immune mechanisms acting in the unique environment of the oral cavity builds a demand for unique therapies that relate to specific immune reactions. Contemporary orthodontic, periodontal, and surgical treatments already face restrictions that weaken their efficacy and patient quality of life, based on recent reports. Breakthroughs in this field would foretell significant improvements on existing dental protocols, which could introduce revolutionary changes in the management of oral health and overall wellness as a whole (Bozec et al., 2023). Aside from this, the integration of new biotechnologies , such as CRISPR-Cas9 and other gene editing technologies, suggests the prospect of breakthrough therapy in immunophysiology. These emerging technologies provide precise alterations at the genetic level, which throw open the gates of regenerative medicine and cellular therapies of high order. With development in immunophysiology further ahead, the necessity to manage inflammatory responses through genetic sensitization and manipulation is increasingly becoming apparent. These developments may find application in therapies that are not only symptom-reducing but also cause-corrective for inflammation, thereby developing a therapeutic strategy that is effective from the inside. Continued research in this area reiterates the hope that further therapeutic options will be developed, essentially changing how we think about and treat both systemic and localized inflammatory illnesses (Bozec et al., 2023).

Test Your Knowledge

1. What are the common classes of anti-inflammatory drugs, and how do they differ in mechanism of action?
2. How do corticosteroids suppress inflammation at the cellular and molecular levels?

SUMMARY

Immunophysiology and inflammation are the best terms to explain the intricate relationship between immune response and physiological processes. Throughout the analysis, it has been evident that inflammation is a crucial adaptive response, but, in dysregulation, can lead to severe pathologies. Regulation of immune signal pathways, particularly by the action of Toll-like receptors like TLR4, illustrates the intricacies of immune adaptation. For example, the study of TLR4 expression in Anatolian ground squirrel testis and epididymis during hibernation shows that immune mechanisms are under dynamic control to consider environmental stimuli, and this is proof of the importance of immunophysiological balance as a means of sustaining reproductive function (Kelley, 1992). The interdependence requires more research to establish the implications of such research towards shedding light on immune-mediated disease. Second, the findings on hepatocyte apoptosis and necrosis in primary sclerosing cholangitis (PSC) underscore inflammation as a central feature of hepatobiliary disease. Elevated serum concentrations of apoptotic markers, namely cytokeratin-18 fragments, indicate close correlation with disease severity and with concomitant inflammatory responses. Such correlation serves to emphasize the direct impact of immunophysiology on disease development and patient outcome and illustrates the potential for modulating such pathways through targeted therapy. The absence of a significant difference in HMGB1 levels between controls and PSC patients again highlights the complexity of inflammatory markers and their relationship with disease conditions (Masuoka et al., 2015). Illuminating these dynamics may provide better diagnostic and treatment methods for hepatobiliary pathologies. To put it simply, the conclusions of the immunophysiology and inflammation findings suggest that even though the immune system has a vital role in protecting the body, when dysregulated, it can bring about many diseases. This provides a framework to enjoy the manner in which physiologic and environmental changes can affect immune responses. With further research, a better understanding of how immune mechanisms correspond with other biological systems will provide new avenues for treatment. Ultimately, these findings speak to the need for multidisciplinary investigation in the field of immunophysiology because it is not merely inflammation but instead more general health repercussions, further highlighting the relevance of this field in contemporary medical research.

When examining the intricate association of inflammation and immunophysiology, certain significant points are revealed that underscore the complexity of the immune response. One prominent point is the role of cytokines, namely IL-17, in modulating the action of cells. IL-17 has been identified to inhibit apoptosis in infected macrophages, which are mainly responsible for keeping bacterial growth at bay, particularly when in relation to Mycobacterium infection. This inhibition is achieved through mechanisms that modulate the p53 pathway signaling, thereby altering the expression of pro- and anti-apoptotic proteins. These processes illustrate how immune modulators can affect the resolution of inflammation as well as the fate of infected cells, implying a delicate balance necessary in effective inflammatory responses and immunity (Cruz et al., 2015). Moreover, the mucosal immune system is a cornerstone when preservation of homeostasis is considered, particularly in the gut. The system can differentiate between innocuous antigens and potential pathogens, showing an innate function to ensure intestinal integrity. Any departure from the said balance may lead to severe inflammatory disorders, including Inflammatory Bowel Disease (IBD). Recent evidence suggests that environmental factors, including diet and exposure to pollutants, are increasingly recognized to trigger and perpetuate these conditions. Such factors can alter the gut microbiota, which is imperative in the regulation of immune responses, thereby enabling local inflammation and disease pathogenesis (Curciarello et al., 2019). Briefly, the crosstalk between cytokines, cell apoptosis, and immune homeostasis in the mucosa captures the sophistication of immunophysiology. The complex mechanisms by which cytokines like IL-17 control immune cell activity demonstrate the amenable nature of these mechanisms to therapeutic manipulation. In parallel, the control of environmental influences on the gut microbiota emphasizes the urgent need to develop a detailed understanding of innate and adaptive immunity to apply accurate measures for the prevention and treatment of inflammatory disease. Thus, the convergence of immune responses and inflammation not only accounts for the complexity of disease mechanisms but also presents significant opportunities for future investigation and drug discovery.

KEY TERMS FROM THIS CHAPTER

- Adaptive immunity
- Antigen
- B lymphocytes (B cells)
- Complement system
- Dendritic cells
- Immunological memory
- Innate immunity
- Antibody
- Autoimmunity
- Chronic inflammation
- Cytokines
- Histamine
- Inflammatory response
- Interleukins (ILs)

CRITICAL THINKING QUESTIONS

1. **Which type of immune cell is primarily responsible for producing antibodies?**
   a. T cells
   b. B cells
   c. Neutrophils
   d. Macrophages
2. **Which of the following is a hallmark sign of inflammation?**
   a. Numbness
   b. Pallor
   c. Swelling
   d. Paralysis
3. **Which cytokine is most associated with initiating the inflammatory response?**
   a. Interleukin-10 (IL-10)
   b. Tumor necrosis factor-alpha (TNF-α)
   c. Interferon-gamma (IFN-γ)
   d. Erythropoietin
4. **The complement system contributes to immunity by:**
   a. Inhibiting antibody production
   b. Killing infected cells directly
   c. Enhancing phagocytosis and lysing pathogens
   d. Suppressing inflammation
5. **Which type of immunity provides a rapid but non-specific response to pathogens?**
   a. Adaptive immunity
   b. Humoral immunity
   c. Cell-mediated immunity
   d. Innate immunity

Short Answer Questions

1. Define innate immunity and name two key components.
2. What is the primary function of macrophages in the immune response?
3. List the four classic signs of inflammation.
4. What role do cytokines play in inflammation?
5. Describe the difference between humoral and cell-mediated immunity.
6. What is the function of the complement system?
7. Name the major types of T cells and their primary functions.
8. How do neutrophils contribute to the inflammatory response?
9. What triggers the activation of the adaptive immune system?
10. What is immunological memory?

Answers to Critical Thinking Questions

1. (b); 2. (c); 3. (b); 4. (c); 5. (d).

REFERENCES

1. Cruz, A., Ludovico, P., Torrado, E., Gama, J. B., Sousa, J., Gaifem, J., Appelberg, R., Rodrigues, F., Cooper, A. M., Pedrosa, J., Saraiva, M., & Castro, A. G. (2015). IL-17A Promotes Intracellular Growth of Mycobacterium by Inhibiting Apoptosis of Infected Macrophages. *Frontiers in immunology*, *6*, 498. https://doi.org/10.3389/fimmu.2015.00498(accessed on 28th June 2025).
2. Aker, J. E. (2016). Regulatory T cell plasticity and its role in the rejection of pancreatic islet allograft tissue. https://core.ac.uk/download/142066287.pdf (accessed on 28th June 2025).
3. Andrews, C., Durum, S. K., & McLean, M. H. (2018). Cytokine tuning of intestinal epithelial function. https://core.ac.uk/download/323303802.pdf (accessed on 28th June 2025).
4. Suzaki, H., Asano, K., Ohki, S., Kanai, K., Mizutani, T., & Hisamitsu, T. (1999). Suppressive activity of a macrolide antibiotic, roxithromycin, on pro-inflammatory cytokine production in vitro and in vivo. *Mediators of inflammation*, *8*(4-5), 199–204. https://doi.org/10.1080/09629359990351(accessed on 28th June 2025).
5. Bakshi, J., Mishra, K. P., & Singh, S. (2024). External factors affecting gastrointestinal barrier and mucosal immunity at high altitude. https://core.ac.uk/download/595878643.pdf (accessed on 28th June 2025).
6. Nakov, D., Hristov, S., Stankovic, B., Pol, F., Dimitrov, I., Ilieski, V., Mormede, P., Hervé, J., Terenina, E., Lieubeau, B., Papanastasiou, D. K., Bartzanas, T., Norton, T., Piette, D., Tullo, E., & van Dixhoorn, I. D. E. (2019). Methodologies for Assessing Disease Tolerance in Pigs. *Frontiers in veterinary science*, *5*, 329. https://doi.org/10.3389/fvets.2018.00329(accessed on 28th June 2025).
7. Marichal T, Boyman O and Reber LL (2020) Editorial: Role of Neutrophils in Inflammatory Diseases. Front. Immunol. 11:627939. doi: 10.3389/fimmu.2020.627939 (accessed on 28th June 2025).
8. Bozec, A., Deschner, J., Galler, K., Jantsch, J., et al. (2023). Advancing oral immunology for improving oral health. https://core.ac.uk/download/574067827.pdf (accessed on 28th June 2025).
9. Masuoka, H. C., Vuppalanchi, R., Deppe, R., Bybee, P., Comerford, M., Liangpunsakul, S., Ghabril, M., & Chalasani, N. (2015). Individuals with Primary Sclerosing Cholangitis Have Elevated Levels of Biomarkers for Apoptosis but Not Necrosis. *Digestive diseases and sciences*, *60*(12), 3642–3646. https://doi.org/10.1007/s10620-015-3805-7 (accessed on 28th June 2025).
10. Curciarello, R., Canziani, K. E., Docena, G. H., & Muglia, C. I. (2019). Contribution of Non-immune Cells to Activation and Modulation of the Intestinal Inflammation. *Frontiers in immunology*, *10*, 647. https://doi.org/10.3389/fimmu.2019.00647(accessed on 28th June 2025).
11. Pérez, C. V., Theas, M. S., Jacobo, P. V., Jarazo-Dietrich, S., Guazzone, V. A., & Lustig, L. (2013). Dual role of immune cells in the testis: Protective or pathogenic for germ cells?. *Spermatogenesis*, *3*(1), e23870. https://doi.org/10.4161/spmg.23870 (accessed on 28th June 2025).
12. V. Nesterova, I., A. Chudilova, G., V. Kovaleva, S., V. Lomtatidze, L., & V. Rusinova, T. (2019). Remodeling of Phenotype CD16 + CD11b + Neutrophilic Granulocytes in Acute Viral and Acute Bacterial Infections. IntechOpen. doi: 10.5772/intechopen.81631(accessed on 28th June 2025).

13. V. Nesterova, I., V. Kovaleva, S., V. Malinovskaya, V., A. Chudilova, G., & V. Rusinova, T. (2021). Congenital and Acquired Interferonopathies: Differentiated Approaches to Interferon Therapy. IntechOpen. doi: 10.5772/intechopen.91723V. Nesterova, I., V. Kovaleva, S., V. Malinovskaya, V., A. Chudilova, G., & V. Rusinova, T. (2021). Congenital and Acquired Interferonopathies: Differentiated Approaches to Interferon Therapy. IntechOpen. doi: 10.5772/intechopen.91723(accessed on 28th June 2025).

14. Braido, F., Scichilone, N., Lavorini, F., Usmani, O. S., Dubuske, L., Boulet, L. P., Mosges, R., Nunes, C., Sanchez-Borges, M., Ansotegui, I. J., Ebisawa, M., Levi-Schaffer, F., Rosenwasser, L. J., Bousquet, J., Zuberbier, T., Canonica, G. W., Cruz, A., Yanez, A., Yorgancioglu, A., Deleanu, D., ... GA2LEN (2016). Manifesto on small airway involvement and management in asthma and chronic obstructive pulmonary disease: an Interasma (Global Asthma Association - GAA) and World Allergy Organization (WAO) document endorsed by Allergic Rhinitis and its Impact on Asthma (ARIA) and Global Allergy and Asthma European Network (GA^{2}LEN). *The World Allergy Organization journal*, *9*(1), 37. https://doi.org/10.1186/s40413-016-0123-2(accessed on 28th June 2025).

15. Kersten, E., Paun, C. C., Schellevis, R. L., Hoyng, C. B., Delcourt, C., Lengyel, I., Peto, T., Ueffing, M., Klaver, C. C. W., Dammeier, S., den Hollander, A. I., & de Jong, E. K. (2018). Systemic and ocular fluid compounds as potential biomarkers in age-related macular degeneration. *Survey of ophthalmology*, *63*(1), 9–39. https://doi.org/10.1016/j.survophthal.2017.05.003(accessed on 28th June 2025).

16. Wallace, J. L., Ianaro, A., & de Nucci, G. (2017). Gaseous Mediators in Gastrointestinal Mucosal Defense and Injury. *Digestive diseases and sciences*, *62*(9), 2223–2230. https://doi.org/10.1007/s10620-017-4681-0 (accessed on 28th June 2025).

17. Gálvez Galán, I., Ortega Rincón, E., & Torres Piles, S. T. (2018). Balneotherapy, immune system, and stress response: A hermetic strategy? https://core.ac.uk/download/304324234.pdf (accessed on 28th June 2025).

18. Kelley, K. W. (1992). The physiology of immunology. https://core.ac.uk/download/75906983.pdf (accessed on 28th June 2025).

THERMOREGULATION AND TEMPERATURE CONTROL

8

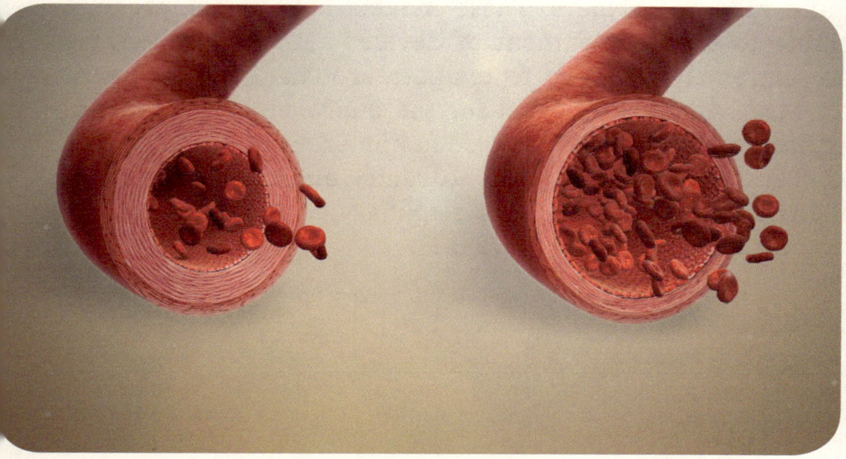

LEARNING OBJECTIVES

After studying this chapter, you will be able to:

1. Discuss the human body's temperature range.
2. Explain the mechanisms of heat production.
3. Discuss the mechanisms of heat loss.
4. Focus on the role of the hypothalamus.
5. Learn about physiological responses to temperature changes.
6. Evaluate the pathophysiological conditions affecting thermoregulation.

Introduction

It is crucial to comprehend temperature control and thermoregulation to be able to value human physiology and its adaptive responses to environmental stress. The core temperature of the human body is maintained quite stable, a function of utmost significance for maximal enzymatic activity and overall metabolic function. Homeostasis is maintained through highly advanced physiological control systems responding to internal and external changes in temperature. These systems not only protect the body against extreme temperatures but also permit cellular processes to proceed unimpeded, illustrating the importance of thermal equilibrium under various physiological states. Knowledge of thermoregulation is particularly valuable in fields ranging from medicine to engineering, specifically in designing systems for high-thermal-stress environments, such as, aerospace or intensive care facilities. As the human body faces changing environmental conditions, it becomes essential for humans to respond physiologically to thermal changes. When humans face heat, for example, they use techniques like sweating and vasodilation to lose excess heat energy. In cold temperatures, on the other hand, shivering and peripheral vasoconstriction are utilized to retain heat. The significance of these responses extends to medical science, whereby proper knowledge of thermoregulation assists in the treatment of diseases that relate to temperature and in enhancing hospital treatment approaches for efficiency (Kaciuba-Uscilko & Greenleaf, 1989). Responses to heat, for instance, are not only crucial to athletes but also to heat-disease patients as well as to individuals requiring special temperature control upon recovery or surgery. Thus, human thermoregulation is an interesting study that gives information about elementary physiology and also valuable applications in medicine. The scientific research in thermoregulation is supported by advances in technology and computational modeling. Computational Fluid Dynamics (CFD) is a significant advancement whereby it is now possible to model heat and mass transfer in many clinical devices , such as incubators and radiant warmers. These models help to comprehend heat transfer mechanisms and contribute to the development of devices aimed at vulnerable populations, namely neonates, who are extremely sensitive to temperature changes (Wrobel et al., 2010). Understanding such transfer mechanisms is relevant for the improvement of thermal protection systems not only in the environment of newborns but also in numerous other fields, e.g., in protective gear for astronauts or workers performing tasks in extreme conditions. Hence, the study of temperature regulation and thermoregulation is a multidisciplinary endeavor, combining fundamental physiology with new technological advances (Figure 8.1).

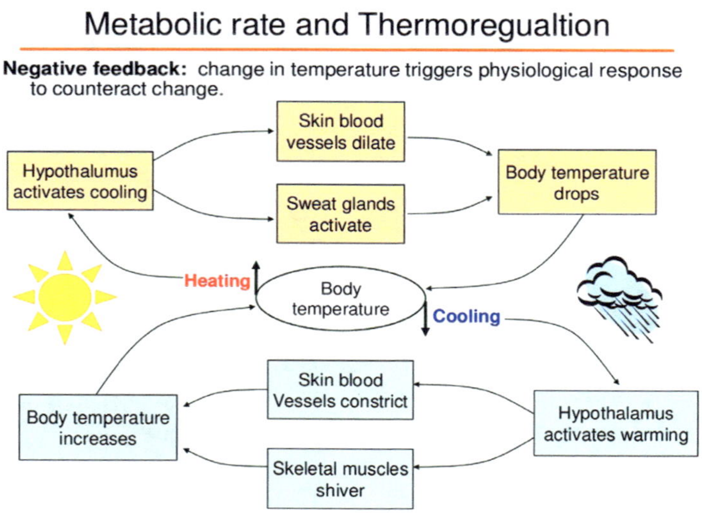

Figure 8.1. Thermoregulation.

Source: https://image.slidesharecdn.com/lec09thermoregulation-13330360448832-phpapp02-120329105250-phpapp02/95/lec-09-thermoregulation-31-1024.jpg?cb=1333540747.

Definition of Thermoregulation

The process of thermoregulation is critical to appreciating how human physiology achieves a constant internal temperature in the face of changing external environmental conditions. Thermoregulation is defined as the physiological mechanisms for controlling body temperature within a narrow range to enable optimal metabolic processes. The human organism is a complex system capable of registering temperature changes and responding with proper physiological mechanisms to either lose heat in hyperthermia or retain heat upon exposure to cold. These mechanisms are crucial as even small deviations from the optimal range can result in impaired cellular function and, by proxy, systemic failure. Thermoregulation is thus a delicate balance, reacting not only to changes in the external temperature but to internal metabolic requirements as well. The secret to thermoregulation lies in the hypothalamus, the body's thermostat. In the brain, this formation takes input from peripheral thermoreceptors found throughout the body and computes this data to produce homeostasis. With the increase in the body temperature, the hypothalamus sends signals to various effectors , such as sweat glands to enhance evaporative loss of heat by sweating and simultaneously leads to the dilation of blood vessels for increased loss of heat. It causes shivering to generate heat and vasoconstriction to retain heat during cold. This intricate feedback process highlights not just the interconnectedness of multiple physiological systems but also the central role played by the hypothalamus in maintaining temperature homeostasis. In addition, as human activity continues to advance and individuals are subjected to heterogeneous environments, an understanding of this control mechanism becomes increasingly important in addressing thermal stress issues. Thermoregulation is an active process, not a passive one; it is regulated by several variables, such as, physical status, acclimatization, and hydration. Individual variability, including differences in metabolic rate, can affect the capacity to effectively thermoregulate. Further, the body's ability to acclimatize to fluctuating external temperatures, either naturally or through artificial means, is of paramount importance to human health, especially for individuals working in extreme environments, such as, sports athletes or space travelers in space exploration. Effective thermoregulation can determine exposure success to extreme environments, ranging from intense training to long-duration stays in space where traditional physiological controls are likely to be reached. An understanding of the nuances of thermoregulation, including balance of energy metabolism and thermal balance under varying activities, as documented in Kaciuba-Uscilko & Greenleaf (1989), is essential in the creation of effective thermal protection systems and countermeasures that can guard human function against temperature extremes.

Importance of Temperature Control in Human Physiology

The relevance of body temperature control in human physiology lies in its essential role in maintaining homeostasis, a balance of internal conditions that are required for proper function. The optimal range for the functioning of the human body is an extremely tight range of approximately 36.1°C to 37.2°C. Moving beyond this range can result in adverse physiological effects, including disruptions in metabolic processes, enzyme activity, and overall cellular function. For instance, increased body temperature upon exercise increases metabolic rate and energy use, which must be compensated for by heat dissipation mechanisms such that heat-related ailments are prevented. Effective thermoregulatory processes, therefore, are basic measures that enable the organism to adapt to changing external conditions while maintaining appropriate internal temperatures, thereby ensuring proper physiological functioning. Besides, the body's thermoregulatory mechanism involves intricate feedback loops involving the hypothalamus, sweat glands, and circulatory system. Through these, humans possess multiple physiological responses , such as vasodilation, sweating, and shivering, through which they can control body temperature to changes in external and internal environments. Disruption of this delicate process can pose harm to health, as demonstrated in patients suffering from conditions , such as multiple sclerosis (MS). Current studies demonstrate that MS patients can be affected by impaired sweating responses and altered thermoregulatory mechanisms, thereby exacerbating their symptoms during heat stress following physical activity. Such data emphasizes the greater role of effective temperature regulation in the context of long-term health and physical capacity, as any impairment leads to severe problems with the management of heat stress and exercise. In addition, temperature regulation and exercise physiology interact to emphasize the necessity for bodies to be kept within a perfect body temperature during exercise. As the bodies engage in hard work, the metabolic heat production rate increases, requiring efficient thermoregulatory mechanisms to avoid heat stress.

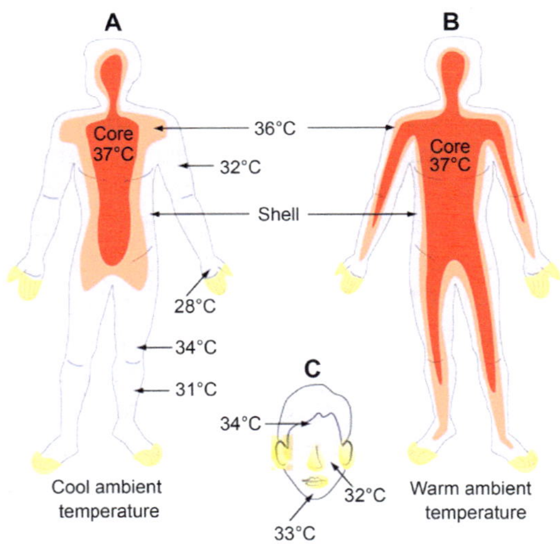

Figure 8.2. Diagrammatic illustration of body temperature in the human body.

Source: https://www.researchgate.net/profile/Matthew-White-25/publication/51178470/figure/fig1/AS:394173648785408@1470989729106/Diagrammatic-illustration-of-body-temperature-in-the-human-body-a-In-cold-environments_W840.jpg.

Research has indicated that individuals with some impairments, such as, those of MS, exhibit reduced sweat production and abnormal skin blood flow on exercise, as their research illustrates compared to healthy subjects (Allen et al., 2018). Such physiological impairments can limit exercise tolerance under thermal stress and highlight the importance of protective interventions and acclimatization strategies, particularly under extreme conditions, for ensuring safety and enhancing the performance of physical activities in healthy and impaired individuals. Thus, understanding and correcting the complexities of thermoregulation is critical in favoring public health intervention and designing preventive interventions against the impact of dysregulation of temperature (Figure 8.2).

8.1. The Human Body's Temperature Range

Learning Outcome

1. Describe the normal body temperature and its variations;
2. ocus on factors influencing body temperature;
3. Learn about the consequences of temperature deviations.

The human body maintains a relatively uniform temperature range of approximately 98.6°F (37°C), although individual temperatures within the range of 97°F to 99°F are typical. This extremely precise thermoregulation is needed for enzymatic function, metabolic reactions, and homeostasis generally. If the body temperature deviates from this norm, essential physiological mechanisms are triggered to restore equilibrium. As an illustration, when faced with heat, the hypothalamus activates such processes as sweating to dissipate heat. In contrast, when faced with cold, shivering can ensue, producing heat through muscle work. This balance between heat production and loss illustrates the intricate regulatory mechanisms of the body to promote optimal functioning in spite of environmental fluctuations. Knowledge of the human body's temperature range is thus paramount to understanding how thermoregulatory mechanisms maintain health and performance in different climates. The mechanism of temperature control is modulated by factors , such as age, gender, environmental conditions, and even psychological status, resulting in variability in baseline temperature among individuals. For example, younger individuals have a slightly increased mean temperature compared to elderly individuals, whose physiological machinery may not be as efficient in preventing heat build-up. In addition, psychological states, including stress and anxiety, can trigger autonomic responses that affect temperature control through processes like increased blood flow or breathing regulation. Research indicates that these distinctions are critical to assess the levels of thermal comfort across different environments, as illustrated by recent studies exploring the effect of thermal discomfort on behavior within home environments during the heating period (Gauthier, 2015). In this way, the multifaceted phenomenon of temperature regulation not only includes physiological processes but also individual characteristics and external influences. The awareness of the human body's thermal range has ramifications extending beyond mere physiology, impacting clinical interventions and energy-saving measures in architecture. An understanding of how humans respond to thermal discomfort, particularly in extreme weather, allows researchers and practitioners to further refine interventions against heat stress or hypothermia. Cutting-edge approaches , such as adaptation strategies for behavior, aim to bring together environmental control and human response in a way that optimizes comfort in the home and work environments (Gauthier, 2015). Additionally, greater sensitivity to how temperature variability affects health and productivity can guide public health policy to mitigate the danger of climate change. Therefore, a general understanding of thermoregulation not only underpins knowledge of human physiology but also real-world answers to improving the quality of life and preserving health in various environments (Figure 8.3).

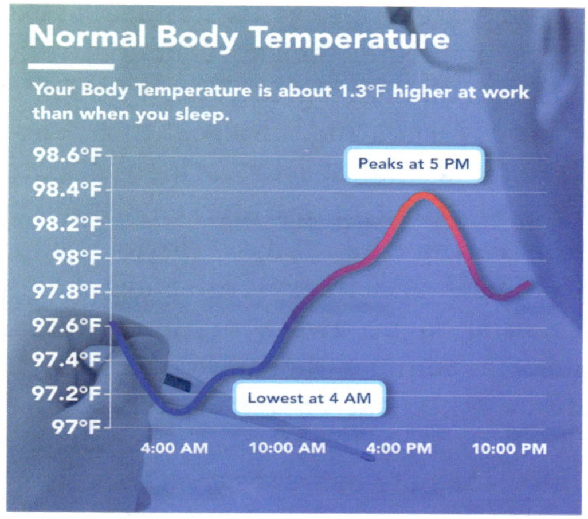

Figure 8.3. The redefinition of human body temperature.

Source: https://www.clearvuehealth.com/i/normaltemp.png.

8.1.1. Normal Body Temperature and Its Variations

It is essential that the internal temperature within the human body is held constant for the proper functioning of physiological processes, typically in the range of 98.6 degrees Fahrenheit (37 degrees Celsius). Nevertheless, the value deviates significantly in accordance with a number of factors like the time of day, age, sex, and individual metabolic rate. For instance, the body temperature is reduced in the morning and increased in late afternoon and evening due to diurnal rhythms. Also, children exhibit a greater body temperature than adults due to their faster metabolic rate and higher production of heat during growth and development. This healthy variation foundation underlies the significance of understanding the principles of thermoregulation, as deviations from the norm can predict a range of health disorders and hence combining temperature regulation with overall health diagnosis. During situations of extreme changes in the environment, the body must dynamically regulate its heat production and dissipation to maintain homeostasis. Muscle activity in exercise also generates heat in excess, which needs greater thermoregulatory reflexes, such as, vasodilation and increased perspiration, to avoid overheating. Interestingly enough, individuals acclimatize to various climates—, such as adjusting to warmer environments—demonstrating the body's flexibility using physiological and behavioral mechanisms. It is essential to be aware of these processes because inadequate thermal control at times of effort or in extreme weather conditions may lead to heat disorders. By exploration of the interface between energy metabolism and thermal balance and definition of physiological responses of the body, scientists are better able to advise mechanisms for avoiding such states in the course of exercise or heat exposure (Kaciuba-Uscilko & Greenleaf, 1989). Beyond typical fluctuations in bodily temperature, medical devices employed for neonatal care likewise indicate the complexity of thermal regulation in different populations. Devices like radiant warmers and incubators utilize complex heat transfer mechanisms to provide optimal temperatures for vulnerable populations, i.e., preterm infants, whose thermoregulatory capacity is often compromised. Computational Fluid Dynamics (CFD) modeling has also proven itself as an effective tool in maximizing these devices, modeling various heat and mass transfer scenarios in a bid to improve patient outcomes. This application of technology illustrates how learning thermoregulation not only aids physiological knowledge but also promotes medical practice innovations, establishing the centrality of temperature regulation in health and in the clinic (Wrobel et al., 2010) (Figure 8.4).

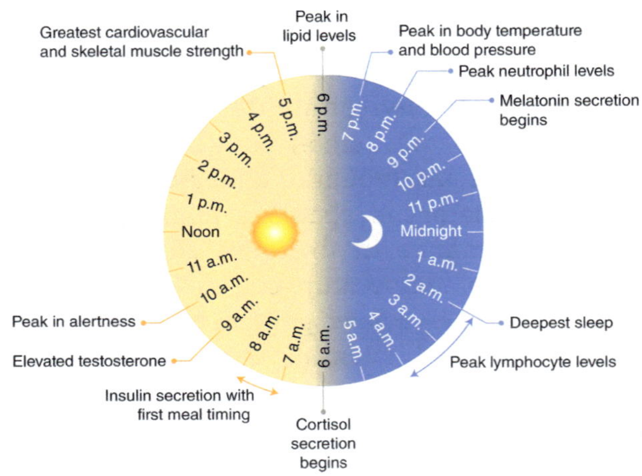

Figure 8.4. Circadian-rhythm.

Source: https://themenshealthclinic.co.uk/wp-content/uploads/2020/04/Circadian-Rhythm.png.

8.1.2. Factors Influencing Body Temperature

The human body possesses a core temperature within a relatively narrow range and is crucial for optimal physiological function. Intrinsic and extrinsic factors play roles in the process of thermoregulation. Metabolic function, general health, and hormonal control are the biotic factors that significantly influence this process. For instance, when there is excessive physical activity, metabolic function is increased, thereby improving body-generated heat. Conversely, environmental factors external to the body, like ambient temperature and humidity, strongly influence how the body dissipates heat. As demonstrated in experiments with lizards in different environments, the thermal characteristics of environments are able to affect physiological processes and constrain activity, evoking the entwinement of habitat and thermal regulation (Smith & Ballinger, 2001). This intricate dynamic of intrinsic and extrinsic factors captures the complexity of homeostasis in human thermoregulation. Other than metabolic and environmental factors, individual differences

, such as body composition, age, and sex also influence the regulation of body temperature. For instance, younger individuals have higher metabolism levels and therefore produce more heat than older individuals with slower metabolic functions. Moreover, percentage and distribution of body fat play equally critical roles because fat tissue is an insulator, both in conserving heat as well as dissipating heat. The variation in thermoregulatory efficiency between women and men—customarily attributed to endocrine regulation and body composition differences—may create measurable variations in temperature regulation, particularly under stress or exercise. From research, it is seen that certain physiological states and lifecycle stages have the potential to alter the sensitivity of thermoregulatory mechanisms, ultimately influencing people's thermal balance and susceptibility to heat and cold injury. Recent technologies , such as infrared thermography (IRT), have provided new methods for the assessment of body temperature change compared to traditional measures. IRT provides a means of non-invasive measurement of skin temperature, possibly reflecting core temperature change during various physiological and environmental states. Standardized protocols for data acquisition using IRT are emerging as significant in sports medicine and exercise to improve diagnostic practice and performance assessment (Moreira et al., 2017). This syncretism of these cutting-edge approaches can not just fortify our understanding of thermoregulation during various activities, but also improve the regulation of heat-related health risks. The comparison of factors influencing body temperature through both biological and technological lenses enables researchers to develop more comprehensive strategies for sustaining effective thermal balance in various populations and environments (Figure 8.5).

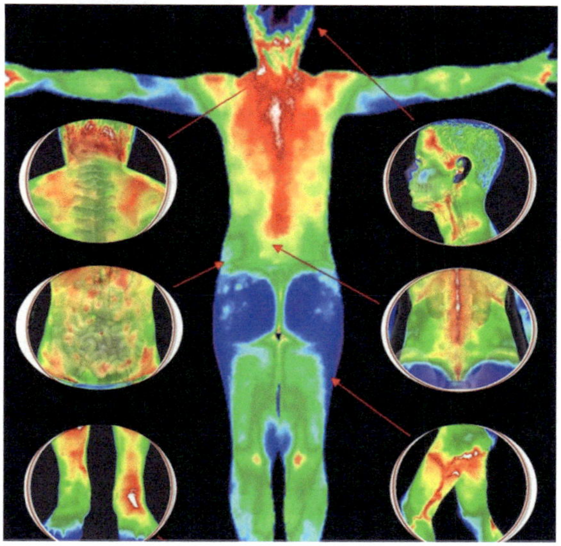

Figure 8.5. Infrared thermography (IRT).

Source: https://i.pinimg.com/originals/24/83/26/24832650896ab91351d007d74293a0a3.jpg.

8.1.3. Consequences of Temperature Deviations

Homeostasis is necessary for the maintenance of physiological function, and temperature deviation has profound health consequences. The body of a human being has a very narrow margin of temperature where the cellular processes best prosper. If exposed to extreme heat or cold, the body has a difficult time sustaining this homeostasis due to hypothermia or hyperthermia. Hypothermia and organ failure result from internal body temperatures below 95°F and lead to slow metabolic processes. Symptoms of confusion, drowsiness, and lethargy are the signs of severe cases. Hyperthermia is found in a cases where body temperature is raised, leading to life-threatening conditions like heat stroke. In both cases, homeostasis is disturbed, and body functions important for life can be affected, demonstrating the significance that effective thermoregulation holds within human physiology. In addition to basic physical well-being, the impact of temperature imbalance reaches as far as hydration and electrolyte balance. Given that water plays a critical role in thermoregulation, extreme alterations in body temperature can lead to dehydration. For instance, over-perspiration in conditions of hyperthermia will deplete body stores of water, interfering with the flow of blood and cellular activities. Comprising 60% of the adult human body, water is important in thermoregulation, the transport of nutrients, and the elimination of waste from the body (Ellis-Lepard et al., 2018). Dehydration will also enhance the pathological impact of temperature extremes, initiating a cycle of amplified effect on physiological stability and the demand for a proper understanding of hydration's role during the course of temperature excursions. Physiological adaptation for the improvement of heat regulation is also required to neutralize the risks of thermal stress. Individuals exposed to heat temperatures can develop heat acclimatization, which improves cardiovascular function and allows for effective sweating mechanisms. However, the effectiveness of such adaptations will vary greatly between individuals depending on factors like genes, age, and fitness. For example, athletes may employ methods like menthol mouth swilling to allow cooling and performance improvement during heat stress conditions. While this might be effective for some, individuals may respond differently to identical interventions, and therefore customized temperature control measures are important (Best et al., 2019). The response variability to temperature deviations highlights the need for more studies to uncover the mechanisms behind this, so that individually adapted procedures for preserving thermoregulation and homeostasis can be developed.

Test Your Knowledge

1. What is the normal range of human body temperature, and how does it vary with age, time of day, and activity?
2. How do fever and pyrogens alter the body's temperature set point during infection or inflammation?

8.2. Mechanisms of Heat Production

Learning Outcome

1. Explain the metabolic processes contributing to heat;
2. Define the role of muscle activity in thermogenesis;
3. Learn about impact of food intake on heat production.

Within the complex scenario of thermoregulation, mechanisms of heat production play a pivotal role in the maintenance of homeostasis within the human body. The basis of heat production rests in metabolic processes, namely cellular respiration, by which nutrients are broken down for energy generation and subsequently produce heat as waste. This heat of metabolism produces heat and is necessary for sustaining fundamental physiological functions, especially during physical exercise or cold exposure. Besides, contractions of the muscles in activities also release a significant amount of heat, contributing further to total thermal balance. As brought out in the research on energy metabolism, understanding these intricate pathways outlines the manner in which the body acclimatizes to changing environmental and inner conditions in a manner that provides efficient thermoregulation (Kaciuba-Uscilko & Greenleaf, 1989). In addition to metabolic processes, the body applies a number of physiological processes for enhancing or reducing the production of heat by means of environmental adjustments. For instance, shivering is a rapid, reflex muscular process that significantly increases heat generation during cold temperatures through high metabolic rates. It is a valuable compensatory process when ambient temperatures are low, enabling the body to be capable of sustaining core temperature despite diminished environmental warmth. Conversely, during heat stress, heat production must be balanced by effective mechanisms of heat loss , such as sweating and dilation of the skin's blood supply. The role of the thermoregulatory system in regulating these responses is central, particularly in conditions like exercise, where metabolic heat production is very much increased. The role of these mechanisms in ensuring effective temperature regulation during varying states of body activity and environmental temperatures is thus established (Kaciuba-Uscilko & Greenleaf, 1989). Furthermore, certain pathologies, for instance, MS, can significantly disrupt normal mechanisms of heat production and thermoregulation. Studies have shown that MS patients possess impaired sudomotor function, which jeopardizes their ability to sweat properly during physical activity. This diminished response to sweating not only augments risk for overheating but also suggests the necessity of immediate adaptive interventions in exercise and activity planning in affected populations. For instance, MS patients are less able to lose heat even though they have the same core temperatures as normal controls during exercise, which indicates a potential alteration of thermoregulatory function. Awareness of these particular difficulties illuminates why some medical conditions are capable of influencing thermoregulation and emphasizes the need for modifying the strategies of heat handling accordingly in order to optimize health and performance (Figure 8.6).

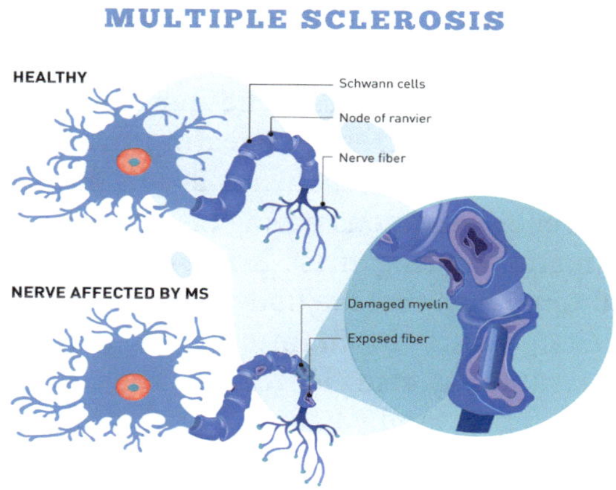

Figure 8.6. Multiple sclerosis.

Source: https://www.compactcath.com/wp-content/uploads/2019/08/Kidney_MS-1.png.

8.2.1. Metabolic Processes Contributing to Heat

Metabolic processes play a crucial role in thermogenesis and heat production in the human body, largely through basal metabolic rate (BMR) and physical exercise. BMR reflects the cost of energy required to maintain rudimentary physiological processes, thereby contributing to heat production even during rest. Thermogenic activity varies greatly with age, sex, and hormonal secretion levels, with higher BMR leading to greater heat production. When exercising, metabolic functions intensify, increasing heat production further. Metabolism of carbohydrates and fats in exercise degrades energy, and it is released as heat energy, demonstrating the dynamic relationship between thermoregulation and metabolism. Thermoregulation by the body thus hinges on the effectiveness and intensity of metabolic processes, and a foundation for research into mechanisms of thermoregulation under various environments can thus be provided. Incidentally, the concept of acclimatization brings out the body's huge responsiveness to different thermal environments in its ability to regulate heat through metabolic adjustments. Acclimatization involves physiological adaptations towards enhancing an individual's capacity to cope with temperature extremes, whether hot or cold. When it is hot, increased sweating and effective heat dissipation mechanisms are utilized, with metabolic adaptations paving the way for energy dissipation during these stressors. Yet, under cold temperatures, the body employs shivering thermogenesis to maintain the core body temperature by using shivering, wherein muscle contractions rapidly happen, producing heat as a product of increased metabolic function.

This understanding of these natural responses and their basis in metabolism is needed in order to design effective thermal protection systems and countermeasures, particularly for astronauts subjected to extreme conditions in intra- and extravehicular activities, as reviewed in Kaciuba-Uscilko & Greenleaf,. (1989). The impact of metabolic processes extends beyond mere heat generation; it includes the complicated interaction between temperature regulation and overall health. For example, energy metabolism is interrelated with water and electrolyte balance, specifically during exercise as the loss of sweat can cause dehydration and compromise thermoregulation.

While athletes perform intense activities, the need for effective energy metabolism becomes greater and requires the perfect balance of fluids and electrolytes to ensure optimal physiological function and avoid heat illnesses. Besides, as explained in Kaciuba-Uscilko & Greenleaf,. (1989), many heat diseases can arise if metabolic responses of the body are overwhelmed by exposure to excess amounts of heat. Therefore, a complete understanding of metabolism is paramount not only for explaining mechanisms of heat production but also for health protection and performance enhancement during crises in temperature control in various environments (Figure 8.7).

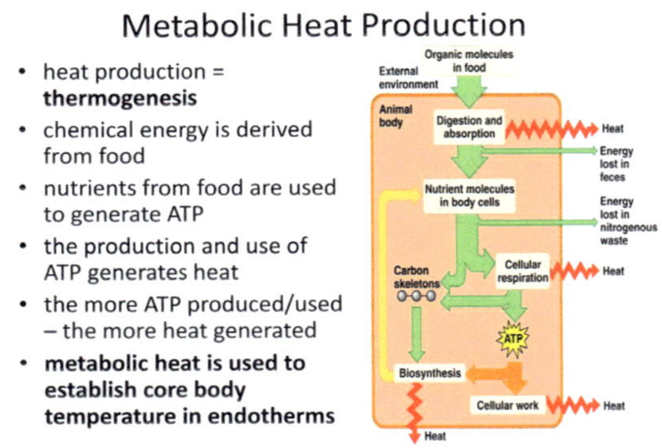

Figure 8.7. Metabolic-heat-production.

Source: https://image1.slideserve.com/2179069/metabolic-heat-production-l.jpg.

8.2.2. Role of Muscle Activity in Thermogenesis

Muscle contraction is also one of the major contributors to thermogenesis, which plays a vital role in maintaining the body's warmth. When muscles contract while exercising, they generate heat as a metabolic byproduct. This is extremely important when in cold temperatures and there has to be a consistent core body temperature for physiological functions. Exercise helps increase the metabolic rate significantly, thus generating more heat. Shivering thermogenesis is a special type of muscle activity that produces involuntary muscle contractions to produce heat without the intent of activity observed with exercise. As noted in acclimatization research on cold exposure, the ability of the body to adapt through muscular activity not only increases thermoregulation but also influences the formation of protective thermal systems in space travelers (Kaciuba-Uscilko & Greenleaf, 1989). Heat generated by muscles, then, is an integral component of the human body's response to thermal stress. In addition to voluntary motion, the process of shivering illustrates an involuntary response to cold, emphasizing the body's ability to generate heat through muscle contraction. Shivering involves repetitive and involuntary contractions of the skeletal muscles, able to increase the body's temperature by about 1 degree Celsius for each subsequent minute of action. This reflexive process is a critical survival reaction in cold temperatures, complementing our inherent thermoregulatory mechanisms. Muscle function and thermogenesis are complemented even further through the inclusion of brown adipose tissue (BAT), which can generate non-shivering thermogenesis. BAT can be stimulated by muscular activity, which generates yet more heat production despite being cold. It indicates how human beings have evolved diverse mechanisms of body temperature regulation, adding to the complexity of our overall physiology (Wilson, 2017). Aside from their role in acute temperature control, muscle activity participates in long-term energy balance and metabolic health. Regular physical activity not only enhances thermogenic response but also muscle mass growth, which is metabolically active tissue. The excess muscle mass comes in the form of a greater basal metabolic rate, which assists in maintaining the body at a suitable temperature while at rest and in reducing reliance on external heat sources. In addition, the impact of muscle osmosis and thermogenic events combined on overall energy expenditure could lead to improved body composition in the long term. Muscle activity is thus a significant aspect of the intricate mechanisms of thermoregulation, encompassing a significant component of how the body can maintain homeostasis under varying thermal environments (Kaciuba-Uscilko & Greenleaf, 1989; Wilson, 2017). (Figure 8.8).

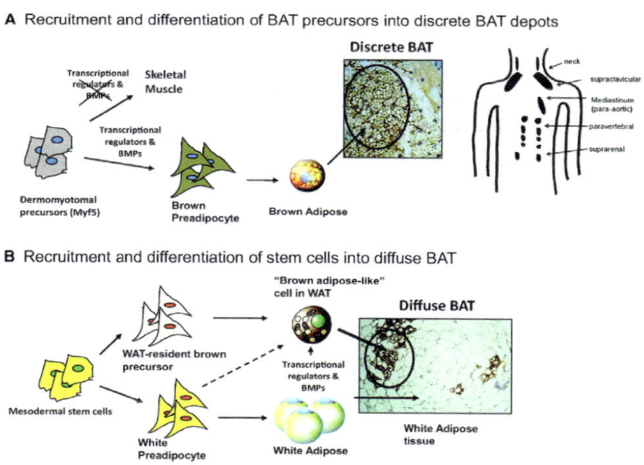

Figure 8.8. Modulation of inflammatory response and pain.

Source: https://www.ahajournals.org/cms/asset/d6337a25-db08-4091-b8fa-80bef02ffe03/zhc0221207840004.jpeg.

8.2.3. Impact of Food Intake on Heat Production

The relationship between food intake and heat production is a basic aspect of human thermoregulation, illuminating how the metabolic process affects body temperature maintenance. When one eats, it undergoes a sequence of biochemical conversions, which metabolize nutrients to generate energy.

In this metabolic process, heat is produced as a byproduct, which aids in maintaining the core body temperature. The thermic effect of food, or the energy expended on digestion, absorption, and storage of the nutrients, contributes significantly to total heat production. High-protein diets, for instance, cause more thermic effect than fats and carbohydrates, suggesting that diet macronutrient composition controls the extent of the heat generated in the body. This process reveals the intricate interconnectedness between dietary behavior and metabolic thermogenesis, emphasizing the significance of food intake in regulating thermal homeostasis. The physiological mechanisms involved in the influence of food intake on heat production are complex and multifaceted. During the ingestion process, the body's metabolic rate increases to address the energy needs of digestion and nutrient absorption. Calorimetric experiments have proven this effect, and differences in food type and quantity have been found to directly affect energy expenditure. Volunteers, for example, who were subjected to controlled calorimetric tests had their metabolism and heat regulation altered, especially after subjecting themselves to specific dietary regimens, such as, those with high protein intake or precisely timed meals. The difference in heat production, as observed from these experiments, illustrates how different nutritional strategies are capable of enhancing or inhibiting the thermal response of the body and thereby affecting not only levels of comfort but also more general physiological processes. This points to the significance of further fine-tuning our understanding of ways in which dietary practices might affect heat production by regulating heat through mechanisms of thermoregulation. Moreover, the interplay between food intake and thermoregulation has significant implications for well-being and health. Where there is excess heat generation—e.g., with exercise or in a hot, demanding thermal environment—the provision of adequate calories becomes significant to preserve energy levels and prevent thermal stress. Insufficient energy intake will compromise the body's ability to handle heat, and it will end up with heat exhaustion. Not only does this act suggest the requirement for the establishment of a proper balance of energy, but it also points towards the role played by diet in optimizing physiological responses to environmental stress. An understanding of the thermoregulatory implications of varying levels of food can be applied in dietetic advice and instruction, particularly for sportspersons or workers who work under extreme conditions. As research advances, elucidating the interconnections between food composition and thermoregulatory adjustments is a valuable direction for the progress of nutritional science (Annis et al., 1974; Cornelissen et al., 2009).

Test Your Knowledge

1. What are the primary sources of heat production in the human body under resting and active conditions?
2. What is non-shivering thermogenesis, and how is brown adipose tissue involved in this process?

8.3. Mechanisms of Heat Loss

Learning Outcome

1. Explain the radiation and its effects on body temperature;
2. Define the evaporation and sweating as cooling methods;
3. Describe the conduction and convection in heat loss.

It is in the context of thermoregulation that it is important to know the mechanisms of heat loss in order to maintain homeostasis of human physiology. Heat is lost by multiple modalities that consist of conduction, convection, radiation, and evaporation. Conduction occurs when heat passes directly from the body to cooler surfaces or objects in contact with it, but convection occurs when air or water moves around the body and increases heat loss because cooler materials replace warmer ones. Notably, these processes are not mutually exclusive; they are prone to intermingle and influence overall thermal balance. For example, an increase in environmental air temperature decreases the efficiency of convective cooling, requiring greater dependence on evaporative cooling, particularly through sweating during physical exertion or exposure to hot environments, and thereby affecting physiological responses to heat stress (Kaciuba-Uscilko & Greenleaf, 1989). Evaporation plays a significant role and accounts for a high proportion of heat loss during exercise and in hot environments.

As sweat evaporates from the skin, it takes heat away from the body, thereby cooling it effectively. The process very much depends on ambient humidity, however. In humid conditions, the air has high water vapor content, therefore inhibiting sweat evaporation, thereby increasing body temperature and even potentially causing heat illnesses. In addition, physiological reactions to increase heat loss, such as, increased sweat gland activity and cutaneous blood flow, are crucial to high-efficiency thermoregulation. Understanding these mechanisms is crucial in developing countermeasures against heat stress, especially in environments where normal mechanisms become compromised (Wrobel et al., 2010). The integration of technology in medicine for monitoring and the maximization of heat loss procedures becomes increasingly relevant, particularly in neonatal therapy. Computational Fluid Dynamics (CFD) studies revealed the dynamics of heat transfer in medical devices like incubators, indicating the degree to which varying designs could affect thermal regulation of vulnerable groups. Simulation of heat and mass transfer can help healthcare practitioners better understand the impact of environmental conditions on patient treatment. Their efficiency is most vital as the devices must offer an appropriate thermally warm climate for neonates that are unable to efficiently self-regulate body temperature. CFD study findings offer significant advice on improvements in device design and ensuring adequate thermoregulation in clinical setups, ultimately improving critical patient care health outcomes (Wrobel et al., 2010) (Figure 8.9).

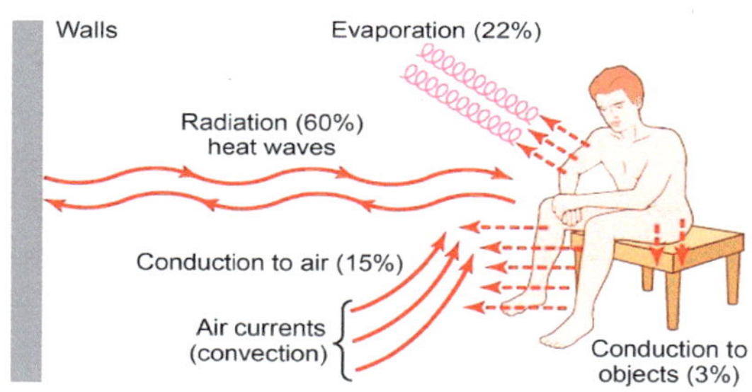

Figure 8.9. Mechanisms for heat transfer.

Source: https://derangedphysiology.com/main/sites/default/files/sites/default/files/CICM%20Primary/R%20Thermoregulation/image%20of%20heat%20transfer%20from%20Guyton%20%26%20Hall.jpg.

8.3.1. Radiation and Its Effects on Body Temperature

The relationship between body temperature and radiation is a key aspect of thermoregulation, especially in environments that are impacted by different amounts of radiant energy. When human skin is subjected to radiant heat sources, such as, the sun or artificial ones, the body responds with physiological mechanisms in an attempt to sustain a constant internal temperature. The skin absorbs such radiation, making the surface warm, and this can, in turn, trigger such reactions as vasodilation. The mechanism enhances the flow of blood to the skin, enabling dissipation of heat by conduction and convection. An inefficiency in such a response not only distracts from thermal equilibrium but can also trigger heat stress and related complications. A knowledge of how exposure to radiation in different environments is necessary for the development of procedures to protect people, such as, astronauts, exposed to extreme heat conditions (Kaciuba-Uscilko & Greenleaf, 1989). Acclimatization to thermal extremes plays a critical role in managing the influence of radiation on body heat. Through research, artificial and natural acclimatization processes have been identified to enhance the ability of the body to handle high temperatures (Kaciuba-Uscilko & Greenleaf, 1989). This is particularly the case for workers who are in hot environments, where the risk of heat illnesses can rise alarmingly. Effective acclimatization entails cardiovascular, endocrine, and thermoregulatory changes that aid in the homeostasis of fluid and electrolytes. For instance, the rate of sweating and efficiency of evaporation, through acclimatization, could be increased, thereby allowing more effective cooling mechanisms when exposed to excessive heat. Including an understanding of these adaptive processes in the development of thermal protection systems could make a substantial difference in safety and performance, especially for space and field applications (Kaciuba-Uscilko & Greenleaf, 1989). Furthermore, the influence of radiation on core body temperature is closely related to general thermal balance and energy metabolism. In environments where subjects are directly exposed to radiation, energy dissipation may increase as the body tries to rid itself of excess heat, besides maintaining core temperature. Thermodynamic equilibrium is critical for metabolic functions directly related to muscle function and endurance. An understanding of the nuances through which diseases of heat are developed in response to radiation can dictate rules on safe operating conditions. The text, including particular bibliographies of key studies, supports the need to explore these relationships further and emphasizes the need to create efficient systems for terrestrial as well as extraterrestrial applications. Ultimately, learning about the interaction of radiation and thermoregulation is central to advancing human health and performance in a broad spectrum of environments (Figure 8.10).

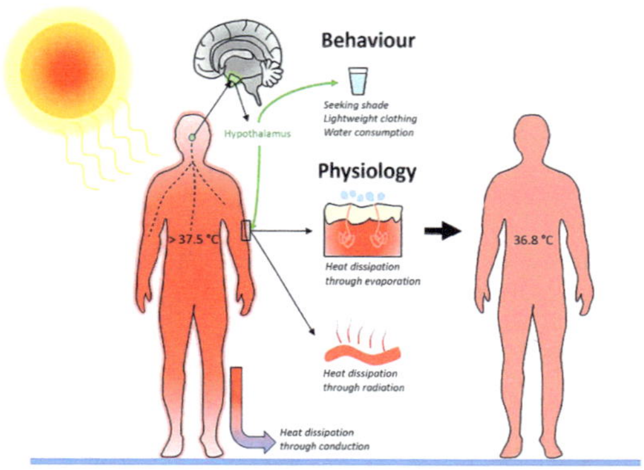

Figure 8.10. Radiation and its effects on body temperature.

Source: https://journals.openedition.org/factsreports/docannexe/image/7652/img-2.jpg.

8.3.2. Evaporation and Sweating as Cooling Methods

The human body employs different mechanisms to attain homeostasis, with sweating and evaporation being rudimentary mechanisms of cooling under thermoregulation. When body temperature increases due to external heat or physical exercise, the hypothalamus stimulates sweat glands to initiate the secretion of perspiration. The sweat, which consists largely of water, accumulates on the skin's surface. The cooling effect occurs because the sweat evaporates; at this liquid-to-vapor phase transition, the latent heat is taken from the skin, and it lowers the body temperature. This process is highly effective in low-humidity conditions, as the water vapor pressure in the air is much lower in such conditions, favoring evaporation. Also, some conditions , such as air flow and exposure to surface area, can further enhance this cooling, and therefore it is important for athletes and physically active individuals to optimize their sweating response under various conditions. Sweating, although a helpful system of cooling, is influenced by a myriad of physiological and environmental factors. Individual variability in sweat rate, depending on genetics, hydration level, and acclimatization to heat, is what makes this system efficient. There are some people who will produce a lot of sweat, whereas others may not produce much sweat, with the latter losing their thermoregulatory efficiency. Measurement of body-area localized sweat rates has taken center stage in research with tools , such as the resistance hygrometer, enabling measurement of both passive and active body areas of sweat. The technology aids in ascertaining how the activity of the sweat glands is associated with thermal loading and intensity of exercise in order to enable an educated approach for ensuring optimal performance in sports and working environments. Critically, as Suga (2025) suggests, the physiological processes involved in the production of sweat are complex and warrant closer scrutiny for an understanding of their implications for the management of heat and successful thermoregulation. Beyond the provision of a cooling effect, sweating also has metabolic and behavioral functions unique to thermoregulation. Perception and performance can be influenced by the sense of cooling through evaporative influences, with its enhancement often being utilized by athletes via methods like the use of menthol, as in Best et al. (2019). Menthol swabbing has been found to be a potential adjunct to traditional sweating, giving a perception of cooling that can trigger sustained physical performance in spite of hot environments. This dynamic interplay between physiological reaction and subjective comfort underscores the importance of an appreciation for individual variability in sensitivity to cooling agents. Through the detailed understanding of sweating and evaporation as cooling mechanisms, we can enhance practice toward the development of more efficient heat management techniques in high-stakes situations, with ultimate benefit to athletic function and overall well-being (Figure 8.11).

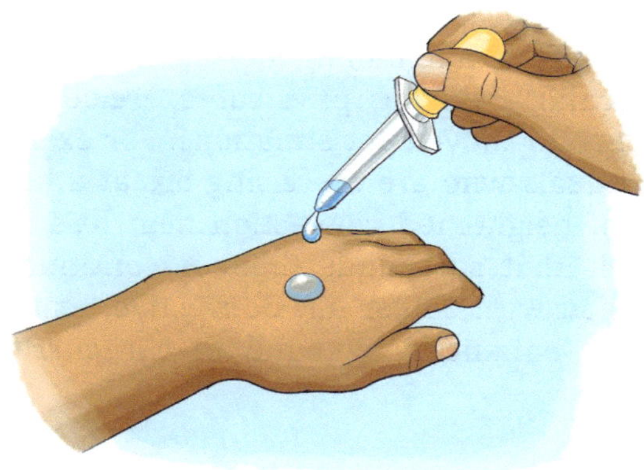

Figure 8.11. Evaporative cooling with liquids.

Source: https://static.scientificamerican.com/sciam/cache/file/993EA105-7F88-4ABB-9D821C38ED974E53_source.jpg?w=1200.

8.3.3. Conduction and Convection in Heat Loss

The heat loss mechanisms of the human body can be critically examined through the conduction and convection mechanisms. Conduction is the movement of heat through direct contact between materials. In thermoregulation, this is evident where the human body, which constantly generates heat as a byproduct of metabolism, comes into direct contact with surrounding cold surfaces. For instance, if one is sitting on a cold surface, conduction transfers heat away from the body, and this can lead to a decrease in core temperature. Conductive heat loss is greater under cold conditions, where body contact with cold materials enhances the rate of heat transfer away from the skin. The efficiency of this heat loss conductive is largely dependent on clothing materials, which are insulating, thereby affecting overall thermal comfort and body temperature regulation, making it crucial to understand clothing physics and heat dynamics (Pan, 2019). Conversely, convection plays an important role in heat loss with the movement of air or fluid that surrounds the body. Because air warms up around the skin due to body temperature, it is lighter and will rise, creating a current where it is pushed by cooler air, thus enhancing heat removal. Convection transfer is significant in maintaining thermal homeostasis, particularly during physical exercise or in varying air movement situations. For example, individuals who are exercising are at a higher risk of heightened convection heat loss since the air that surrounds them is continuously supplied with colder air. Convective heat loss is also enhanced by wind or air currents; thus ambient conditions also contribute significantly to determining the capability of body to maintain its temperature. They highlight the importance of environmental and body positioning variables in thermoregulation and propose that further investigation is necessary to comprehend their subtlety (Shungu, 1991). The interplay between conduction and convection illustrates the adaptive nature of physiological thermoregulation. When both processes are taken together, it is evident that they do not work separately; instead, they are dependent on each other, and together they affect the body's capacity to regulate a constant internal temperature in the face of external changes. The layered nature of clothing, for instance, can concurrently impact conduction as well as convection by acting as an insulator and decreasing air movements against the skin. In addition, the best-configured clothing can mitigate conductive heat loss and offer evaporative cooling through sweating during thermoregulatory processes. Considering these factors, creating a deeper understanding of these processes is crucial to enhancing more efficient measures in clothing design and environmental acclimatization for enhancing human thermal comfort and efficiency in varied environments (Pan, 2019).

Test Your Knowledge

1. What are the four primary mechanisms of heat loss in the human body, and how do each function?
2. Describe how vasodilation and sweating help regulate body temperature during heat exposure.

8.4. The Role of the Hypothalamus

Learning Outcome

1. Identify the structure and function of the hypothalamus;
2. Define the hypothalamic set point for temperature regulation;
3. Describe the feedback mechanisms in thermoregulation.

The hypothalamus is a central integrator of numerous facets of body temperature homeostasis and a primary determinant of thermoregulation. Located at the base of the brain, it is a small complex structure that contains populations of neurons that sense changes in the body's thermal state. Cued by numerous peripheral temperature receptors, the hypothalamus can quantify internal changes in temperature and effect related responses. For instance, the hypothalamus regulates sweating and the adjustment of blood supply to the skin, functions critical to thermoregulation, particularly under hypothermia or hyperthermia conditions. Moreover, it can modulate activities , such as the seeking of lower temperatures or different amounts of physical exercise, thanks to its interaction with other parts of the brain, ensuring proper reaction to thermal danger and homeostasis. In addition to its direct regulatory functions, the hypothalamus also regulates longer-term reactions to temperature changes via its function within the endocrine system. The hormones released from the hypothalamus affect metabolic rate and heat production and thus play a crucial role in thermoregulation and energy balance. For example, during caloric restriction or fasting, the hypothalamus can drive metabolic responses, as evidenced by circadian rhythm experiments. Such studies have shown that the body's circadian system has an incredible role in thermoregulation, particularly for people under fasting. For instance, reduced body temperature was a significant response during the light phase, suggesting that hypothalamic signals activate the circadian system to modulate thermogenic responses according to environmental cues and feeding state (Nagashima et al., 2009). Hence, the hypothalamus has a major role not only in acute temperature control but also in general adaptive response.

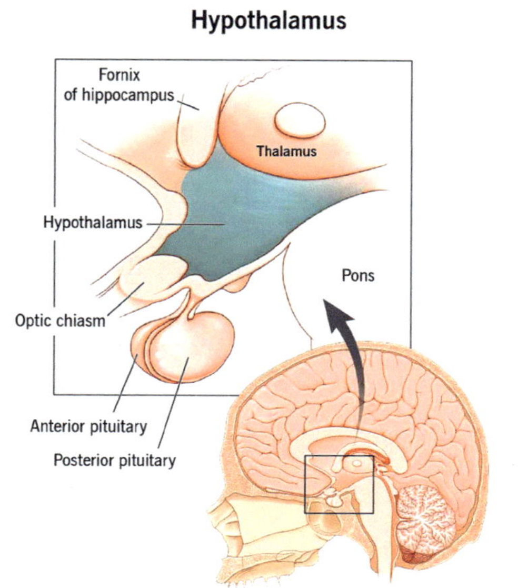

Figure 8.12. Hypothalamus.

Source: https://my.clevelandclinic.org/-/scassets/images/org/health/articles/22566-hypothalamus.

The temperature control by the hypothalamus is further integrated with behavior and social factors, attesting to the complex nature of thermoregulation in human physiology. Disorders that induce thermal stress, such as, severe exercise or unregulated heat exposure, illustrate how the hypothalamus regulates both physiological and subjective adaptations. Research has uncovered that participants wearing protective sporting attire, for example, in men's lacrosse, experience heightened thermal feeling and perceived exertion while undertaking physical exercise due to the thermal load provided by the attire. This underscores the point that the hypothalamus must integrate sensory feedback on both internal states and external environmental conditions (Glasgow, 2019). Thus, understanding the intricate operations of the hypothalamus in thermoregulation is key to comprehending how to optimize athletic performance as well as prevent heat illnesses and thus reflects its significance in the broader area of human physiology (Figure 8.12).

8.4.1. Structure and Function of the Hypothalamus

The hypothalamus, a critical brain region, is the master control of most of the body's homeostatic processes, including temperature regulation. Lying below the thalamus and consisting of numerous nuclei, the hypothalamus is informed about the temperature of the body and regulates the body's physiologic activities to generate thermal homeostasis. The hypothalamus contains specialized neurons that are sensitive to temperature and serve as thermoreceptors. When the body temperature deviates from the set point, these neurons start processes to either lose heat during hyperthermia or conserve heat during hypothermia. This regulation is critical in the avoidance of thermal stress, which leads to severe health complications. Apart from its function in thermoregulation, the hypothalamus also regulates most of the behavioral and hormonal reactions that contribute to thermoregulation. It controls the autonomic nervous system, stimulating sweat gland function in heat and inducing shivering to generate body heat in cold. Moreover, the hypothalamus influences hunger and thirst so that dehydration or lack of nutrients does not impair the body's ability to thermoregulate properly. This unification of several physiological processes speaks to the integrative role of the hypothalamus in preserving homeostasis. Appreciation of its form and function introduces the complexity of thermoregulation, emphasizing the necessity for an optimal internal climate for overall health. Research has further illuminated the complex interaction between circadian rhythm and hypothalamic function in thermoregulation. It has been proposed that the suprachiasmatic nucleus (SCN), part of the hypothalamus, plays a role in temperature control through regulation of metabolic production of heat in response to the light-dark cycle. For instance, calorie restriction in mice results in fluctuating temperatures of the body that are contingent upon their circadian phases, indicating that the hypothalamus will have to adjust its thermoregulatory responses based on environmental and behavioral factors. The nervous tracts connecting the SCN with other hypothalamic nuclei are the cause of these fluctuations, illustrating how time of day can make a significant impact on thermoregulation. These findings underscore the multifunctional roles of the hypothalamus in thermoregulation, which emphasize the need for further research on comprehension of the processes involved in human physiology (Nagashima et al., 2009; Glasgow, 2019) (Figure 8.13).

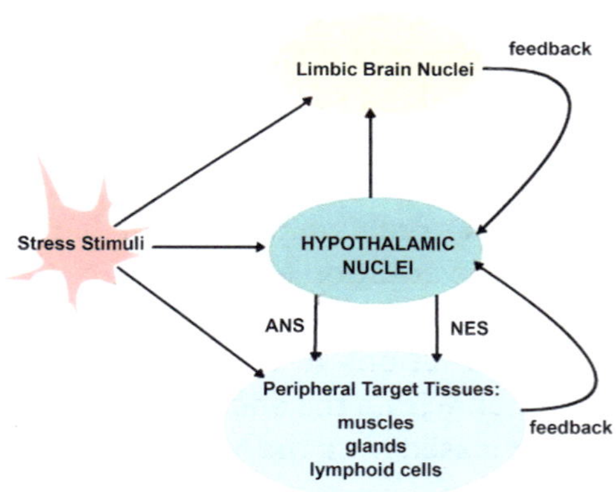

Figure 8.13. Hypothalamus: structural organization.

Source: https://nba.uth.tmc.edu/neuroscience/m/s4/images/copyright_marked_images/html5/1-1_NEW.jpg.

8.4.2. Hypothalamic Set Point for Temperature Regulation

The hypothalamic temperature set point is a critical control mechanism for maintaining homeostasis in the human body. In the brain, the hypothalamus is the master regulator of physiological responses to temperature changes. The sensitive organ receives input from thermoreceptors scattered throughout the body and thus provides a real-time assessment of body temperature. Whenever the temperature deviates from the set point predetermined, usually 37 degrees Celsius, the hypothalamus triggers adaptive body responses. These may be in the case of vasodilation, profuse sweating if too warm, or vasoconstriction and shivering to generate heat in the case of cold. Understanding the intricacies of this regulation system is fundamental to the identification of the kinds of disruptions that lead to states of hyperthermia or hypothermia, thereby situating the hypothalamus' role beyond a simple temperature regulator, but as an integral part of the balance of the physiological states in general. Thermoregulation is also influenced by various extrinsic factors that modify the hypothalamic set point. For example, acclimatization to intense environmental conditions, i.e., excessive heat or cold, requires physiological adaptations that recalibrate this set point. Research informs us that both naturally occurring acclimatization and artificially created adaptations are essential for maximizing thermal performance in humans, especially in strenuous conditions , such as intense physical activity or space travel (Kaciuba-Uscilko & Greenleaf, 1989). As the body acclimatizes, processes like altered metabolic rates, alterations in sweat gland function, and behavioral alterations all aid the acclimatization. Recognizing the role of the hypothalamus in acclimatization processes underlines the necessity of a malleable set point in a position to respond suitable to stressors, so the body can remain in balance despite external variation. Interestingly, the circadian rhythm also interacts with the hypothalamic set point, further intertwining thermoregulation. Circadian effects can affect daytime body temperature, with various patterns being observed in the production of metabolic heat depending upon the external environment and time (Nagashima et al., 2009). The suprachiasmatic nucleus (SCN) of the hypothalamus is at the center of this, triggering changes in specific light and dark cycles and determining thermodynamic reactions. As an illustration, fasting during the daytime can lead to a reduction in core body temperature through reduced metabolic heat generation, whereas nighttime feeding maintains temperatures constant (Nagashima et al., 2009). Comprehending these interactions between circadian rhythms and hypothalamic regulation can lend richness to our knowledge of thermoregulation, suggesting that body temperature regulating systems are not merely reactive but actively governed by rhythmic biological processes (Figure 8.14).

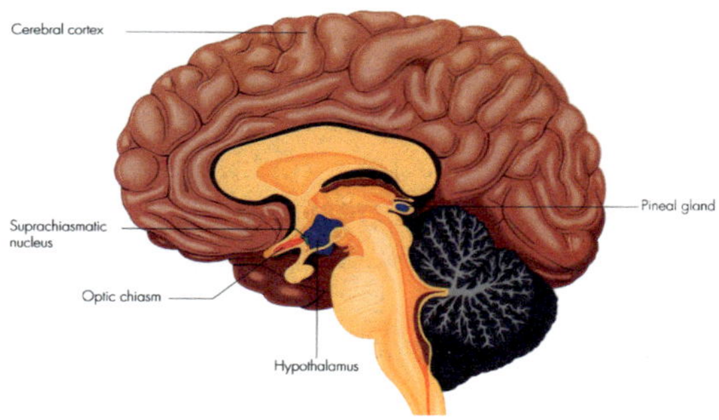

Figure 8.14. Suprachiasmatic nucleus (SCN) within the hypothalamus.

Source: https://upload.wikimedia.org/wikipedia/commons/8/80/Suprachiasmatic_Nucleus.jpg.

8.4.3. Feedback Mechanisms in Thermoregulation

The human body can maintain a stable internal temperature through a series of intricate feedback mechanisms that demonstrate the operations of homeostasis. Central to this mechanism are thermoreceptors, which detect changes in body temperature and pass on this information to the body's thermostat, the hypothalamus. On receiving this feedback indicating deviations from the set point, the hypothalamus initiates physiological mechanisms to restore balance. For instance, when the body temperature rises, responses , such as vasodilation and sweating are initiated to result in heat loss. When the body temperature drops, shivering and vasoconstriction take place to preserve heat. These feedback mechanisms constitute prototypical illustrations of a negative feedback system, in which the output acts to reverse the initial change to stabilize the internal environment and enable the body to function optimally in spite of fluctuating external conditions. Impressive thermoregulation is especially important under the force of extreme environmental stress, as in the case of exposure to hot temperatures or intense physical exertion. On such occasions, feedback integration assumes the highest priority. As has been discussed in acclimatization to heat, the body's metabolic adaptations go through remarkable modifications to improve thermal tolerance. For sports persons or workers in hot climates, the capacity to dissipate heat and maintain fluid equilibrium efficiently assumes utmost importance. Consequently, compensations , such as increased sweat rates and greater peripheral blood flow to the skin surface occur to enhance cooling. In addition, electrochemical balance is promoted in their role, since dehydration will greatly impair thermoregulatory function. This occurs in the form of dynamic interaction between more than one system, indicating the complexity and importance of feedback mechanisms for efficient temperature regulation under elevated demands. Moreover, knowledge of thermoregulatory feedback mechanisms has direct implications for thermal protection system design in aerospace engineering, among other areas. When scientists observe human physiological reactions to hostile environments, it is evident that countermeasures must be designed so that human function remains preserved under stress. Research on energy metabolism with exercise shows how thermoregulation is altered in various conditions, providing useful information to engineers who are designing space suits for astronauts (Kaciuba-Uscilko & Greenleaf, 1989). By learning from these feedback mechanisms, designers can construct systems that accept human acclimatization and performance when exposed to extreme thermal conditions. Finally, these findings point to the significant intersection of biomedical science and engineering, promising innovations that facilitate human survivability in hostile environments.

Test Your Knowledge

1. What are the key functions of the hypothalamus in maintaining homeostasis?
2. How does the hypothalamus regulate body temperature through feedback mechanisms?

8.5. Physiological Responses to Temperature Changes

Learning Outcome

1. Identify the vasodilation and vasoconstriction;
2. Define the shivering and non-shivering thermogenesis;
3. Describe the behavioral adaptations to temperature fluctuations.

The physiological responses to temperature variations in the human body are multifaceted and necessary in order to provide stable homeostasis. When exposed to warmer temperatures, the body initiates several mechanisms for cooling the body, primarily through vasodilation and sweating. Sweating provides for evaporative cooling; as sweat evaporates from the body surface, it radiates heat away, thereby helping to regulate core body temperature. Besides, vasodilation raises blood flow to the skin to release excess heat into the environment. These reactions are highly important during exercise or in hot ambient temperatures because they help in preventing heat illnesses , such as heat exhaustion and heat stroke. In particular, the interaction between thermoregulation and hydration status is also significant, since dehydration will blunt sweat function and thermoregulatory capability, leading to a cascade of physiological impairments that enhance the risk of heat illness. In addition to these acute physiological compensations, adaptive responses to thermoregulation can also develop over time through a process known as acclimatization. Acclimatization is with physiological adaptations that increase a person's level of tolerance to hot temperatures, such as, increased sweat secretion and altered electrolyte status. These adaptations lessen the perceptual responses to heat stress and exhaustion and allow individuals to perform more efficiently in hot conditions. For instance, research has proven that individuals who are acclimatized can tolerate high temperatures better due to improved effectiveness in thermoregulation (Kaciuba-Uscilko & Greenleaf, 1989). This adjustment is of specific significance to athletes and workers in the hot environment, where heat illness threats are enhanced. Understanding these adjustments allows for more effective training programs and protective measures to counteract heat stress.

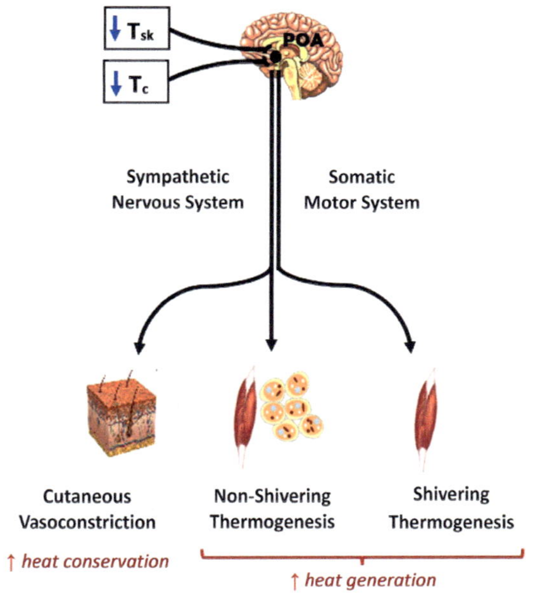

Figure 8.15. Regulation of physiological thermosensor responses to cold exposure.

Source: https://www.researchgate.net/profile/John-Castellani/publication/351841954/figure/fig1/AS:1027326087274498@1621945034682/Regulation-of-physiological-thermoeffector-responses-to-cold-exposure-Decreases-in-mean.png.

Finally, the body's responses to temperature are not absolute across all humans; they are controlled by different factors like age, gender, and composition. For example, research indicates that protective gear can affect thermal perception and induce extra stress when exercising in the heat. Participants who wear particular protective equipment can develop higher thermal perceptions and ratings of perceived exertion (Glasgow, 2019), which can hinder performance and increase the risk of overheating. Therefore, it is essential to pay attention to the interaction between environmental factors, individual characteristics, and external equipment when researching thermoregulation. This systematized strategy emphasizes the multifaceted character of human body reactions to changes in temperature, demonstrating that successful heat stress control necessitates comprehension of these complex physiologic processes (Figure 8.15).

8.5.1. Vasodilation and Vasoconstriction

Vasodilation and vasoconstriction are imperative physiological responses involved in the role of thermoregulation, which enables the maintenance of core body temperature independent of changing environmental conditions. Vasodilation refers to the dilation or widening of the blood vessels, which enhances the circulation of blood to the surface of the skin to facilitate heat dissipation from the body through convection and radiation. This mechanism is particularly crucial during conditions of elevated body temperature or heat stress, in which it enables increased heat dissipation, a vital parameter in preventing overheating. As the literature explained, autonomic control over cutaneous circulation, most notably during hyperthermic conditions, highlights the value of active vasodilation in the effective management of heat stress. The equilibrium between these mechanisms ensures that the inside temperatures are maintained and cellular activities continue unbroken even during poor thermal conditions (Smith & Johnson, 2016). Alternatively, vasoconstriction, in which the blood vessels tighten, prevents loss of body heat through a reduction of blood supply to the outermost parts. This is essential during cold weather when core body temperature must at all times be conserved. This process is centrally controlled by the sympathetic nervous system, in that vasoconstriction protects vital organs against thermal stress by limiting peripheral heat loss. During the last century, studies have proven that sympathetic vasoconstrictor action functions simultaneously across various body regions, essentially coordinating a protective response to cold (McNabb, 2021). The regulatory mechanisms involve complex neurovascular interactions, where vasoconstriction can favor the flow of warmer blood to core organs at the expense of peripheral regions. Such a complicated process highlights the balance the body achieves between vasodilation and vasoconstriction in maintaining homeostasis with varying thermal stresses. In conclusion, the dynamic interaction between vasodilation and vasoconstriction is at the core of thermoregulatory mechanisms that govern human physiology. These mechanisms, in addition to regulating body temperature as a response to environmental thermal conditions, are also a method of ensuring maximum operation at the cellular and systemic level. An understanding of these responses highlights the intricacies of the autonomic regulation of blood flow and emphasizes the need for additional research into the neural and physiological pathways involved. These can potentially be utilized for clinical purposes concerning autonomic dysfunction and its impact on thermoregulation, and they can uncover potential remedies and interventions for (Smith & Johnson, 2016) (Figure 8.16).

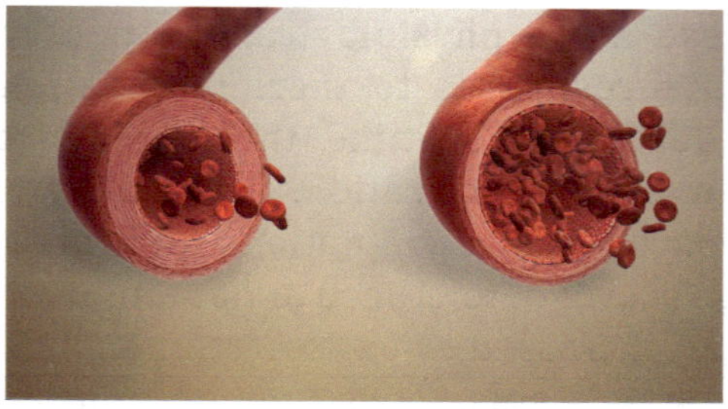

Figure 8.16. Vasodilation.

Source: https://upload.wikimedia.org/wikipedia/commons/2/2d/Vasodilation.jpg.

8.5.2. Shivering and Non-Shivering Thermogenesis

The ability of the body to maintain core temperature in the face of environmental stresses is a key aspect of thermoregulation. Two fundamental mechanisms that serve this purpose are shivering and non-shivering thermogenesis. Shivering, a reflex contraction of skeletal muscle, generates heat through increased metabolic rate. This reflex phenomenon comes into action when the body's temperature has dropped and is particularly valuable in the acute reaction to cold exposure. The effectiveness of shivering varies depending on many factors, including the individual's overall health status, body composition, and even the presence of brown adipose tissue (BAT). Although shivering is able to raise body temperature rapidly, it remains energetically costly and not a very good long-term means of thermoregulation, particularly in neonates, whose maintenance of thermoneutrality has unique challenges (Bienboire-Frosini et al., 2023). Non-shivering thermogenesis, though, is a more energy-efficient system of heat production. It occurs primarily in brown adipose tissue, a necessary part of thermoregulation, especially in infants at risk for hypothermia. Uncoupling proteins in brown fat enable the release of energy as heat rather than storage in the form of chemical energy. The induction of BAT during cold stress unveils a crucial adaptation for body temperature maintenance regardless of the energy expense of shivering. The magnitude of non-shivering thermogenesis has been reported to vary among species and be gene-, biochemistry-, and environment-dependent. By enabling a cleaner form of thermoregulation, non-shivering thermogenesis addresses the complexities of body temperature regulation in human physiology (Bienboire-Frosini et al., 2023). However, the impact of such thermogenic activities extends beyond the control of temperature. Non-shivering and shivering thermogenesis may have beneficial effects on overall health, as demonstrated in tests of cold water immersion (CWI) treatment. Even though there is more work to be done, preliminary findings are that repeated cold exposure may lead to beneficial changes in adipose tissue structure in the body, which can lower the risk of cardiovascular disease. Although the effects vary between individuals and the worldwide impact on health needs to be explored further, the interaction between these thermoregulatory phenomena and global health puts into perspective the importance of body temperature regulation in human well-being. Thus, shivering and non-shivering thermogenesis not only play a vital role in the regulation of temperature for the short term but may also play a part in long-term metabolic well-being (Figure 8.17).

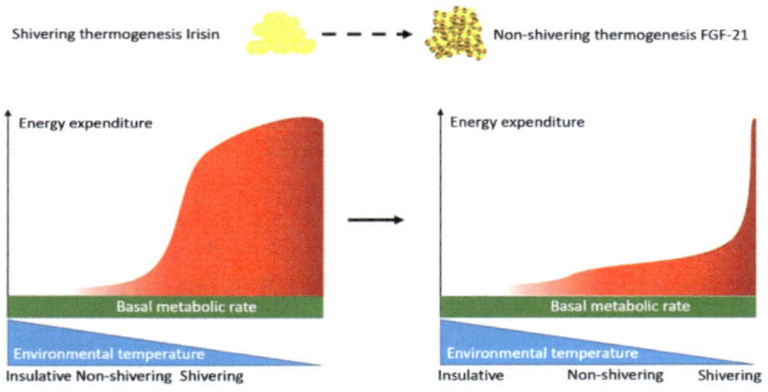

Figure 8.17. Model of interplay between shivering and non-shivering thermogenesis.

Source: https://www.researchgate.net/publication/323619727/figure/fig1/AS:601715053195264@1520471456360/Model-of-interplay-between-shivering-and-non-shivering-thermogenesis-Exposure-to-cold.png.

8.5.3. Behavioral Adaptations to Temperature Fluctuations

In the context of thermoregulation, human beings have several behavioral adaptations to deal with temperature changes. These adaptations are essential in ensuring homeostasis and entail alterations in activity level, dress, and interactions with the environment. For example, during cold climates, one may boost energy expenditure due to physical activity to produce body heat, while at the same time getting shelter to reduce exposure to low temperatures. Conversely, when exposed to excessive heat, behaviors , such as seeking shade, restricting physical activity, and increasing the intake of fluids conducive to hydration become the norm. These behavioral adaptations are reflective of the body's physiological adaptations when it reacts to temperature change, since they allow for the maintenance of optimal core temperatures requisite for metabolic activity and general well-being. The interface of behavior with thermoregulation is not only a survival response but also demonstrates the nuances of human adaptability to extremes in the environment. In addition, the function of energy allocation strategies is disclosed in untangling the sensitivities of temperature variability in behavioral adaptations. Energy is a restricted commodity, and individuals are compelled to partition behaviors maximizing energy acquisition and minimizing expenditure in stressful thermal environments. For example, the physiological response to cold environmental temperatures has a tendency to trigger hormone responses that impact both metabolic and behavioral strategies. Under conditions where food is scarce, organisms can exhibit energy-conserving behavior, thereby modifying their activity budgets in a way to sustain levels of energy. This adjustment is particularly crucial as it assists in survival under cold stress or heat extremes, thus reaffirming the role of behavioral responses as facilitatory factors in thermoregulation. Through such computed adjustments, human beings manage to cope with the complexities of temperature fluctuations, keeping their energy balance steady in the face of shifting environmental states (Touitou, 2021). As human populations continue to feel the effects of global climate change, understanding behavioral adaptations to temperature shifts becomes increasingly critical. Rising global temperatures and weather-related events demand more than physiological adaptation, though. Adaptive behavioral adjustments are necessary to minimize heat stress and maximize health. Research points out that individuals can also enhance adaptive capacities through community-based schemes that educate good coping strategies, such as, dressing appropriately for varying temperatures and enhancing everyday activity based on climatic conditions. Social interaction also plays a pivotal role, with group behavior among communities having the potential to foster common strategies for withstanding extreme temperatures, thereby improving measures for thermoregulation. This heightened perception of behavioral adaptations not only renders humans more able but also promotes resilience by way of a collective means for dealing with adversity caused by climate change, advancing the understanding of thermoregulation in human physiology (Lenasi & Šijanec, 2023).

Test Your Knowledge

1. How does the body respond physiologically to cold exposure to maintain core temperature?
2. What are the mechanisms activated during heat exposure to prevent overheating?

8.6. Pathophysiological Conditions Affecting Thermoregulation

Learning Outcome

1. Describe the hyperthermia and its causes;
2. Define hypothermia and its implications;
3. Discuss the disorders affecting thermoregulation.

The human body maintains a stable internal temperature through the process of thermoregulation, which is mediated by various physiological mechanisms. However, a number of pathophysiological disorders can impair this ability and lead to dysregulation of body temperature. These diseases may be due to intrinsic or extrinsic etiologies, such as, genetic mutations or metabolic disturbances, or environmental toxins or infections. A very good example is hypothyroidism, where there are insufficient thyroid hormones to lead to a decreased metabolic rate, hindering production of heat and inducing hypothermic responses. Also, neurodegenerative diseases can disrupt hypothalamic centers that initiate thermogenic responses, causing faulty thermal perception in the victims. Infections are also a serious issue to thermoregulation, particularly those infections that induce fever as a response to an immunity process. Fever occurs when pyrogens activate the hypothalamus to raise the body's temperature set point, hence initiating immune processes. However, high fever or prolonged exposure to higher temperatures may bring about negative effects , such as heat exhaustion or heat stroke, especially among vulnerable groups , such as the elderly. Pathologies , such as severe sepsis or meningitis may further complicate this response to generate an ineffective thermoregulatory capacity. These disorders are particularly dangerous because they disrupt the delicate balance between heat production, storage, and loss, leading to possibly lethal consequences. Disorders of the autonomic nervous system are also significant contributors to thermal dysregulation. Disorders , such as diabetic neuropathy can prevent the proper functioning of involuntary mechanisms that increase sweating and vasodilation, crucial mechanisms for thermoregulation. Thus, the individuals who are afflicted with such disorders are most likely to become unable to dissipate heat, hence prone to hyperthermia, particularly in tropical conditions or when engaged in physical activities. The influence of neurological disorders can even be observed on peripheral and central systems that are involved in thermoregulation, which further prevents a person from being capable of dealing with fluctuating temperatures. Given these complexities, understanding how pathophysiological conditions affect thermoregulation is essential for developing tailored therapeutic interventions (Figure 8.18).

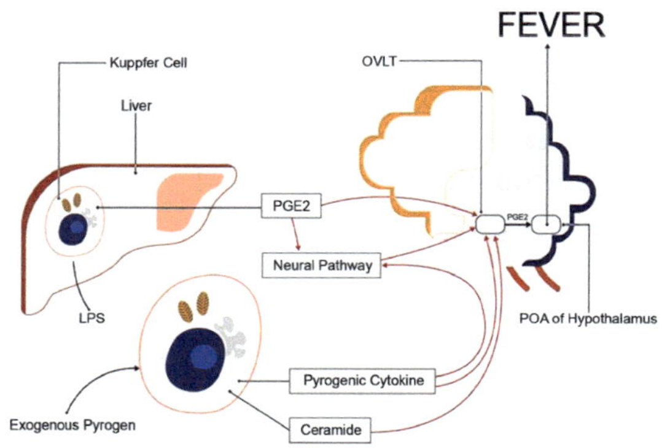

Figure 8.18. A polypeptide produces fever by metabolic changes.

Source: https://res.cloudinary.com/onio/image/upload/v1632644940/onio-website/c914c5f03158e986a80cb9b443c0218b.jpg.

8.6.1. Hyperthermia and Its Causes

It is vital to comprehend hyperthermia in order for it to be capable of comprehending the subtlety of human thermoregulation. Hyperthermia is caused by the body's temperature regulating mechanism failing, leading to an abnormal rise in core body temperature. Hyperthermia can be caused by a variety of environmental factors, such as, exposure to high ambient temperatures, particularly when exercising heavily. The body regulates its temperature through mechanisms , such as sweating and increased blood flow to the skin. However, when these processes become over-stimulated, for example, in states of excessive heat or prolonged exertion without adequate fluid replacement, hyperthermic states can develop. A comprehensive understanding of such processes is essential to useful intervention in settings ranging from sporting events to occupational medicine.

Furthermore, understanding the physiological response of the body to heat stress allows for efficient engineering of effective cooling systems to prevent hyperthermia in the course of operations that expose individuals to high temperatures (Kaciuba-Uscilko & Greenleaf, 1989). Aside from weather conditions, physiological and psychological factors may lead to hyperthermia. Personal responses to heat also vary significantly with age, acclimatization, water status, and overall physical fitness. For instance, youngsters or heat-inexperienced athletes can easily develop a more rapid onset of hyperthermia compared to seasoned players used to hot conditions. Fluid administration is crucial in the maintenance of body temperature and inadequate fluid replacement can hinder the body's effective dissipation of heat. These are behavioral factors that point to the importance of public awareness of heat safety precautions and the imperative for preventive actions during heat conditions. Thus, the knowledge of the multiple causes of hyperthermia allows for enhanced preparedness and response actions in varying contexts, therefore safeguarding individuals against heat-related illnesses (Kaciuba-Uscilko & Greenleaf, 1989). Besides, the impacts of hyperthermia extend beyond physical considerations, intersecting with areas like sporting performance and occupational health. Elevated body temperatures impair cognitive function, diminish physical performance, and make individuals vulnerable to heat disorders like heat exhaustion and heat stroke. In competitive sporting settings, teams must include efficient rehydration practices and flexibility to maximize performance and safeguard athletes' health. The use of cooling aids, such as, ice vests or menthol preparations, has been proposed as a potential intervention for regulating body temperature during exercise. As studies explore various forms of cooling, an advanced comprehension of the way these interventions affect distinctive physiological responses will be crucial in formulating recommendations for optimal performance and heat-stressed defense during high-intensity exercise. Combined, these findings of hyperthermia and its causes identify open discussion of heat management practices in the workplace, sport, and daily life (Figure 8.19).

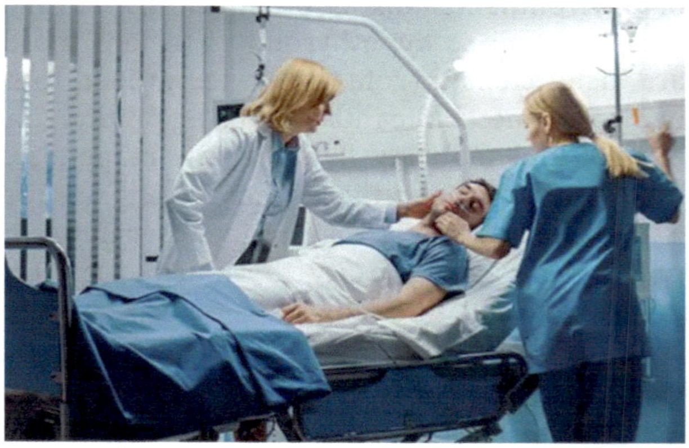

Figure 8.19. Causes of hyperthermia.

Source: https://external-content.duckduckgo.com/iu/?u=https%3A%2F%2Fimages.medicinenet.com%2Fimages%2Farticle%2Fmain_image%2Fmalignant-hyperthermia.jpg%3Foutput-quality%3D75&f=1&nofb=1&ipt=5741549766dfc2ac88ad44b3fb8ad604ba83e9c03ac58c3d2bc974c73445a08a.

8.6.2. Hypothermia and Its Implications

The state of hypothermia is a critical failure in thermoregulation in humans, where body temperature drops below normal, typically due to exposure to cold for an extended duration. Reduction in core temperature disrupts cellular and metabolic processes, leading to the malfunction of body functions. The body initially attempts to counteract the cold by mechanisms , such as shivering thermogenesis, where heat is generated because of muscular activity. However, as the core temperature falls, the above responses become ineffective, causing confusion, drowsiness, or unconsciousness. Hypothermia does not bring about only immediate physiological alterations but also severe sequelae of prolonged exposure, resulting in cardiac arrest or irreversible damage. An awareness of this becomes vital for individuals living or working in cold regions, making appropriate heat-retaining measures to prevent hypothermic accidents all the more important. From the point of view of modern medicine, recognition of hypothermia is extremely important for hospital personnel, particularly in the departments of emergencies and intensive care. Hypothermia, in addition to being difficult to diagnose and treat acute cases of, also needs to be resolutely protected against and cured. For instance, the use of technology , such as Computational Fluid Dynamics (CFD) is essential when developing medical devices used for maintaining core temperature among vulnerable populations, such as, neonates. The results of the CFD simulation provide information about various heat transfer mechanisms, such that patient care can be enhanced by medical practitioners through enhanced design of incubators and radiant warmers, which provide controlled thermal conditions to patients susceptible to hypothermia (Wrobel et al., 2010). Thus, the degree of hypothermia care translates into thermal protection design in which people who spend time exposed to hazardous conditions are well guarded against cold exposure. Cold acclimatization varies significantly among people, based on different factors like age and physiological acclimatization. Research has demonstrated that the elderly are most likely to be affected by hypothermia due to a poor thermoregulatory function and reduced subcutaneous insulation (Kaciuba-Uscilko & Greenleaf, 1989). ulation in human physiology (Figure 8.20).

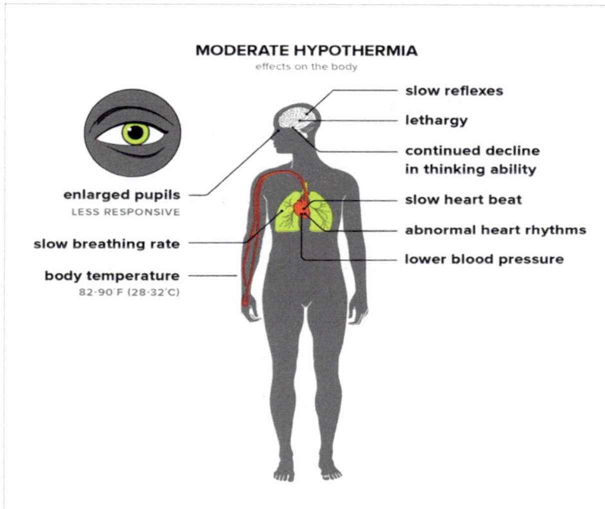

Figure 8.20. Hypothermia: symptoms, treatment, stages.

Source: https://post.medicalnewstoday.com/wp-content/uploads/sites/3/2021/11/moderate_hypothermia-1024x1024.png.

This vulnerability among populations necessitates tailored interventions in patient care and public health interventions to reduce the incidence of hypothermia during cold weather. Effective preventive education regarding symptom detection early and protective gear can mitigate risk in populations that are vulnerable. Additionally, understanding the body's reaction to cold can inform strategies for staying thermally comfortable, especially in individuals with compromised homeostatic mechanisms. Overall, the connotations of hypothermia demonstrate the necessity of an interdisciplinary approach consisting of clinical practice, engineering technology, and public health programs to enhance thermoregulation and temperature reg

8.6.3. Disorders Affecting Thermoregulation (e.g., Fever, Heat Stroke)

Thermoregulatory illnesses are significant in human physiology, particularly in the case of fever and heat stroke. Fever, commonly induced by infections, is a voluntary rise in body temperature as a protective mechanism in response to pathogens. This is coordinated by the hypothalamus, which increases the set point of body temperature. These alterations in thermoregulation are responsible for many other physiological alterations, including an increase in metabolic rate and vascular response alterations. It is indicative of the body's attempt to create an unfavorable environment for microorganisms, yet inappropriately high or prolonged fever can lead to complications , such as dehydration or febrile seizures. Monitoring and controlling fever dynamics are crucial to successful clinical management, particularly in pediatric or critically ill patients, where temperature control may increasingly become compromised. Another acute disorder of thermoregulation is heat stroke, in which mechanisms for heat dissipation by the body are overpowered so that there is an appreciable increase in core temperature. Characteristically precipitated by high environmental temperatures and intense physical exertion, particularly in susceptible , such as athletes or the elderly, heat stroke may result in multi-organ failure and profound morbidity if it is not treated urgently. The presentation may consist of altered mental status, confusion, and potential neurological damage. Prevention measures against heat stroke are proper hydration, acclimatization to increasing heat, and early recognition of heat illness signs. A study on horses highlighted the importance of continuously monitoring body core temperature while exercising outdoors to prevent heat-related disease and underscored the significance of effective thermoregulation in exercising and overall populations (Verdegaal, 2022). In disorders of thermoregulation, conditions like multiple sclerosis (MS) demonstrate the complexity of thermoregulation in specific patient populations. One of the typical phenomena of MS is Uhthoff's phenomenon, whereby a raised body temperature exacerbates neurological symptoms, thus complicating the patient's condition. This is largely due to a reduced thermoregulatory response in individuals who are heat-sensitive, such that core temperatures increase during exercise or in warm environments. Research indicates that such patients may experience fatigue and impairment of intellect as their central temperatures rise and therefore, effective targeted interventions are called for in order to enable them to cope effectively. It is important to understand the physiological mechanisms underlying such conditions as Uhthoff's phenomenon so as to develop strategies for improving the quality of life among those whose lives are affected, given that temperature regulation is of critical significance when dealing with their overall well-being (Chaseling, 2018).

Test Your Knowledge

1. What are the causes, symptoms, and consequences of hyperthermia and hypothermia?
2. How do fever and pyrogenic cytokines alter the body's thermoregulatory set point?

SUMMARY

The intricate mechanism of thermoregulation demonstrates the body's extraordinary ability to maintain homeostasis in the face of changing environmental temperature and bodily requirements. A knowledge of these mechanisms, particularly the operation of sweating and vasodilation, is essential for a comprehensive understanding of human physiological responses to physical exercise or heat exposure. Of special interest are the findings in multiple sclerosis (MS), illustrating how diseases can decrease thermoregulatory efficiency, such as, the diminished sweating during exercise in MS patients compared to normal individuals doing the same exercises (Allen et al., 2018). Such findings not only illustrate the challenges faced by persons with the diseases but also illustrate the way that tailored interventions need to supplement their unique thermoregulatory responses. Further, thermal regulation emphasizes the importance of integrating more than one sensory stimulus into performance improvement mechanisms. The employment of menthol, for instance, offers an intriguing method for improving exercise performance through the use of cooling sensations that potentially enhance endurance and heat stress tolerance. This hedonic response, compounded by physiological mechanisms, could potentially grant athletes an edge in clever and cunning situations and therefore encourages further research into such cooling strategies (Best et al., 2019). The success of menthol treatment is witnessing a growing understanding of how sensory inputs are able to impact cardiovascular and thermoregulatory outcomes and represents a significant field in science and application. Lastly, advancing our understanding of thermoregulation paves the way for interventions with the ability to maximize performance during heat stress and improve the quality of life in patients with thermoregulatory dysfunction. The disparity between results from studies of multifaceted physiology underlines the complexity of temperature regulation in human physiology. With continued research into the interaction of exercise, environment, and genetics, subsequent research should endeavor to shed light on the complexities of thermoregulation across varying populations. Greater knowledge and evidence-based interventions will not only enhance our physiological knowledge base but will also have profound impacts on health, exercise performance, and overall well-being in a rapidly thermally stressed world.

A comprehensive concept of thermoregulation is a cornerstone of human physiology since it interprets the body's mechanisms to maintain internal temperature in variable outer environments. The key processes of heat production, heat loss, and behavioral adaptations, including sweating, shivering, and altering clothing, are implications of how complex this regulatory mechanism is. Furthermore, thermoregulation is instructed within a range of applications extending from sport performance to medical treatments for heat disease. For instance, in a study of lacrosse athletes, scientists found that protective equipment strongly influenced perceptual stress related to thermal sensation and effort, illustrating the complex interaction between physical environment and biological control (Glasgow, 2019). These findings form the basis of how protective gear not only influences performance but also alters athletes' physiological acclimatization to heat and form the basis of our wider understanding of thermoregulation in high-intensity exercise. Furthermore, advances in technology , such as infrared thermography (IRT) are enhancing our capability to quantify skin temperature and examine thermoregulation in sports and clinical settings. Standardization of consensus-based IRT data gathering protocols is a crucial step toward harmonization in sports and exercise medicine practice. It has been established that consensus-based guidelines encourage extensive assessments, which enable better detection of thermoregulatory responses between populations (Moreira et al., 2017). The existence of the Thermographic Imaging in Sports and Exercise Medicine

(TISEM) checklist indicates a trend towards enhancing methodologies used with skin temperature testing, resulting in more precise and usable accuracy with thermal tests. By establishing uniform methods of data collection and analysis, researchers can increase reliability within research studies on thermoregulation, again shaping intervention practice and performance improvement. Finally, the use of thermoregulation extends far beyond the ivory tower to practical arenas like sport science, occupational medicine, and environmental physiology. Accurate understanding of thermoregulation is key for athletes, trainers, and physicians—to enable them to adopt effective methods for reducing heat stress and optimizing performance. For instance, knowledge of enhanced perceived thermal sensation among lacrosse players with protective gear informs hydration and rest interval modification to prevent heat-related illness (Glasgow, 2019). Moreover, with ongoing developments in IRT as a normative tool for the assessment of thermoregulatory response, its inclusion in training and Medicare protocols may lead to enhanced heat exposure surveillance and control. Consequently, ongoing investigation into thermoregulation not only enhances theoretical frameworks but also enables practitioners to be in possession of information that can inform sheltered and effective practice in fluctuating thermal conditions.

KEY TERMS FROM THIS CHAPTER

- Behavioral thermoregulation
- Brown adipose tissue
- Cold exposure
- Core body temperature
- Evaporation
- Fever (pyrexia)
- Heat loss mechanisms
- Heat production
- Heat stroke
- Homeostasis
- Hypothalamus
- Non-shivering thermogenesis
- Peripheral temperature sensors
- Radiation
- Set point
- Shivering
- Sweating
- Thermoreceptors

CRITICAL THINKING QUESTIONS

1. **What is the primary organ responsible for regulating body temperature?**
   a. Liver
   b. Hypothalamus
   c. Kidneys
   d. Pituitary gland
2. **Which physiological response helps increase body temperature when exposed to cold?**
   a. Vasodilation
   b. Sweating
   c. Shivering
   d. Panting
3. **How does vasodilation contribute to temperature regulation?**
   a. It reduces heat loss by constricting blood vessels.
   b. It increases heat loss by widening blood vessels near the skin.
   c. It produces heat through muscle contractions.
   d. It conserves heat by increasing metabolism.
4. **Which mechanism is the most effective way for humans to lose excess heat during hot weather?**
   a. Radiation
   b. Conduction
   c. Evaporation (sweating)
   d. Convection
5. **What term describes the body's ability to maintain a stable internal temperature despite external temperature changes?**
   a. Homeostasis
   b. Metabolism
   c. Thermogenesis
   d. Adaptation

Short Answer Questions

1. What is thermoregulation and why is it important for the human body?
2. Which part of the brain acts as the body's thermostat?
3. Name three physiological responses to cold exposure.
4. How does sweating help cool the body?
5. What role does vasoconstriction play in temperature control?
6. Define hypothermia and mention one symptom.
7. What is the difference between fever and hyperthermia?
8. How does shivering generate heat?
9. What is meant by the term "set point" in body temperature regulation?
10. Describe the role of brown adipose tissue in thermogenesis.

Answers to Critical Thinking Questions

1. (b); 2. (c); 3. (b); 4. (c); 5. (a).

REFERENCES

1. Moreira, D. G., Costello, J. T., Brito, C. J., Adamczyk, J. G., Ammer, K., Bach, A. J. E., Costa, C. M. A., Eglin, C., Fernandes, A. A., Fernández-Cuevas, I., Ferreira, J. J. A., Formenti, D., Fournet, D., Havenith, G., Howell, K., Jung, A., Kenny, G. P., Kolosovas-Machuca, E. S., Maley, M. J., Merla, A., ... Sillero-Quintana, M. (2017). Thermographic imaging in sports and exercise medicine: A Delphi study and consensus statement on the measurement of human skin temperature. *Journal of thermal biology*, *69*, 155–162. https://doi.org/10.1016/j.jtherbio.2017.07.006 (accessed on 28th June 2025).
2. Allen, D., Chaseling, G., Davis, S., Huang, M., et al. (2018). Impaired thermoregulatory function during dynamic exercise in multiple sclerosis. https://open.bu.edu/bitstream/2144/32925/3/AllenDR-MSExerciseThermoreg-Manuscript-R2.pdf (accessed on 28th June 2025).
3. Annis, J. F., Troutman, S. J., & Webb, P. (1974). Cycles in metabolism and heat loss. Prepared under Contract No. NAS9-12683 by Webb Associates, Inc. Yellow Springs, Ohio 45387 https://core.ac.uk/download/pdf/42896135.pdf (accessed on 28th June 2025).
4. Pan N. (2019). Unique Thermal Properties of Clothing Materials. *Global challenges (Hoboken, NJ)*, *3*(7), 1800082. https://doi.org/10.1002/gch2.201800082(accessed on 28th June 2025).
5. Bailón Luesma, R., Valderas Yamuza, M. T., & Vallverdú Ferrer, M. (2019). Characterization of the autonomic nervous system response under emotional stimuli through linear and non-linear analysis of physiological signals. https://core.ac.uk/download/324149571.pdf (accessed on 28th June 2025).
6. Smith, G. R., & Ballinger, R. E. (2001). THE ECOLOGICAL CONSEQUENCES OF HABITAT AND MICROHABITAT USE IN LIZARDS:: A REVIEW. *Contemporary Herpetology*, *1*, 1-28. https://doi.org/10.17161/ch.vi1.11957(accessed on 28th June 2025).
7. Russ Best, Martin Barwood , Jason Gillis, Owen Jeffriese(2019). Oral application of L-menthol in the heat: From pleasure to performance. The 18th International Conference on Environmental Ergonomics ICEE2019 https://core.ac.uk/download/287723714.pdf (accessed on 28th June 2025).
8. Bienboire-Frosini, C., Domínguez-Oliva, A., Gazzano, A., Gómez-Prado, J., et al. (2023). The role of brown adipose tissue and energy metabolism in mammalian thermoregulation during the perinatal period. https://core.ac.uk/download/599310023.pdf (accessed on 28th June 2025).
9. Chaseling, G. (2018). Physiological considerations of heat intolerance in people with multiple sclerosis. https://core.ac.uk/download/212696489.pdf (accessed on 28th June 2025).
10. Cornelissen, J. M. R., van Dixhoorn, I. D. E., & Groot Koerkamp, P. W. G., et al. (2009). Brief of requirements of the dairy cow. ISSN 1570 - 8616 https://core.ac.uk/download/pdf/29251363.pdf (accessed on 28th June 2025).
11. Ellis-Lepard, K. (2018). Does hydration impact memory: A systematic review. https://core.ac.uk/download/215462394.pdf (accessed on 28th June 2025).
12. Espeland, D. (2021). The beneficial health effects of voluntary exposure to cold water – A continuing subject of debate. https://core.ac.uk/download/489822790.pdf (accessed on 28th June 2025).
13. Wrobel, L. C., Ginalski, M. K., Nowak, A. J., Ingham, D. B., & Fic, A. M. (2010). An overview of recent applications of computational modelling in neonatology. *Philosophical transactions.*

Series A, Mathematical, physical, and engineering sciences, *368*(1920), 2817–2834. https://doi.org/10.1098/rsta.2010.0052(accessed on 28th June 2025).

14. Gauthier, S. M. S. (2015). Developing a method to monitor thermal discomfort response variability. https://core.ac.uk/download/78076816.pdf (accessed on 28th June 2025).
15. Wilson Stuart P. 2017Modelling the emergence of rodent filial huddling from physiological huddlingR. Soc. Open Sci.4170885
16. http://doi.org/10.1098/rsos.170885 (accessed on 28th June 2025).
17. Glasgow, A. (2019). The effects of men's lacrosse protective equipment on thermoregulation and perceptions during exercise heat stress. https://core.ac.uk/download/215464062.pdf (accessed on 28th June 2025).
18. Hanna Kaciuba-Uscilko and John E. Greenleaf (1989). Acclimatization to heat in humans. (EASA-TB- 10 10 12) NASA Technical Memorandum 101 01 2 43 p CSCL 06s https://core.ac.uk/download/pdf/42827514.pdf (accessed on 28th June 2025).
19. Lenasi, H., & Šijanec, J. (2023). The physiology of thermoregulation in exercise: A brief review. https://core.ac.uk/download/580130030.pdf (accessed on 28th June 2025).
20. McNabb, L. (2021). Quantifying the relationship of bilateral blood flow in glabrous skin at rest and during sympathetic perturbations. https://core.ac.uk/download/480267682.pdf (accessed on 28th June 2025).
21. Nagashima, K., Tokizawa, K., & Uchida, Y. (2009). The circadian system alters thermoregulation depending on the time of day and feeding condition. https://core.ac.uk/download/pdf/288329.pdf (accessed on 28th June 2025).
22. Smith, C. J., & Johnson, J. M. (2016). Responses to hyperthermia. Optimizing heat dissipation by convection and evaporation: Neural control of skin blood flow and sweating in humans. *Autonomic neuroscience : basic & clinical*, *196*, 25–36. https://doi.org/10.1016/j.autneu.2016.01.002(accessed on 28th June 2025).
23. Petersen, L. M., & Tisa, L. S. (2012). Influence of temperature on the physiology and virulence of the insect pathogen *Serratia* sp. strain SCBI. https://core.ac.uk/download/215530903.pdf (accessed on 28th June 2025).
24. Shungu, K. (1991). Temperature regulation post hemorrhagic shock in rats: A theoretical analysis. https://core.ac.uk/download/622134485.pdf (accessed on 28th June 2025).
25. Suga, T. (2025). Use of an electrical resistance hygrometer to measure human sweat rates. https://core.ac.uk/download/pdf/42861786.pdf (accessed on 28th June 2025).
26. Touitou, S. (2021). Energetics in wild female Assamese macaques (*Macaca assamensis*): A behavioral and physiological approach. https://core.ac.uk/download/477734542.pdf (accessed on 28th June 2025).
27. Verdegaal, L. E. J. M. M. (2022). Thermoregulation in exercising horses: Aspects of temperature monitoring during field exercise. https://core.ac.uk/download/553758458.pdf (accessed on 28th June 2025).

EXERCISE PHYSIOLOGY AND ADAPTATIONS

9

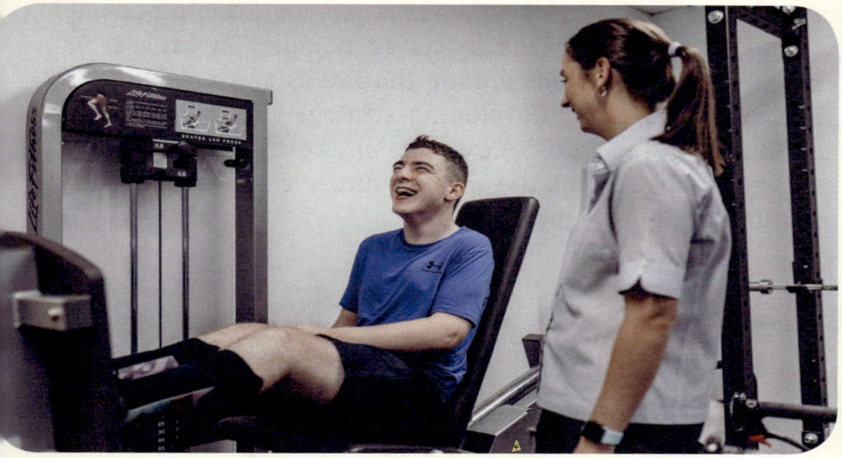

LEARNING OBJECTIVES

After studying this chapter, you will be able to:

1. Discuss the energy systems in exercise.
2. Explain the cardiovascular responses to exercise.
3. Discuss the muscular responses to exercise.
4. Focus on respiratory responses to exercise.
5. Learn about hormonal responses to exercise.
6. Evaluate the factors influencing exercise adaptations.

Introduction

Exercise physiology is essential to the understanding of adaptation and response of the body to physical exercise. It is the study of physiological occurrences that occur with exercise, including cardiovascular, muscular, and metabolic responses. Through the study of how the body reacts to various intensity and modality exercises, exercise physiologists can better understand how to optimize performance and maximize health overall. For instance, the dynamic between aerobic and anaerobic pathways during high-intensity exercise not only informs training practice but also guides recovery strategy development. This conceptual knowledge is foundational, as it explains why specific training programs can lead to improvements in physiological parameters , such as maximal oxygen consumption, cardiac output, and muscle strength, all of which are crucial for athletic performance and health maintenance (Hurst, 2014). Moreover, exercise physiology also allows the examination of different training modalities and the particular impact that they produce on the body. For example, it has been shown that Sprint Interval Training (SIT) can produce similar improvements in aerobic function to those of Endurance Training (ET), but in a more time-efficient manner. The ability of the physiological systems to adapt to novel training stimuli is perhaps the best representation of the necessity of periodizing exercise programs. When the various forms of training are done together, say SIT and ET, the impact is synergistic and usually has a positive effect on performance and on health outcomes. This serves to underscore not only the value of individualized exercise protocols but also the value of the application of exercise physiology in directing effective training programs that honor individual limitations and fitness levels (Ferguson et al., 2013). The inclusion of exercise physiology research findings further underscores the importance of evidence-based practice in fitness and rehabilitation. The physiological changes achieved with structured exercise programs, such as, improved cardiovascular function and metabolic economy, show the body's remarkable ability to adapt to stressors. This adaptability is important for the athlete seeking maximum performance as well as the individual seeking health-related benefits in fitness. As exercise physiologists continue to investigate the interactions among the intensity, duration, and recovery of exercise, what they learn becomes a basis for developing strategies that operate to achieve optimal health and performance. Ultimately, the study of exercise physiology not only adds to our understanding of the body's capability but also forms the way for future research in sports science and health promotion to evolve (Hurst, 2014) (Figure 9.1).

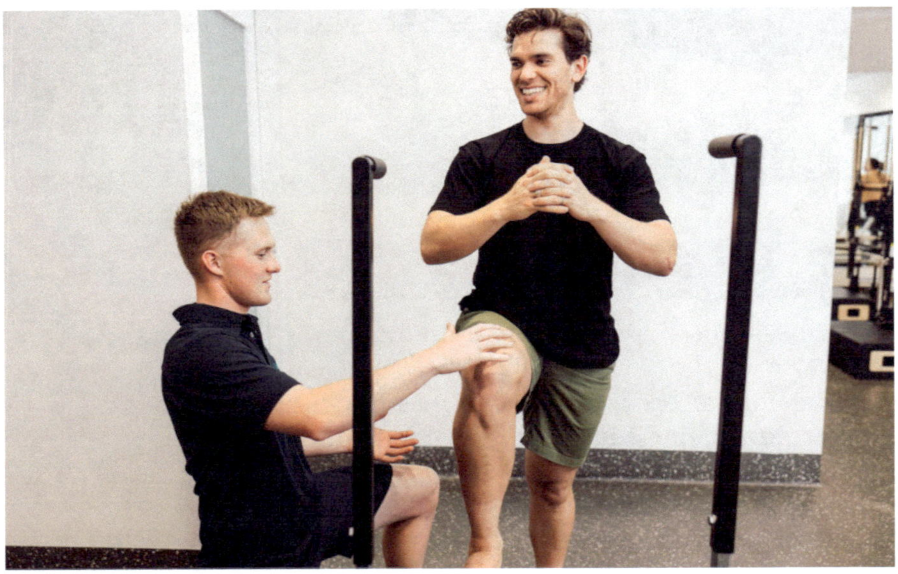

Figure 9.1. Exercise physiology.

Source: https://tidalhealth.com.au/wp-content/uploads/2023/10/66A8383-scaled.jpg.

Definition of Exercise Physiology

It takes an in-depth examination of how the body responds to and reacts to movement. It is a field of science that bridges biological sciences with health, focusing on the physiological processes of various exercise forms. Exercise physiology examines such fields as cardiovascular conditioning, muscle strength of muscles, and energy metabolism, essentially examining how such changes influence athletic performance and overall health. Most relevant are the responses to different kinds of exercise, which reflect the body's incredible plasticity, enabling a person to shape his/her physical potential. It includes structural and biochemical adaptations that are responsible for improving performance as well as preventing injuries, being compulsory knowledge for trainers, athletes, and physicians. The essence of exercise physiology lies in the understanding of muscular power, which is one of the most powerful predictors of sports performance. Due to the force and speed, it has a factor of speed that differentiates it from naked strength. The ability to generate power can sometimes be the deciding factor in the success of athletes in various sports. New evidence offers inconsistent findings regarding training protocols for the development of muscular power, including isotonic, isokinetic, and plyometric training protocols, describing volumes on how challenging the adaptations within this area are. The efficacy of different speeds of contraction is something yet to be explored, with considerations for optimal training. This ongoing study not only attempts to simplify the existing paradigms but also identifies the potential of novel training modalities in being capable of yielding better performance outcomes, as seen in investigations on the inertial loading techniques, which are of significant importance to the future of exercise physiology (Brenneman, 2016). Additionally, the exercise timing within the day can also influence physiological reaction and performance response. Indeed, there was evidence that showed morning resistance-based training can enhance afternoon performance due to the variation in hormones, particularly salivary testosterone levels. This circadian response accentuates the specific interaction between exercise timing, hormonal regulation, and physical performance. Moreover, empirical findings based on the study of sub-elite track sprint cyclists show that morning weight programs may lead to enhanced performance in subsequent activities, pointing to the necessity for structured training programs. Although physical alterations resulting from such practices are complex, they speak of an advanced interaction between training timing and physiological responses, providing avenues for additional understanding of exercise physiology in the context of athlete preparation and performance (McDonald & Maulder, 2018).

Importance of Studying Exercise Physiology

The physiology of exercise is of foremost significance in understanding how the human body reacts and adapts to physical training. By examining the underlying physiological mechanisms involved in exercise, researchers and professionals can gain secrets regarding the optimization of performance and improvement in health outcomes. Research in this field of study encompasses many topics like the energy system, muscle adaptations, and cardiovascular reactions, which matter the most for athletes and sports enthusiasts. Besides, exercise physiology aids the design of efficient training programs tailored to the needs of the individual, enhancing performance while minimizing the risk of injury. This is particularly relevant in competitive sports, as awareness of muscular strength and its induction by training methods has a direct bearing on success. The uses, thus, of exercise physiology extend beyond sports, incorporating rehabilitation, management of health, and overall physical well-being. Another imperative role of exercise physiology study is its role in promoting health and preventing chronic disease. Physical exercise has also been shown to be the basis for improving cardiovascular, metabolic, and musculoskeletal health. The physiological foundation of these processes enables clinicians to develop interventions promoting physical exercise in myriad populations, such as, those with pre-existing conditions. Further, exercise physiology informs public health to foster a healthy lifestyle and preventive behaviors. Such inputs gain additional significance in the aftermath of global sedentary living habits and associated health issues. Incorporating principles of exercise physiology within health education enables individuals to be guided towards exercising choice over physical activity to yield improved quality of life and increased lifespan. Lastly, the study of exercise physiology propels sports science applications with sporting implications directly for performance. Training modality research inquiries , such as changes in contraction velocities and impact on muscle adaptation for power, enhance our understanding of optimal training models. According to Brenneman (2016), particularly important for achieving maximum performance in the majority of sport is the force-velocity relationship. Also, the novel examination of training techniques, such as, inertial loading, offers promising avenues for future research to continue maximizing power and general athletic proficiency. Empirical research focus is paramount within the ever-evolving discipline of sports science, as it delivers evidence-based interventions for coaches and athletes alike. Thus, the relevance of exercise physiology extends beyond individual performance to enhance sport methodologies in general and to enhance the sporting experience (Figure 9.2).

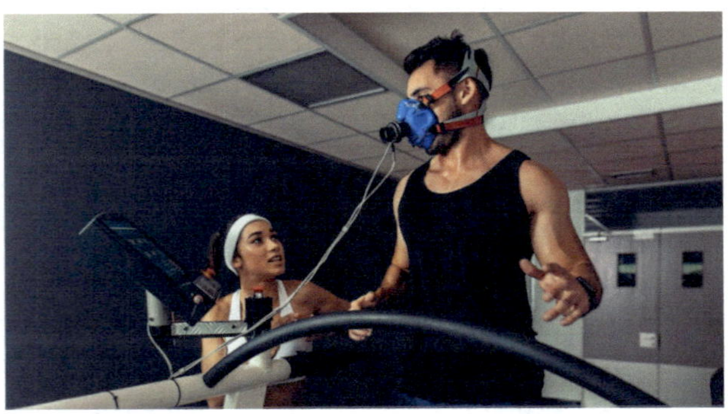

Figure 9.2. Importance of studying exercise physiology.

Source: https://mncalliedhealth.com/wp-content/uploads/2024/01/What-is-Exercise-Physiology-1-1-1200x675.jpg.

9.1. Energy Systems in Exercise

Learning Outcome

1. Describe the ATP production;
2. Focus on anaerobic vs. aerobic energy systems;
3. Learn about role of energy systems in different types of exercise.

Being aware of energy systems employed during exercise is at the heart of the field of exercise physiology, particularly in respect to training-induced adaptations. Three energy systems are primarily employed by the human body to fuel physical activity, viz., the phosphagen system, anaerobic glycolysis, and aerobic metabolism. Each of the energy systems has a distinct function based on the intensity and duration of the exercise. The phosphagen system provides immediate energy through the hydrolysis of creatine phosphate and adenosine triphosphate (ATP) for brief periods of high-level activity of a duration of around 10 seconds. Anaerobic glycolysis provides energy for moderate to high intensity exercise of 30 seconds to a duration of approximately two minutes, producing energy quickly at the cost of the build-up of lactate. Finally, aerobic metabolism is crucial to sustaining long-term exercise, enabling the conveyance of energy from carbohydrate and fat oxidation to support endurance activity as well as overall metabolic function. Emerging evidence on varied training protocols, for example, Sprint Interval Training (SIT), demonstrates how these systems of energy can be utilized optimally to enhance physical capacity and physiological adaptation. SIT combines brief periods of high-intensity exercise with active recoveries, primarily stimulating the anaerobic and aerobic systems, thus achieving an equivalent amount of aerobic improvement to conventional ET (Hurst, 2014). Significant studies have established the efficacy of SIT in conferring significant health gains, i.e., improved cardiorespiratory fitness measures and metabolic profiles, but involving less cumulative time than ET. By employing both energy systems, SIT may potentially offer a more efficient means of training, ultimately providing better health and performance outcomes. Full research is necessary, however, to contrast and compare SIT with other training modes to optimize the potential of these energy systems. In addition to the Speed-tolerable duration relationship, new data on high-intensity interval training (HIIT) further elucidate the intricacy of energy system utilization in exercise. The hyperbolic relationship defines how long individuals can sustain exercise at varying levels of intensity and has important exercise design implications (Ferguson et al., 2013). By specific protocols, evidence indicates that optimally designed intervals of HIIT facilitate maximum use of both anaerobic and aerobic systems to provide the most efficient level of energy and performance gains. By examining disparate work rates and time intervals, scientists are beginning to derive optimal HIIT parameters for the optimization of physiological adaptations. This emerging understanding emphasizes the utility of tailored exercise programs in creating deep adaptations in cardiorespiratory capacity and muscular endurance, ultimately culminating in a comprehensive appreciation of energy systems across various forms of physical activity (Figure 9.3).

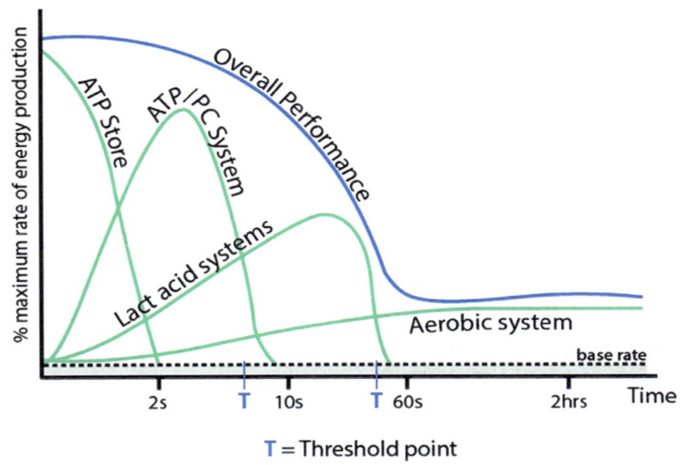

Figure 9.3. Energy systems and their application to training principles.

Source: https://lh6.googleusercontent.com/proxy/44_ZvHJsdwsh0U_daCb0RbTuT0P5hL3EzWiKrldVxHydUrwUe2floHmyQCljvmeltfmgbeGqD8bb0ALK0oTGTbswVNK3H9P9xEy3_7gR8AmgBBy-Q-W1RYa9NXA1KCPnbj0W5kSUmwZ5lGwM9YYytYs7EffeyqzzEP310zT6-JmUH2mcPfobGhFdIzCsu8wbpuo.

9.1.1. Overview of ATP Production

Adenosine triphosphate (ATP) is the primary biological currency of energy that enables cellular processes responsible for exercise physiology. ATP generation occurs through various metabolic mechanisms, including the phosphagen system, glycolysis, and oxidative phosphorylation. During maximal exercise, the phosphagen system maximally reconstitutes ATP from adenosine diphosphate (ADP) and inorganic phosphate (Pi) through the substrate creatine phosphate. This form of ATP creation is instant but holds energy demands for a very brief period, typically around 10 seconds.

It is thus vital for fast, explosive movements, but will eventually have to switch to glycolysis or oxidative metabolism to sustain exercise, particularly with prolonged exercise. As the duration of exercise prolongs, glycolysis is then the dominant mechanism for ATP production, especially during exercises at moderate intensity. This anaerobic reaction is glucose cleavage to produce ATP without oxygen, yielding energy rapidly but also lactic acid, which can contribute to muscle fatigue. Glycolysis is effective in producing ATP for 30 seconds to 2 minutes of all-out effort. The body is thereafter more reliant on aerobic metabolism, or the utilization of oxygen to convert substrates—, such as carbohydrates and fats, into ATP.

Through glycolysis and subsequent oxidative phosphorylation, a prodigious supply of ATP is generated, making it essential for sustaining long-term aerobic workouts. The efficiency and production level of this process are greatly enhanced, yielding approximately 36 molecules of ATP per molecule of glucose, thereby highlighting its importance during endurance activities. Coordinating various mechanisms of ATP production highlights the adaptability of human physiology in managing diverse exercise demands. For example, research has identified that sprint interval training (SIT) will elicit comparable aerobic capacity adaptations to traditional endurance training (ET), with the implication of the importance of maximizing pathways of energy production to enhance performance (Hurst, 2014). Endurance training has also been linked with increased mitochondrial biogenesis, which enhances the oxidative capacity and overall energy efficiency of the muscle (Craig et al., 2015). Such accommodations illustrate the active cross-talk between mechanisms of ATP production and training modalities, which is indicative of how the body can maximize its energetic output to meet specific demands. As athletes undergo various training protocols, such an understanding of metabolic tactics is of prime importance in maximizing procedures towards enhanced performance and recovery in various sporting environments (Figure 9.4).

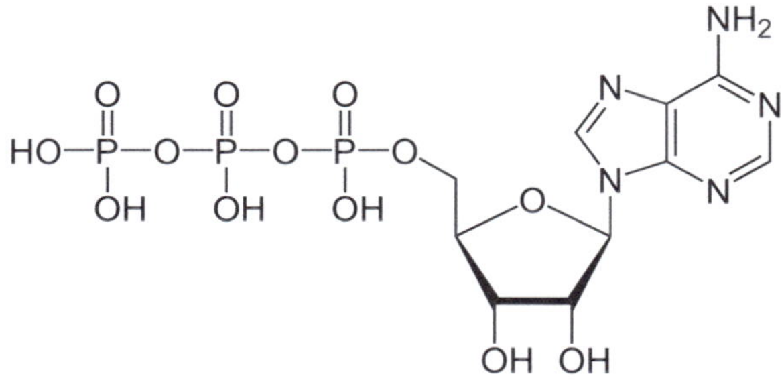

Figure 9.4. Adenosine triphosphate (ATP).

Source: https://upload.wikimedia.org/wikipedia/commons/thumb/3/31/Adenosintriphosphat_protoniert.svg/1200px-Adenosintriphosphat_protoniert.svg.png.

9.1.2. Anaerobic vs. Aerobic Energy Systems

The difference between anaerobic and aerobic energy systems is core to the examination of exercise physiology and adaptations. Anaerobic metabolism occurs in the absence of oxygen and is primarily employed with brief spikes of high-intensity activities , such as sprinting or weight training. This system relies predominantly on the energy from muscle glycogen, producing adenosine triphosphate (ATP) effectively but at a quick rate. Conversely, aerobic metabolism is observed in the presence of oxygen and supports extended, low-level activities. It allows for the breakdown of carbohydrates and fats to generate ATP in a manner that returns increased energy over an extended period. Knowledge regarding these processes makes it possible to maximize performance and enable adapting training programs to the individual needs of various sports disciplines. Research on specific training modalities allows considerable diversity in the efficacy of anaerobic versus aerobic training. SIT, for example, has emerged as a time-efficient alternative to traditional endurance training ET, with comparable improvements in aerobic capacity with reduced training time. Studies indicated that optimal combinations of ET and SIT possess the ability to enhance various physiological variables , such as resting heart rate and blood cholesterol levels (Hurst, 2014). This indicates the importance of not only identifying the individual energy systems but also applying their capabilities in order to maximize performance outcomes. As coaches and athletes learn to value divergent training practices, the utilization of anaerobic and aerobic systems in conditioning programs has emerged as a focal point for attaining athletic adaptations. On the backdrop of emphasis on aerobic and anaerobic training, it is also appropriate to consider the unique physiological requirements inherent in non-traditional sports, such as, dance. Dancers are often engaged in choreography, which, while not completely aerobic in content, may fail to offer sufficient aerobic stimuli to initiate significant adaptations to fitness. This insufficiency emphasizes the necessity for further fitness training to increase aerobic power, muscular balance, and status for fitness status, like other sportsmen (Koutedakis & Jamurtas, 2007). Failure to address these considerations exposes dancers to the risk of injury and restricts their functional capacity to function. Through the addition of special aerobic and anaerobic conditioning to dance rehearsals, teachers are able to encourage improvements in important indices of fitness without compromising on the artistic quality of performances, which ultimately leads to enhanced sporting performance and health in participating dancers (Figure 9.5).

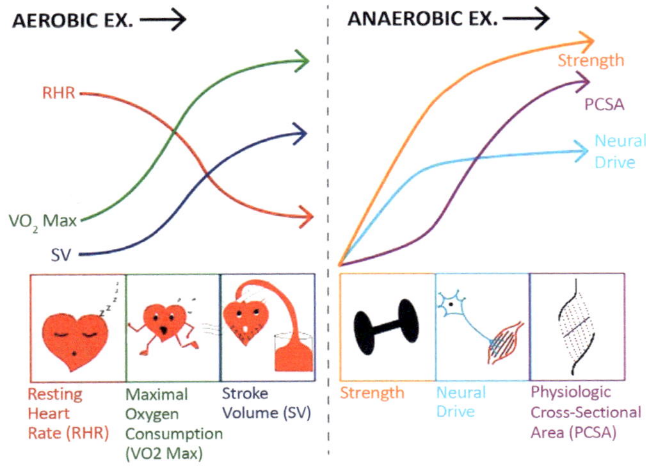

Figure 9.5. Anaerobic exercise.

Source: https://www.physio-pedia.com/images/thumb/1/17/Aerobic_Anaerobic_Exercise_Adaptations.jpeg/450px-Aerobic_Anaerobic_Exercise_Adaptations.jpeg.

9.1.3. Role of Energy Systems in Different Types of Exercise

Classification of exercise into different modalities necessitates a good understanding of the energy systems that supply energy for movement. The body predominantly utilizes three energy systems: the phosphagen system, the glycolytic system, and the oxidative system. They are called upon depending on the intensity and duration of the exercise. For short bursts of high work rates, i.e., sprinting or weightlifting, the phosphagen system is in control, relying on stored ATP and creatine phosphate for instant energy requirements. At the other extreme, during moderate-intensity sessions, e.g., steady jogging, the glycolytic system becomes operative, breaking down glucose to produce ATP through anaerobic metabolism. This transition reflects the ways in which various energy systems work together to power an athlete's performance, supporting the dynamic nature of human physiology in adapting to multiple training stimuli. With prolonged exercise, reliance on oxidative metabolism becomes essential to maintain energy supply. The oxidative system provides ATP via the aerobic breakdown of carbohydrates and fats, particularly for long, steady-state efforts like marathon running. This process is particularly significant as it facilitates sustained energy production and glycogen storage protection. Adaptations due to long-term aerobic exercise include elevated mitochondrial density and increased cardiovascular effectiveness, resulting in increased aerobic capacity and endurance performance. Furthermore, the incorporation of different training modes, as illustrated in studies, demonstrates that integrating aerobic and anaerobic components is responsible for optimizing physiological adaptations and consequently results in enhanced overall exercise performance and health benefits. Such adaptations not only optimize sporting performance but also enhance metabolic health, which signifies the systemic importance of varied energy systems. In addition to inherent physiological adaptations involving energy-related systems, certain new research suggests that the modification of strategies , such as nutritional interventions or sensory stimulation, can also enhance performance during exercise. For instance, substances , such as menthol can be utilized to optimize the exercise session through the delivery of coolness and probable work capacity augmentation by sensory modulation. This adds an interesting dimension to the role of energy systems, where the interaction between nutritional or psychological intervention and physiological functioning is essential. Lastly, practitioners working in sports environments have the flexibility to tailor such interventions based on responses to maximize performance and endurance. The results acquired through such studies identify the significance of acquiring and applying energy system knowledge in the areas of curriculum planning as well as in competition settings, thereby influencing physiological reactions to different exercises (Best et al., 2019).

Test Your Knowledge

1. What are the three main energy systems used during exercise, and how do they differ in duration and intensity of activity?
2. Describe the role of the ATP-PCr (phosphagen) system in short, high-intensity activities.

9.2. Cardiovascular Responses to Exercise

Learning Outcome

1. Explain the heart rate and stroke volume changes;
2. Define the blood flow distribution during exercise;
3. Understand the long-term adaptations of the cardiovascular system.

The cardiac system plays a vital role in exercise response, enabling oxygen and nutrient delivery to contracting muscles and the elimination of waste products. During exercise, there is augmented stroke volume and heart rate with increased cardiac output, which is described as the volume of blood per minute ejected by the heart. This physiological adaptation is tasked with sustaining elevated workloads and maximizing performance. Exercise intensity, duration, and individual fitness levels all play a key role in these cardiovascular adaptations. Interestingly, as the body adapts to regular exercise, there are cardiovascular adaptations like increased capillary density, improved blood flow regulation, and improved cardiac efficiency within the cardiovascular system. All of these enhancements enhance overall cardiovascular fitness and exercise tolerance, establishing a key link between cardiovascular health and exercise that falls under the broad umbrella of exercise physiology. Apart from heart rate and stroke volume alterations, exercise blood pressure responses yield valuable insight into cardiovascular health. With moderate to high intensity exercise, systolic blood pressure tends to rise in response to blood flow requirements, while diastolic blood pressure is relatively constant or can also exhibit minor alterations. Elevation of systolic blood pressure signals augmented cardiac output and peripheral resistance due to vasodilation within contracting muscle masses. Significantly, regular involvement in exercise, particularly aerobic training, is associated with long-term reductions in resting blood pressure, hence avoiding hypertension and other cardiovascular disease-related conditions.

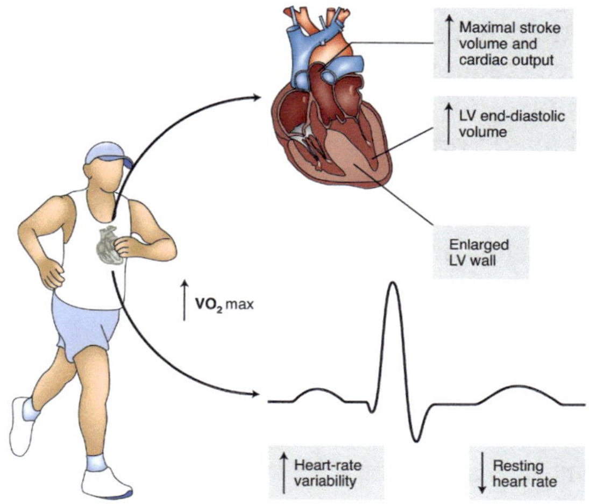

Figure 9.6. Cardiovascular responses to exercise.

Source: https://media.springernature.com/m685/springer-static/image/art%3A10.1038%2Fs42255-020-0262-1/MediaObjects/42255_2020_262_Fig1_HTML.png.

The interplay between exercise intensity and blood pressure responses emphasizes the exercise potential as a non-pharmacological intervention in the improvement of cardiovascular health outcomes, greatly enhancing cardiovascular responses in exercise physiology and adaptation knowledge. Further, the type of exercise performed could play an important role in cardiovascular adaptation. Sprint interval training (SIT) has been researched to give equal gains in aerobic capacity with endurance training, but in a fraction of the time spent. As suggested by existing literature, the combination of SIT and endurance training has been proven to produce notable effects in various physiological parameters, including resting heart rate, blood pressure, and metabolic factors like cholesterol and blood glucose concentration levels (Hurst, 2014). This indicates the plasticity of the cardiovascular system because it can respond effectively to various types of training. In addition, high-intensity training-induced adaptations are used to signify the cardiovascular system's ability for plasticity in response to various exercise stimuli. It is consequently essential to understand these responses for maximizing training regimens as well as for retaining cardiovascular health and functional ability on a long-term basis, revealing certain connections between particular exercise approaches and overall well-being (Figure 9.6).

9.2.1. Heart Rate and Stroke Volume Changes

The relationship between stroke volume and heart rate is a critical element of cardiovascular adaptation with exercise and reflects the ability of the body to maintain with increased demands for oxygen and nutrients. Heart rate increases dramatically with exercise to permit increased blood flow, and stroke volume—amount of blood the heart ejects per beat—also increases. Evidence indicates that adaptations in these ways are imperative for enhancing cardiovascular efficiency and performance, particularly in endurance training situations. For instance, compared to traditional endurance training (ET), sprint interval training (SIT) has also been found to provide similar enhancements in aerobic capacity, thereby demonstrating its promising potential for optimizing heart rate and stroke volume responses during exercise. Not. Surprisingly, successful training programs that can modulate these cardiovascular parameters can be associated with a significant improvement in overall health capacity for exercise, leading to salutary health effects and enhanced athletic performance (Hurst, 2014). Moreover, the physiological adaptation of stroke volume and heart rate is not only restricted to endurance exercise, but also reach even high-intensity interval training methods. With the greater workload to which the heart adapts, mechanisms , such as increased myocardial contractility and blood volume changes contribute to increased stroke volume. Such adaptations are classically observed in subjects undergoing well-designed exercise regimens, significant reductions in resting heart rate commonly being linked with augmented stroke volume. Such adaptations translate to improved general cardiovascular function and fitness levels.

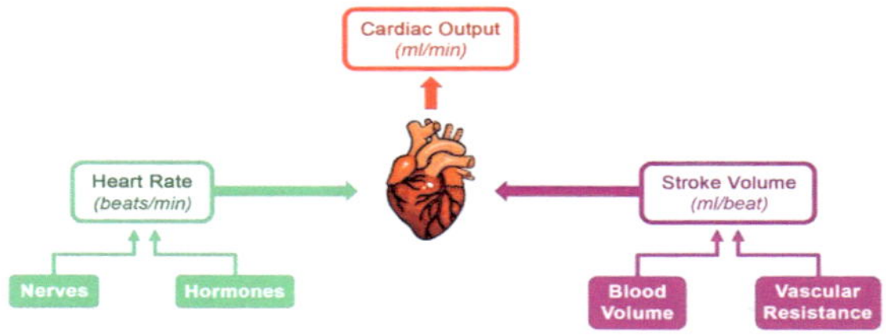

Figure 9.7. Cardiac output.

Source: https://old-ib.bioninja.com.au/_Media/cardiac-output_med.jpeg.

Prominently, the changes are observed across all age groups, suggesting that training protocols, either SIT- or ET-based, are capable of producing wide-ranging cardiovascular adjustments regardless of the subject's initial fitness status. Heart rate and stroke volume management assume significance as training intensity advances, finally enhancing the exercise performance quality (Liang et al., 2019). Finally, understanding the intricacies of heart rate and stroke volume changes is an observation that provides guidance for designing training courses to improve physiological response. Employing varied training methods, including combining sprint and endurance exercises, can initiate maximal adaptations in heart rate and stroke volume with respect to applying single methods. The results indicate that the subjects following combined training courses exhibit significant improvement in resting heart rate and capacity for exercise. This affirms the legislation that varied and regular stimulation of cardiovascular tissues through diverse training protocols can lead to greater cumulative gains. Hence, this evidence affirms the relevance of proper exercise prescription for eliciting acute and chronic adaptations in cardiovascular health, affirming the need for certain training protocols to utilize the interaction between stroke volume and heart rate (Hurst, 2014) (Figure 9.7).

9.2.2. Blood Flow Distribution During Exercise

The human body also undergoes vast physiological changes under exercise, the most significant of which is blood distribution in the circulation to provide satisfaction for the metabolic demands. Initially, blood circulation is redirected from non-vital organs to skeletal muscle, resulting in augmented perfusion into areas engaged in high-intensity exercise. Such discrimination is regulated by vasodilation of contracting muscles and vasoconstriction in areas , such as the gastrointestinal tract. The autonomic nervous system is also crucial, releasing neurotransmitters that control vascular resistance, thereby permitting increased flow where it's needed most. Thus, maximizing oxygen and nutrient delivery to contracting tissues enhances performance and endurance, making clear the importance of understanding this special physiology of exercise adaptations. The intricate control of blood distribution during exercise also involves the interaction of various factors, including exercise intensity and duration. Intense efforts, like sprinting or circuit training, demonstrate greater blood flow redistribution than low-intensity, steady-state exercise. During high-intensity exercise, the body at its disposal possesses a specialized mechanism whereby working muscles can potentially receive almost doubled blood supply. This acute response is important to sustain prolonged efforts that demand the quick production of energy. Identification of these mechanisms not only informs us about training programs but also informs us about how exercise adaptations can improve vascular function and general athletic performance. Examination of this responsiveness in the cardiovascular system allows for specifically targeted training protocols, which can contribute profoundly to increasing performance outcomes and eventually result in successful exercise prescription (Minett & Costello, 2015). Apart from the severity of exercise, the nature of the training program is also critical to establish long-term changes in the distribution of blood flow. Studies have shown that interval training, involving repeated succession of high and low-severity exercise with brief rest periods, can further optimize the economy of blood flow during exercise and recovery. This method allows for increased cardiovascular requirement without undue metabolic cost. Specifically, the resultant Speed-tolerable duration (S-tLIM) formed in these high-intensity bouts can dictate the training effectiveness parameters and adaptations (Ferguson et al., 2013). With variations in intensity and duration, trainers can optimize the efficiency of cardiovascular systems and trigger adaptations that lead to improved exercise capacity. Last but not least, an understanding of the physiology behind blood distribution during exercise is important in formulating maximally effective training programs that are compatible with each athlete's needs.

9.2.3. Long-Term Adaptations of the Cardiovascular System

The long-term adjustments of the cardiovascular system with regular exercise are profound, resulting in improved efficiency and performance. Endurance exercise is particularly effective in facilitating these adjustments, including increased stroke volume and cardiac output during rest and exercise. This is largely due to the ability of the heart to expel more blood with each beat, a process known as myocardial remodeling. This reorganization enables the left ventricle to contain more blood, resulting in improved delivery of oxygen to the body. These physiological changes are required to sustain prolonged exercise and reduce the risk of cardiovascular disease. The individual adaptations reflect not only the capacity of the heart to enlarge but also its responsiveness to chronic stressors, thereby uncovering a remarkable level of plasticity under the impact of chronic exercise exposure. Daily exercise enables various hemodynamic adjustments to take place, which are responsible for long-term cardiovascular system change. Notably, exercise training leads to decreases in resting heart rate, lowering of blood pressure, and increased vascular compliance. These changes augment the cardiovascular system's efficiency in order to secure improved perfusion of exercising tissues during exercise. Furthermore, increased capillary density within the skeletal muscle facilitates improved oxygen extraction and delivery of nutrients, which are foundational for improving exercise performance.

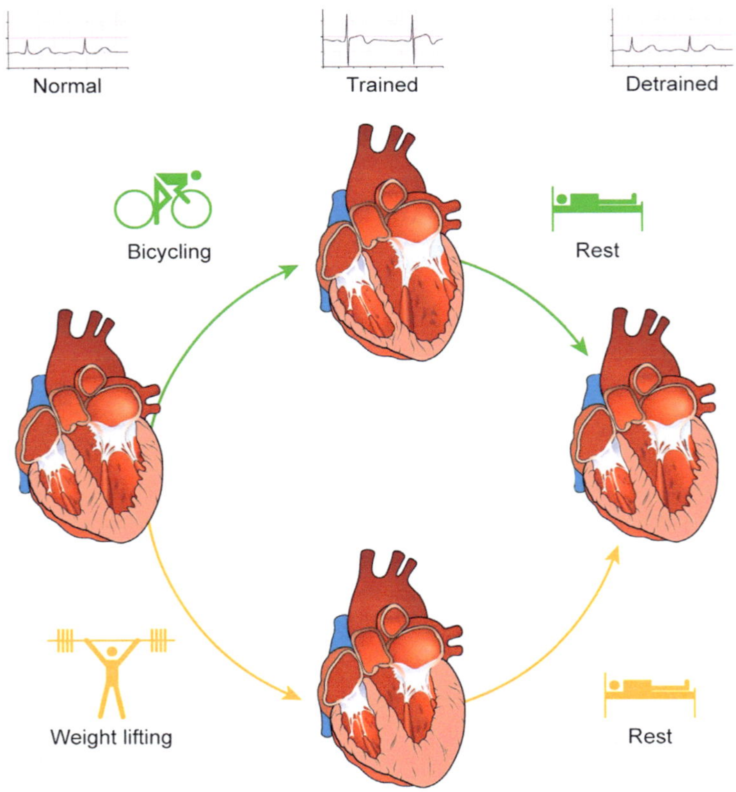

Figure 9.8. Cardiovascular adaptation in athletes.

Source: https://ars.els-cdn.com/content/image/1-s2.0-S1050173815001188-gr1.jpg.

These changes are conducive to cellular metabolism and energy production, which is important in maintaining the ability to sustain exercise for extended periods. Basically, these adaptations highlight the intricate relationship between sustained physical activity and cardiovascular well-being, reaffirming the advantages of sustained exercise in helping achieve maximal cardiovascular performance throughout life. While the benefits of cardiovascular adaptations to training are well documented, differentiation of these physiological changes from potential underlying pathologies is required. The athlete's heart phenomenon has morphological characteristics that overlap with cardiac conditions at risk of sudden cardiac death. Sensitive evaluation is needed to distinguish between normal adaptations and potential cardiac disease. As disseminated in recent publications, an interdisciplinary approach combining history, clinical evaluation, and sophisticated imaging techniques is needed in this respect. Through the use of techniques , such as echocardiography and ECG, physicians can effectively diagnose the athletes who could fall into the grey zone between adaptive physiological changes and incipient cardiac disease. Thus, both exercise elicits adaptive long-term changes within the cardiovascular system and while they intensify physiological enhancement, their caution and vigorous assessment still reign supreme in safeguarding athlete health and preventing undesirable outcomes, evidence of the excellent physiological gain/pathological risk equilibrium (McGuire et al., 2018; Baggish et al., 2023) (Figure 9.8).

Test Your Knowledge

1. What mechanisms regulate blood flow distribution to active muscles during exercise?
2. Explain the role of the autonomic nervous system in controlling cardiovascular function during physical activity.

9.3. Muscular Responses to Exercise

Learning Outcome

1. Explain the muscle fiber types and their functions;

Define the hypertrophy and strength adaptations;

Describe the role of neuromuscular adaptations in performance.

The muscle reactions to exercise are crucial in understanding the broader scheme of exercise physiology and adaptations. During physical stress, skeletal muscles possess a range of acute and chronic reactions aiming to enhance efficiency and performance. Among the acute reactions to exercise are increased recruitment of additional muscle fibers and greater rates of energy production, which are fueled primarily by enzymatic muscle cell activity. This initial response also causes the release of certain hormones, such as, testosterone and growth hormone, that assist in the repair and development of muscle. With prolonged training, muscles learn to adapt through mechanisms like hypertrophy, where muscle fibers become enlarged, and changes in myofibrillar density, to ultimately achieve an overall capacity of the muscle to generate force and power. One of the underlying concepts behind these muscular adaptations is grounded in the theory of specific training stimuli. Different types of training—resistance training, aerobic exercise, plyometrics—elicit varying muscle adaptations in anticipation of specific athletic performances. By way of example, isotonic training with variable resistance has been shown to improve strength and power through the optimization of muscle contraction velocities, according to recent studies. Conversely, isometric and isokinetic exercises provide opposing means directed at muscle stabilization and endurance. Despite the plurality of training practices, not all are as effective in their application; therefore, the understanding of the complexity of exercise modalities in creating effective training programs to elicit muscular reactions is paramount (Brenneman, 2016). Additionally, the methodological process via periodization is vital in optimizing training efficacy and efficiency. Periodization is the process of smartly changing the variables of resistance training over a period to efficiently optimize physiological adaptations. Periodization was initially employed in Russia and considers volume, intensity, and recovery time to prevent staleness and provide ongoing performance improvement. Periodized programs, as research proves, can significantly outperform non-periodized programs in terms of muscle gain and fat loss (Yanes, 2019). As such, trainers and coaches have to use periodization principles, always modifying their athlete training programs so as to induce intended muscular responses. Through acknowledging and implementing the principles of muscular physiology, such as, acute responses and adaptations of different methods of training, practitioners can develop improved athletic performance (Figure 9.9).

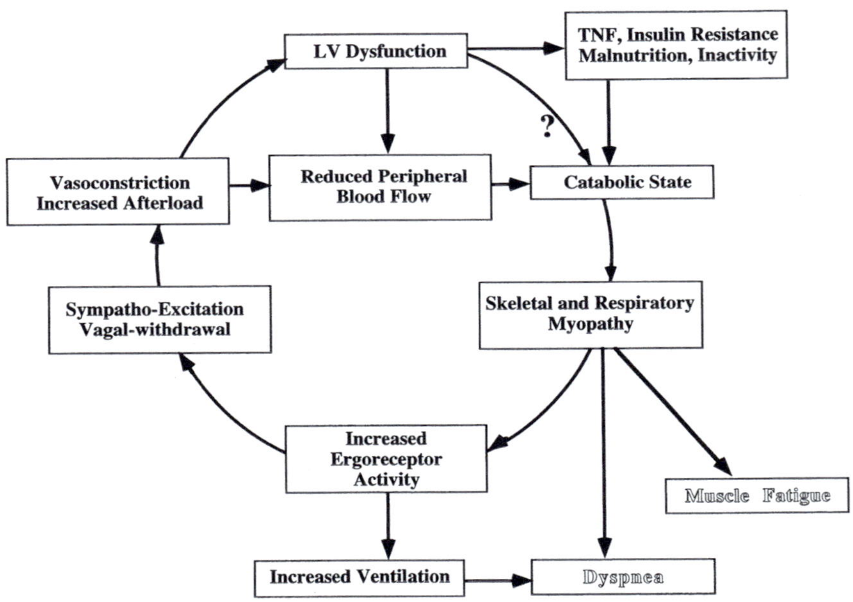

Figure 9.9. Muscular responses to exercise.

Source: https://www.ahajournals.org/cms/10.1161/01.CIR.93.5.940/asset/150399a1-c3bc-48cd-8443-4973026f141c/assets/graphic/hc0561357006.jpeg.

9.3.1. Muscle Fiber types and Their Functions

Understanding the different types of muscle fibers is crucial for appreciating their respective functions and the adaptive responses to different forms of exercise. Human skeletal muscle consists predominantly of two types of fibers: Type I fibers, also slow-twitch fibers, and Type II fibers, or fast-twitch fibers. Type I fibers are highly oxidative, richly endowed with mitochondria and blood supply, and hence highly resistant to fatigue. Such fibers are sufficiently able to sustain long-term activities , such as running or cycling over a distance. On the contrary, Type II fibers are themselves split into Type IIa and Type IIb fibers, of which Type IIa has a hybrid function for oxidative and glycolytic metabolism and Type IIb has its primary source of anaerobic pathways for explosive power. The difference reflects the specificity of muscle fibers, which is a reflection of their unique functions in exercise physiology as well as performance effects differences. The distribution of muscle fibers between individuals can also play an important role in exercise adaptations and sports performance. Genes, training regimens, and even physiological demands dictate muscle fiber content. For instance, endurance athletes who are well-trained possess a higher percentage of Type I fibers, which enhances their aerobic capacity and endurance. Conversely, sprinters will have a prevalence of Type II fibers, as these are needed for the rapid, forceful movements inherent in sprinting events. Recent research indicates that endurance training has the effect of increasing the oxidative capacity of both Type I and Type II fibers so that their mitochondrial density is increased in the muscle tissue. This adaptation is most important for enhancing overall function during extended physical activity since it reflects directly on improved utilization of energy in exercise (Craig et al., 2015). Furthermore, functional aspects of muscle fiber types encompass clinical applicability outside of the sporting performance context. For example, musculoskeletal disorder patients or rehabilitating patients can be given a special procedure of training emphasizing specific adaptations in the muscle fibers to improve the recovery and functional ability. Moreover, exercise-stimulated mitochondrial biogenesis, particularly in Type I and IIa fibers, is critical for metabolic health. Enhanced mitochondrial function sustains augmented oxidative metabolism and may influence the risk of chronic diseases related to active living. With this improved understanding of muscle fiber types and their functions comes the potential to create interventions that utilize exercise to enhance muscle health and fitness, with the emphasis placed on the role of physical activity in every population (Dickson et al., 2025) (Figure 9.10).

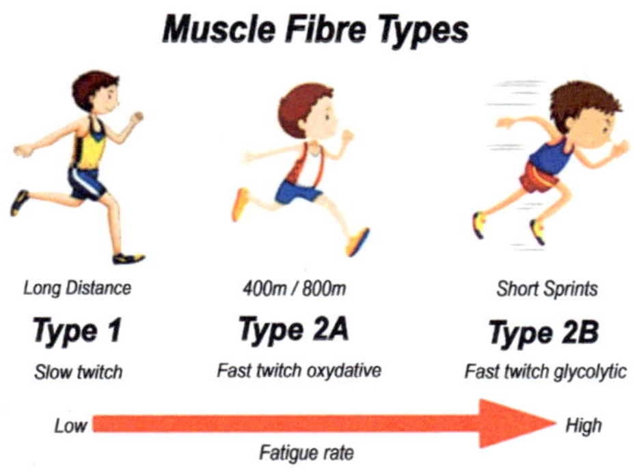

Figure 9.10. Muscle fiber type review.

Source: https://atpplusct.com/wp-content/uploads/2017/06/Muscle-Fiber-type.jpg.

9.3.2. Hypertrophy and Strength Adaptations

The interaction of hypertrophy with strength adaptation is central in the physiology of exercise. Hypertrophy is the growth in muscle size due to resistance training, which most people who want to improve their appearance or function desire. It takes place mostly through muscle fiber recruitment, protein synthesis, and hormone action. Because muscles are stressed when working out, microtears are created, which invite the body to initiate a repair process that thickens the muscle fibers. This physiological adaptation is intimately linked to strength gain because larger muscles may be capable of exerting more force. However, it must be clarified that hypertrophy and strength are not exact synonyms. While larger muscle size tends to provide the foundation for greater strength, rate of force production and neuromuscular coordination also act on the expression of strength in sporting performance with significant effects. Exercise adaptation research focuses especially upon training modalities for optimal hypertrophic and strength gains. A powerful technique of increased muscular power, involving both force and velocity, has been explored in a variety of investigations. For instance, isotonic, isokinetic, and plyometric training methods have been applied to determine their influence on muscular power adaptations. Notably, muscular power is distinct from mere strength, placing priority on rapid force utilization, which is integral to sporting excellence. Although the present literature is in disagreement regarding the effectiveness of differing training velocities for maximal power improvement, it emphasizes the demand for further research. More specifically, the study of inertial loading as an exercise method has been identified as a promising direction to optimize both power and strength adaptations in a prescribed exercise protocol (Brenneman, 2016). Lastly, the history of aging cannot be overlooked when it comes to discourse on hypertrophy and strength adaptations. Sarcopenia, or the decline in muscle mass and strength with increasing age, poses a significant hindrance to maintaining functional abilities in older persons. Exercise has been a promising intervention to counteract these declines, improving muscle function and preserving overall quality of life. Studies have demonstrated that resistance training can induce beneficial adaptations in the elderly, though the process of anabolic resistance—the lowered efficacy of muscle protein synthesis in aging—has a persistent nagging concern. Forefront studies with progressive resistance training have reported excellent strength, muscle, and neuromuscular functioning gains in both young and elderly subjects, thus illustrating the importance of strength adaptations across life (Graber et al., 2019). The intricate relationship between aging, hypertrophy, and strength adaptations requires the implementation of age-specific exercise protocols to enhance health and mobility among older populations (Figure 9.11).

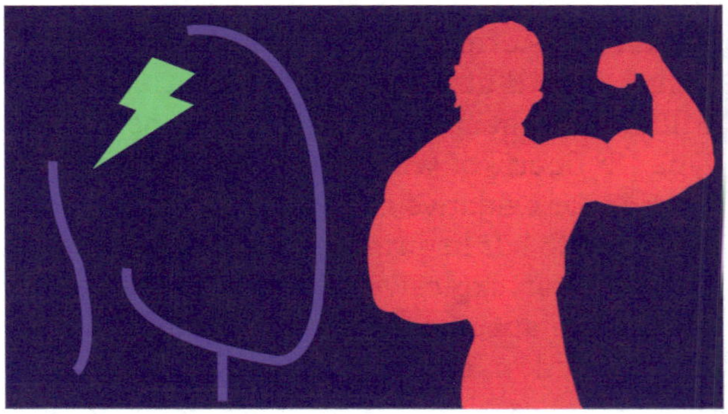

Figure 9.11. The effect of stress on muscle and strength adaptations.

Source: https://houseofhypertrophy.com/wp-content/uploads/2022/07/stress-and-strength-muscle.png.

9.3.3. Role of Neuromuscular Adaptations in Performance

The role that neuromuscular adaptations play in sporting performance is a crucial area of study in exercise physiology. As athletes continually train, their bodies develop in significant ways at the muscular and nervous system levels in order to enhance their sports performance capability. Among the rises in strength of muscles, production of power, and coordination, all of the necessary components for optimal sporting performance are encompassed. For instance, resistance training, particularly with eccentric modalities, has been shown to improve force development and muscular economy and thus result in enhanced athletic performance. The training benefits individuals of all ages since it has been established that young athletes can accumulate significant strength and injury tolerance through certain eccentric training regimens (Drury et al., 2019). These adjustments not only improve measures of performance but also lead to long sport careers by reducing the risk of injury. While neuromuscular adjustments occur, it is important to understand their mechanisms, namely how exercise affects muscle fiber type and neural drive. Present studies indicate that training can lead to alterations in muscle fiber types, with a substantial increase in fast-twitch fibers vital for explosive movement. On top of that, neuromuscular efficiency also improves, allowing for better synchronization of motor units at high intensities of exercise. Synchronization is particularly important in sports with rapid and explosive movements, such as, sprint running or weightlifting. Additionally, the process of aging complicates the maintenance of these adaptations because older adults are more likely to develop sarcopenia, characterized by a decrease in muscle mass and muscle strength (Graber et al., 2019). It is therefore necessary to develop personalized training programs that not only utilize neuromuscular adaptation but also meet the specific needs and limitations of different populations. Neuromuscular training methods integrated into exercise programs present a promising path towards the enhancement of athletic performance in different groups. Eccentric resistance training has been found to significantly improve their physical qualities and contribute towards establishing required movement patterns in young athletes (Drury et al., 2019). In the meantime, for aging persons who experience age-related muscle loss, specified exercises can reduce functional impairments related to sarcopenia, rendering physical exercise an essential intervention in the preservation of quality of life (Graber et al., 2019). Such strategies underscore the need to commit to physical training throughout the lifespan, optimized to meet personal requirements, such that neuromuscular adjustments not only occur but also remain maintained throughout. Lastly, gaining an appreciation for these adaptations serves to optimize performance potential and minimize the risk of injury across the lifespan in athletes and coaches.

Test Your Knowledge

1. How do skeletal muscles adapt acutely during aerobic and anaerobic exercise?
2. What are the metabolic changes in muscle cells during sustained physical activity?

9.4. Respiratory Responses to Exercise

Learning Outcome

1. Identify the changes in breathing rate and depth;

Define the gas exchange efficiency during exercise;

Describe the long-term adaptations of the respiratory system.

The respiratory system plays a vital role in meeting the augmented body demand for oxygenation during exercise. As an individual starts exercising, the body initiates a sequence of respiratory adaptations that enhance oxygen delivery to contracting muscles. It involves an augmentation in tidal volume and respiratory rate, which are respectively the depth and frequency of breathing. These changes enable increased ventilation, thereby increasing the oxygen and carbon dioxide exchange in the alveoli. Again, between the intensity of exercise and respiratory response, there could be no straightforward relationship; for example, as the intensity of the exercise goes up, there is a coordinated rise in respiratory rate to match the enhanced need for oxygen supply and the elimination of carbon dioxide, ultimately enabling effective energy production through aerobic metabolism. This compensatory respiratory reaction is required to sustain long-duration exercise and indicates the fitness of the individuals. In the accompanying respiration musculature, there comes the adaptation with the rise in ventilation during exercise. Regular endurance training can induce physiological changes within the respiratory system that maximize its structure and function. For instance, endurance exercise stimulates the formation of oxidative fibers in muscle, increases capillary density, and mitochondrial biogenesis in respiratory musculature. Greater diaphragmatic and intercostal muscle capacity increases the efficiency of inspiration and expiration, allowing improved gas exchange rates during augmented physical activity. With endurance activities being prolonged, studies show that such adaptations result in a heightened overall capacity for gas exchange, allowing for enhanced endurance and performance in sports activities (Craig et al., 2015). Therefore, the respiratory adaptations are indicative of the body's capacity to adapt its systems so as to meet the physiological demands brought about by regular exercise. Moreover, the confluence of endurance and high-intensity training paradigms could have deep breathing implications, highlighting the potential of systemic adaptations in exercise physiology. For instance, studies on SIT have shown that such a time-efficient protocol can produce improvements in aerobic capacity comparable to traditional endurance training (Hurst, 2014). The repeated bout of exercise with recovery periods challenges the respiratory system in an alternative manner and can produce desirable adaptations similar to those from endurance training at steady state. This emphasizes the importance of diverse training modalities for optimizing respiratory function and overall cardiovascular health. By. The incorporation of exercise strategies can make an immersive experience of enhanced respiratory efficacy, which will ultimately lead to global performance and health, articularly in relation to measurements like maximal oxygen uptake, which is crucial for sustained exercise (Figure 9.12).

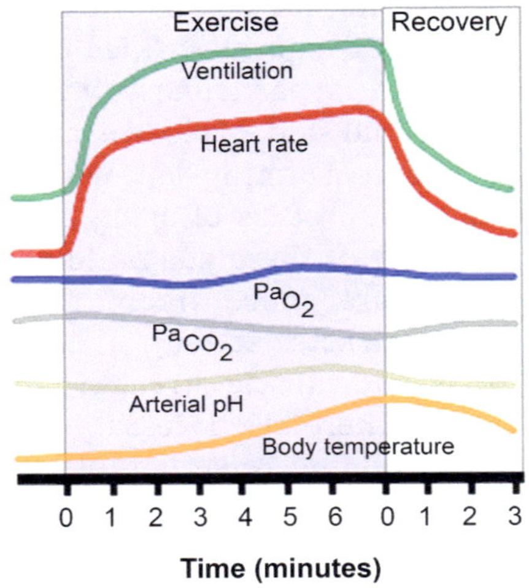

Figure 9.12. Exercise physiology: respiratory contribution.

Source: http://www.medicine.mcgill.ca/physio/vlab/exercise/img/vent_cycling.gif.

9.4.1. Changes in Breathing Rate and Depth

The relationship between exercise intensity and changes in breathing rate and depth is well-documented in exercise physiology. As physical activity escalates, the body's demand for oxygen increases, necessitating alterations in respiratory patterns. Typically, during both aerobic and anaerobic exercises, the ventilatory response increases to accommodate the rising production of carbon dioxide and the need for oxygen. This adaptation is evidenced by an increase in the frequency of breaths and the amount of each inhalation and exhalation, referred to as tidal volume. These adjustments ensure proper gas exchange at the level of the alveoli to more effectively deliver oxygen to the blood and remove metabolic waste products. The physiological requirement of alteration in respiratory patterns is regulated primarily by the central nervous system, which continuously monitors the blood gas concentrations, so that immediate alterations in respiratory mechanics can be enabled to allow sustained physical activity. Additionally, individual variations in the extent of increase in rate and depth of breathing can also be accounted for by variations in fitness level, surroundings, and the nature of exercise. Well-trained athletes will have a more efficient respiratory response, with less steep rises in breathing rates compared to untrained individuals subjected to the same loads. This efficiency is significant because it decreases the onset of fatigue and maximizes performance. Environmental factors , such as higher altitudes or humidity, may also necessitate further adjustments in breathing methods to ensure adequate oxygenation. This exchange between exercise requirements and human capabilities underscores the need for individually prescribed training programs that consider both the environmental and physiological determinants influencing respiratory adaptation during exercise. Of particular interest is that respiratory adaptation not only enhances oxygen uptake but also metabolic processes regulated by carbon dioxide levels. Efficient ventilation plays an important role in acid-base balance within the body during exercise. Increased depth and frequency of breathing allow for the greater removal of carbon dioxide, a metabolic byproduct of increased muscular activity. Failure to maintain proper control of carbon dioxide levels leads to hypercapnia, which impairs mental function and overall exercise performance. The manner in which the body finely tunes respiratory responses during exercise yields guidance for enhancing training sessions and performance outcomes. As has been intimated in recent literature, close observation of breathing mechanics during exercise can also enhance interventions to maximize sporting performance, pointing to an evolving arena of exercise physiology research (Best et al., 2019; Conkin et a;., 2019).

9.4.2. Gas Exchange Efficiency During Exercise

The efficiency of gas exchange during exercise is an important factor in determining overall athletic performance and physiological adaptation. As exercise intensity increases, so does the oxygen demand, which necessitates increased respiratory and circulatory changes. During exercise, the ability of the body to exchange gases, primarily oxygen and carbon dioxide, takes precedence. The respiratory function adjustments—e.g., increased tidal volume and breathing rate—allow for greater oxygen uptake and delivery to contracting muscles. The cardiovascular system also plays a vital role by increasing blood flow and oxygen transmission, thereby maximizing gas exchange efficiency. It has been ascertained through research that properly formatted training protocols can lead to significant gains in VO2 max, a popular parameter of aerobic fitness that represents the metabolism of oxygen by the body during strenuous exercise (Hurst, 2014). Such coordination of respiratory and cardiovascular adjustments is crucial for improved performance and endurance in sportswomen and sportsmen. Besides this, the gas exchange economy can be adjusted depending on the type of exercise. High-intensity interval training (HIIT) has also emerged as an effective strategy not just to enhance aerobic capacity but to optimize gas exchange. Research indicates that shorter, more intense periods of work with recovery intervals can be just as effective as endurance training, but with shorter duration (Hurst, 2014). The strategy maximizes recruitment of muscle fibers as well as elevated mitochondrial density, thus promoting improved utilization of oxygen. It is noteworthy that the physiological adaptation to different training modalities can result in adaptations differing from one another to affect gas exchange efficiency to enable the athlete to perform at their best under different intensities and exercise durations. Additionally, the environment under which exercise takes place has the potential to significantly affect gas exchange efficiency. For example, high-altitude conditions pose special challenges because of lowered oxygen levels, forcing the body to adapt via physiological adaptation to ensure performance levels are maintained. Birds that migrate at high altitudes are a classic example of such an adaptive mechanism, with changes in morphological and kinematic aspects of their flight behavior to ensure optimized performance under thinner air conditions. These changes, while specific to avian physiology, reflect the body's response to altitude in humans, with acclimatization found in elevated red blood cell production and enhanced pulmonary ability. An understanding of the ways in which the environment affects gas exchange is helpful in athlete training at altitude or competing in varied conditions. The studies on these changes inform training methodology and recovery modalities, which ultimately result in improved athletic performance and endurance (Figure 9.13).

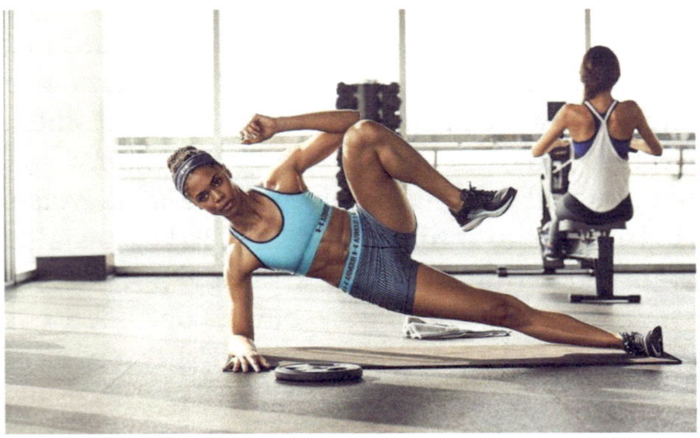

Figure 9.13. High-intensity interval training (HIIT).

Source: https://ocsportsandrehab.com/wp-content/uploads/2022/10/High-Intensity-Interval-Training-1024x643.jpg.

9.4.3. Long-Term Adaptations of the Respiratory System

The long-term adjustments of the respiratory system play a crucial role in facilitating improved overall exercise performance as well as cardiovascular health. A cascade of physiological adjustments follows regular aerobic exercise, specifically enhancing the lung capacity and efficiency. As one participates in prolonged physical activity, one can find a significant rise in tidal volume and respiratory rate to facilitate more oxygen exchange during rest and exercise. This adaptation is particularly important in endurance sports, which predominantly rely upon efficient oxygen utilization to support prolonged efforts. In addition, respiratory muscles like the diaphragm and intercostals hypertrophy from training, causing improved ventilatory endurance. These adjustments not only optimize performance at physical labor but also minimize the risk of respiratory disease, supporting the merit of a healthy lifestyle in attaining long-term respiratory health. As a correlate of enhanced lung function, long-term adjustments within the respiratory system also act to demonstrate improvement in the economy of gas exchange. With frequent exercise training, there is more density of pulmonary capillaries in the vicinity of the alveoli with augmented oxygen diffusion into the bloodstream. The enhanced perfusion with increased alveolar surface area enhances the overall capacity to provide oxygen to exercising muscle. The efficiency of carbon dioxide removal is also improved, since the blood pH adaptations and bicarbonate buffering system enable athletes to exercise for longer at higher intensities without the detrimental effects of acid accumulation. This is noted in studies showing that athletes exhibit lower respiratory rates during sub-maximal exercise levels, as a sign of an optimally adapted respiratory system capable of meeting metabolic demands with less effort (Craig et al., 2015). These adaptations tell us how frequent exercise influences respiratory physiology and general athletic capacity. Besides, respiratory system long-term adaptations highlight the interlinked character of respiratory and metabolic processes with sustained physical activity. Augmented mitochondrial biogenesis, orchestrated by endurance training, also plays a pivotal role outside the context of skeletal muscle endurance; it carries over to increased oxidative capacity in the respiratory system itself. Improved mitochondrial function in respiratory tissues can contribute to more effective energy metabolism, supporting the maintenance of respiratory muscles during prolonged activity. Cooperative effects of training-induced respiratory changes lead to reduced perceived exertion, allowing athletes to uphold higher intensities for longer durations with reduced fatigue effects. This shift not only provides the respiratory system's role in sporting performance but also illustrates the broader health implications of chronic aerobic exercise, highlighting the importance of exercise to achieve maximum oxygen utilization with the passage of time (Hurst, 2014).

Test Your Knowledge

1. How do ventilation rate and tidal volume change during various intensities of exercise?
2. Explain how gas exchange in the lungs adapts to meet increased oxygen demands during exercise.

9.5. Hormonal Responses to Exercise

Learning Outcome

1. Describe the role of hormones in energy metabolism;
2. Define the acute hormonal responses during exercise;
3. Discuss how to chronic adaptations of the endocrine system.

The interaction between exercise and the endocrine response lies at the heart of understanding training adaptations of the physiological responses. The body releases various hormones like epinephrine, norepinephrine, and cortisol during exercise that play critical roles in stress response and energy metabolism. The body's ability to perform at higher levels is increased through acute exercise through the action of these hormones to release energy substrates stored within. This acute reaction redirects metabolic processes to the use of carbohydrates and fats, achieving peak performance levels. Changes in hormonal reactions with habitual exercise over a period can make energy utilization more efficient and decrease fatigue. Enhanced regulation of hormones contributes substantially to increased physical performance and overall training program effectiveness, demonstrating the central role played by endocrine systems in the physiology of exercise. In dealing with the effects of prolonged or excessive training, hormonal responses can be used as markers of possible syndromes of overtraining, which usually manifest both physically and psychologically. Surprisingly, diseases like elevated levels of cortisol are usually associated with overtraining and consequently have negative impacts on performance and recovery. It is characterized by not only physical breakdown but also mood, motivation, and fatigue changes, pointing to the interconnectedness of the endocrine system and central nervous system function. Overtraining has been shown to result in hormonal dysfunctions as well as compromised physiological functioning, which can be reflective of symptoms seen in other stress disorders, for instance, those seen in astronauts undergoing prolonged space travel. Thus, hormonal profile regulation can be an important strategy for overtraining prevention and optimal athletic performance in various conditions (Hackney, 2025).

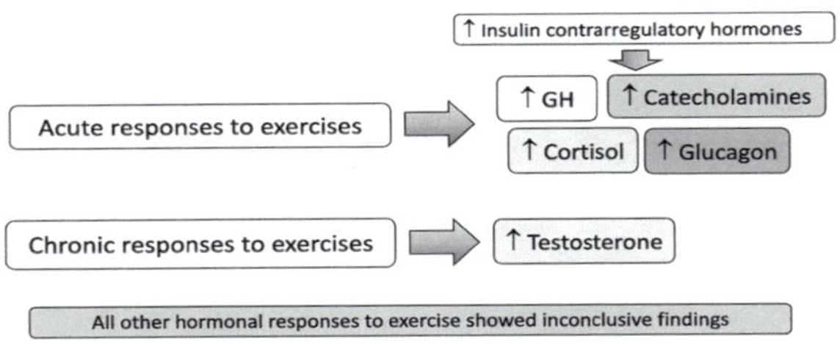

Figure 9.14. Hormonal responses to exercise.

Source: https://www.researchgate.net/publication/336967950/figure/fig1/AS:962817465282562@1606564980917/Current-knowledge-on-hormonal-responses-to-exercises.png.

Knowledge of the endocrine system's exercise response adaptation is essential to design effective training regimens and countermeasures, particularly under specific conditions like microgravity. Musculoskeletal response to weightlessness is a classic illustration of the need for hormonal adaptation to maintain physiological integrity during stress. For instance, the reduction of gravitational loading in flight reduces musculoskeletal function, particularly relevant to knowledge of hormonal responses to exercise as possible countermeasures. Through investigation of the relationship between exercise-induced hormonal adaptation and musculoskeletal adaptation to unloading, scientists expect to find measures for counteracting the negative impact of weightlessness. This can guarantee not only the health of astronauts during flight but also yield information that can be applied to earthly sports performance and rehabilitation (Conkin et al., 2019) (Figure 9.14).

9.5.1. Role of Hormones in Energy Metabolism

The interplay between hormones plays a very crucial role in regulating energy metabolism, particularly during physical activity. The key hormones of insulin, glucagon, and cortisol play a central role in determining the body's energy level and fuel utilization. Insulin released from the pancreas stimulates glucose uptake by muscle cells, increasing glycogen synthesis, which is a finite storage of energy. Conversely, glucagon acts to free energy stores by activating gluconeogenesis in the liver when blood glucose levels are low in order to maintain the body in a state of homeostasis during prolonged activity. Cortisol, a stress hormone, regulates energy metabolism by increasing gluconeogenesis with the added effect of changing fat and protein breakdown to provide energy for exercise. Understanding these hormonal responses lies at the heart of exercise physiology because not only do they impact sport performance, but also training-induced adaptations in metabolic pathways. Adaptation of skeletal muscle to exercise is integrally related to hormonal signaling, where exercise-stimulated hormonal changes are responsible for alterations in metabolism. For instance, exercise has been determined to enhance the metabolic power of skeletal muscle, which equates to improved energy homeostasis. This is partially mediated through the transcriptional regulation of the metabolic enzymes, which is regulated primarily by the class II family of histone deacetylase (HDAC) transcriptional repressors. HDAC5, specifically, plays a critical role in this regard;

its phosphorylation and inhibition by kinases , such as AMPK and protein kinase D increase the expression of genes involved in energy metabolism. As a result, understanding these molecular mechanisms reveals how adaptations in skeletal muscle and hormonal control of exercise are closely related and provide effective energy utilization and enhanced performance through training adaptation (McGee, 2007). Furthermore, dysregulation of hormones can dramatically influence exercise responses and energy metabolism. For instance, conditions like anorexia nervosa (AN) illustrate the ill effects of extreme caloric deprivation on hormone pathways, namely those which regulate energy metabolism and reproductive processes. Abnormalities in the hypothalamic-pituitary-ovarian axis occur in AN women, leading to functional amenorrhea and abnormal reproduction due to endocrine adjustments. These disruptions underscore the significance of endocrine regulation not just for temporary energy metabolism during exercise but also for long-term physiological wellness and steadiness. These sentiments signify the worth of proper nutrition and hormonal balance in effective energy metabolism, particularly in populations engaging in high-intensity sports. Control of these aspects assists in preventing dangers and promoting enhanced exercise physiology and adaptations (Poterasu et al., 2020) (Figure 9.15).

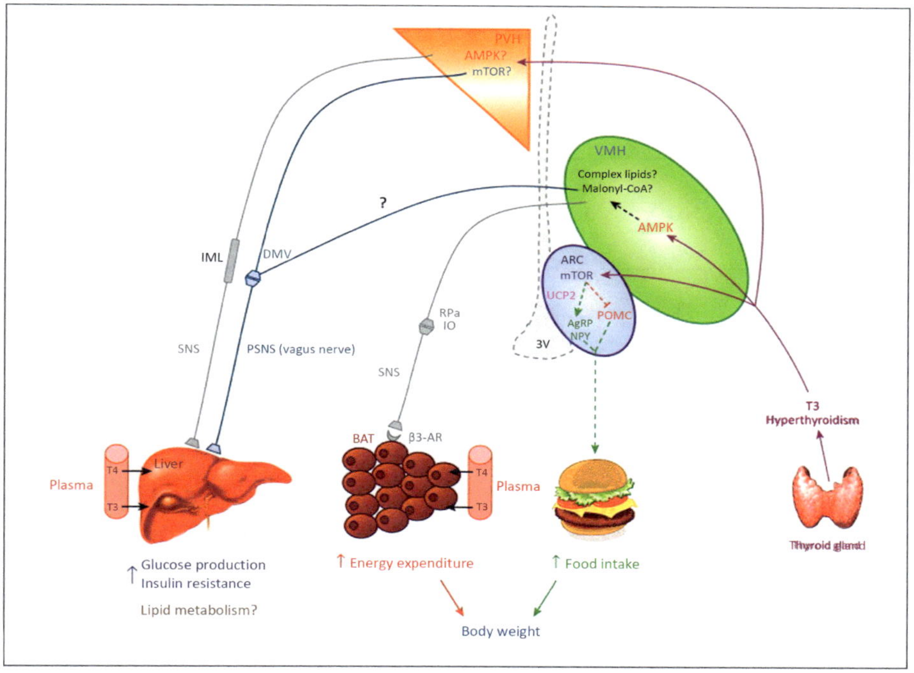

Figure 9.15. Hormones in energy metabolism.

Source: https://www.cell.com/cms/attachment/2007958663/2030600616/gr3.jpg.

9.5.2. Acute Hormonal Responses During Exercise

The acute endocrine responses produced by exercise play an important role in regulating numerous physiological adjustments induced by physical exercise. When the body exercises, the endocrine system responds by secreting hormones , such as cortisol, epinephrine, and norepinephrine, which facilitate energy metabolism, cardiovascular actions, and mobilization of substrates to be used as fuel. With increasing intensity of exercise, the release of such hormones is quicker, facilitating heightened glycogenolysis and lipolysis, significant processes in terms of keeping energy levels steady. In addition, the interaction between such hormones not only facilitates short-term responses to somatic stressors but also lays the groundwork for long-term adaptations in the form of increased muscular strength and endurance. Understanding these hormonal mechanisms is necessary in order to optimize training protocols and enhance athletic performance, thereby emphasizing their relevance to the exercise physiology environment as a whole. In addition to the acute hormonal reactions, hydration status during acute exercise also has an important role in altering the endocrine milieu and physiological load. A short-term heat acclimation study demonstrated that dehydration caused by exercise provided elevated plasma aldosterone levels, which were linearly correlated with plasma volume expansion and thus suggested that fluid management can influence hormonal responses. This response was clearly demonstrated when dehydrated and hydrated conditions were contrasted, illustrating the qualitative relationship between hydration status and regulation through hormones during exercise.

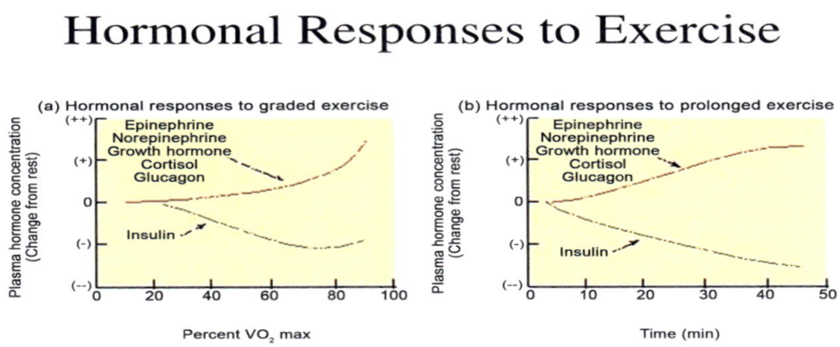

Figure 9.16. Hormonal responses to exercise.

Source: https://image1.slideserve.com/1871051/hormonal-responses-to-exercise1-l.jpg.

These results underscore the importance of hydration strategies for training programs, particularly in athletes performing sustained or high-intensity exercise. Proper hydration can conceivably enable athletes to utilize hormonal mechanisms to improve endurance and overall performance more efficiently and decrease risks associated with dehydration-induced performance impairments (Armstrong et al., 2014). Also, the variation in men's and women's hormonal adaptations to resistance training attests to the intricacies of the gender differences in exercise physiology. Current research has argued that while men tend to record higher absolute strength gains following resistance training, men and women alike exhibit equivalent relative changes in strength. The implication here is one of a shared hormonal adaptive response to resistance training despite differing baseline values. The temporary peak of anabolic hormones, such as, testosterone and growth hormone, following exercise may be the reason for these adaptations, although the extent and effectiveness of these responses may vary between genders. An understanding of these phenomena is important for the development of gender-specific training programs that optimize hormonal responses and muscle adaptation. By tailoring resistance training protocols to specific hormonal responses, practitioners can achieve maximum physical training outcomes in diverse populations, making important contributions to exercise physiology and adaptation science (Bottaro et al., 2016) (Figure 9.16).

9.5.3. Chronic Adaptations of the Endocrine System

The long-term adaptations of the endocrine system due to repeated exercise are comprehensive and multidimensional, acting on a broad range of physiological processes that enhance athletic performance. Through sustained physical activity, the body initiates a cascade of hormonal responses that assist in muscle growth, metabolism, and overall energy homeostasis. Levels of testosterone and HGH rise through resistance training to promote protein synthesis and muscle hypertrophy. Moreover, adrenal cortex acclimatization generates altered cortisol reactions, essential for post-exercise recovery from exercise stress. Endocrine alterations not only optimize metabolic routes for energy generation but also are instrumental in body composition control, vital for an athlete aiming for maximal performance. These endocrine changes illustrate the relevance of training programs with high quality that consider hormonal response, as periodization can optimize such long-term adaptations (Lewis et al., 2015).

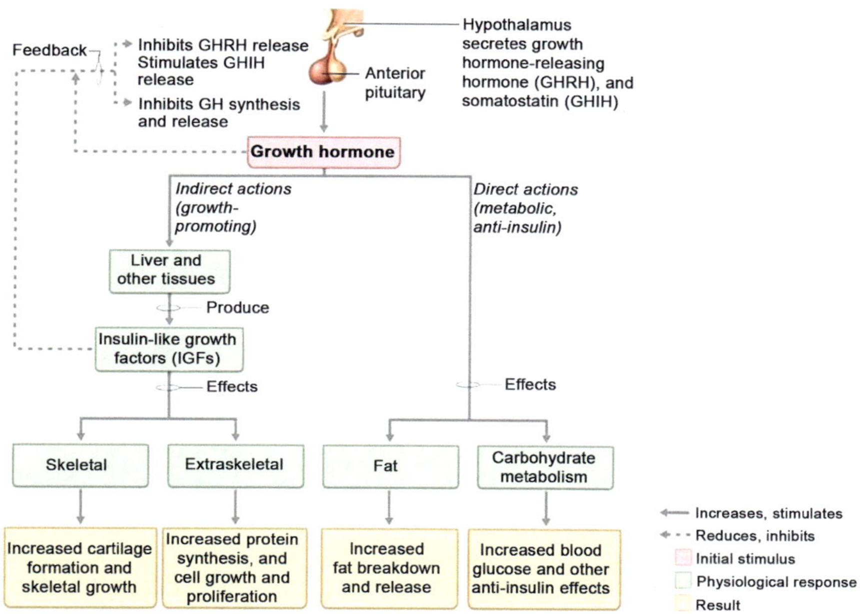

Figure 9.17. Pathophysiology of the endocrine system.

Source: http://image.slidesharecdn.com/endocrine1med2013-130411104108-phpapp01/95/pathophysiology-of-the-endocrine-system-general-adaptation-syndrome-violation-of-hypophysis-and-adrenal-glands-39-638.jpg?cb=1430146359.

Another significant aspect of chronic endocrine adaptations is the relationship between exercise and insulin sensitivity. Regular exercise enhances muscle sensitivity to insulin, facilitating glucose entry and reducing the prevalence of insulin resistance, particularly in avoiding conditions , such as type 2 diabetes. With augmented action of insulin, endurance training produces modifications in the release of glucagon and other hormones involved in glucose control. These systemic adjustments facilitate increased utilization of fat as a substrate for fuel during prolonged exercise. Such adaptation is not limited to high-level athletes; even minimal exercise can precipitate beneficial endocrine adjustments favoring metabolic health. Understanding these mechanisms is significant as it illustrates how exercise on a daily basis enhances glucose homeostasis and overall metabolic health, thereby serving essential public health and disease prevention significance (Carter et al., 2019). Endocrine adaptations of the system also involve alterations in stress hormone profiles, primarily cortisol, that can be favorable or unfavorable depending on the balance of training. Long-term exposure to high cortisol levels, which may be caused by poor recovery or training overloads, can lead to maladaptations , such as the unexplained underperformance syndrome (UUPS). UUPS calls for a comprehensive strategy to training that encompasses recovery as well as training. This is disputed by taking into consideration not only the physiological adaptations but also psychological and environmental factors influencing an athlete's performance. By employing a multidisciplinary approach that incorporates the views of nutrition, physiology, and psychology, athletes, as well as coaches, can design more efficient training programs that steer clear of the risks of chronic stress reactions and maximize endocrine adaptations for improved athletic performance (Lewis et al., 2015) (Figure 9.17).

Test Your Knowledge

1. Which hormones are released during exercise, and what are their primary physiological effects?
2. Describe the roles of insulin and glucagon in regulating blood glucose levels during exercise.

9.6. Factors Influencing Exercise Adaptations

Learning Outcome

1. Describe the genetics and individual variability;
2. Define nutrition and its impact on performance;
3. Describe the training modalities and their effectiveness.

The adaptation process to exercise is regulated by many factors, and each contributes in significant ways to determining the extent to which one adapts for improved physical performance. Among the contributing factors is the type of training stimulus employed. Resistance training, for instance, usually leads to muscle hypertrophy and improved strength through mechanisms , such as muscle fiber recruitment and changes in hormone levels. Specifically, strength-testing exercises , such as weightlifting may maximize testosterone levels, particularly when performed in the morning, as demonstrated through studies using cycling and weight-based regimens in which testosterone trends are decisive for afternoon performances. Therefore, exercise category and timing have significant effects on physiological changes resulting from training schedules, highlighting the fine interaction between exercise type and hormone response in sport participants (McDonald & Maulder, 2018). Individual difference is also a significant determinant of exercise adaptations that include genetic composition, fitness level, and psychological toughness. The aforementioned differences between individuals require individualized training programs that can maximize performance outcomes. For instance, national Under 18 field hockey players were analyzed employing GPS technology to quantify the various demands on players based on their respective positions, indicating how targeted conditioning can be translated into improvements in adaptations. Midfield players had differentiated running demands from strikers, indicating that positional training was important in order to optimize each player's performance potential. These findings emphasize the importance of personalized training interventions and highlight that understanding an athlete's unique physiological and psychological landscape can inform more effective exercise strategies that elicit effective adaptations (Merwe, 2018). Moreover, environmental factors can strongly influence exercise adaptations to contribute to the effectiveness of training, along with the recovery process. Conditions , such as altitude, temperature, and even humidity can all have impacts on the physiological reactions of athletes during exercise, which will subsequently determine adaptation results. Altitude, for example, induces adaptations , such as red blood cell production increases to compensate for reduced oxygen levels and therefore improve aerobic capacity over time. In contrast, the very extreme temperatures can impose stress that would compromise performance and recovery if poorly managed. Lastly, an understanding of environmental demands and exercise adaptation interactions can aid in creating holistic training programs that not only address physiological needs but also permit the ambient conditions players are subjected to while training and competing (Figure 9.18).

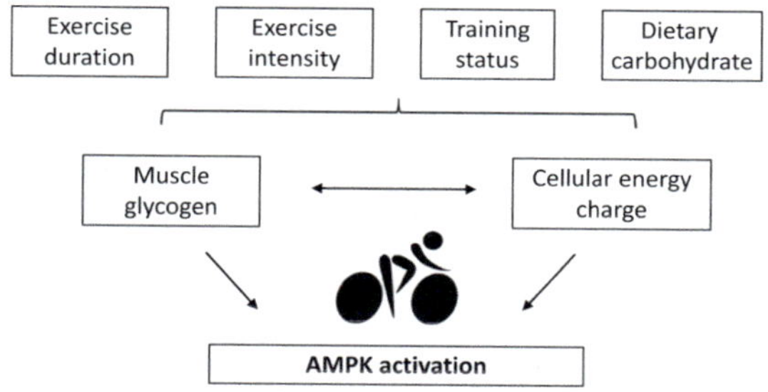

Figure 9.18. Factors influencing endurance training adaptation.

Source: https://external-content.duckduckgo.com/iu/?u=https%3A%2F%2Fwww.eatsleep.fit%2Fwp-content%2Fuploads%2FAMPK-factors-1024x512.png&f=1&nofb=1&ipt=cc3ffb0e6bfa0f788e13af0144b0fe08fdebc98e07a0125912e59f67f6e1c70d.

9.6.1. Genetics and Individual Variability

The study of genetics and intra-person variation has profoundly impacted the understanding of exercise physiology, particularly how individuals respond to training stimuli. Research demonstrates that genetics plays a significant role in much of the variability in adaptation to exercise. Genetics, in turn, can account for up to 50% of the difference in individuals' responses to endurance training in terms of cardiovascular fitness. This genetic influence is important in the regulation of baseline fitness levels, responsiveness to training interventions, and adaptations in general. The identification of individual genetic variation, therefore, emphasizes the importance of individualized training programs that consider these variations, thereby achieving maximum performance and health gains. Additionally, while genetic tendencies have a large amount of control over exercise impacts, methodological factors also have a large amount of contribution to intersubject variability. The parameters of endurance training—type, volume, and intensity—have been found to have a significant effect on individuals' response to exercise. Recent evidence suggests that approximately 20% of individuals might not respond significantly to cardiorespiratory fitness with the conventional training protocols. However, by optimizing training protocols to the physiological ceiling of each individual, investigators have found that elucidates higher rates of response in adaptations in cardiorespiratory fitness. This adaptability underscores the need to integrate individualized training approaches to counterbalance the limitation brought about by genetic variability and enhance physiological adaptation in various populations (Meyler et al., 2021).

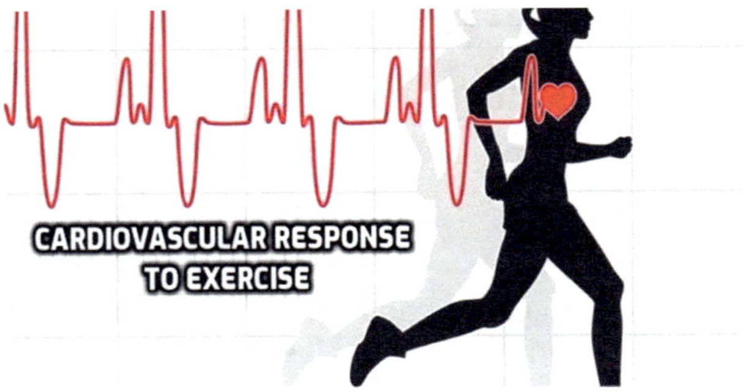

Figure 9.19. Cardiovascular response to exercise.

Source: https://bodybuilding-wizard.com/wp-content/uploads/2019/09/cardiovascular-response-to-exercise-351x185@2x.jpg.

With ongoing advancements in the exercise physiology field, our future research needs to aim at explaining the connection between genetic predispositions and training modalities. It is crucial to know whether increased response rates are primarily achieved as a result of decreased variability or greater mean changes in fitness adaptations. This study may elicit trends in chronic adaptations that may further influence training protocols. It is equally crucial that funding program-supported studies, which include Grant VP1-3.1-ŠMM-07-K-02-057, contribute to further analyzing the interaction between exercise response and genetics. By examining such subtleties, researchers are able to design more efficient, evidence-based exercise programs tailored to an individual's genetics, promoting greater physical function and health in diverse populations (Kvedaras et al., 2017) (Figure 9.19).

9.6.2. Nutrition and Its Impact on Performance

Nutrition is fundamental to athletic performance since it has repercussions on energy, endurance, and recuperation. A balanced meal rich in carbohydrates, proteins, healthy fats, vitamins, and minerals provides the body with the nutrients used by both anaerobic and aerobic energy systems. Carbohydrates, for instance, are the primary fuel for high-intensity effort, and proteins are central in muscle repair and development following effort. Optimizing nutrition's strategic timing can also enhance performance; pre- and post-exercise carbohydrate intake can optimize glycogen replenishment and support accelerated recovery times. As discussed in current research, as their body will adapt to training regimens, so too may their nutritional needs, thus necessitating a tailored dietary strategy approach specific to their individual purposes and physiological adaptations. Recent studies have illuminated the intricate dynamic between nutritional interventions and exercise performance. For example, if components of the OPTIMAL Theory, such as, Enhanced Expectancies and Autonomy Support, were applied while conducting a cycle exercise under simulated altitudes, the participants exhibited clear improvement in performance measures , such as cycling time and wattage output (Ugale, 2019). This indicates that not only do macronutrients play a vital role, but also psychological aspects, on the basis of proper nutrition, influence athletes' belief in their potential and thus enhance performance outcomes. It seems evident that the best system of nutrition, along with motivational strategies, can affect exercise efficacy in a positive way, thereby upholding the significance of meal planning in sports training. Moreover, the mode and timing of nutritional intake could have an impact on hormonal response to performance. A study involving sub-elite track sprint cyclists demonstrated the effect of morning resistance training on testosterone and its influence on subsequent afternoon cycling time trial performance (McDonald & Maulder, 2018). The observation underscores the necessity for exploring macronutrient composition as well as the timing of intake in relation to training modes. Nutritional interventions not only enable physiological adjustments but might also enhance hormonal states conducive to maximal sporting performance. Thus, coaches and athletes must be cognizant of the multi-factorial contribution of nutrition in crafting total training programs maximizing body and mind for competitive sport (Figure 9.20).

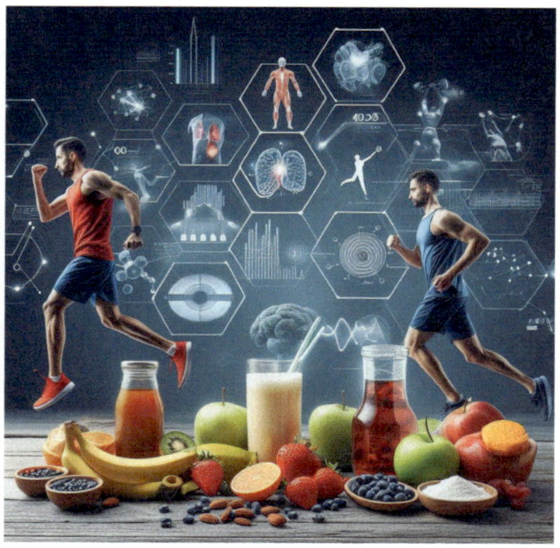

Figure 9.20. Nutrition and its impact on performance.

Source: https://miro.medium.com/v2/resize:fit:1024/0*4_Rc7sgv5hgM2ueg.jpg.

9.6.3. Training Modalities and Their Effectiveness

The effectiveness of training modalities on athletic performance and physiological adaptation improvement is a crucial branch of research in exercise physiology. All training modalities, from resistance training to high-intensity interval training, promote different adaptations, which can influence the abilities of an athlete. For instance, resistance training, which includes isotonic and isometric exercises, is primarily focused on muscular strength and power enhancement. But in recent studies, it was found that alterations in contraction velocity greatly affect power production, illustrating that explosive movements can create greater performance benefits in sports requiring sudden energy bursts. The evaluation of these different training protocols is significant as it contributes to the tailoring of programs to fulfill the distinct needs of the athlete, thus maximizing training efficacy and efficiency and complementing any documented performance gaps in literature (Brenneman et al., 2016). In contrast to traditional endurance training, SIT has gained popularity due to its time efficiency and efficacy for improving aerobic capacity. Experiments demonstrate SIT can cause physiological adaptations consistent with those achieved with longer, more conventional endurance training regimens. SIT works on the repeated episodes of exhaustive effort with recovery or submaximal exercise to challenge the body's metabolic systems. Of significant importance is the fact that it was established that a comparison of SIT and endurance training provided considerable elevations in cardiovascular indexes, such as, resting blood pressure and heart rate, speculating that SIT might be a viable substitute for time-scarce athletes. Not only does this technique enhance aerobic performance, but it also maximizes significant health indicators, stating that strategic modality combinations during training can optimize overall athletic function (Hurst, 2014). The study of mixed training modalities, such as, pairs of endurance and sprint interval training, is an interesting new field of exercise physiology. It has been theorized that by combining different modes of training, synergistic effects may occur and produce more effective adaptation than single modality treatments. For example, when a recent study was conducted, the subjects participating in a combined mode of training demonstrated significant increases in both aerobic power and muscular endurance than individuals who trained in a single modality. Varying the training stimuli enables sportsmen to experience more neuro-muscular coordination and economy of metabolism. Thus, identifying the interconnected nature of different training modalities improves an athlete's schedule as well as puts more focus on employing a multi-method approach towards training in an attempt to thrive and improve health gains (Hurst, 2014; Brenneman et al., 2016).

Test Your Knowledge

1. How do age, gender, and genetics influence an individual's response to exercise training?
2. What role does nutrition play in enhancing or limiting exercise-induced physiological adaptations?

SUMMARY

Exercise physiology and adaptation research reveal that various training modalities have powerful influences on physiological outcomes and increases in performance. Sprint Interval Training (SIT), for instance, has been reported to elicit aerobic capacity adaptations comparable to standard Endurance Training (ET) but requiring much less time commitment. This efficiency is critical with the busy lifestyle of today, wherein maximizing exercise return within a limited time is often the objective for individuals who are engaging in exercise programs. Knowing, then, the interplay among different training types is crucial in stressing the importance of maximizing exercise prescriptions for personal goals in health and functional capacity. As demonstrated through research, the inclusion of SIT in training programs has been found to contribute significantly to major cardiovascular health indicators, confirming that finely targeted, high-intensity sessions can be life-altering for individuals from all age groups (Hurst, 2014). Additionally, the application of high-intensity interval training tenets challenges traditional notions regarding endurance exercises by demonstrating that long-duration, high-intensity efforts are capable of generating exemplary physiological adaptations. The speed-tolerable duration (S-tLIM) relationship is educative with regard to how individuals can make efficient travels and break thresholds of exertion during training. By normalizing training intensity in terms of intervals, work capacity can be enhanced and adaptative reactions beneficial for improved performance can be triggered. The findings of studies on fixed workload HIIT and maximal HIIT protocols suggest that well-designed sessions can be a source of relatively large improvements not only in the athletic performance of individuals but also in several measures of health, such as, blood pressure and metabolic markers (Ferguson et al., 2013). Thus, the appropriate application of the above techniques overcomes the challenges typically encountered by traditional techniques. Overall, this analysis of exercise physiology and resulting adaptations of training modes of exercise underscores the value of scientifically driven and individually adapted fitness. The synthesis of SIT and ET as interval training protocols provides valuable information for creating efficient workout plans that respond to the individual. Athletic trainers, coaches, and recreational athletes may use this information to improve physical capabilities while also addressing health challenges. More research needs to to explore the physiological implications of combined training techniques, ultimately enhancing our understanding and exercise science implementation. Thus, the evolution in exercise methods continues to yield superior benefits on health and performance, reaffirming that strategic shifts in training can yield precious payoffs for a wide range of individuals looking to enhance their physical well-being (Ferguson et al., 2013; Hurst, 2014). Exercise physiology research reveals valuable knowledge of how the body reacts to various forms of training and, in turn, improves overall performance and well-being. One such discovery demonstrates the efficacy of SIT compared to traditional ET. Research indicates that SIT can evoke equivalent improvements in aerobic capacity and thus suggests that time-efficient approaches , such as these, can effectively augment physical work capacity and initiate good adaptations. As noted in studies, the incorporation of SIT in training protocols allows one to achieve significant physiological adaptations, such as, increased oxygen use and cardiovascular performance, offering a useful alternative for individuals with limited time to devote to exercise (Hurst, 2014). Moreover, the intricacy of strength training further underlines the importance of individualized exercise protocols. Nautilus Sports/Medical Industries owner Arthur Jones advocated for some training techniques for maximizing muscular growth through intense focus , such as training to volitional fatigue. In opposition to conventional norms, which recommend multiple sets and programs, the Jones method indicates that performing a single set on a particular exercise can be sufficient to allow for dramatic increases in strength and power. This perspective counters traditional training ideologies and highlights the need for functional methods that yield effective results in both athletic and non-athletic groups (Smith & Bruce-Low, 2004). Ultimately, the compounded evidence concerning training modalities illustrates the interaction of exercise type and variation of response. The findings report that a combined training program, incorporating both endurance training and strength training elements, may be more advantageous to health in the long term. The test subjects exhibited significantly better key physiological variables, including resting heart rate and blood pressure, through a varied range of training programs emphasizing aerobic and anaerobic conditioning equally. These results confirm the plasticity of the human body since they validate the proposition that particular training methodologies will bring about significant changes in indicators of health, emphasizing the role of exercise physiology in developing appropriate fitness programs (Hurst, 2014).

KEY TERMS FROM THIS CHAPTER

- Aerobic metabolism
- Anaerobic metabolism
- Capillarization
- Cardiac output
- Endurance training
- Heat acclimatization
- Hormonal responses
- Lactic acid
- Mitochondrial biogenesis
- Muscle fatigue
- Muscle hypertrophy
- Neuromuscular adaptations
- Oxygen debt
- Respiratory rate
- Strength training
- Stroke volume
- Type I muscle fibers (slow-twitch)
- Type II muscle fibers (fast-twitch)

CRITICAL THINKING QUESTIONS

1. **What does VO2 max measure?**
   a. Maximum heart rate during exercise
   b. Maximum oxygen uptake during intense exercise
   c. Maximum strength of muscles
   d. Maximum lactate production
2. **Which energy system provides immediate energy for high-intensity, short-duration exercise (about 10 seconds)?**
   a. Aerobic glycolysis
   b. Oxidative phosphorylation
   c. ATP-PCr (phosphocreatine) system
   d. Anaerobic glycolysis
3. **What is a common cardiovascular adaptation to regular endurance training?**
   a. Increased resting heart rate
   b. Decreased stroke volume
   c. Increased capillary density in muscles
   d. Decreased blood volume
4. **During intense exercise, lactic acid is produced primarily due to:**
   a. Aerobic metabolism
   b. Anaerobic glycolysis
   c. Oxidative phosphorylation
   d. Fat metabolism
5. **How does regular aerobic exercise typically affect resting heart rate?**
   a. It increases resting heart rate
   b. It decreases resting heart rate
   c. It has no effect on resting heart rate
   d. It causes irregular heart rate

Short Answer Questions

1. What is VO2 max and why is it important in exercise physiology?
2. Define anaerobic and aerobic metabolism.
3. Name two major cardiovascular adaptations to regular endurance training.
4. What role does lactic acid play during intense exercise?
5. How does regular exercise affect resting heart rate?
6. Describe the physiological mechanisms behind muscle fatigue and recovery.
7. Explain how resistance training leads to muscle hypertrophy and strength gains.
8. Discuss the acute and chronic hormonal responses to exercise.
9. Describe the role of heat production and thermoregulation during exercise.
10. Write the effects of exercise on body composition and metabolic health.

Answers to Critical Thinking Questions

1. (b); 2. (c); 3. (c); 4. (b); 5. (b).

REFERENCES

1. Conkin, J., Downs, M., et al. (2019). Evidence-based approach to establish space suit carbon dioxide limits. NASA/TP-2019-220202 https://core.ac.uk/download/pdf/323104209.pdf (accessed on 28th June 2025).
2. Craig, D. M., Ashcroft, S. P., Belew, M. Y., Stocks, B., Currell, K., Baar, K., & Philp, A. (2015). Utilizing small nutrient compounds as enhancers of exercise-induced mitochondrial biogenesis. *Frontiers in physiology*, *6*, 296. https://doi.org/10.3389/fphys.2015.00296(accessed on 28th June 2025).
3. Liang, J. N., Lee, Y. J., Akoopie, E., Kleven, B. C., Koch, T., & Ho, K. Y. (2019). Impaired H-Reflex Adaptations Following Slope Walking in Individuals With Post-stroke Hemiparesis. *Frontiers in physiology*, *10*, 1232. https://doi.org/10.3389/fphys.2019.01232(accessed on 28th June 2025).
4. Alkhatib, A. (2017). Exercise intensity for health and sports performance: Recent updates. https://core.ac.uk/download/322335862.pdf (accessed on 28th June 2025).
5. Altshuler, D. L., & Dudley, R. (2006). The physiology and biomechanics of avian flight at high altitude. https://core.ac.uk/download/4887664.pdf (accessed on 28th June 2025).
6. Meyler, S., Bottoms, L., & Muniz-Pumares, D. (2021). Biological and methodological factors affecting V̇O2max response variability to endurance training and the influence of exercise intensity prescription. *Experimental physiology*, *106*(7), 1410–1424. https://doi.org/10.1113/EP089565 (accessed on 28th June 2025).
7. Armstrong, L. E., Armstrong, N., Ashenden, M., Bergeron, M. F., Borg, G., Brandenberger, G., Brandenberger, G., et al. (2014). Short-term heat acclimation is effective and may be enhanced rather than impaired by dehydration. https://core.ac.uk/download/151156551.pdf (accessed on 28th June 2025).
8. Baggish, A., Biffi, A., Bossone, E., Castelletti, S., Cavarretta, E., Cavigli, L., D'Andrea, A., et al. (2023). Athlete's heart: A cardiovascular step-by-step multimodality approach. https://core.ac.uk/download/622823217.pdf (accessed on 28th June 2025).
9. Russ Best, Martin Barwood , Jason Gillis, Owen Jeffriese(2019). Oral application of L-menthol in the heat: From pleasure to performance. The 18th International Conference on Environmental Ergonomics ICEE2019 (accessed on 28th June 2025).
10. Drury, B., Ratel, S., Clark, C. C. T., Fernandes, J. F. T., Moran, J., & Behm, D. G. (2019). Eccentric Resistance Training in Youth: Perspectives for Long-Term Athletic Development. *Journal of functional morphology and kinesiology*, *4*(4), 70. https://doi.org/10.3390/jfmk4040070(accessed on 28th June 2025).
11. Bottaro, M., Castanheira, R. P. M., Gentil, P., Paoli, A., et al. (2016). Comparison of upper body strength gains between men and women after 10 weeks of resistance training. https://core.ac.uk/download/53528349.pdf (accessed on 28th June 2025).
12. Brenneman, M. T. (2016). Training for muscular power adaptations: The role of contraction type and velocity. https://core.ac.uk/download/211333301.pdf (accessed on 28th June 2025).
13. Smith D, BruceLow S. JEP (2004). Strength training methods and the work of Arthur Jones. Journal of Exercise Physiology 2004;7(6):52-68..
14. Carter, C. S., Justice, J. N., & Thompson, L. (2019). Lipotoxicity, aging, and muscle contractility: Does fiber type matter? https://open.bu.edu/bitstream/2144/40625/7/carter_justice_thompson_Lipotoxicity_paper_04302019.pdf (accessed on 28th June 2025).

15. Poterasu, M., Rowland, D. L., Ciobanu, C., & Fica, S. (2020). Anorexia Nervosa and Reproduction: Connecting Brain to Gonads. *Journal of Mind and Medical Sciences*, *7*(1), 1-8. https://doi.org/10.22543/7674.71.P18 (accessed on 28th June 2025).

16. Lewis, N. A., Collins, D., Pedlar, C. R., & Rogers, J. P. (2015). Can clinicians and scientists explain and prevent unexplained underperformance syndrome in elite athletes: an interdisciplinary perspective and 2016 update. *BMJ open sport & exercise medicine*, *1*(1), e000063. https://doi.org/10.1136/bmjsem-2015-000063(accessed on 28th June 2025).

17. Minett, G. M., & Costello, J. T. (2015). Specificity and context in post-exercise recovery: it is not a one-size-fits-all approach. *Frontiers in physiology*, *6*, 130. https://doi.org/10.3389/fphys.2015.00130(accessed on 28th June 2025).

18. Dickson, K. J., Hess, E. L., Powers, J. V., Wallace-Robinson, J., et al. (2025). Publications of the space physiology and countermeasures program, Musculoskeletal Discipline: 1980–1990. https://core.ac.uk/download/pdf/42810681.pdf (accessed on 28th June 2025).

19. Graber, T. G., Fandrey, K. R., & Thompson, L. V. (2019). Novel individualized power training protocol preserves physical function in adult and older mice. *GeroScience*, *41*(2), 165–183. https://doi.org/10.1007/s11357-019-00069-z (accessed on 28th June 2025).

20. Kvedaras, M., Minderis, P., Fokin, A., Ratkevicius, A., Venckunas, T., & Lionikas, A. (2017). Forced Running Endurance Is Influenced by Gene(s) on Mouse Chromosome 10. *Frontiers in physiology*, *8*, 9. https://doi.org/10.3389/fphys.2017.00009(accessed on 28th June 2025).

21. Hackney, A. C. (2025). Overtraining and exercise motivation: A research prospectus. https://core.ac.uk/download/pdf/42823203.pdf (accessed on 28th June 2025).

22. McGuire, S., Horton, E. J., Renshaw, D., Jimenez, A., Krishnan, N., & McGregor, G. (2018). Hemodynamic Instability during Dialysis: The Potential Role of Intradialytic Exercise. *BioMed research international*, *2018*, 8276912. https://doi.org/10.1155/2018/8276912(accessed on 28th June 2025).

23. Hurst, R. A. (2014). The effects and differences of sprint interval training, endurance training and the training types combined on physiological parameters and exercise performance. https://core.ac.uk/download/29841767.pdf (accessed on 28th June 2025).

24. Koutedakis, Y., & Jamurtas, A. (2004). The dancer as a performing athlete: physiological considerations. *Sports medicine (Auckland, N.Z.)*, *34*(10), 651–661. https://doi.org/10.2165/00007256-200434100-00003(accessed on 28th June 2025).

25. McDonald, K. & Maulder, P. S. (2018). The effects of morning preconditioning protocols on testosterone, cortisol and afternoon sprint cycling performance [conference presentation]. Annual Conference, 26-27 October 2018 Otago Museum, Dunedin https://core.ac.uk/download/187724674.pdf (accessed on 28th June 2025).

26. McGee, S. L. (2007). Exercise and MEF2–HDAC interactions. http://hdl.handle.net/10536/DRO/DU:30025017 (accessed on 28th June 2025).

27. Ferguson C, Wilson J, Birch KM, Kemi OJ (2013) Application of the Speed-Duration Relationship to Normalize the Intensity of High-Intensity Interval Training. PLoS ONE 8(11): e76420. https://doi.org/10.1371/journal.pone.0076420 (accessed on 28th June 2025).

28. Ugale, C. B. (2019). Optimizing cycle exercise performance during normobaric hypoxia exposure. https://digitalscholarship.unlv.edu/cgi/viewcontent.cgi?article=4697&context=th

esesdissertations (accessed on 28th June 2025).

29. Van der Merwe, F. H. (2018). GPS analysis of a team competing at a national under 18 field hockey tournaments. https://core.ac.uk/download/187724717.pdf (accessed on 28th June 2025).

30. Yanes, B. L. (2019). Periodization for massive strength gains. https://core.ac.uk/download/286697632.pdf (accessed on 28th June 2025).

NEUROENDOCRINE INTEGRATION AND STRESS RESPONSE IN PHYSIOLOGY

10

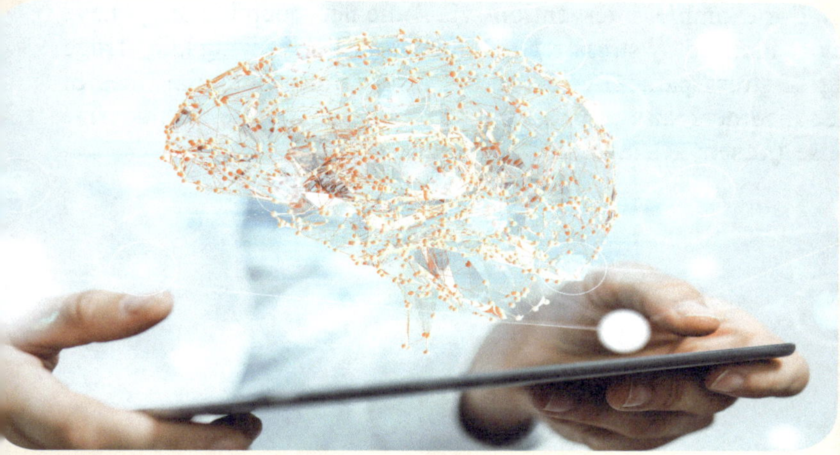

LEARNING OBJECTIVES

After studying this chapter, you will be able to:

1. Understand the neuroendocrine system.
2. Explain the functions of the cell membrane.
3. Discuss the mechanisms of stress response.
4. Identify the effects of chronic stress.
5. Determine the neurotransmitters and hormones in stress.
6. Evaluate the coping mechanisms and stress management.

Introduction

The intricate interaction of the neuroendocrine system with the physiological stress response has been of great concern in physiological research. This interaction is marked by a complex reciprocal relationship between hormones, neurotransmitters, and a variety of physiological systems combining to regulate adaptive responses to stress. Notably, the hypothalamic-pituitary-adrenal (HPA) axis is central to this system, regulating the release of stress hormones , such as cortisol. Disruptions along this axis may yield a range of physiological and psychological disorders, and as such underscores the necessity for an integrated understanding of neuroendocrine integration responding to stress. This introduction sets the stage for the discussion of how these biological underpinnings influence functional outcomes of health and illness, particularly in cases where stressors overwhelm biological capacity and yield maladaptive processes. As another elucidation of the neuroendocrine integration process, recent studies have given increased attention to metabolic and structural changes as a response to some stressors, e.g., drought in plants.

To illustrate, research on sainfoin (Onobrychis viciaefolia) shows that resistance against drought stress leads to extensive anatomical and physiological modifications in leaves of plants. The assessment of drought-resistant lines indicates that anatomical features, such as, increased epidermal and palisade tissue thickness, relate to lower levels of reactive oxygen species and increased protection metabolites. By demonstrating the physiological adaptation to environmental stressors, this research belongs to the broad subject of learning about adaptation mechanisms in other organisms exposed to stress, emphasizing the necessity of an integrated strategy for neuroendocrine response in other biological systems (Yao et al., 2024). The modulatory function of neuropeptides in stress response also emphasizes the significance of neuroendocrine regulation. Recent findings reveal corticoliberin, as a primary neuropeptide, to be a key regulator of the HPA axis in controlling the synthesis of adrenal hormones during stress. Studies on neuropeptides' influence on corticotropin-releasing hormone and corticosterone levels have demonstrated them to reverse stress-induced disruptions. For example, interventions via some neuropeptide drugs have successfully inhibited hormonal hyperactivity induced by stress-related illnesses. This growing knowledge base not only clarifies our understanding of stress pathophysiology but also defines potential lines of therapy for the modulation of stress-related disorders, and emphasizes the requirement of neuroendocrine integration in physiological stress response (Yasenyavskaya, 2024) (Figure 10.1).

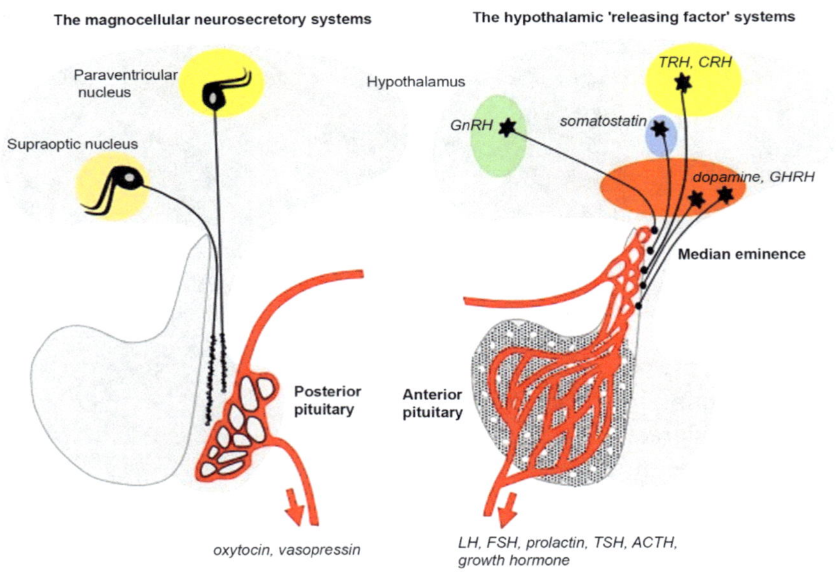

Figure 10.1. Neuroendocrine System.

Source: https://ars.els-cdn.com/content/image/1-s2.0-S0025556418302578-gr1.jpg.

Definition of Neuroendocrine Integration

Neuroendocrine integration plays a key concept in the coordination of nervous and endocrine systems to regulate physiological reactions, particularly under stress. Neuroendocrine integration is the coordination of the brain neurons with the endocrine glands that secrete hormones into the blood. Neuroendocrine integration allows the body to attain homeostasis under various physical and psychological stresses. For instance, following a stressor, the hypothalamus releases corticotropin-releasing hormone (CRH), which stimulates the anterior pituitary gland to release adrenocorticotropic hormone (ACTH). The sequence ultimately results in secretion of cortisol by the adrenal cortex, a critical hormone facilitating mobilization of energy and control of immune responses (Sies et al., 2017). Thus, integration of the neuroendocrine is a necessary avenue through which the body reacts to stress in a manner that assures both short-term and long-term stability at the physiological level. Integration between neuroendocrine systems is also necessary to modulate the body's redox state, or oxidation to reduction reactions ratios at the cellular level. Oxidative stress, if not regulated, can lead to cell damage; however, the neuroendocrine response is also responsible for managing this balance through redox signaling pathways. Current evidence suggests the role of oxidative eustress, where minor oxidative provocation can enhance redox signaling and promote resilience in physiological processes (Sies et al., 2017). Neuroendocrine integration, therefore, not only involves stress responses but also the control of redox states by molecular means, impacting cellular function and health. It is, therefore, important to understand neuroendocrine integration in physiological and pathological processes, particularly how the body would respond to stressors. The influence of neuroendocrine integration extends beyond the immediate modulation of stress; it also has a vital bearing on long-term health effects. Dysregulation of neuroendocrine mechanisms can lead to chronic stress, which is linked to various health disorders, including metabolic disorders and cardiovascular diseases. For instance, prolonged elevation of cortisol can result in metabolic changes, while dysregulation of stress responses can have negative impacts on cognition and mood (Lovallo, 2016). From the study of the mechanisms of neuroendocrine integration, researchers can gain insights into prevention and treatment of stress-related conditions. This convergent perspective highlights interdisciplinary approaches to understanding the interactions between the nervous system, endocrine function, and the body's stress response, offering possible integrative strategies for facilitation of resilience and overall health in the context of chronic stressors (Figure 10.2).

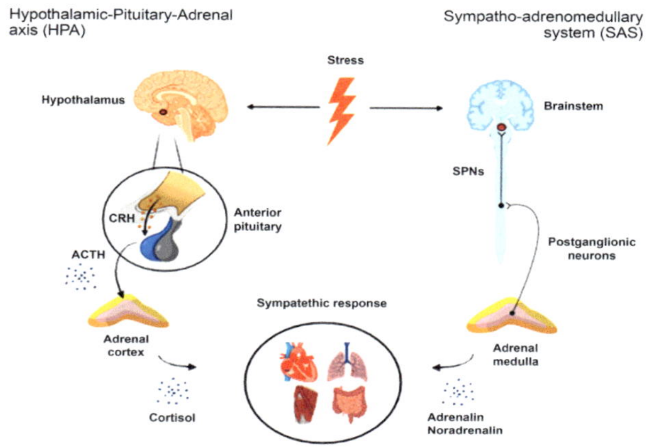

Figure 10.2. Stress adaptation and the brainstem with focus on corticotropin-releasing hormone.

Source: https://www.mdpi.com/ijms/ijms-22-09090/article_deploy/html/images/ijms-22-09090-g001.png.

Importance of Stress Response in Physiology

Stress response is a critical physiological mechanism that allows organisms to respond to environmental stressors and maintain homeostasis. Controlled centrally by the hypothalamic-pituitary-adrenal (HPA) axis, it controls the release of glucocorticoids, led by cortisol, in reaction to stress. Corticotropin-releasing hormone (CRH) plays a critical role in initiating this cascade of hormone release, both in the HPA axis and in extrahypothalamic pathways, to modulate behavioral consequences. Significantly, the identification of CRH signaling, particularly through its G protein-coupled receptors, has provided insight into how the organism organizes adaptive reactions to stress at the cellular and molecular levels. This information is essential for the development of therapeutic interventions aimed at mitigating the detrimental effects of chronic stress on health and thus emphasizing the significance of the stress response to overall physiological function (Inda et al., 2017). The impact of stress extends beyond short-term physiology to long-term well-being and health. Chronic stress can also lead to pathophysiological conditions like anxiety disorders and metabolic syndromes due to the continuous activation of the stress response. Recent studies have established that chronic stress can alter neural circuits involved in emotional regulation and social behavior, thereby making individuals vulnerable to psychiatric illnesses. The case of the linkage between social vigilance and stress illustrates how adaptive behaviors in situations that are chronic in nature can result in maladaptive outcomes. With the complexity of social environments growing, the prevalence of stress-related disorders rises, with a focus on developmental stages , such as adolescence. It is important to possess knowledge regarding the neuroendocrine integration of stress responses at such pivotal moments for reasons of effective prevention and treatment (Wright et al., 2020). The neuroendocrine stress response also highlights the interactive sophistication between internal physiological mechanisms and external stimuli. As the body is subjected to stressors, hormonal messengers like adrenaline and cortisol not only activate physiological systems for immediate response but also shape behavioral responses through routes in neural circuitry. This integration enables vital adaptations, like a rapid heart rate and enhanced alertness, to help survival in adverse circumstances. But two-edged aspects of these reactions—protective as well as risky—indicate the value of fine-tuning. Disruption of such signaling mechanisms can lead to maladaptive stress responses that make significant contributions to numerous diseases , such as chronic inflammation and mood disorders. The understanding of the physiological meaning of the stress responses thus fosters a global dialogue of its function towards guaranteeing short-term adaptation as well as long-term resistance to health (Inda et al., 2017).

10.1. The Neuroendocrine System

Learning Outcome

1. Describe the components of the neuroendocrine system;
2. Focus on the role of the hypothalamus;
3. Learn about the interaction between the nervous and endocrine systems.

The neuroendocrine system plays a key role in maintaining homeostasis within the body, particularly in response to stressors. It is a complex system that includes interaction between the nervous system and the endocrine glands in order to facilitate immediate responses to internal and external stimuli. The hypothalamic-pituitary-adrenal (HPA) axis is one of the primary components of the system, which regulates the production of stress hormones like cortisol. When exposed to stress, the hypothalamus releases corticotropin-releasing hormone (CRH) that stimulates the pituitary gland to release adrenocorticotropic hormone (ACTH). ACTH stimulates the adrenal glands to release cortisol, facilitating various physiological adaptations in stress coping. This neuroendocrine coordination is necessary to study the function of hormonal regulation of acute and chronic stress responses and their implications for overall health and well-being. Dysregulation of the neuroendocrine axis under conditions of early adversity has significant long-term effects on stress response. It has been found that adversity in early life may alter the functioning of the HPA axis, leading to chronic changes in stress reactivity and susceptibility to mental illness. Specifically, extended separation of rodents from mothers has shown that prolonged stress can lead to an overactive adrenal response, causing heightened corticosterone levels—the rodent version of cortisol. Conversely, brief separations appear to foster resilience, as evidenced by a blunted adrenal response to stress. Thus, the neuroendocrine system is not only crucial in stress coping in the instant but is also a key contributor to a person's susceptibility or resistance toward stress-related disorders in the future (Rivarola & Renard, 2014). During stress, the CRH-mediated signaling pathways are of greater significance. CRH acts as a neuromodulator in both hypothalamic and extrahypothalamic circuits, regulating adaptive endocrine and behavioral responses to stress. The binding of CRH to its G protein-coupled receptors (GPCRs), CRHR1 and CRHR2, triggers a cascade of intracellular signaling that brings about a variety of physiological responses. Recent findings have documented other CRH signaling nuances, such as, new mechanistic processes involved in the generation of cAMP and ERK1/2 activation that are pivotal in mediating the adaptive reactions of the body to stress. Knowledge of these pathways is critical in discovering potential pharmacological treatments for the neuroendocrine system to counteract the consequences of stress-related diseases, ultimately advancing therapeutic approaches (Inda et al., 2017) (Figure 10.3).

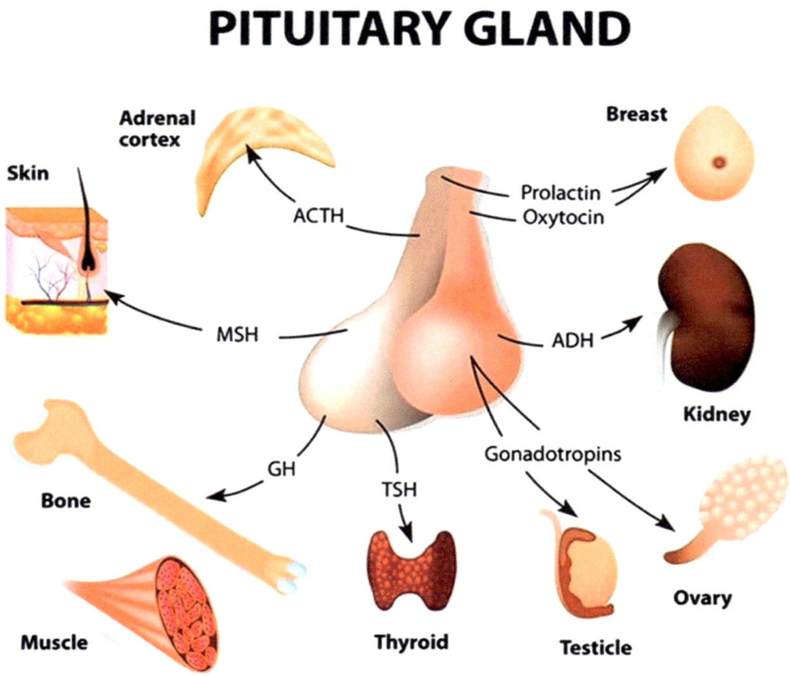

Figure 10.3. Pituitary gland hormones and functions.

Source: https://www.news-medical.net/image-handler/picture/2018/5/shutterstock_189972851.jpg.

10.1.1. Components of the Neuroendocrine System

In demystifying the components of the neuroendocrine system, one needs to consider the intricate dynamics of the hypothalamic-pituitary-adrenal (HPA) axis, an important regulatory pathway for stress response. At the core of this axis is corticotropin-releasing hormone (CRH), which initiates the stress response by stimulating the anterior pituitary gland to release adrenocorticotropic hormone (ACTH), which subsequently induces the adrenal cortex to release glucocorticoids, spearheaded by cortisol. Besides its classical role in the HPA axis, CRH is involved in a number of extrahypothalamic pathways where it functions as a neuromodulator to influence behavioral and physiological responses to stress. Experiments have indicated that the signaling by CRH might be more complex than was initially thought, establishing important molecular components and cell processes , such as G protein-coupled receptor activation and subsequent processes like cAMP generation and ERK1/2 activation, confirming its critical relevance in neuroendocrine function (Inda et al., 2017). The neuroendocrine system also includes the convergence of immune responses, as in the emerging idea of immune-neuroendocrine phenotypes (INPs). Immune-neuroendocrine heterogeneity across populations has gained increasing attention, with researchers laying out certain INP profiles that are able to influence the response to stressors. For instance, findings from avian research, that of domestic hens, indicate that chronic stress can affect the profile of these INP profiles such that it skews the balance between innate and adaptive immune response. This immunoneuroendocrine modulation reflects a sophisticated adaptability within the system in that even under selective pressure, populations are capable of a multi-aspect response to environmental pressures. These findings emphasize the cross-talk between immune response and stress, suggesting that the neuroendocrine system is not only a regulating mechanism but also an active participant in physiological resilience (Nazar et al., 2017). Furthermore, research on the neuroendocrine axis illustrates its intricate role in regulating both stress responses and metabolic homeostasis. Some of the other important factors are the thyroid gland, which releases hormones that influence metabolic activity, and the pancreas, which regulates blood glucose levels through the release of insulin and glucagon. All of these factors combined are involved in an organism's response to external and internal stressors. Their effects are profound, as they not only respond to CRH signals but also play a part in its effect. For instance, chronic stress can initiate dysregulation of thyroid function, worsening the metabolic problems and making the response to stress more complicated. Appreciation of these integrated factors is necessary in order to realize the integrative nature of the neuroendocrine system, as they together orchestrate the physiological stress responses, underscoring the fine-tuning required for health and homeostasis (Figure 10.4).

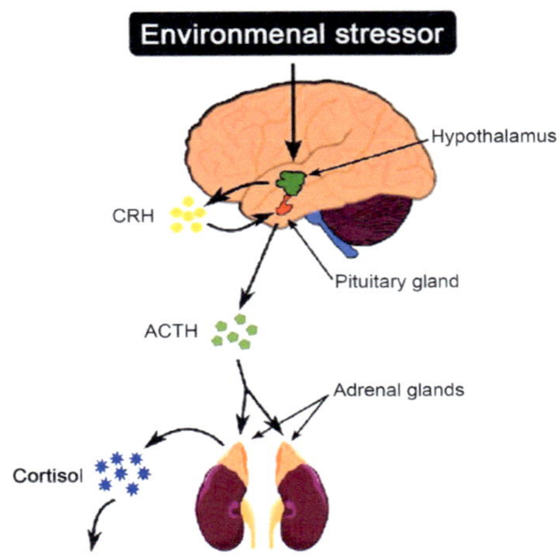

Figure 10.4. Hypothalamic-pituitary-adrenal (HPA) axis.

Source: https://www.researchgate.net/profile/Pierrich-Plusquellec/publication/261951085/figure/fig1/AS:614264893100046@1523463571394/Hypothalamic-pituitary-adrenal-HPA-axis-Experiencing-an-environmental-stressor-as.png.

10.1.2. Role of the Hypothalamus

The hypothalamus plays an important role in neuroendocrine integration by acting as an essential link between the endocrine system and the nervous system and thereby regulating various physiological reactions to stress. The small but complex structure is located at the base of the brain and comprises several nuclei, one of which is the paraventricular nucleus and its role in initiating the stress response. Under stressors, hypothalamic neurons release corticotropin-releasing hormone (CRH) into circulation, which in turn stimulates the anterior pituitary gland to release adrenocorticotropic hormone (ACTH). This is achieved through a process that activates the hypothalamic-pituitary-adrenal (HPA) axis, leading to the release of adrenal cortex glucocorticoids, which control metabolism, immunity, and behavior during stress, further entrenching the role of the hypothalamus in playing a pivotal role in homeostasis under stress (Sukhareva, 2021). Beyond the integration of neuroendocrine signals, the hypothalamus also coordinates autonomic and behavioral responses through its intricate neural circuitry. The extrahypothalamic brain areas where CRH is found emphasize the ubiquitous influence of the neuropeptide beyond the traditional HPA axis. These regions are concerned with the modulation of emotional and behavioral reactions required for survival. For instance, the CRH action at its specific receptors assists in the modulation of numerous mediator systems for stress-related behaviors like anxiety and fear reactions. Dysregulation of the CRH system can result in pathological conditions like anxiety disorders and depression, illustrating the importance of the hypothalamus for physiological functions and stress-related mental illness pathophysiology (Sukhareva, 2021). At a more general level, neuroendocrine mechanisms in the stress response are studied beyond mammals, with informative data presented by comparative studies of physiology. This study reveals that teleost fish, like terrestrial vertebrates, possess equivalent neuroendocrine mechanisms to confront stress, using the hypothalamic-pituitary-interrenal axis as an operational counterpart to the HPA axis. Coordination among neuroendocrine and immune responses in fish establishes the evolutionary conservation of mechanisms to handle stress. Stress-induced alterations in this integrated system not only interfere with homeostasis but also represent an example of a dynamic interaction between immune function and neuroendocrine signals, illustrating the integrating role of the hypothalamus in responding to physiological challenge across species (Figure 10.5).

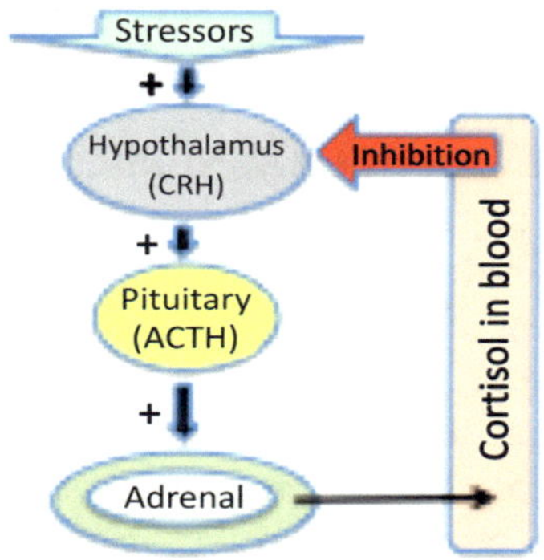

Figure 10.5. Adrenocorticotropic hormone.

Source: https://vivo.colostate.edu/hbooks/pathphys/endocrine/hypopit/acth.png.

10.1.3. Interaction Between the Nervous and Endocrine Systems

The interaction between the nervous and endocrine systems is key to homeostasis and adaptation to stressors. Central to its coordination is the hypothalamic-pituitary-adrenal (HPA) axis, a critical neuroendocrine loop. When one is stressed, the hypothalamus releases corticotropin-releasing hormone (CRH), which triggers the pituitary gland to release adrenocorticotropic hormone (ACTH). The hormone subsequently causes the adrenal glands to release cortisol, a steroid hormone that is involved in many physiological processes, including metabolism and immune response. The balance between the nervous system's rapid signaling and the slow, though long-lasting, effects of endocrine signaling illustrates the complexity of the body's stress response mechanisms, which are crucial for survival in unfavorable environments. Additionally, the impact of early experience on HPA axis function can have significant long-term differences in stress response. It has been demonstrated through experiments that aversive experiences , such as extended maternal separation, can alter fundamentally endocrine responses to stress, typically leading to either increased or decreased hormonal responses depending on the duration of separation. These findings evidence environmental impact on neuroendocrine integration. Specifically, studies have found that short separation leads to blunted stress response, whereas prolonged separation elicits exaggerated responses, suggesting that these early life experiences have a long-term impact on the behavioral as well as physiological components of stress regulation. These developmental trajectories explain how early mother-infant interaction shapes the neuroendocrine terrain and determines mental health outcomes in later life (Rivarola & Renard, 2014). Moreover, the sex difference in stress responses demonstrates the complexity of the interactions between neuroendocrine. Affective and anxiety disorders are more prevalent in women, and the variability in activity of the HPA axis has been proposed to be involved in these differences. Notably, the literature suggests that maternal separation may exert sexually dimorphic influences on the HPA function, which might modulate the stress reactivity differently in males and females. This discrepancy reflects the role of environmental and biological factors in stress responsiveness through neuroendocrine pathways. Because stress affects physical as well as emotional health throughout a person's life, it is important for caregivers to adopt a more holistic approach, taking into consideration the interdependent nature of the endocrine and nervous systems to stress management and wellness at large (DeLisle & Estrine, 2006).

Test Your Knowledge

1. What is the neuroendocrine system, and how does it integrate the nervous and endocrine systems to regulate body functions?
2. Describe the role of the hypothalamus and pituitary gland in coordinating neuroendocrine responses.

10.2. Mechanisms of Stress Response

Learning Outcome

1. Explain the fight-or-flight response;
2. Define the hormonal changes during stress;
3. Describe the activation of the sympathetic nervous system.

The mechanisms of stress responses involve intricate interactions between neuroendocrine systems that are of crucial significance to human physiology. Upon stress, the hypothalamic-pituitary-adrenal (HPA) axis is activated, leading to the release of corticotropin-releasing hormone (CRH) from the hypothalamus. CRH initiates a cascade that activates the anterior pituitary gland, which releases adrenocorticotropic hormone (ACTH). ACTH subsequently leads to the secretion of glucocorticoids by the adrenal cortex, mainly cortisol, which helps in mobilizing energy stores and suppressing non-essential processes to survive in the short term. CRH signaling nuances are more than the release of hormones; they are highly complex mechanisms that regulate behavioral responses to stress and illustrate how psychological and physiological dimensions exist intertwined in stress episodes (Inda et al., 2017). Understanding of such mechanisms is central to the discovery of potential interventions for stress disorders. Further research reveals the modulatory function of immune-neuroendocrine phenotypes (INPs) in regulating responses to stress among various populations. There is an indication that there are various INPs with variations in immune-neuroendocrine interactions that can influence individuals' response to stress. For example, studies into chronic stress effects on home hens reveal that the coexistence of polarized INP—LEWIS-like and FISCHER-like—shows different results in immune and hormonal functioning (Nazar et al., 2017). Such data suggest not only that stress affects physiological processes but also that it causes a change in the immune-neuroendocrine profile distribution, thus pointing to the dynamic adaptability of biological behavior towards unfavorable conditions.

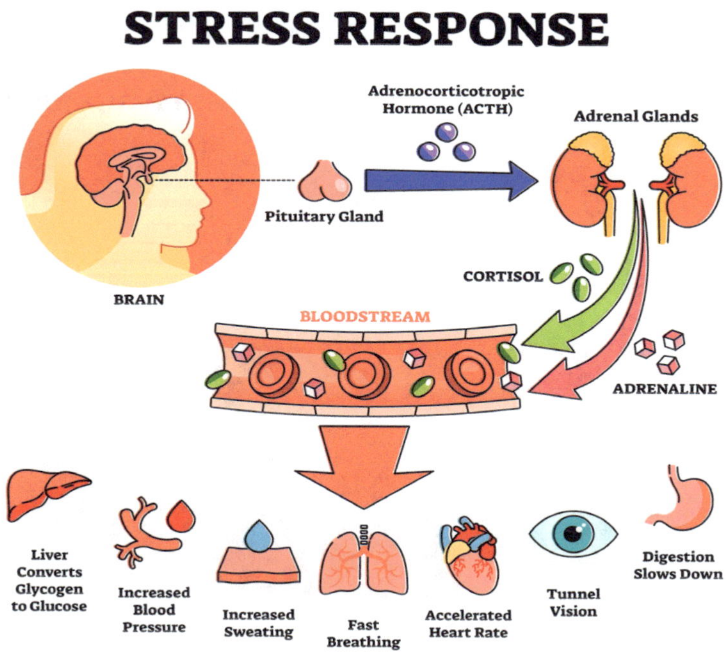

Figure 10.6. HPA-stress-response.

Source: https://www.simplypsychology.org/wp-content/uploads/hpa-stress-response.jpeg.

Analysis of these subgroups has the promise of advancing the boundaries of personalized medicine, as it can gain a greater understanding of the individual stress response and its implications. Finally, the integration of neuroendocrine responses is a key to understanding the body's ability to cope with stress. Neuroendocrine communication and immune competence interaction exhibits a multifaceted mode of stress modulation involving hormonal mechanisms regulating physiological change and immune processes responding to varying levels of stress exposure. Adaptation processes observed among different populations suggest some level of biological preparedness for stress that can inform future treatment. An appreciation for the intricacy of these interactions lies at the heart not only of appreciating stress-related conditions but also of laying the groundwork for integrated interventions for health and well-being (Inda et al., 2017; Nazar et al., 2017). In short, stress response mechanisms involve an integrated conceptualization of somatic and psychological interactions that describe the human body's complex design in handling adversity (Figure 10.6).

10.2.1. The Fight-or-Flight Response

Fight-or-flight is a fundamental physiological reaction that enables organisms to react swiftly to dangers with a view to surviving potentially dangerous circumstances. The neuroendocrine system, which involves the hypothalamus, pituitary gland, and adrenal glands, initiates the response. Upon sensing a danger, the hypothalamus stimulates the activation of the sympathetic nervous system, and this leads to catecholamine release in the form of adrenaline and noradrenaline. Such hormones prepare the body for action, resulting in increased heart rate, increased blood pressure, and heightened levels of blood glucose.

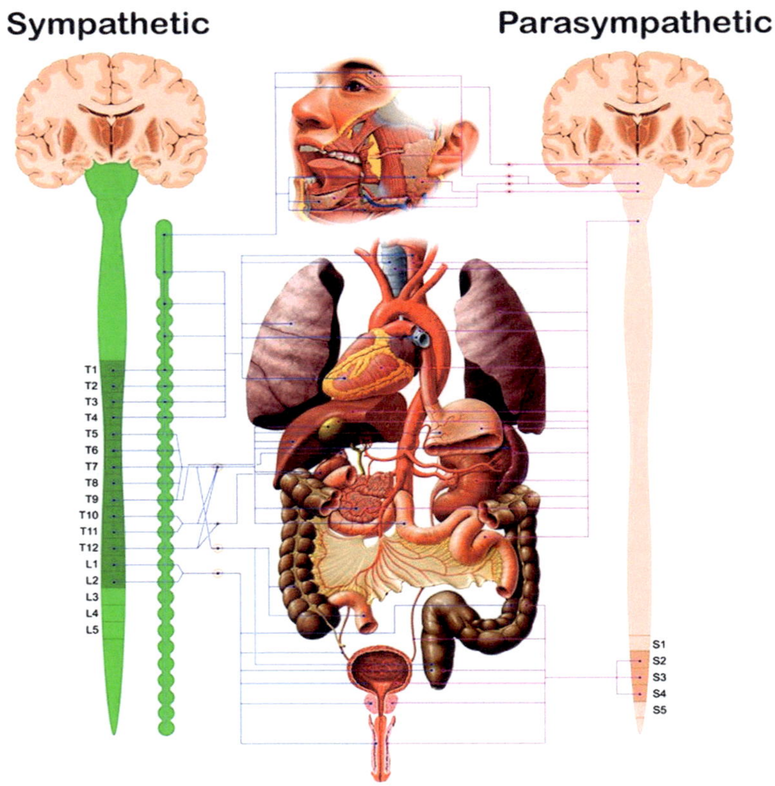

Figure 10.7. Sympathetic nervous system.

Source: https://www.kenhub.com/thumbor/Q9Pm7Bl0UvqzCdePojka-qjA0GY=/fit-in/800x1600/filters:watermark(/images/logo_url.png,-10,-10,0):background_color(FFFFFF):format(jpeg)/images/library/14062/gnEvUC2kgTFXvmrjP39Yw_Sympathetic_nervous_system.png.

These adjustments improve physical performance and focus, allowing individuals to avoid or confront dangers successfully. This biological preparedness is the foundation for the core role of fight-or-flight in the context of acute stressors, as a survival technique developed over thousands of years to protect one from the environment. In addition to short-term physiological adaptations, fight-or-flight involves intricate endocrine-nervous system interactions, emphasizing the importance of neuroendocrine coordination in stress coping. When a stressor is identified, the HPA axis is triggered, leading to the secretion of CRH and then ACTH from the pituitary gland.

This chain ultimately leads to the secretion of cortisol, a glucocorticoid responsible for the regulation of energy and immunosuppression. While cortisol serves to conserve energy reserves for heightened activity, repeated exposure to stressors is harmful to health, including metabolic dysregulation and immune suppression. Understanding these neuroendocrine processes highlights the sophistication of stress responses and the necessity of maintaining hormonal balance for overall well-being (Lovallo, 2016). In addition, the integration of stress response systems and emotional regulation during fight-or-flight response plays a crucial role in efficient coping mechanisms. The limbic system, particularly the amygdala, plays a pivotal role in emotional appraisal and threat response.

It processes environmental stimuli, triggering the neuroendocrine changes for the possibility of a fight-or-flight response. Notably, the intensity of the response and emergent coping strategies have been discovered to be determined largely by psychological and social factors, such as, variation in stress perceptions and resilience. Such stressors initiating the response may also be multifaceted, embracing not only physical dangers but also emotional and psychological ones. Consequently, a holistic interpretation of the fight-or-flight response entails considering these emotional factors and their potential impact on mental and physical health consequences (Cryan et al., 2019) (Figure 10.7).

10.2.2. Hormonal Changes During Stress

The neuroendocrine response to stress involves a highly coordinated interaction between multiple of the hormone axes, particularly the hypothalamic-pituitary-adrenal (HPA) axis. After detection of a stressor, the hypothalamus releases corticotropin-releasing hormone (CRH), which stimulates the pituitary gland to release adrenocorticotropic hormone (ACTH). This process ultimately leads to the release of glucocorticoids, primarily cortisol, by the adrenal glands. These hormones play a critical role in allowing the body to respond to stress by controlling metabolism, immune status, and homeostasis. Recurrent exposure to stress can lead to dysregulation of the HPA axis that manifests as elevated cortisol and has been found to be associated with numerous types of stress-related pathology, such as, depression and anxiety. An understanding of the intricacies of these hormonal changes is key to the design of therapeutic regimens for stress-related pathologies. Research indicates that early life experience significantly affects the regulatory mechanisms of the HPA axis and the resulting hormonal response to stress. For instance, maternal separation in rodents demonstrates how brief separations reduce adrenal responses, leading to lower corticosterone secretion. Longer separations, however, have been associated with an overactive response of the HPA axis. These findings suggest the possibility that early-life stressors can influence the basis for long-term alterations in stress responsivity and potentially predispose to anxiety and affective disorders later in life. Gender also emerges here, as the prevalence of affective disorders is higher in women than in men due to sexually dimorphic effects on HPA axis function. By exploring these parameters, one is able to better explain the impact that hormonal fluctuations during development stages have on stress reactivity throughout life (Rivarola & Renard, 2014). Another consideration of steroid hormones better explains the intricate dynamics of stress reactions, as they play an important role in neuroendocrine functions. Hormones , such as estrogens and testosterone exert influences that extend beyond reproductive health, contributing to stress-related behaviors and physiological mechanisms as well. For instance, progesterone is said to be neuroprotective against neurodegenerative disease, with its role in the neuroendocrine system in stress responses. The function of these hormones speaks volumes for the intricacy of the integration process of the neuroendocrine system, with the hormonal programming able to influence not only stress reactivity but also metabolic and cognitive processes. A knowledge of how these hormones interact can provide vital information on intervention development to counteract the damaging effects of stress on mental and physical health (Zubeldia-Brenner et al., 2016) (Figure 10.8).

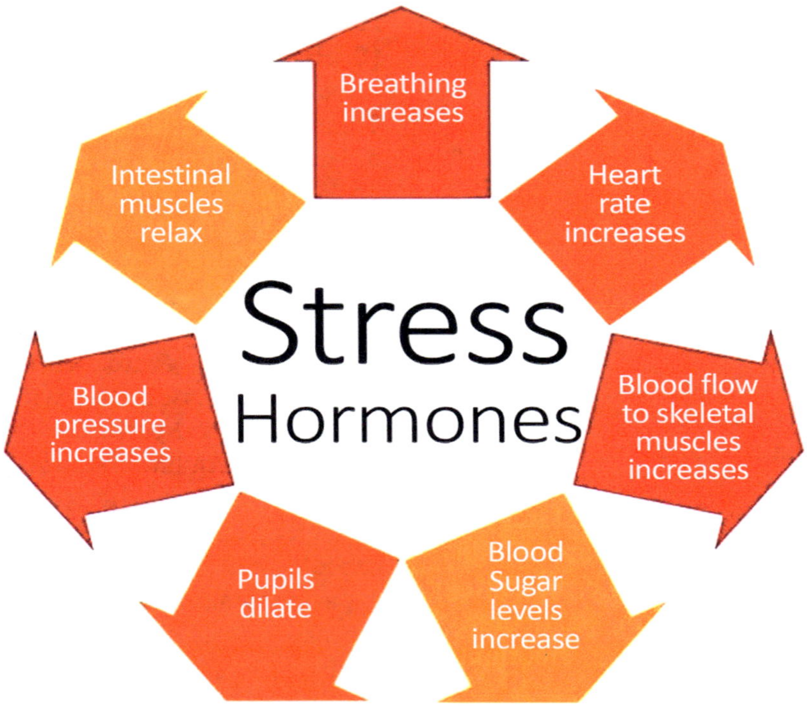

Figure 10.8. Stress hormones.

Source: https://mountaintrek.com/wp-content/uploads/2016/03/Stress-Hormones.jpg.

10.2.3. Activation of the Sympathetic Nervous System

Sympathetic nervous system (SNS) activation is a major component of the body's stress response as part of the integrated neuroendocrine system. The system is activated upon detection of threat or challenge, and a series of physiological reactions takes place to ready the body for immediate action, or fight or flight response. The most important neuroendocrine components, including catecholamines, epinephrine and norepinephrine, are released into the bloodstream, triggering increased heart rate, increased blood pressure, and augmented peripheral flow to skeletal muscle. Sympathetic activation not only supplies instantaneous body responses but also influences metabolic functions, allowing mobilization of energy reserves. The synergy between sympathetic activation and hormonal mechanisms attests to the complexity of the body's stress responses, illustrating the SNS's essential function in maintaining homeostasis under heightened emotional and physical stress. In addition to immediate physiological effects, the influence of sympathetic nervous system activation also has implications for longer-term health effects. Repeated SNS activation can lead to a state of chronic stress, which adversely affects various systems within the body. For instance, neuroendocrine dysregulation has been implicated in the pathogenesis of anxiety, depression, and cardiovascular disorders. Of special interest is that major depressive disorder (MDD) has been associated with heterogeneous endocrine profiles, which highlights the dynamic interplay between stress, the SNS, and mental health. Studies have determined that the different subtypes of depression have been seen to present with differing metabolic features, and again, an overall understanding of how SNS activation interacts with neuroendocrine functioning needs to influence the health course of the patient. This may be able to inform more specific treatment protocols in the treatment of stress-related disorders (Lang & Borgwardt, 2013). In addition to physical and mental health effects, sympathetic nervous system activation has a profound connection to the gut-brain axis, which regulates microbiome-central nervous system communication. With current data, gut microbiota play an essential role in shaping the immune system, metabolism, and stress response. Stress and its physiological equivalents can influence microbiota composition, hence have an impact on neurodevelopmental disorders as well as mental health. As a result, microbial metabolites can also regulate the activation of glial cells in the brain, thereby controlling neural processes , such as neurogenesis. The connection between the sympathetic nervous system and the gut-brain axis provides evidence of the complex network of interactions, proving that stress has an impact on mental well-being through direct regulation of neurotransmitter systems and indirectly through microbial activity. This is a reflection of a multi-dimensional model of neuroendocrine integration, which is required to comprehend the overall implications of stress on the physiology of the body (Cryan et al., 2019) (Figure 10.9).

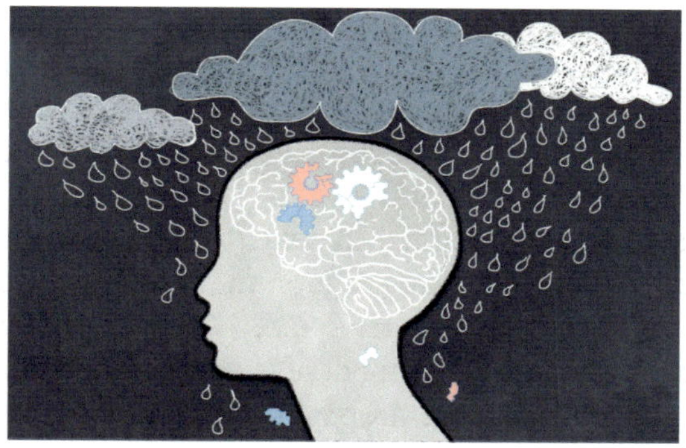

Figure 10.9. Major depressive disorder: symptoms & treatments.

Source: https://atlanticbehavioralhealth.com/wp-content/uploads/2024/06/understanding-mdd.webp.

Test Your Knowledge

1. What are the major components of the stress response system, and how are they activated during acute stress?
2. Describe the role of the hypothalamic-pituitary-adrenal (HPA) axis in mediating the hormonal response to stress.

10.3. The Hypothalamic-Pituitary-Adrenal (HPA) Axis

Learning Outcome

1. Explain the structure and function of the HPA axis;
2. Define the role of cortisol in stress response;
3. Describe the feedback mechanisms regulating the HPA axis.

The HPA axis is a crucial regulatory process within the body's stress response, integrating neural and endocrine input to provide homeostasis. It begins with the release of CRH from the hypothalamus, which leads to the release of ACTH from the anterior pituitary gland. The latter causes the adrenal cortex to release glucocorticoids, most notably cortisol in humans. These biochemical interactions are important as they not only prepare the body to respond to stress but also govern many physiological processes like metabolism, the immune system, and mood. Dysregulation of this delicate system can lead to critical health outcomes. It is for this reason that it is important to be aware of the HPA axis so that one can recognize how chronic stress can present itself in physical as well as psychological disorders. Research has indicated that early life events strongly program the HPA axis function, leading to long-term effects on the stress response of the individual. For example, research has shown that brief maternal separation in rodents induces a blunted adrenal response to stress, which is a sign of adaptation and resilience. On the other hand, prolonged separations can result in a robust sensitization of the HPA axis, as evidenced by abnormally increased cortisol release upon exposure to stress. These findings suggest that formative form-offspring interactions are central in determining later-life reactivity to stress (Rivarola & Renard, 2014). Identification of the role played by such experiences in early life reveals the neurobiological processes that render an individual vulnerable to stress-related disease, highlighting the HPA axis as a dynamic modulator of environmental effects on health. HPA axis dysregulation is invariably associated with a spectrum of stress-related diseases, including PTSD and major depressive disorder, proving the role of the axis in mental health. Alterations in cortisol regulation may be indicative of deeper disruptions in the neuroendocrine system, where the interaction among CRH, ACTH, and cortisol is compromised. Theoretical models have explained typical and pathological HPA axis states, illustrating how alterations in the amplitude and timing of stress can yield diverse health outcomes (Chou et al., 2016). This knowledge underlines the idea that maladaptive stress exposure can alter the stress response circuitry of the brain, supporting the need for functional therapeutic processes to mend the disrupted pathways. It is against this background that the therapeutic utility of psychotherapeutic interventions, such as, exposure therapy, emerges as a way to restore balance between dysregulation and re-establish homeostasis of the HPA axis (Figure 10.10).

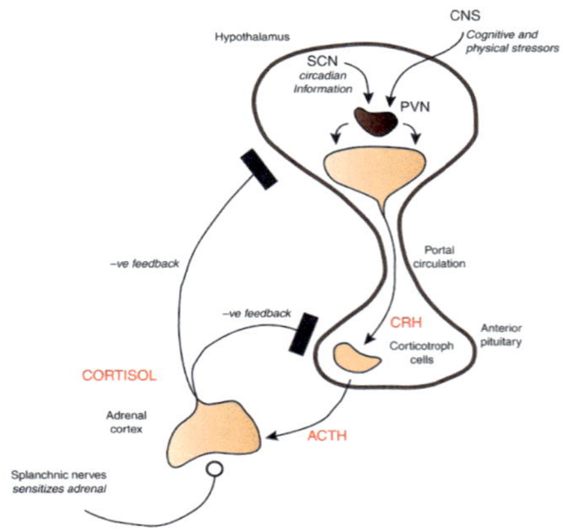

Figure 10.10. Hypothalamic-pituitary-adrenal (HPA) axis.

Source: https://www.bjanaesthesia.org.uk/cms/10.1093/bja/aet077/asset/e2b55f64-2e6c-4cb0-b106-dece47a3f5ec/main.assets/gr1_lrg.jpg.

10.3.1. Structure and Function of the HPA axis

The hypothalamic-pituitary-adrenal (HPA) axis is a complex system that regulates the body's response to stress. It begins with the secretion of corticotropin-releasing hormone (CRH) from the hypothalamus, which causes the secretion of adrenocorticotropic hormone (ACTH) by the pituitary gland. The ACTH in turn causes the adrenal glands to secrete glucocorticoids, primarily cortisol in the human body. This systemic release of cortisol plays several roles, mostly assisting in the regulation of metabolism, modulation of the immune response, and the general adaptational responses of the body to stress. Notably, the HPA axis has a self-regulating feedback mechanism in which increased cortisol levels allow for inhibition of CRH and ACTH, hence ensuring homeostasis. But under conditions of chronic stress, this feedback mechanism can become impaired and lead to maladaptive behavioral and physiological traits that are responsible for some of the stress disorders. It has been established by research that early life events, particularly stressful ones, can result in long-term changes in the function of the HPA axis. For instance, rodent models of experiment reveal that prolonged maternal separation increases the adrenal stress response and cortisol secretion. In comparison, brief intervals of separation can elicit a blunted response, showing the plasticity to multiple stressors.

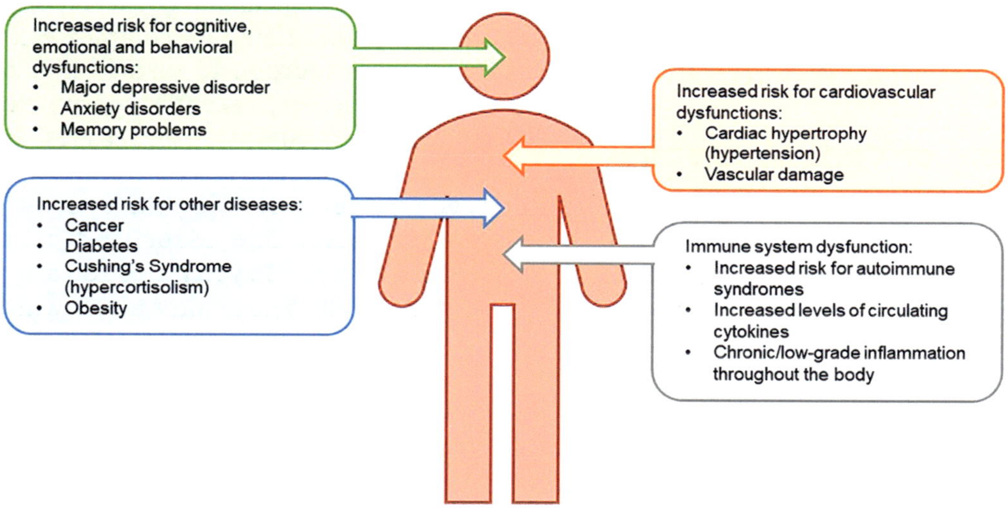

Figure 10.11. Structure and function of the HPA axis.

Source: https://www.frontiersin.org/files/Articles/601939/fnbeh-14-601939-HTML/image_m/fnbeh-14-601939-g001.jpg.

All such differences highlight the significance of environmental conditions and interactions with the mother in building up the development of neuroendocrine systems. Additionally, the association of HPA axis dysregulation with an increased risk for psychological illness, particularly among females, highlights the absolute significance of the knowledge of gender-specific responses. The consequences of these early experiences are that they can long-lastingly remodel behavioral outputs via alterations of the body's hypothalamic-pituitary-adrenal communication pathways, which have been linked to anxiety and affective disorders (Rivarola & Renard, 2014). The dynamics of the HPA axis are also described through mathematical modeling, which describes its behavior as being under the control of intricate interactions between physiological components. In particular, the gradual process of cortisol-mediated CRH biosynthesis and immediate synaptic effects together determine the axis response to stressors. Such models are illustrative of how the timing, duration, and magnitude of exposure to stress can induce switching between stable states of the HPA axis, likely giving rise to diseases like post-traumatic stress disorder (PTSD) or major depressive disorder. Disorders in this axis are more likely to be associated with chronic states of dysfunction of the feedback mechanisms. This highlights the important role not only in short-term responses to stress but also in longer-term outcomes of traumatic exposures. Thus, an understanding of these dynamics is essential in providing critical insights into treatment approaches, like exposure therapy, which are aimed at re-establishing normal functioning of the HPA axis and minimizing physiological correlates of stress disorders (Chou et al., 2016) (Figure 10.11).

10.3.2. Role of Cortisol in Stress Response

The role of cortisol in stress response is a primary one for neuroendocrine integration as an essential mediator for the way organisms react to stressors. Upon experiencing a stressful stimulus, the hypothalamus activates theHPA axis, releasing ACTH. The hormone triggers the release of cortisol by the adrenal glands, typically referred to as the stress hormone. Greater cortisol levels prepare the body to confront challenges, affecting a wide range of physiological processes, including metabolism, immune response, and even mental processes. Owing to its multi-tasking role, cortisol enables mobilization of energy stores, suppression of non-essential activities, and alertness of the brain, which are essential for survival in the instant. But chronic hypercortisolism as a result of prolonged exposure to stress can introduce negative health effects, illustrating the fine equilibrium present in the system for response and stress. And beyond the direct physiological responses, cortisol's influence permeates to invade realms of behavior and regulation of emotions. From observations in the study of attachment theory, cortisol levels can shed insight into understanding between human relationships and the health effects of stress. Cortisol change due to stress may affect individuals' capacity to develop secure attachments, central to emotional well-being. This suggests a two-way relationship where cortisol change not only indicates physiological readiness for immediate reaction but also affects interpersonal and social interactions. Precisely, fluctuating cortisol levels may distort decision-making mechanisms, potentially developing risk-taking behavior as individuals cope with stressors. Hence, cortisol may be central to connecting physiological reactions with psychological and social experience under stress, emphasizing its complex role in human health. In addition to further illuminating the role of cortisol, recent research examines its function in cognitive processes and health-relevant behaviors, positioning it within an even larger physiological context. Exposure to a stressor and associated cortisol surge influence neural systems of reward processing and learning. These alterations will then affect decision-making strategies, shifting choices in favor of habitual actions over adaptive learning. Such studies highlight the complexity of stress response because they involve physiological pathways with psychological implications, such that comprehensive treatment for demystifying stress-related behavior is critical. In light of the above, as the demand for further research in this area indicates, offering integrative models describing the relationship between cortisol, neurobiology, and behavior is critical. By combining these sciences, researchers can design interventions aimed at preventing the detrimental effects of stress that are cortisol-mediated, underscoring its significance in health and chronic disease prevention (Robles & Kane, 2014; Porcelli & Delgado, 2017) (Figure 10.12).

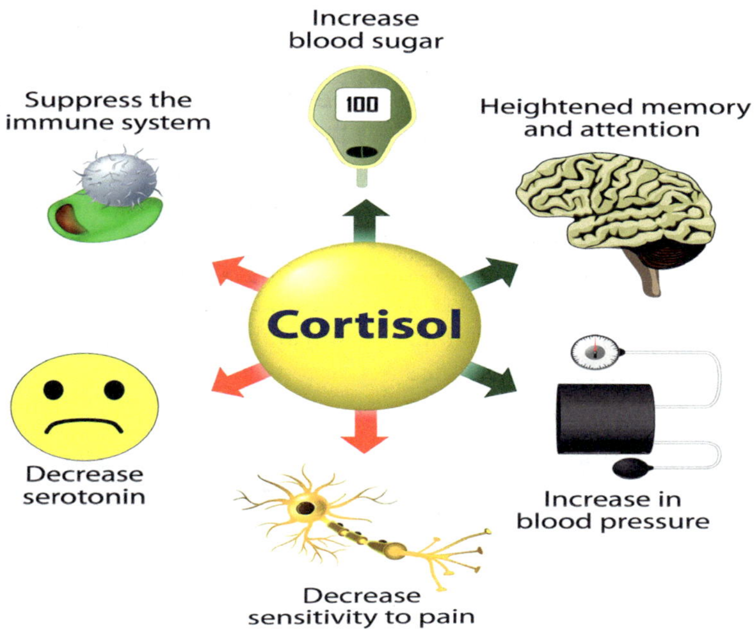

Figure 10.12. Role of cortisol in the stress response.

Source: https://cdn.ausmed.com/ausmed-blog-images/2017/12/20171218_body.jpg.

10.3.3. Feedback Mechanisms Regulating the HPA Axis

The negative feedback systems regulating the hypothalamo-pituitary-adrenocortical (HPA) axis are central components of the body's stress response system, enabling an optimal physiological stress response to stressors. Activation of the HPA axis results in the release of CRH from the hypothalamus, stimulating the anterior pituitary to release ACTH. ACTH, in turn stimulates the adrenal cortex to secrete glucocorticoids, of which cortisol is the most important glucocorticoid. The action of glucocorticoids is not just the mobilization of energy resources but also includes negative feedback actions that help to regulate the HPA activity. By inhibiting receptors in the pituitary gland and hypothalamus, glucocorticoids inhibit further release of CRH and ACTH, effectively terminating the stress response and stopping the system from being overactivated, which would lead to maladaptive effects. This feedback loop emphasizes the intricate homeostasis that the body attains as a response to stressors. The significance of feedback loops governing the HPA axis is best realized when appreciating the bodily effects of prolonged stress. Stimulation of the HPA axis for long periods of time may initiate a state of hypercortisolism, in which the glucocorticoid levels remain high at the cost of several bodily systems. Individual variability, such as, genetics, early life history, and environmental stressors, can influence individuals to respond differently to stress, resulting in varying profiles of HPA axis regulation. Not only does chronic stress impact the feedback sensitivity of the HPA axis, which could lead to the failure to downregulate hormonal responses, but it has also been demonstrated to alter stress response neural circuits. Thus, insight into these feedback mechanisms is key to understanding how chronic stress can predispose individuals to a multitude of pathologies, including depression and anxiety disorders, which are often defined by dysregulated HPA axis function

(Herman et al., 2016). Furthermore, current developments center around the intersection between the microbiota-gut-brain axis and the feedback control mechanisms of the HPA axis, informing new knowledge about their functions in stress response and regulation of physiology. The gut microbiota plays a significant role in the body's neuroendocrine response and can influence HPA axis function through several mechanisms of biochemistry. To illustrate, microbial metabolites , such as short-chain fatty acids, have been determined to influence the production of certain neurotransmitters and hormones that can enhance or impair the stress response. This linkage suggests that gut health is at the core of healthy HPA axis function, particularly in terms of feedback sensitivity and stress resilience. Examining these linkages, researchers aim to uncover possible therapeutic choices for stress disorders on the basis of the primary function of feedback mechanisms to facilitate neuroendocrine integration and overall physiological health (Cryan et al., 2019).

Test Your Knowledge

1. How does negative feedback regulate hormone levels within the HPA axis?
2. What are the effects of chronic HPA axis activation on metabolism, immunity, and brain function?

10.4. Effects of Chronic Stress

Learning Outcome

1. Identify the physiological consequences of prolonged stress;
2. Define the impact on mental health;
3. Describe the long-term effects on the immune system.

Chronic stress outcomes are revealed within the neuroendocrine system of the body, altering physiologic processes and overall health. When stress is sustained over a prolonged period of time, the neuroendocrine response is deregulated, leading to sustained elevations of stress hormones , such as cortisol. Such hyperactivation can contribute to a broad spectrum of disease states, such as, metabolic disease, cardiovascular disease, and psychiatric illness , such as depression and anxiety. Chronic exposure to high levels of cortisol has been linked to impaired cognitive functioning, including memory loss and information processing deficits, that are detrimental to academic and work performances. Furthermore, these physiological changes are a foundation of understanding the mechanisms by which chronic stress leads to long-term health complications, particularly in the context of the dynamic between stress and other physical factors impacting health that are the foundation of resilience and vulnerability among different populations (Duffee et al., 2021). During childhood development, the consequences of chronic stress are profoundly important given the criticality of early neurodevelopment. Adverse childhood experiences, such as, abuse or neglect, have significant effects on the development of the neuroendocrine system, modifying basal stress reactions and biasing towards lifelong physical and psychological morbidity. Empirical research has demonstrated that individuals exposed to chronic stress during early developmental periods typically exhibit brain development and function alterations, resulting in enhanced responsiveness to stressors during the adult period. This neurodevelopmental model emphasizes the necessity for trauma-informed care practices that promote resilience and buffer against the deleterious effects of stress experienced during early childhood. Healthcare professionals can intervene on these adverse experiences and implement interventions that promote healthy neuroendocrine integration, enhancing the capacity of individuals to regulate stress through the course of their lives (Kuntz, 2020). Moreover, the dynamic interplay of chronic stress, resilience, and health results requires comprehensive approaches integrating trauma-informed policies into healthcare and education settings. These steps not only recognize the intense impact of toxic stress on neuroendocrine activity but also strive to construct environments that enhance protective strengths and social support systems. By instituting a trauma-informed model, the practitioner can better assess and respond to the chronic stressors that are impacting individuals and foster relational health and resilience. Literature indicates constructing strong relationships and safe, supportive environments as countermeasures to the potentially dangerous effects of chronic stress on health outcomes. Therefore, it is crucial to address the intricate aspects of stress during childhood and adulthood to promote overall well-being and develop greater resilience towards the challenges of life (Duffee et al., 2021) (Figure 10.13).

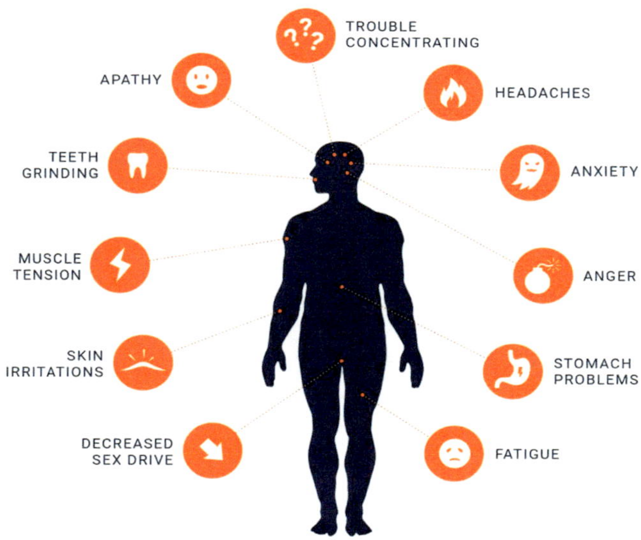

Figure 10.13. Chronic stress.

Source: https://www.grwhealth.com/wp-content/uploads/2023/04/60c2763f34f3187342484d82_what-is-stress.jpg.

10.4.1. Physiological Consequences of Prolonged Stress

Chronic stress evokes a complex pattern of physiological effects that engage many systems of the body, particularly those governed by the HPA axis. With repeated exposure to stressors, the HPA axis becomes hyperactive with increased secretion of glucocorticoids, for instance, cortisol. Cortisol is a central hormone involved in the body's stress response by mobilizing energy and controlling many biological processes, including immunity and metabolism. However, chronic elevation of cortisol levels can have deleterious health effects, including impairment of cognitive functioning, increased vulnerability to pathogens, and changes in metabolic homeostasis. Significantly, this pathology highlights the need to examine individual variation in resistance and vulnerability to stress, particularly in relation to how chronic stress impacts hormonal regulation and metabolic function in long-term contexts (Rivarola & Renard, 2014).

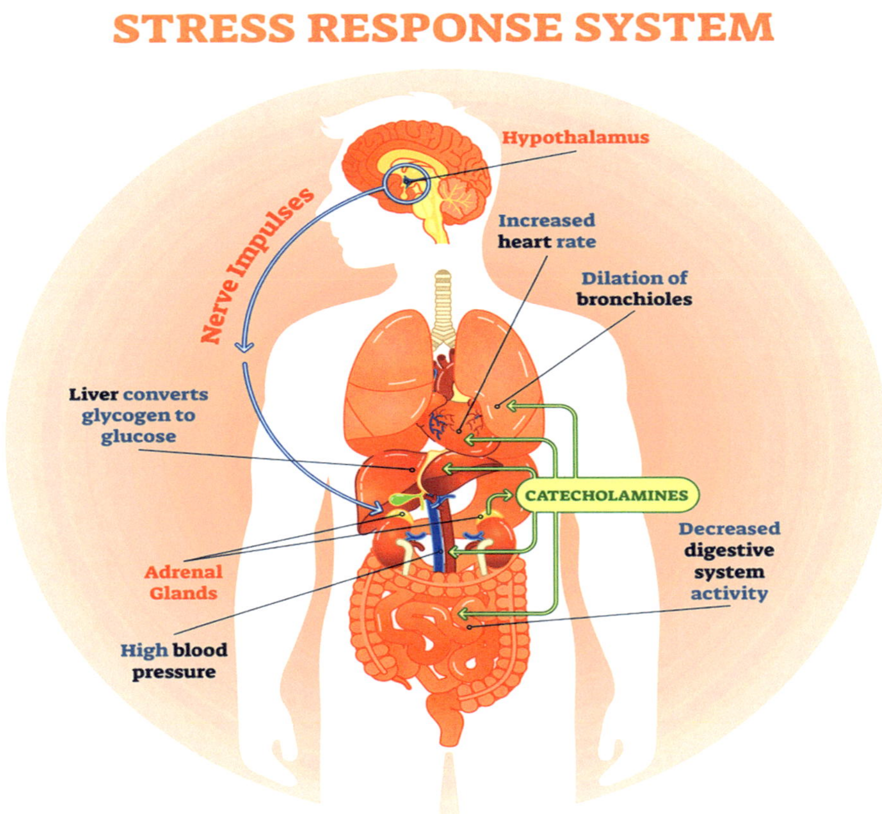

Figure 10.14. Effects of stress on the body.

Source: https://cdn.painscale.com/cms/imgs/dd6452d0-4bb7-11eb-87d5-15e76591973e.jpg.

The physical effects of chronic stress also include widespread reorganization of neural function and behavior, largely mediated by stress hormones like CRH. CRH plays a crucial role in initiating stress through its action on the HPA axis and has been shown to play a role in stress-related illness. Repeated exposure to high CRH levels has also been demonstrated to result in changes in neurotransmitter systems and neuroplasticity, thus influencing mood and behavior. Dysregulation of CRH signaling, for instance, may result in enhanced anxiety and depression, further indicating the role of neuroendocrine integration in stress-related disorder pathology. These endocrine changes increase the necessity to respond to the temporal dynamics of stress responses, especially when developing interventions that would reverse such impacts on mental health (Inda et al., 2017). Additionally, the physiological effects of chronic stress extend beyond stress responses to address potential long-term alterations in health outcomes. Chronic stress is associated with an increased risk of developing a range of disorders, from cardiovascular disease to metabolic syndromes and psychiatric illness. The complex correlation arises from the combined effect of repeated exposure to increased stress hormones, chronic inflammation, and mitochondrial injury, which can impair overall health and longevity. Evidence indicates early life stressors could have the potential to predispose individuals to these chronic diseases, in addition to emphasizing the importance of early experiences in influencing neuroendocrine function and pathways to health. Understanding these relationships has the potential to guide preventative intervention methods since the two-way interaction between stress and health is critical in promoting resilience and well-being for populations exposed to chronic stress (Rivarola & Renard, 2014) (Figure 10.14).

10.4.2. Impact on Mental Health

The intricate dynamics of stress and mental health are increasingly recognized in the neuroendocrine integration context. Chronic exposure to stress activates the HPA axis, and glucocorticoid concentrations increase, leading to significant alterations in the neural connection circuitry. Specifically, it has been shown that chronic stress affects the interaction between the amygdala and the prefrontal cortex, areas largely responsible for emotional processing and decision-making. This dysregulation is believed to be accountable for enhanced anxiety and depression, as prolonged exposure to glucocorticoids can induce neuroinflammatory responses within the central nervous system, exacerbating mental disorders. The complexity of such interaction warrants the necessity of a general understanding of how neuroendocrine responses directly affect psychological states, illustrated in novel clinical approaches targeted towards managing the psychosomatic relation felt in chronic stress conditions (Shuja, 2025). Adolescents are particularly susceptible to the development of social rejection and stress-related mental health disorders. Recent research highlights that the transformations that take place at adolescence age make the population highly vulnerable to the negative effects of social exclusion. These transformations result in alterations of brain regions involved in stress responses, such as, the medial prefrontal cortex and the hypothalamic paraventricular nucleus. Stimulation of these regions has been shown to regulate behavioral response to stress and regulate autonomic nervous system activity. In addition, social solitude during this phase of critical development has also been shown to lead to enduring emotional maladjustment and cardiovascular disorder, illustrating an intimate association between environmental experience and neurobiological change. Understanding of these processes will be crucial to the development of preventative strategies and interventions for reducing the adolescent burden on mental health (Yao et al., 2025). The impacts of chronic social isolation and stress extend beyond single mental health to affect public health concerns at large. As loneliness levels and associated mental health disorders rise in today's society, particularly during times of crisis , such as pandemics, there is an evident necessity for treatments that address both the psychological and the physiological aspects.

Treatments that combine behavior therapy with pharmacological interventions are potentially capable of lowering the detrimental effects of stress, and thus, evidence indicates a symbiotic effect whereby improved mental health can significantly alleviate stress symptoms. In addition, comprehending the role of lifestyle determinants and environmental conditions, including stress and support systems in society, becomes essential in the multidimensional approach to mental illness. This holistic approach would enhance resilience among individuals subjected to the ill effects of stress, thereby leading to a high quality of life and mental health (Shuja, 2025) (Figure 10.15).

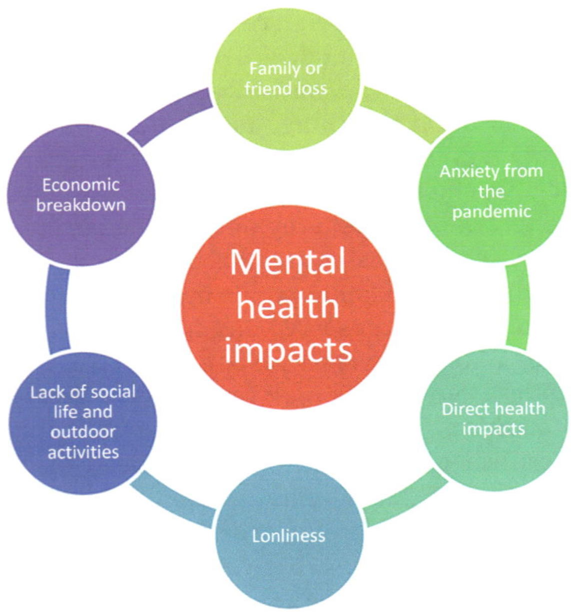
Mental health impacts
Family or friend loss
Anxiety from the pandemic
Direct health impacts
Lonliness
Lack of social life and outdoor activities
Economic breakdown

Figure 10.15. Mental health impacts.

Source: https://html.scirp.org/file/3-1950726x2.png?20220517090000458.

10.4.3. Long-Term Effects on the Immune System

The long-term impact of stress on the immune system is significant and multifaceted, illustrating the cross-talk between the neuroendocrine and immune systems. Stress triggers the release of a myriad of hormones, of which cortisol is notable, that, while essential for short-term reactions, can undermine immune homeostasis when released in bulk over prolonged periods. Chronic stress states, whether elicited through socioeconomic stress or trauma, can engender a cascade of immune dysfunction leading ultimately to heightened susceptibility to infection and autoimmune disease. Individuals who are exposed to chronic stress will often show altered cytokine profiles, which reflect a tendency towards a state of pro-inflammation that has been associated with numerous chronic diseases. It is important to understand mechanisms through which stress impinges on immune responses, as such information offers the promise of understanding potential therapeutic interventions capable of reversing the detrimental effects of chronic stress on immune function (DeLisle & Estrine, 2006). Furthermore, early life stress can have long-term implications for the immune system, laying the groundwork for a host of stress-related diseases later in life. Research has indicated that adverse experiences in early life, such as, maternal separation, can irreversibly influence the HPA axis and immune mechanisms. These experiences place individuals in a heightened state of reactivity to stress and unique immune response patterns, which can make them susceptible to pathologies , such as anxiety and depression. Significantly, gender differences in these stress responses occur due to factors like genetic and hormonal changes that result in different ways males and females experience stress. The long-term effects of early stressors emphasize the need to attend to emotional and psychological adjustment from childhood since these interventions can build immune resilience and promote long-term health benefits (Rivarola & Renard, 2014). The intersection of stress, the immune system, and chronic disease points to the need for an integrated health care model that integrates psychological as well as physiological elements. Traditional health care generally deals with physical and mental wellness separately, without taking the two-way interactions between the systems into account. Therefore, adopting a more holistic model that recognizes the central role played by stress in regulating immune function is imperative. By connecting neuroendocrine responses to immune health, healthcare practitioners can create tailored interventions that address the fundamental causes of chronic stress and its immune implications. These holistic methods not only aim to fix present symptoms but also aim to encourage long-term health by enhancing resilience to psychological stressors and their debilitating effect on immune function (DeLisle & Estrine, 2006).

Test Your Knowledge

1. How does chronic stress affect the endocrine, immune, and nervous systems over time?
2. What are the long-term consequences of sustained elevated cortisol levels on metabolism and mental health?

10.5. Neurotransmitters and Hormones in Stress

Learning Outcome

1. Describe the role of adrenaline and noradrenaline;
2. Define the influence of serotonin and dopamine;
3. Discuss how to interaction of hormones in stress modulation.

The communication between hormones and neurotransmitters is at the heart of understanding the body's response to stress. Stressors activate the HPA axis, with the release of CRH and ACTH. The sequence ends with the release of cortisol from the adrenal glands, a major player in controlling energy metabolism and immune function. While this is happening, neurotransmitters , such as norepinephrine and serotonin control mood and arousal level, dictating people's experience and reaction to stressors. The integration of hormonal and neurotransmitter activities is responsible for a coordinated response that prepares the body for an instant response, which speaks volumes about the complexity of neuroendocrine signaling in the stress response. Moreover, chronic stress has been very much related to the alteration of neurotransmitter levels, particularly with regard to mood and cognition. Chronic exposure to stress has been demonstrated to lead to dysregulation of neurotransmitter systems, such as, reduced levels of serotonin and dopamine, which are highly linked to anxiety and depression. Such dysregulation tends to worsen physical illness, since persistent stress is bound to impair body function and make individuals susceptible to several diseases. This realization emphasizes the importance of treating both the psychological and physiological aspects of stress in the realm of health care, so as to bridge the gap between neurological and endocrine. To this end, both hormones and neurotransmitters play a crucial role as players in the complex dance of stress-related health outcomes and direct potential therapeutic options. Finally, stress effects on sexual health also merit attention, demonstrating how stress-mediated changes in neurotransmitter and hormone levels can disrupt sexual function. Evidence indicates that fluctuations in sex hormone levels and access to neurotransmitters can lead to various sexual dysfunctions in terms of desire, arousal, and orgasm phases. For instance, fluctuations in dopamine and norepinephrine levels may decrease sexual arousal, and the changes in testosterone levels may influence libido. Kumar et al (2009) illustrate the complexity of sexual function and the way in which physical and psychological elements blend during stress responses. This multidimensional component to sexual health also supports further demands for an integrative approach to clinical practice that addresses both the neuroendocrine effect of stress and the psychological dimensions of sexual health. Through the recognition of the multifactorial influence of stress, doors are opened to more integrative treatment approaches, which include both mental and physical considerations (Figure 10.16).

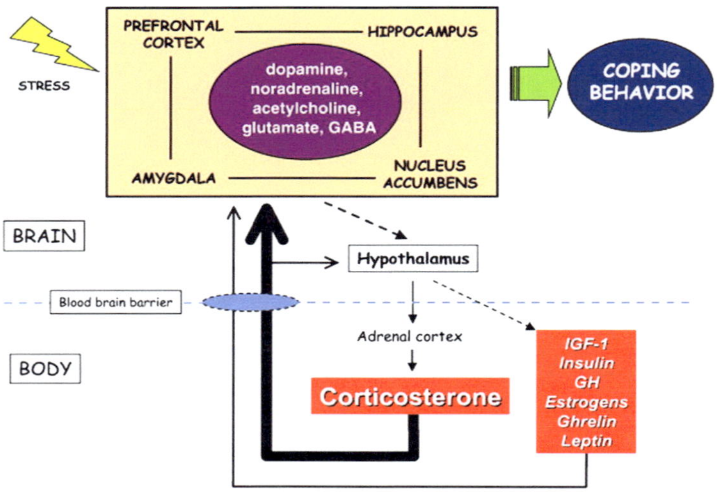

Figure 10.16. Stress, neurotransmitters, corticosterone and body–brain integration.

Source: https://ars.els-cdn.com/content/image/1-s2.0-S0006899311023183-gr1.jpg.

10.5.1. Role of Adrenaline and Noradrenaline

The role of adrenaline and noradrenaline in the neuroendocrine stress response is essential in the preservation of homeostasis within the body. Both the catecholamines are synthesized in the adrenal medulla and are integral mediators of the fight-or-flight response. With the presentation of a stressor, signals from the hypothalamus trigger the discharge of these hormones into a cascade of body changes. It increases heart rate, speeds up glucose metabolism, and supplies blood to skeletal muscles faster, readying the organism to take action quickly. In contrast, noradrenaline functions primarily as a neurotransmitter in the central nervous system to heighten alertness and focus. The intricate signaling displays the mechanism of adaptation that organisms use to counteract stressors, indicating how adrenaline and noradrenaline are components in the overall stress response system. Recently, the interaction between physical activity and chronic stress has attracted serious interest, especially with regard to catecholamine metabolism. It is revealed by studies that regular exercise may significantly affect the action and synthesis of such hormones. For instance, in a certain study, the effect of exercise on gene expression for catecholamine biosynthesis was investigated, and it was discovered that levels of exercise in rats subjected to chronic stress significantly boosted noradrenaline as well as adrenaline levels (Gavrilović et al., 2017). The findings show that exercise not only increases catecholamine levels but also suppresses oxidative stress induced by chronic stressors. The consequent balance in catecholamine concentrations can augment neuroendocrine function, increasing stress resistance. This suggests an interaction of sophistication between lifestyle variables and neuroendocrine status and illustrates the ability of exercise to reverse endocrine responses favorably. Furthermore, subject variation in responsiveness to stress might be partly attributable to variations between the amounts of adrenaline and noradrenaline in susceptible individuals. Personality theories suggest that such individual differences are likely to generate varying behavioral and emotional reactions to stress (Armario & Nadal, 2013). For example, individuals with a higher adrenaline reaction would be more sensitive to stressors, so it might lead to anxiety disorders or other psychiatric illnesses. However, an adjustment of the noradrenaline response can be protective in that it allows cognitive clarity and emotional regulation. These variations underscore the importance of valuing the intricate roles of these catecholamines within acute stress response as well as long-term psychological well-being. With additional growth in research, therapeutic potential for manipulation of catecholamine pathways is an emerging and potential avenue for enhancing stress resistance and overall mental health (Figure 10.17).

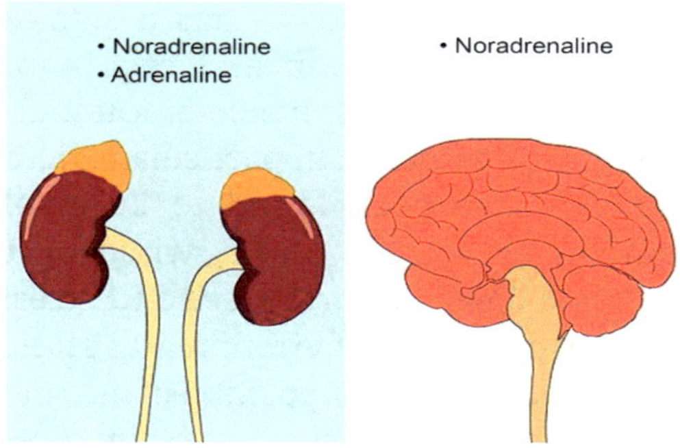

Figure 10.17. Role of adrenaline and noradrenaline in the neuroendocrine response to stress.

Source: https://www.wikihow.com/images/thumb/b/bf/What-Is-Noradrenaline-Step-2.jpg/v4-460px-What-Is-Noradrenaline-Step-2.jpg.

10.5.2. Influence of Serotonin and Dopamine

The equilibrium between serotonin and dopamine is crucial in the regulation of physiological responses to stress, influencing mood and cognitive function. Serotonin, or the feel-good neurotransmitter, plays a significant role in stabilizing emotions and overseeing various neuroendocrine operations. Dopamine, on the other hand, is a component of the brain's reward system and influences motivation and pleasure response. These neurotransmitters interact with the HPA axis, an integral part of the body's stress response. Serotonin and dopamine imbalance have been associated with several mood and anxiety disorders, where heightened stress reactivity can translate to exaggerated physiological outcomes. Understanding these mechanisms not only teaches us about normal stress physiology but also indicates where therapeutic approaches to relieving stress-related disorders may target, emphasizing the critical function of neurochemical balance to overall well-being. The gut-brain axis is a crucial pathway by which serotonin and dopamine exert their actions on neuroendocrine integration and stress response. There is new evidence that indicates the gut microbiota has a significant impact on the production and regulation of these neurotransmitters, hence emotional and psychological well-being. In particular, microbial metabolites have been found to be involved in modifying serotonin levels, which in turn may regulate cognitive processes and stress. In addition, as observed, environmental stressors and diet influence the composition of microbiota, suggesting that these aspects are involved in mental health outcomes. Such findings highlight the need for an interdisciplinary approach in neuroscience and psychology since they reveal the intricate way the health of the gut interacts with neurochemical mechanisms. Such interaction opens new possibilities for treatments for both the microbiome and the neuroendocrine system to treat stress disorders and general health (Cryan et al., 2019). Also, the functions of serotonin and dopamine in disease conditions, such as, migraine, also establish their critical role in the neuroendocrine process. The evidence indicates that serotonin has a central role in the pathophysiology of migraine, namely through controlling vascular reactivity and pain processing. The trigeminal system, which is activated during migraines, is controlled by serotonin pathways, and this supports the neurotransmitters' dual role in mood modulation and pain mediation. Similarly, dopamine's contribution to migraine may be understood in terms of its actions within sensory processing during an attack, with fluctuations in the sign of dopamine signaling having the potential to modulate pain perception threshold. A complete comprehension of serotonin and dopamine dynamics thus adds not only to demystifying the neurobiological causes of migraines but also emphasizes their broader contribution to the processing of emotional and physiological stress. Recent studies promise much for novel therapeutic strategies involving these neurotransmitter systems to mitigate the burden of stress-related illness, scrutinizing their full spectrum of action on human health (Goadsby et al., 2017) (Figure 10.18).

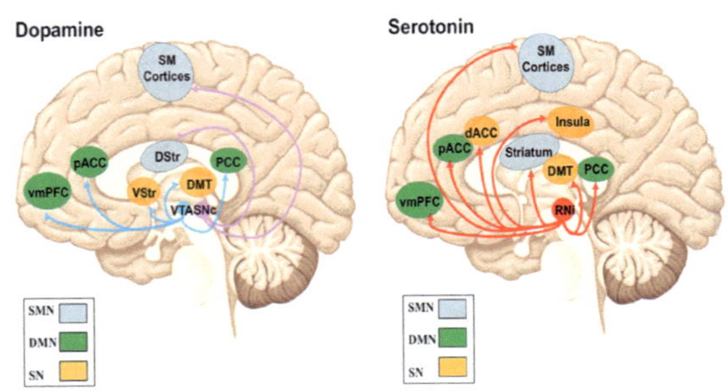

Figure 10.18. Opposite effects of dopamine and serotonin on resting-state networks.

Source: https://media.springernature.com/full/springer-static/image/art%3A10.1038%2Fs41380-019-0406-4/MediaObjects/41380_2019_406_Fig1_HTML.png.

10.5.3. Interaction of Hormones in Stress Modulation

The interaction between hormones is significant in governing the stress response, serving as a primary mechanism through which the body reacts to challenge. Central to this interaction is the HPA axis, which governs glucocorticoid discharge, particularly cortisol, in response to stressors. Hormones , such as CRH, ACTH, and cortisol interact within this axis to initiate a cascade of physiological processes that will act to counteract the effect of stress. CRH is a neuromodulator, which influences both behavioral and humoral responses, and is controlled by many factors , such as emotion states and external stimuli. Recent studies have pushed the understanding further on the molecular mechanisms of CRH signaling, claiming its role in stress responses as well as psychiatric disorders and thereby necessitating an expansion of research on CRHRs towards potential treatments (Inda et al., 2017). Moreover, early life experience leaves a permanent mark on the hormonal interaction involved in stress modulation, indicating the long-term relevance of developmental adversity here. Experiments indicate that adverse conditions at critical early periods have the potential to trigger long-lasting changes in the function of the HPA axis that modulate both endocrine and behavioral stress responses later in life. For instance, brief maternal separation of rodents tends to reduce adrenal sensitivity, while prolonged separation triggers excessive stress responses. These findings point to the subtle effects early experience may have on an individual's stress response system since environmental context plays a strong role in determining the product of hormone interaction. Notably, gender differences have also been cited, wherein women are found to be more vulnerable to disease from stress. These variations further illustrate the manner in which stress hormones are not only reactive but a part of the intricate system of behavior and psychological health deserving of extensive research (Rivarola & Renard, 2014). It is required to explore the intricate web of hormonal interactions underpinning the mode of stress to advance our knowledge of stress pathologies. Stress hormones and behavior exhibit an active relationship that is more than a mere physiological response. For instance, chronic stress can lead to dysregulation of CRH and cortisol, resulting in heightened vulnerability to mental illness , such as depression and anxiety. Thus, unraveling the mechanisms of hormone interaction not only elucidates adaptive stress response but also maladaptive ones that can form chronic illnesses. The potential research should also expound on such hormonal mechanisms, that is, in various settings encompassing development stages, gender differences, and individual susceptibility to stressors. Such an effort has the potential to inform therapeutic strategies aimed at hormone systems in the management of stress disorders, thereby enhancing overall mental health outcomes (Rivarola & Renard, 2014; Inda et al., 2017).

Test Your Knowledge

1. 1. Which key neurotransmitters are involved in the stress response, and what roles do they play in the brain and body?
2. How do hormones like cortisol, adrenaline, and noradrenaline function during acute and chronic stress?

10.6. Coping Mechanisms and Stress Management

Learning Outcome

1. Describe the psychological strategies for stress reduction;
2. Define the physiological approaches to managing stress;
3. Describe the importance of lifestyle changes in stress management.

Coping strategies are critical components of managing stress, which influence reactions to the stressors and their physiological effects. Coping styles can be illustrated, frequently differentiating between active and passive responses. Those who are active will display low heart rate variability (rHRV), thereby demonstrating a constant, high-energy level reflecting their approach to managing challenges. This high level of energy output, while indicative of an assertive coping style, also incorporates the potential for overextension and burnout. Reactive individuals, characterized by higher rHRV, employ a more flexible style and can adjust their energy expenditures in line with situational requirements. This heterogeneity not only influences their short-term stress coping but also significantly influences their long-term well-being and health, as has come to be realized through longitudinal studies of energy management mechanisms across various species, for example, grey seals, in confirming that coping mechanisms are highly dependent on individual physiological profiles (Shuert et al., 2025). Coping mechanisms are also understood when they are analyzed for how they respond to stress on a biochemical level, specifically how they impact one's neuroendocrine system. Stress triggers the HPA axis, which leads to an increase in cortisol, playing an important role in the body's response to stress and energy mobilization. Elevated cortisol levels can enhance an individual's ability to cope in the short run, but chronic exposure tends to generate adverse health effects , such as immune suppression and metabolic dysregulation. Such a combination of stress response and coping activity is an interactive process between psychological drivers and physiological mechanisms. Plants also exhibit coping behavior when exposed to environmental stresses , such as heat, by altering various morphophysiological traits and biochemical processes. These adaptations not only enhance tolerance to stress but also reflect the adaptive strategies observed in animals and in humans, showing a general need for efficient stress regulation in a very broad array of various biological systems (Khanzada et al., 2025). Finally, healthy coping mechanisms and stress management are essential to overall health under adversity. Individuals capable of identifying their coping styles might be capable of accessing their strengths and evading their weaknesses, thereby providing enhanced psychological and physiological outcomes. Self-knowledge improvement and efficient coping skills training will help individuals cope with stress, hence decreasing the likelihood of chronic stress disorders. Moreover, integrating both human and animal stress responses information will make interventions possible that will attend to coping mechanisms' physiological needs. For example, understanding how energy management strategies influence stress resistance can encourage whole health modalities aimed at the achievement of balance in the application of physical as well as mental health. With ongoing research into the nuances of neuroendocrine integration in stress response, the need for personal coping strategies becomes increasingly apparent, guiding therapeutic interventions as well as personal development initiatives in stress coping (Khanzada et al., 2025; Shuert et al., 2025) (Figure 10.19).

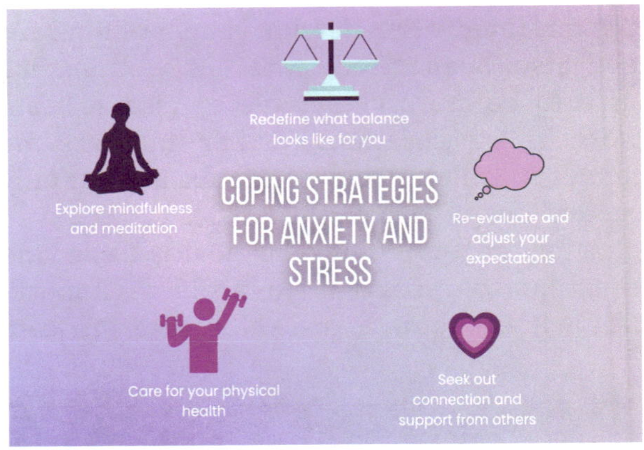
COPING STRATEGIES FOR ANXIETY AND STRESS
Redefine what balance looks like for you
Explore mindfulness and meditation
Re-evaluate and adjust your expectations
Care for your physical health
Seek out connection and support from others

Figure 10.19. Coping techniques for stress and anxiety.

Source: https://thebuzznepal.com/wp-content/uploads/2024/04/645cfb305e096946599ddf4b_coping-strategies-stress-and-anxiety-1024x685.jpg.

10.6.1. Psychological Strategies for Stress Reduction

In stress management, psychological approaches have become key factors for effective intervention. Cognitive-behavioral therapy (CBT) is an example, allowing people to identify and challenge maladaptive patterns of thinking that contribute to stress. By enhancing adaptive coping styles, CBT allows restructuring of perceptions surrounding stressors and eventually redirects the physiological stress response. This shift reflects the intricate interaction between psychological and neuroendocrine conditions, as stress has been shown to induce hormonal imbalances that negatively impact general well-being. It has been found that successful psychological interventions create resistance to stress, maintaining balance in the neuroendocrine system and reversing stress-induced neural deficits. Thus, incorporating these practices into stress management programs not only improves psychological health but also improves physiological health by balancing the body's stress response system. Meditation and mindfulness exercises are yet another critical component of psychological stress reduction techniques. These exercises encourage individuals to reach a higher state of consciousness, giving them informative feedback regarding their emotional and physiological responses to stress. Through a focus on the present moment, mindfulness exercises are able to successfully counteract the predominant influences of past anxieties or future uncertainties, facilitating a calmer state of mind. This exercise has been found to induce significant reductions in cortisol levels, thereby modulating the neuroendocrine response to stress. Also, neuroimaging studies have indicated that mindfulness meditation on a regular basis can alter brain function and structure, enhancing regions of the brain that are responsible for emotional control and reducing the amygdala's reactivity – a core component of the stress response. Thus, the integration of mindfulness in daily life not only provides immediate psychological relief but also favorable outcomes on underlying neuroendocrine processes, resulting in long-term resilience to stress. The role played by social support to psychological therapies of stress cannot be overestimated. Social interaction within a social network assures emotional support, with others sharing experiences and mutual understanding in moments of stress. Psychological work points out the significance of perceived support since it can serve as a buffer to prevent the damaging effects of stressful experience and create an adaptive neuroendocrine response. Social interactions have been shown to induce the release of oxytocin, a stress-reducing hormone linked with increased well-being. Facilitating healthy relationships and social interaction thus not only appears as a psychological necessity but also as a physiological one. Social support, in this case, can thus be viewed as a highly effective form of stress resilience that interacts with psychological interventions that facilitate increased mental and physical health. By emphasizing the resilience of the community, these strategies provide a nonreductive philosophy for stress management within the broader framework of neuroendocrine integration (Figure 10.20).

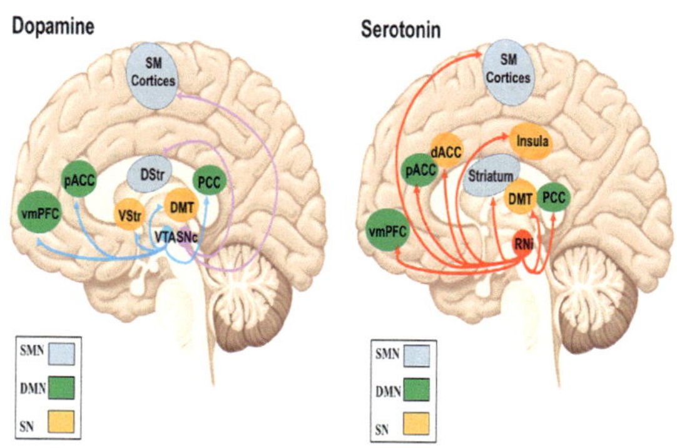

Figure 10.20. Reduce stress and improve well-being.

Source: https://www.verywellhealth.com/thmb/_zdHPRT3b9Y92Yim-OdtH7ly_dU=/1500x0/filters:no_upscale():max_bytes(150000):strip_icc()/how-to-reduce-stress-5207327_FINAL-907db114a640431ba1e8ecbb9e81b77f.jpg.

10.6.2. Physiological Approaches to Managing Stress

Physiological stress management emphasizes the dynamic interaction between the neuroendocrine system and the body's response to stress. The HPA axis is at the center of the process, with its impact on cortisol and other stress hormone release. The process is initiated by perceived threat, demonstrating how the brain organizes physiological functions to prepare fight or flight responses. However, prolonged stress can result in dysregulation of the HPA axis, producing chronic states like depression and anxiety. Understanding these physiological processes allows for the development of targeted interventions that aim to restore balance. Interventions , such as mindfulness, exercise, and respiratory therapy have been shown to not just decrease the short-term effect of stress but also to give long-term health benefits by controlling hormonal responses and enhancing general well-being (DeLisle & Estrine, 2006). The use of physiological strategies of stress management is predominantly through enhancing the body's built-in resilience through lifestyle modification. There is evidence that suggests that consistent physical exercise can dampen stress response by lessening HPA axis activity and encouraging the release of endorphins, which play a pivotal role in mood regulation. In addition, nutritional strategies, including omega-3 fatty-acid-rich diets, are responsible for enhanced neuroendocrine functioning and stress-induced inflammation reduction in the body. Stress-reduction interventions like tai chi and yoga have been effective in not just reducing physiological markers of stress but also improving psychological well-being. These kinds of holistic interventions address the body and mind and show that the interplay between the physiological and psychological aspects is relevant in achieving optimal health outcomes (N/A). Ultimately, the treatment of stress with physiological methods needs an entire system that takes into account environmental and biological variables. Chronic exposure to stress may disrupt the subtle equipoise of neuroendocrine systems and may lead to significant health disparities. To counter this, public health measures need to include stress management education, for instance, encouraging individuals to engage in regular physical activity, adopt healthy dietary habits, and utilize mindfulness. A proactive approach may allow individuals to control their stress responses and improve their quality of life. By blending physiological interventions with psychological counseling, we can make provision for a more efficient way of managing stress, which is commensurate with the holistic nature of human health and well-being (DeLisle & Estrine, 2006) (Figure 10.21).

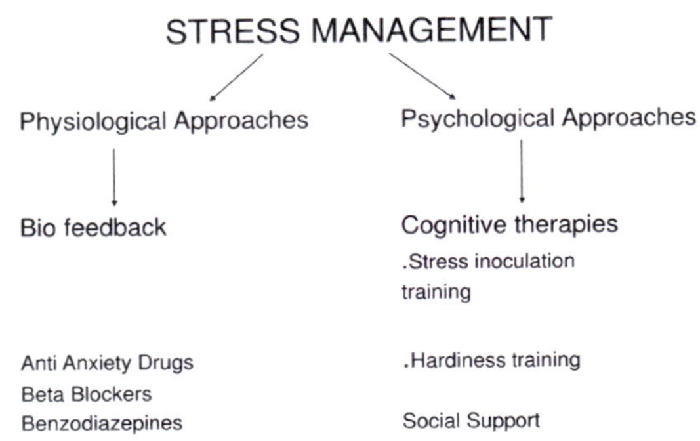

Figure 10.21. Physiological approaches to managing stress.

Source: https://image.slideserve.com/434972/slide30-l.jpg.

10.6.3. Importance of Lifestyle Changes in Stress Management

Empirical findings show that lifestyle changes are an essential component of handling stress effectively, a fundamental element of maintaining neuroendocrine health. The HPA axis and autonomic nervous system interactions demonstrate how stress responses are directly correlated with physiological mechanisms. Engaging in regular exercise has been shown to dampen stress-induced variability in both systems to create improved mood and cognitive function. Exercise acts as a natural stress antidote by reducing the levels of cortisol, the body's primary stress hormone, and thereby enhancing general psychological well-being. Moreover, the development of standard sleep patterns and nutrition changes can also enhance further resistance to stressors. By developing such lifestyle patterns, individuals can significantly enhance their body's ability to handle stressors and lead both physical and mental well-being. The emotional distress in modern society has been proven to lead to severe health complications like cardiovascular diseases (CVD), which are currently known as a leading global cause of mortality. The interlinkages of CVD and stress demonstrate how lifestyle changes become imperative in reducing the risk brought about by psychosomatic diseases. Findings have indicated that chronic stress is not healthy for the cardiovascular system, leading to increased morbidity and reduced quality of life among the affected individuals. Therefore, lifestyle parameter management by means of healthy diets, physical activity, and stress-reducing techniques , such as yoga or mindfulness, becomes the preference. These lifestyle changes not only maximize cardiovascular well-being but also bring long-term mental equanimity, establishing a clinically relevant connection between day-to-day habits and overall health outcomes. As literature highlights, this mutual relationship is indicative of the importance of pre-emptive management of stress by way of lifestyle change (Suciu & Cristescu, 2017). Lastly, creating an atmosphere of support is also a vital but oftentimes overlooked factor in initiating effective lifestyle change. Social networks and support can also very much strengthen a person's adherence to stress-reducing changes. When individuals do activities with other people, even group exercising, stress reduction seminars, or even cooking with others, it creates a sense of belongingness, which further decreases stress. It has been reported that social support can directly affect stress physiological response through the regulation of HPA axis function. Moreover, regular communitarian and relationship-building activities as part of one's routine can build a strong emotional reserve, providing strong buffers against subsequent stressors. Because the body metabolizes stress in an integrated complex manner, emphasizing these lifestyle changes puts people not only in control of stress but in a position to perform exceptionally well in many disparate environments, revealing the far-reaching influence of holistic health practices on physiological reactions (DeLisle & Estrine, 2006).

Test Your Knowledge

1. How do behavioral techniques like exercise, meditation, and breathing exercises help in reducing stress?
2. What role does cognitive restructuring play in coping with psychological stress?

SUMMARY

In combining the intricate interactions between neuroendocrine integration and stress response, there is no doubt that these processes are essential to the study of physiological disease and health. Stress, acute or chronic, triggers diverse responses governed by neuroendocrine mechanisms, further emphasizing the importance of these interactions in maintaining homeostasis. Greater allostatic load (AL), as indicated through various biomarkers, will have a detrimental impact on patient populations, particularly those being treated for chronic disease , such as cancer. Our literature review demonstrates that chronic stress directly impinges on treatment outcomes and overall health, calling for a mandate for healthcare professionals to prioritize stress assessment as part of patient care. This requires further research into the neuroendocrine system's involvement in stress responses, particularly in complex clinical settings where physiological and psychological stimuli converge (Miranda et al., 2024). Furthermore, the function of neuroendocrine change extends not merely to the health of the individual but to wider healthcare practice. For instance, in chronic myeloid leukemia (CML) patients, the association of high AL and poorer survival rates illustrates how stress operates to decline disease prognosis. Interestingly, unraveling these associations can guide clinical interventions because monitoring and regulating allostatic load can enhance treatment efficacy. Clinicians have to adopt a holistic approach that incorporates neuroendocrine factors along with mainstream medicine. By controlling the psychological and physiological ramifications of stress, healthcare professionals can maximize not only survival rates but also overall quality of life for patients with chronic illnesses. Thus, a more integrated concept of patient care must be fostered (Xu et al., 2022). Finally, the intricate interaction between neuroendocrine reactions and physiological stress indicates the necessity for interdisciplinarity in health sciences studies. Researchers and professionals must collaborate to disentangle the biochemical phenomena involved, above all as they relate to disease conditions characterized by elevated stress levels, such as, cancer. The findings underscore the need for the inclusion of neuroendocrine testing as part of routine clinical evaluation so that specific interventions can be made to reverse the detrimental effects of chronic stress. Understanding the mechanisms better will allow future research to improve treatments and promote resilience in patients. As we progress in this line of research, the intent will be to take our growing body of knowledge and make it into actionable strategies that can be implemented effectively within the health systems, thereby ultimately leading to improved outcomes for patients (Miranda et al., 2024).

The neuroendocrine integration and the stress physiological response are primarily controlled by the HPA axis. Central to the response is CRH, which is the principal molecule in initiating basal and stress-evoked responses. CRH exerts its effects on cells and tissues via its action on G protein-coupled receptors (GPCRs) CRHR1 and CRHR2. Recent studies have underlined the complexity of CRH signaling pathways, with particular emphasis on the importance of cAMP generation and ERK1/2 activation in the context of physiological conditions. This sophisticated understanding of the roles of CRH not only promotes our knowledge of stress-induced adaptive behavioral responses but also underscores the potential to design pharmacological treatments to reverse particular neuroendocrine disorders that arise from disrupted stress response (Inda et al., 2017). Further, attachment theory as a construct permits a dramatic framework for investigating the convergence of stress physiology and health. Individual differences in attachment style are shown to bear strongly upon stress-related physiological processes and thus on health outcomes. Research shows that the attachment behavioral system is not only implicated in the regulation of emotional and social processes but also converges with biological processes that have the potential to shape stress response and health. The method of recent research is to believe that physiological changes that are linked to stress could be acting to enable adaptive functions of the attachment system, such as, enhancing cognitive and emotional regulation during stress. By tracing these correlations, researchers can see how attachment influences health behavior and chronic disease, suggesting further exploration of these relationships (Robles & Kane, 2014). In summary, neuroendocrine integration, as manifested by the activity of CRH and its receptors, plays a critical role in regulating the stress response and influencing resultant health outcomes. The interconnection between neuroendocrine signaling and psychological constructs like attachment underscores the intricate nature of stress physiology. Clarification of these relationships is valuable for the identification of new therapeutic agents developed to modify stress responses and abrogate concomitant health ailments. As research continues, it highlights the need for biologically realistic models that can systematically describe the effect of neuroendocrine mechanisms on health and ultimately contribute to interventions that enhance physiological resilience under conditions of stress (Robles & Kane, 2014).

KEY TERMS FROM THIS CHAPTER

- Adrenal cortex
- Adrenocorticotropic hormone (ACTH)
- Allostatic load
- Catecholamines (epinephrine, norepinephrine)
- Corticotropin-releasing hormone (CRH)
- Fight or flight response
- HPA axis (Hypothalamic-Pituitary-Adrenal axis)
- Negative feedback
- Stress hormones
- Adrenal medulla
- Allostasis
- Autonomic nervous system
- Chronic stress
- Cortisol
- Glucocorticoids
- Mineralocorticoids
- Psychoneuroimmunology
- Sympathetic nervous system

CRITICAL THINKING QUESTIONS

1. **Which gland is primarily responsible for initiating the endocrine stress response?**
   a. Pituitary gland
   b. Adrenal cortex
   c. Hypothalamus
   d. Thyroid gland
2. **The hypothalamic-pituitary-adrenal (HPA) axis results in the release of which hormone from the adrenal cortex?**
   a. Epinephrine
   b. Aldosterone
   c. Cortisol
   d. Growth hormone
3. **What is the primary function of cortisol during stress?**
   a. Increase immune system activity
   b. Promote glucose storage
   c. Suppress inflammation and increase blood glucose
   d. Lower blood pressure
4. **Which part of the adrenal gland releases epinephrine and norepinephrine during the acute stress response?**
   a. Adrenal cortex
   b. Adrenal medulla
   c. Zona glomerulosa
   d. Zona reticularis
5. **Which of the following is a major effect of the sympathetic nervous system during stress?**
   a. Decreased heart rate
   b. Pupil constriction
   c. Increased gastrointestinal activity
   d. Bronchodilation

Short Answer Questions

1. What is the hypothalamic-pituitary-adrenal (HPA) axis, and what is its role in stress response?
2. Name the primary hormones released by the adrenal medulla during stress.
3. How does cortisol affect glucose metabolism during stress?
4. What is the role of corticotropin-releasing hormone (CRH) in the stress response?
5. List two physiological effects of sympathetic nervous system activation during acute stress.
6. What is the function of ACTH (adrenocorticotropic hormone)?
7. Differentiate between acute and chronic stress in terms of hormonal responses.
8. Describe the integration of the autonomic nervous system and the endocrine system during a stress response.
9. Explain the phases of the general adaptation syndrome (GAS) and the physiological changes that occur in each phase.
10. Explain the short-term (acute) and long-term (chronic) physiological effects of stress on different body systems.

Answers to Critical Thinking Questions

1. (c); 2. (c); 3. (c); 4. (b); 5. (d).

REFERENCES

1. Robles, T. F., & Kane, H. S. (2014). The attachment system and physiology in adulthood: normative processes, individual differences, and implications for health. *Journal of personality*, *82*(6), 515–527. https://doi.org/10.1111/jopy.12052(accessed on 28th June 2025).
2. Inda, C., Armando, N. G., Dos Santos Claro, P. A., & Silberstein, S. (2017). Endocrinology and the brain: corticotropin-releasing hormone signaling. *Endocrine connections*, *6*(6), R99–R120. https://doi.org/10.1530/EC-17-0111(accessed on 28th June 2025).
3. Armario, A., & Nadal, R. (2013). Searching for biological markers of personality: Are there neuroendocrine markers of anxiety? https://core.ac.uk/download/322421410.pdf (accessed on 28th June 2025).
4. Wright, E. C., Hostinar, C. E., & Trainor, B. C. (2020). Anxious to see you: Neuroendocrine mechanisms of social vigilance and anxiety during adolescence. *The European journal of neuroscience*, *52*(1), 2516–2529. https://doi.org/10.1111/ejn.14628(accessed on 28th June 2025).
5. Chou, T., D'Orsogna, M. R., & Kim, L. U. (2016). Onset, timing, and exposure therapy of stress disorders: Mechanistic insight from a mathematical model of oscillating neuroendocrine dynamics. https://core.ac.uk/download/323078037.pdf (accessed on 28th June 2025).
6. Suciu, M. ., & Cristescu, C (2017). Psychosomatic interrelations in cardiovascular diseases and their consequences on patient's quality of life. DOI: 10.5772/intechopen.69699 https://core.ac.uk/download/322432620.pdf (accessed on 28th June 2025).
7. Cryan, J. F., O'Riordan, K. J., Cowan, C. S. M., Sandhu, K. V., Bastiaanssen, T. F. S., Boehme, M., Codagnone, M. G., et al. (2019). The microbiota-gut-brain axis. *Physiological Reviews, 99*, 1877–2013. https://doi.org/10.1152/physrev.00018.2018 (accessed on 28th June 2025).
8. Porcelli, A. J., & Delgado, M. R. (2017). Stress and Decision Making: Effects on Valuation, Learning, and Risk-taking. *Current opinion in behavioral sciences, 14*, 33–39. https://doi.org/10.1016/j.cobeha.2016.11.015 (accessed on 28th June 2025).
9. Duffee, J. H., Szilagyi, M., Forkey, H., & Kelly, E. T. (2021). Trauma-informed care in child health systems. *Pediatrics, 148*. https://doi.org/10.1542/peds.2021-052579 (accessed on 28th June 2025).
10. Lisa DeLisle Judith Estrine (2006). Stress: Putting the brain back into medicine. An Interdisciplinary Workshop of the INTERNATIONAL LONGEVITY CENTER–USA https://core.ac.uk/download/71356692.pdf (accessed on 28th June 2025).
11. Nazar, F. N., Estevez, I., Correa, S. G., & Marin, R. H. (2017). Stress Induced Polarization of Immune-Neuroendocrine Phenotypes in Gallus gallus. *Scientific reports*, *7*(1), 8102. https://doi.org/10.1038/s41598-017-08733-0(accessed on 28th June 2025).
12. Gavrilović, L., Pajović, S. B., Pavlović, I., Pejić, S., et al. (2017). Animal models for chronic stress-induced oxidative stress in the spleen: The role of exercise and catecholaminergic system. https://core.ac.uk/download/322432294.pdf (accessed on 28th June 2025).
13. Goadsby, P. J., Holland, P. R., Martins-Oliveira, M., Hoffmann, J., Schankin, C. J., & Akerman, S. (2017). Pathophysiology of migraine: A disorder of sensory processing. *Physiological Reviews, 97*, 553–622. https://doi.org/10.1152/physrev.00034.2015 (accessed on 28th June 2025).

14. Zubeldia-Brenner, L., Roselli, C. E., Recabarren, S. E., Gonzalez Deniselle, M. C., & Lara, H. E. (2016). Developmental and Functional Effects of Steroid Hormones on the Neuroendocrine Axis and Spinal Cord. *Journal of neuroendocrinology*, *28*(7), 10.1111/jne.12401. https://doi.org/10.1111/jne.12401(accessed on 28th June 2025).
15. Anil Kumar, M. N., Pai, N. B., Rao, S., Rao, S., & Goyal, N. (2009). Biology of sexual dysfunction. *Online Journal of Health and Allied Sciences*, *8*(1), 1-7.(accessed on 28th June 2025).
16. Herman, J. P., McKlveen, J. M., Ghosal, S., Kopp, B., Wulsin, A. C., Makinson, R., Scheimann, J. R., et al. (2016). Regulation of the hypothalamic-pituitary-adrenocortical stress response. *Comprehensive Physiology*. https://doi.org/10.1002/cphy.c150015 (accessed on 28th June 2025).
17. Khanzada, A., Yan, K., Hu, W., Malko, M., Khan, K. A., Bao, Y., Elboughdiri, N., et al. (2025). Heat stress response mechanisms and resilience strategies in wheat. *Journal of Agronomy and Crop Science*. https://www.semanticscholar.org/paper/45063265c4aa932c1ad891409c3b9423f1790074 (accessed on 28th June 2025).
18. Kuntz, J. (2020). Resilience in times of global pandemic: Steering recovery and thriving trajectories. *Applied Psychology, 70*, 188–215. https://doi.org/10.1111/apps.12296 (accessed on 28th June 2025).
19. Lang, U. E., & Borgwardt, S. (2013). Molecular mechanisms of depression: Perspectives on new treatment strategies. *Cellular Physiology and Biochemistry, 31*, 761–777. https://doi.org/10.1159/000350094 (accessed on 28th June 2025).
20. Lovallo, W. R. (2016). *Stress and Health: Biological and Psychological Interactions*. https://doi.org/10.4135/9781071801390 (accessed on 28th June 2025).
21. Miranda, M., Tjioe, K., Sharara, M., McKenzie, M., Keruakous, A. R., Bryan, L., Jillella, A. P., et al. (2024). Clinical assessment of cumulative stress via allostatic load in chronic myeloid leukemia patients: Implications for treatment outcomes. *Blood*. https://www.semanticscholar.org/paper/589a6a9e446cfd04985c574a1978193f1b410d95 (accessed on 28th June 2025).
22. Rivarola, M. A. ., & Renard, G. M (2014). Qué sabemos sobre las consecuencias a largo plazo de la separación materna temprana y la respuesta neuroendocrina al estrés. https://core.ac.uk/download/159291663.pdf (accessed on 28th June 2025).
23. Shuert, C., Pomeroy, P. P., & Twiss, S. (2025). Stress-coping styles are associated with energy budgets and variability in energy management strategies in a capital breeder. *Proceedings. Biological Sciences, 292*(2046), 20241787. https://www.semanticscholar.org/paper/c1cbf7795f7ac5a6907b975f2d93261a8bfa08da (accessed on 28th June 2025).
24. Shuja, N. (2025). Unraveling the psychophysiological nexus–The impact of stress and mental health on chronic pain and gastrointestinal disorders. *Developmental Medico-Life-Sciences*. https://www.semanticscholar.org/paper/ef8b5b97ff5a26b832e8fd810d03d8ff9c730fa9 (accessed on 28th June 2025).
25. Sies, H., Berndt, C., & Jones, D. P. (2017). Oxidative stress. *Annual Review of Biochemistry, 86*, 715–748. https://doi.org/10.1146/annurev-biochem-061516-045037 (accessed on 28th June 2025).

26. Sukhareva, E. (2021). The role of the corticotropin-releasing hormone and its receptors in the regulation of stress response. *Vavilov Journal of Genetics and Breeding, 25*, 216–223. https://www.semanticscholar.org/paper/23eb7c1c63591133583df5530e6b6291fa492871 (accessed on 28th June 2025).

27. Xu, D., Sun, L., & Qin, X. (2022). Waterless live transport degrades the flesh quality of *Litopenaeus vannamei* by disturbing neuroendocrine response: Based on physiology and metabolomics. *Journal of the Science of Food and Agriculture*. https://www.semanticscholar.org/paper/b9bc0a1d07bb786877ad321283e0b84b5e10f87e (accessed on 28th June 2025).

28. Yao, Y., Nan, L., Wang, K., Xia, J., Ma, B., & Cheng, J. (2024). Integrative leaf anatomy structure, physiology, and metabolome analyses revealed the response to drought stress in sainfoin at the seedling stage. *Phytochemical Analysis: PCA*. https://www.semanticscholar.org/paper/cbd9813f18f7da130ec38623922d0ce3399e6749 (accessed on 28th June 2025).

SLEEP PHYSIOLOGY AND CIRCADIAN RHYTHMS

11

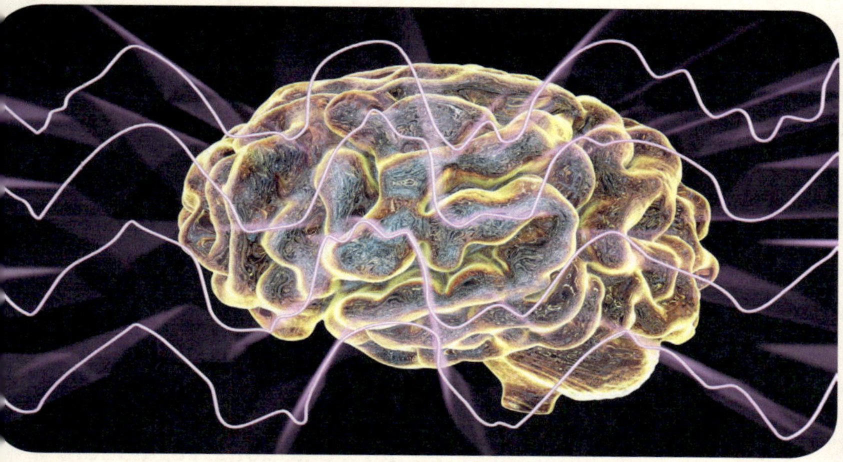

LEARNING OBJECTIVES

After studying this chapter, you will be able to:

1. Discuss the stages of sleep.
2. Explain the biological mechanisms of sleep.
3. Discuss the circadian rhythms explained.
4. Focus on sleep disorders.
5. Discuss the impact of light on sleep.
6. Evaluate the sleep and health.

Introduction

Sleep physiology and circadian rhythm are crucial components of human health and well-being. Both regulate not only the sleep-wake cycle but also our general metabolic processes, including behavior, cognitive function, and physical health. As research expands in the field of sleep, it has been increasingly evident how interconnected the two are. Circadian rhythms, regulated by internal biological clocks, govern the time course of numerous physiological processes, one of which is the sleep-wake cycle. When disturbed, either due to lifestyle or external factors , such as shift work, its impact on health can be dramatic. This association gives insight into interventions for enhancing the quality of sleep and synchronizing biological processes with nature, resulting in enhanced health benefits. Further, research has also been carried out to understand how disrupted sleep and circadian disruption may influence metabolic disease, including diabetes. Current workshops, such as, one held at the National Institute for Diabetes and Digestive and Kidney Diseases, have noted significant correlations between sleep disruptions and energy balance disturbances. These findings point to the necessity of interdepartmental research collaboration between metabolic health researchers and sleep researchers. By conducting comprehensive studies that integrate sleep evaluations with traditional metabolic profiling, researchers are able to uncover the molecular processes of diseases like pre-diabetes and obesity. This data is crucial for formulating targeted interventions that could transform public health policies on circadian and sleep-induced metabolic illnesses (Arble et al., 2015). Adding to this complexity is the fact that circadian rhythms are not always defined in terms of human physiology; they can be used to describe a wider spectrum of living forms. For instance, experiments have established that various species of insects undergo a circadian change in susceptibility to insecticides.

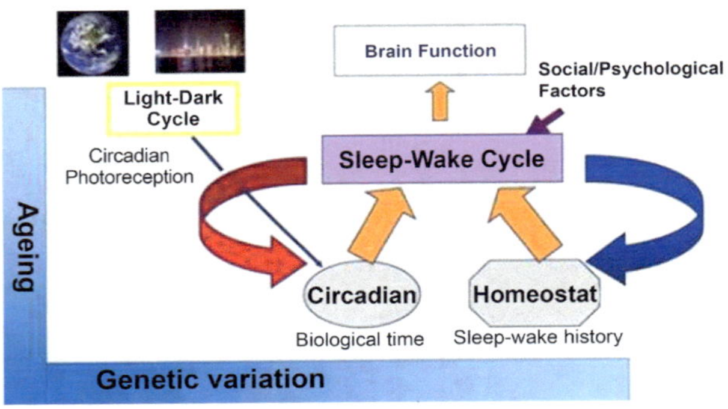

Figure 11.1. Sleep physiology and circadian rhythms.

Source: https://external-content.duckduckgo.com/iu/?u=https%3A%2F%2Ftse4.mm.bing.net%2Fth%3Fid%3DOIP.1KVKh32mZPSk_2DP9tld2AHaEM%26r%3D0%26pid%3DApi&f=1&ipt=b066647f9d39f87aecbf95893522a3716c01add7597ff39b6a2aa48e7d1046eb.

This is a demonstration of the influence of circadian rhythms not just on behavior but also on biochemical processes crucial for survival. Awareness of these patterns applies in pest management, where the timing of insecticide application can greatly determine effectiveness. Within non-human organisms, studies also shed light on circadian rhythms' evolutionary significance, demonstrating the ubiquity of this biological process across taxa. This interdisciplinary research informs us better about the broader implications of sleep physiology for health and ecological dynamics (Khalid et al., 2019) (Figure 11.1).

Definition of Sleep Physiology

Sleep physiology describes the complex biological processes and mechanisms involved with sleep states that are essential for health and well-being. The term sleep physiology refers to the observation of interactions between various physiological parameters, including neurological, hormonal, and metabolic functions in a person in clear sleep stages. Crucially, this science entails an understanding of physiological variations that occur during rapid eye movement (REM) sleep and non-REM sleep. Both stages possess specific brainwave, muscle tonicity, and autonomic activity patterns required for the consolidation of memory, emotional regulation, and restoration of body energy. Since sleep occupies an essential position in human life, studying its physiology reflects the intricate interplay among internal biology and external environments, illustrating its importance in making sleep disorders and treatments meaningful through time. Furthermore, sleep physiology is closely related to the circadian rhythm, which is a foundation stone of human physiology that governs the sleep-wake cycle. This internal clock mechanism operates on roughly a 24-hour cycle, controlled by external factors , such as light and temperature, and governs physiological processes , such as hormone secretion, body temperature, and sleep-wake cycle. At the cell level, circadian rhythms are a product of interconnected transcription and translation feedback loops, reflecting their pervasive effect on utilization of multiple biological systems. As a case in point, Boden et al. (2013) describe how circadian rhythms shape central reproductive physiology functions, and once more, that synchronization of sleep with the circadian rhythm is paramount in attaining optimal health. Their disruption can cause a variety of health issues, and as such, an understanding of sleep physiology is crucial in the development of interventions that will restore circadian synchrony and improve healthcare outcomes. Aside from its function of regulation for sleep, knowledge of sleep physiology unveils larger biological processes, including metabolic processes and cardiovascular function. Sleep disturbances can facilitate alterations in metabolic rate and cardiovascular risks, bridging the gap between sleep physiology and diseases like obesity and hypertension. Experiments have shown that insufficient sleep could deregulate the release of hormones , such as cortisol and insulin, further accelerating these conditions. In addition, as Bailly et al. (2011) indicates, biological rhythms are under a sophisticated regime beyond linear representations of time, presenting the dynamic nature of sleep and its interaction with other physiological cycles. Upon understanding the complexity of sleep physiology and its interaction with circadian rhythms, scientists could target new treatments and presentational interventions for sleep disorders, hence enhancing overall health and encouraging well-being in society (Figure 11.2).

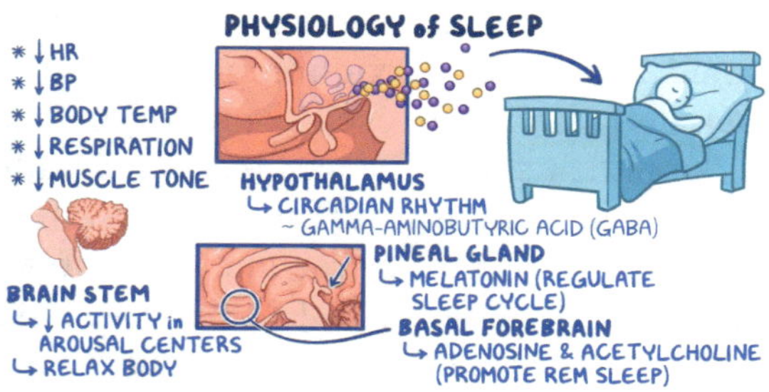

Figure 11.2. Sleep physiology.

Source: https://osmose-it.s3.amazonaws.com/ec_RSmLyRMWJKIuAtwXPirv-SZSsOB_d/_.jpg.

Importance of Studying Sleep

The significance of understanding sleep extends beyond mere curiosity; it plays a crucial role in the comprehension of overall health and wellness. Sleep is a complex process of physiology governed by circadian rhythms, which regulate thousands of aspects of biological function. Disruption of the rhythms has unwanted effects, including metabolic diseases and mental disorders. Quality of sleep and the duration of sleep are known to be associated with increased disease risks , such as diabetes and obesity. Enhanced coordination among sleep and metabolic researchers, as noted in recent workshops on sleep disturbances, is required to unravel the intricate mechanisms between sleep patterns and metabolic health. This intersectional approach emphasizes the need for comprehensive studies that assess both metabolic and sleep function in order to further establish more potent public health policy and interventions for improving sleep quality (Arble et al., 2015). In addition to its metabolic importance, sleep is of broad relevance in the context of mental health. Mental illnesses , such as Seasonal Affective Disorder (SAD) illustrate the impact of circadian rhythms on psychological health, which is why research in this area is essential. Designation of SAD as a psychological illness demonstrates that studying sleep and its effects can generate particular treatments , such as light therapy that targets specific derangements of the circadian rhythm. This validates the observation that sleep is not only a restorative phase but also a building block of psychiatric diagnosis and treatment plans. Through study of these phenomena, it is possible for researchers to bridge the gap between sleep physiology and mental illness and thus contribute to an integrated approach towards treatment for mood disorders and enhance the quality of life for individuals suffering from them (Overy & Tansey, 2014). Ultimately, the understanding of sleep is significant in solving bigger public health problems, particularly during an era when sleep disturbances are more rampant than ever. Sleep research aimed at circadian disruption has provided us with important correlations between the patterns of sleep and chronic disease, and it calls for ongoing investigation. For instance, understanding how sleep apnea and related conditions affect diabetic patients can guide more targeted interventions. The need for further investigations involving heterogeneous populations is highlighted by the ongoing discussions on the potential contribution of chronic adaptations to sleep disruption. By highlighting more the role that circadian rhythms play in systemic health, we can better appreciate the importance of integrating sleep studies into healthcare models. Interdisciplinarity will ultimately result in effective countermeasures against the growing epidemic of sleep disorders (Arble et al., 2015).

Overview of Circadian Rhythms

Circadian rhythms, endogenous biological processes regulating the sleep-wakefulness cycle, are characterized by approximately 24-hour periods governed by environmental stimuli , such as light and temperature. Circadian rhythms are regulated by an endogenous biological clock at the level of the suprachiasmatic nucleus (SCN) of the hypothalamus, which harmonizes physiological processes with the day-night cycle. The interaction between the SCN and peripheral oscillators in numerous body tissues provides a guarantee of coordinated hormonal releases, metabolic activities, and behavioral patterns with environmental stimuli. A human being's circadian rhythm may contribute significantly to sleep patterns, which, in turn, influence overall health. Disruptions of these rhythmic cycles, such as, those experienced through shift work or excessive exposure to artificial light, can lead to sleep disorders, metabolic syndrome, and increased susceptibility to chronic disease, which underscores the importance of rhythmically entrained lifestyles. Circadian misalignment has been increasingly associated with a variety of health risks in research studies, suggesting an important site for intervention and investigation. Specifically, workshops at places , such as the National Institute for Diabetes and Digestive and Kidney Diseases signaled a call for focused research exploring the influence of sleep and circadian disruption on metabolic well-being. Those workshops underscored the need for collaborative efforts in interdisciplinary work between sleep researchers and researchers in metabolism to convert basic research into an applicable public health advantage. Interdisciplinary research is essential to investigating how disturbances of the circadian rhythms are most likely to increase the risk of diabetes and influence other metabolic diseases. Besides, screening for sleep irregularity in longitudinal studies may provide valuable information on their long-term impact on health measures, which in turn may guide clinical practice towards more personalized care regarding sleep and the circadian rhythms (Arble et al., 2015). Additional studies have shown circadian rhythms to go beyond human health and affect different organisms in the animal kingdom. As an example, research on the common bed bug *Cimex lectularius* has illustrated daily fluctuations in susceptibility to insecticides associated with circadian rhythms. The expression of the metabolic detoxification gene of these insects had rhythmic characteristics corresponding to susceptibility to specific insecticides, which suggests that an ecological role and function in pest control are present for circadian cycles. Identifying how other organisms, like insects, exhibit circadian sensitivity can enable further understanding of ecological rhythms, as insight into potential problems with pest control is delivered. This increasing understanding must encourage more universal research approaches that consider circadian biology across different species, ultimately making the scientific underpinning for tackling issues related to sleep, metabolism, and even agriculture even more robust (Khalid et al., 2019).

11.1. The Stages of Sleep

Learning Outcome

1. Describe the non-REM sleep stages;
2. Focus on REM sleep characteristics;
3. Learn about sleep cycle duration and patterns.

Sleep stages are the mandatory components of sleep physiology that have characteristic patterns of brain activity and physiological alteration. Sleep is generally classified into two broad categories: non-REM (NREM) and REM sleep. NREM sleep is further subdivided into three stages: N1, N2, and N3, each comprising different depths of sleep. Stage N1 is the period between wakefulness and sleep and is defined by a decrease in muscle activity and slower brain waves. As individuals transition into Stage N2, there is further relaxation as well as a considerable decrease in heart rate and body temperature. Stage N3 or deep sleep is crucial for restorative functions when the body has engaged in significant cell repair and reconstruction. Proper cycling through these stages is required for overall psychological and physical health, and interruption is responsible for a multitude of health issues. In addition to the rejuvenating effects of NREM sleep, REM sleep also plays a crucial part in cognitive functions, particularly in memory consolidation and emotion regulation. Occurring approximately every 90 minutes throughout the night, REM sleep is also characterized by high brain activity, vivid dreams, and rapid eye movement. REM sleep is associated with the rebuilding and consolidation of knowledge acquired while awake, learning, and creativity. Notably, the presence of REM sleep is significant in the facilitation of emotional equilibrium because it aids in processing and integration of emotional experience. Studies have established that interruptions of REM sleep cause cognitive dysfunction and mood disorders, highlighting the need for uninterrupted sleep cycles. The complex interdependence of the different stages composes a full system that regulates various physiological and psychological processes necessary for well-being. Circadian rhythms regulate the structure of sleep by timing the stages of sleep. The hypothalamic suprachiasmatic nucleus (SCN) is the principal circadian clock, responding to light-dark environmental rhythm and controlling sleep-wakefulness by means of behavioral and hormonal signals. Coordination needs to be maintained to keep well-balanced vigilance and sleep potential, with disruption leading to complaints like insomnia or hypersomnia. Furthermore, circadian mismatches, most often brought about by irregular light exposure or nighttime shifts, may lead to internal desynchronization, and the quality of sleep and overall wellness is affected. Correcting such circadian mismatches has the potential to significantly improve sleep phases and create healthier body states. Understanding the intricate interaction between sleep phases, the circadian rhythm, and overall well-being allows tailored interventions that optimize sleep hygiene and mental health, desperately needed in contemporary society (Holley et al., 1981; Plano et al., 2017) (Figure 11.3).

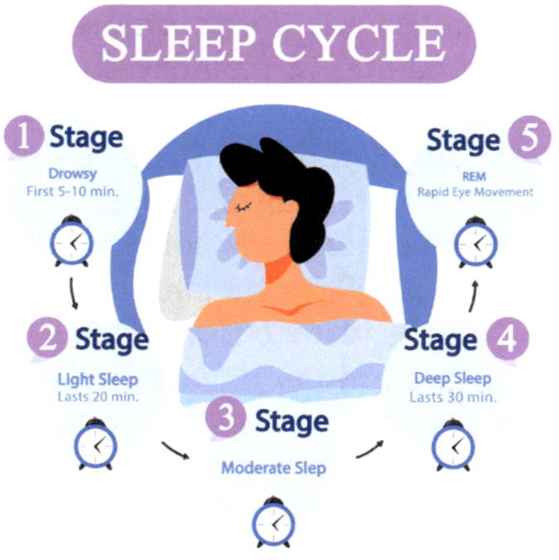

Figure 11.3. Stages of sleep.

Source: https://www.thesleepjudge.com/wp-content/uploads/2019/09/image1.jpg.

11.1.1. Non-REM Sleep Stages

It is necessary to value the stages of non-REM (NREM) sleep in interpreting the sleep structure and its physiological importance overall. NREM sleep consists of three distinct stages—N1, N2, and N3—each of which serves specific responsibilities that assist in restoration work in the mind and body. The initial stage, N1, is the stage of transition from wakefulness to deeper sleep with light sleep and reduced physiological activity. This stage allows for the slowing down of disengagement with the external environment, a necessity for effective entry into higher states of sleep. In stage N2, the body further decelerates heart rate and temperature, aiding better recovery. This stage occupies approximately 50% of total sleep duration and is crucial in memory consolidation and learning; therefore its importance in cognitive function and wakefulness during the day. The most profound stage of non-REM sleep, N3 or slow-wave sleep (SWS), is in charge of extensive recovery and physiological repair. The brain demonstrates delta wave activity during N3, which is a state of deep relaxation. This stage is primarily associated with physical restitution processes , such as tissue repair, protein production, and immune system enhancement. Furthermore, N3 sleep is also instrumental in memory consolidation, particularly for declarative memories—trivia and knowledge that can be consciously recalled. The NREM stages, especially N3, also have serious implications for overall health; research has established that the absence of this stage can lead to chronic brain damage, stress, and disruptions in metabolic function. Thus, adequate NREM sleep, particularly deep sleep, is crucial in order to maintain overall wellness and cognitive function. Circadian rhythms profoundly influence the timing and character of non-REM sleep stages, emphasizing the intricate interdependence between sleep physiology and environmental synchronizers. Circadian rhythms regulate the sleep-wake cycle, and disruptions may induce desynchronies in sleep architecture, particularly in subjects who are subjected to altered light conditions, such as, astronauts on space flights. Research shows that sleep timing alterations will lead to physiological disturbances in alertness and cognition (Samel et al., 1991). Additionally, circadian rhythm integrity is fundamental to peak performance as deviations will lead not only to impaired sleep quality but also increased fatigue and sleepiness (Holley et al., 1981). Therefore, the understanding of the circadian rhythms' function in the regulation of non-REM sleep stages underscores their significance in optimizing sleep quality and enhancing overall health, which implies that future research is required to investigate the means through which the debilitating consequences of circadian misalignments may be avoided (Figure 11.4).

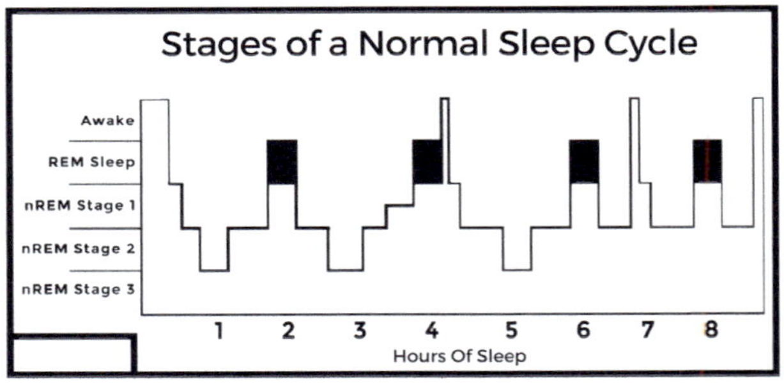

Figure 11.4. Non-REM sleep.

Source: https://external-content.duckduckgo.com/iu/?u=https%3A%2F%2Fcdn.shopify.com%2Fs%2Ffiles%2F1%2F1041%2F4674%2Ffiles%2FHours_1024x1024.png%3Fv%3D1494952388&f=1&nofb=1&ipt=3f029e5ba7e8710644f3ea5f4f74542bd690d5c757e39db58a42d833c47fd9bb.

11.1.2. REM Sleep Characteristics

Rapid Eye Movement (REM) sleep is a distinct phase of the sleeping cycle that is characterized by having distinct physiological and neurological features. During this phase, which typically follows about 90 minutes of sleep, the brain maintains wakefulness levels of activity, with increased neuronal firing and dominance by beta waves. REM sleep is also associated with vividness of dreams, which is facilitated by heightened cerebral blood flow and metabolic activity in various areas of the brain, including the visual association cortices and limbic system. Such abundance of dreaming suggests a significant role for REM sleep in emotion regulation and memory consolidation, creating connections that can be employed to facilitate learning. Therefore, studying the REM sleep dynamics becomes important to know about the functions that it exhibits in cognitive processes and mental health, helping researchers unravel the sleeping physiology complexities as well as control mechanisms in the perspective of circadian regulation. The regulation of REM sleep is very intertwined with neurophysiological networks , such as the hypothalamus and brainstem, being a complex interface of inhibitory and excitatory neurotransmitters. The flip-flop system of sleep-wake regulation describes this interaction, in which unique populations of neurons alternate enhancing wake and sleep. Cholinergic neurons are especially significant during REM sleep in that they maintain the state by increasing release of acetylcholine, which can be viewed to vary arousal and vigilance levels. REM sleep dynamics are also circadian-modulated, such that alteration of endogenous circadian rhythms can bring about alteration of the patterns of REM activity between species. These results underscore the importance of exploring such neurobiological models because they are the foundation of comprehension of how interruptions in REM sleep can lead to some sleep disorders and cognitive dysfunctions, as manifested in diseases like Alzheimer's disease and autism (Grossberg, 2017). Moreover, the physiological functions of REM sleep go beyond the aspect of mere dreaming to involve essential physiological functions vital to overall health. For example, REM sleep has a function in synaptic plasticity, which consolidates the neural connections formed during the day. Consolidation of synapses is necessary for learning and memory, which implies that REM sleep can contribute to the integration of new information into the existing knowledge frameworks. The homeostatic sleep drive also plays a critical role in the regulation of the dynamics of REM sleep, which are necessary to maintain optimal brain functioning. Circadian rhythms also control the timing and character of REM sleep, illustrating just how inextricably these physiological processes are tied up with overall well-being and health. As such, awareness of REM sleep properties improves our broader knowledge of sleep physiology, and their exploration remains vital to understanding the increased prevalence of sleep disorders in contemporary society (Behn & Booth, 2012) (Figure 11.5).

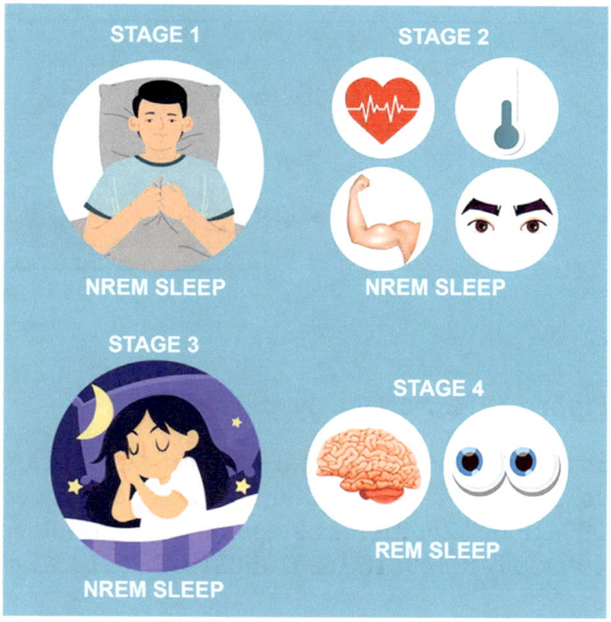

Figure 11.5. REM sleep.

Source: https://cdn.shopify.com/s/files/1/0255/9777/1885/files/an-infographic-chart-showing-stages-of-sleep.jpg?v=1672918060.

11.1.3. Sleep Cycle Duration and Patterns

The dynamics of the length of sleep cycles and stages affect overall health, performance, and well-being substantially. Historically, sleep is apportioned into two broad forms: REM sleep and NREM sleep, which in turn breaks down into stages. These cycles often last between 90 and 120 minutes and occur multiple times during the night, with differences in length and frequency depending on factors like age, lifestyle, and environmental factors. Disruption of these cycles can lead to impaired cognitive function, emotional distress, and a range of metabolic derangements. An understanding of how these cycles of sleep operate can aid in better ways of optimizing sleep quality, especially in specific groups, such as, sports performers who may be able to enhance performance and recovery by maximizing sleep practice. The presence of circadian rhythms also plays a crucial role in the regulation of sleep cycle patterns and sleep duration. Biological clocks make sleep-wake cycles get synchronized with the natural light-dark cycle, with eventual impacts on secretions of sleep and wakefulness hormones. These cycles are controlled by the suprachiasmatic nucleus (SCN) through environmental feedback, primarily light exposure, which possesses an excellent ability to modify metabolic and physiological processes.

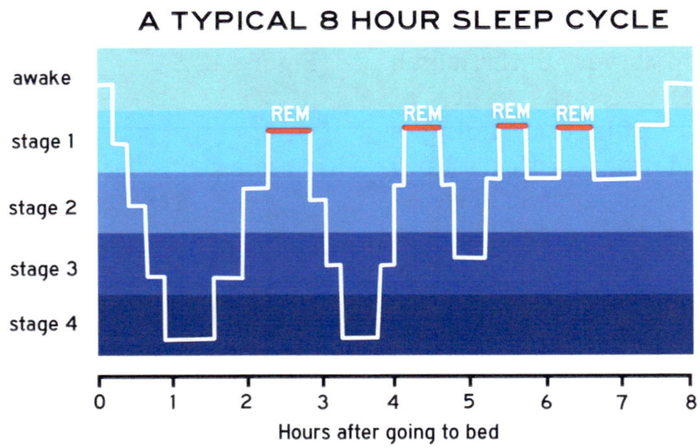

Figure 11.6. Normal sleep pattern.

Source: https://external-content.duckduckgo.com/iu/?u=https%3A%2F%2Fwww.scienceabc.com%2Fwp-content%2Fuploads%2Fext-www.scienceabc.com%2Fwp-content%2Fuploads%2F2019%2F08%2Fdifferent-steps-of-the-night-sleep-cycledesdemona72s.jpg-.jpg&f=1&nofb=1&ipt=cac400e8de7c83e9c1ff3e2c79583cc8301310c12d7b007e850391781c078eba.

When these rhythms are synchronized with environmental cues, they ensure maximal function, but disruptions, such as, those owing to shift work and lifestyle changes, can disrupt sleep quality and undermine metabolic health. Appreciation of the interaction between circadian rhythms and sleep architecture can be critical in avoiding sleep disorders and therefore improving the quality of life of most individuals with sleep disorders (Plano et al., 2017). More studies on the interdependence between sleep cycle duration and circadian rhythms show the need for personalized approaches in optimizing sleep. Young athletes, for instance, can have distinct sleep characteristics tied to their training program, indicating varying levels of performance based on the time of day. A comparative analysis with adolescent competitive swimmers found that although relative performance was constancy regardless of time, physiological variables differed widely, testifying to circadian rhythms' influence on energy states and mood. Trainers and sportsmen must therefore consider the fine role played by sleeping hours in recovery and performance (Grant & Glen, 2018). Through the union of physiological knowledge with actuality, improving not just athletic performance but overall health gains through more profound sleep habits is achievable (Figure 11.6).

Test Your Knowledge

1. What are the different stages of sleep, and how are they classified into REM and non-REM categories?
2. Describe the key physiological characteristics of each sleep stage

11.2. The Biological Mechanisms of Sleep

Learning Outcome

1. Explain the role of neurotransmitters;
2. Define the hormonal influences on sleep;
3. Identify the brain structures involved in sleep regulation.

Understanding the biological mechanisms of sleep is key to appreciating its physiological significance and contribution to overall health. Sleep is regulated by complex interactions among a number of neurochemical players and the body's internal rhythms, which dictate the sleep-wake cycle. Indeed, neurotransmitters , such as gamma-aminobutyric acid (GABA) and serotonin are crucial in promoting sleep. Additionally, the SCN of the hypothalamus is considered to be the master clock, which controls circadian rhythms by responding to extrinsic signals like light. Coordination such that sleep and wakefulness have proper timing is essential in maintaining homeostasis. Disturbances of this strongly integrated system, including exposure to artificial light at night, could disrupt sleep and lead to many forms of illness. With scientists becoming increasingly familiar with these mechanisms, the hope of designing targeted interventions to cure sleep disorders becomes increasingly vivid. Metabolic processes and how they relate to sleep are also a key area of research that serves to illuminate the biological mechanisms of sleep. The influence of circadian rhythms on energy balance and glucose metabolism has become a point of interest in recent work. Alteration of these rhythms, most commonly found with shift work or non-conventional sleep patterns, has been linked to an increased risk of metabolic conditions , such as diabetes. The significance of the link was emphasized during a workshop at the National Institute for Diabetes and Digestive and Kidney Diseases, where scientists promoted an interdisciplinary initiative to examine how sleep and circadian disruption affect metabolic health. This dialogue between sleep physiology and metabolism scientists can be a source of necessary information. By incorporating sleeping measurements in available research on diabetes risk, researchers can identify chronic adaptations as metabolic regulation pathways rendering sleep an essential factor in disease prevention and treatment. The medical profession also now begins to appreciate the necessity of incorporating circadian science into clinical practice. With the advent of widespread research on the molecular basis of circadian rhythms, there is the potential to individualize treatment regimens in terms of someone's biological clock.

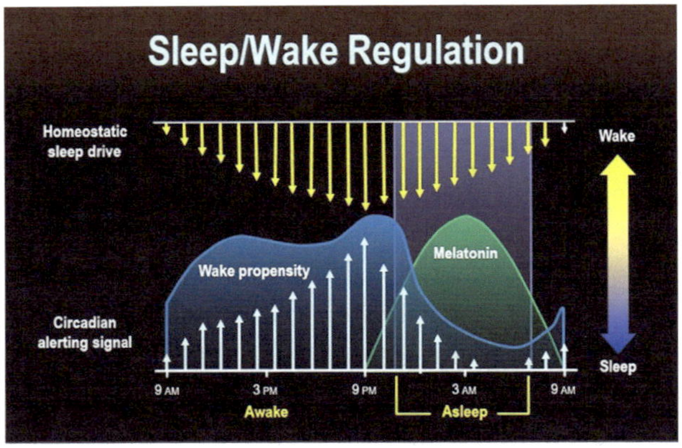

Figure 11.7. Biological mechanisms of sleep.

Source: https://static.wixstatic.com/media/855ada_95eb0ad0707c47b88a4e96acd6bdd98a~mv2.jpg/v1/fill/w_846,h_566,al_c,lg_1,q_85/855ada_95eb0ad0707c47b88a4e96acd6bdd98a~mv2.jpg.

For example, the timing of drug administration can actually be optimized for efficacy and reduced side effects when aligned with the body's innate rhythms. In addition, treatments like continuous positive airway pressure (CPAP) therapy in patients with obstructive sleep apnea have become popular as possible interventions to postpone the onset of diabetes. These results reinforce the importance of further investigation into the complex interplay between sleep, circadian biology, and metabolic health. By examining these linked domains, researchers can ultimately make a larger contribution to the understanding of sleep's biological processes and its implications to human health, as exemplified by the growing consensus of experts in the field (Arble et al., 2015; Field et al., 2021) (Figure 11.7).

11.2.1. Role of Neurotransmitters

Of particular significance in the physiology of sleep is the function of neurotransmitters as the determining force to regulate sleep-wake cycles. Neurotransmitters , such as gamma-aminobutyric acid (GABA), serotonin, and norepinephrine play a crucial role in regulating both the onset and continuation of sleep. GABA, the primary inhibitory neurotransmitter, is responsible for sustaining non-REM sleeping stages through relaxation and inhibition of neuronal excitability. On the contrary, serotonin is involved with circadian regulation, influencing the transition from sleep to wakefulness. The extremely delicate balance between these neurotransmitters enables the brain to respond as per the environment's requirements, thereby enhancing the quality of sleep and general well-being. Thus, understanding the intricate interactions between these chemical messengers illuminates the broader implications for sleep disorders and pharmacological effectiveness in managing sleep behaviors. The interaction of neurotransmitters with circadian rhythms is supplemented by the existence of a sleep-wake regulatory network within the brain. Neuroanatomical studies reveal that neuronal populations across the brainstem and hypothalamus coordinate the control of sleep and wakefulness in intricate synaptic interactions. These encompass both fast synaptic transmissions and slower homeostatic and circadian processes, which reflect the intricacy of sleep regulation. For instance, the dynamics of the sleep-wake regulatory network are by their nature, tied to metabolic parameters, which portray the association between metabolic health and neurotransmitter function. In line with what has been discovered, the circadian system not only controls sleep timing but also coordinates various physiological processes, illustrating how neurotransmitters act as regulators and responders of circadian signals. It is this holistic process that explains how circadian disturbances in neurotransmitter signaling can be disruptive to sleep, thus providing potential avenues for therapeutic intervention that restores circadian rhythms as well as induces quality sleep (Albrecht, 2012). In order to better clarify the role played by neurotransmitters in the physiology of sleep, mathematical modeling of the sleep-wake network reveals dynamics involved in the regulation of REM and non-REM sleep. The mathematical model depicts the interactions between the different populations of neurons, demonstrating how disparate neurotransmitter activity impacts sleep stages. Simulation experiments demonstrate that REM-facilitatory neuron activation is indistinguishably correlated with homeostatic sleep drives and hence an imbalance in neurotransmitter signaling is responsible for dysregulating sleep architecture. For instance, changes in the level of neurotransmitters can lead to variations in REM dynamics, from suppression to irregular cycling, reflecting the intricacy of circadian modulation. This dialogue highlights the significance of neurotransmitters not only in inducing sleep but also in generating a rhythmic and symmetrical sleep pattern, thus underlining their significance in sleep physiology and circadian rhythms (Behn & Booth, 2012) (Figure 11.8).

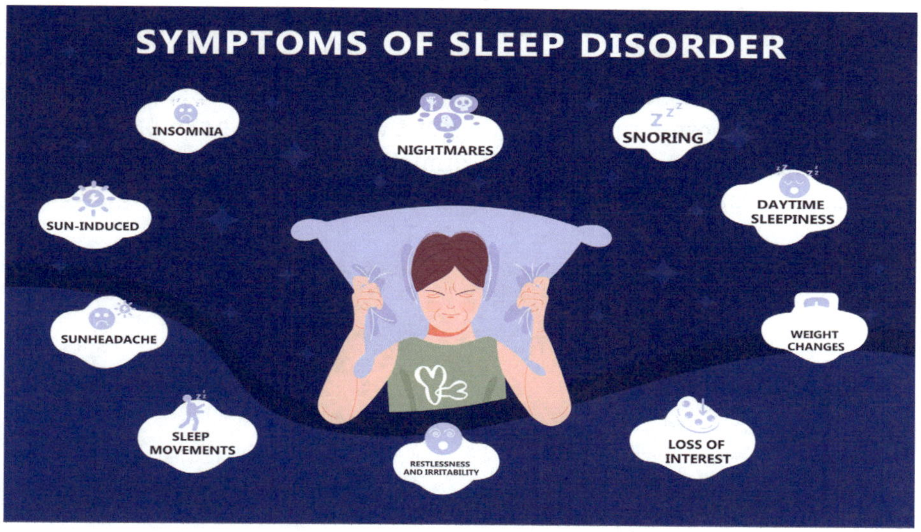

Figure 11.8. Symptoms-of-sleep-disorder-mental-health-problems.

Source: https://www.hemlock.co.ke/wp-content/uploads/2024/03/symptoms-of-sleep-disorder-mental-health-problems.jpg.

11.2.2. Hormonal Influences on Sleep

The intricate interaction between sleep physiology and hormones is a part of circadian rhythm regulation. The hormones melatonin, cortisol, and growth hormone play a central role in regulating sleep patterns so that the internal clock of the body is coordinated with external environmental signals. Melatonin, which is popularly known as the sleep hormone, is secreted by the pineal gland during darkness, promoting sleep onset and maintenance. Its light-sensitive synthesis does make it a central component of the circadian rhythm. Melatonin release aberrations, either induced by exposure to artificial lighting or irregular patterns of sleep, can lead to an enormous array of sleep disorders and decreased overall health, emphasizing the need for normal environmental lighting to preserve endocrine function. An understanding of this interaction is central to the development of techniques that will undo sleep disorders and maximize overall well-being. Cortisol, an adrenal hormone, also has a large impact on sleep-wake patterns. Cortisol would normally have a peak in the early morning to prepare for wakefulness and taper over the course of the day to help with falling asleep at night. This daytime-to-nighttime variation is directly correlated with the circadian rhythm, which coordinates all the bodily processes, including endocrine secretion. Nevertheless, chronic stress and nonrhythmic sleep architecture can disrupt cortisol regulation, leading to sleep disturbances , such as insomnia and disrupted sleep architecture. As highlighted in contemporary studies, the effects of cortisol on sleep, excluding its contribution to the quality of sleep, also could lead to metabolic dysregulation and mood disorders, highlighting the importance of an equilibrium hormonal state for healthful sleep. Identification of such relationships can be utilized in order to develop more effective therapeutic interventions in sleep-disturbed individuals. The interplay between circadian rhythms and hormonal homeostasis also has complex feedback controls that regulate physiological processes, as documented in various studies. The SCN of the hypothalamus serves as the master circadian clock, regulating peripheral oscillators that influence hormonal function and sleep. Disruption of these rhythms, such as, shift work or jet lag, can result in desynchronization of hormone secretion and sleep patterns, with adverse effects on health. For instance, desynchrony of metabolic hormones has been implicated in the pathogenesis of obesity and diabetes as documented in studies examining the impact of disrupted light-dark cycles on energy metabolism. Thus, a better understanding of the action of hormones on sleep can unlock the intricate relationships between circadian rhythmicity, hormonal regulation, and overall welfare and guide future plans towards the prevention and treatment of sleep disorders (Figure 11.9).

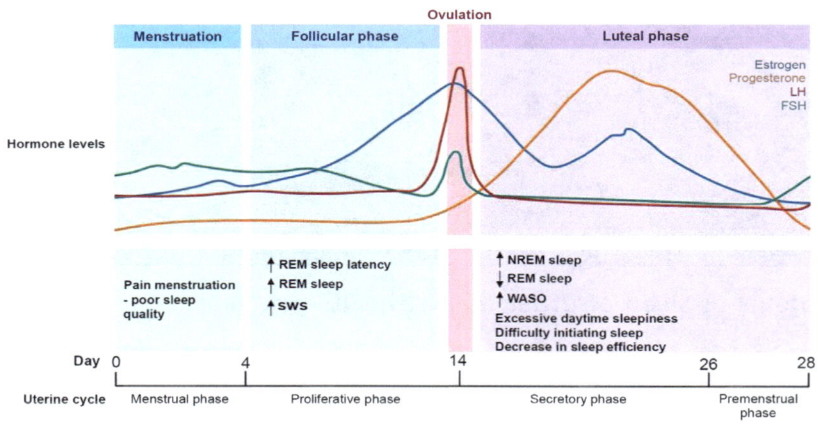

Figure 11.9. Hormonal influences on sleep.

Source: https://www.frontiersin.org/files/Articles/1271827/frsle-02-1271827-HTML-r1/image_m/frsle-02-1271827-g001.jpg.

11.2.3. Brain Structures Involved in Sleep Regulation

Sleep is controlled by the interaction of many brain structures, with the hypothalamus perhaps most critical, namely the , the body's internal circadian clock. This is a small group of cells that receives direct input from the retina in order to synchronize physiological rhythms with light-dark cycles in the environment. The SCN regulates the timing of different sleep-wake cycles by influencing downstream neural and hormonal pathways and consequently influences behaviors , such as feeding and energy consumption. Notably, disruptions to the function of SCNs can lead to a multitude of health issues, including sleep disorders and metabolic dysregulation, highlighting its importance in circadian homeostasis maintenance and health (Plano et al., 2017). Apart from the hypothalamus, sleep regulation also involves the brainstem and other neurotransmitter systems outside of it. More specifically, the reticular activating system which contains tracts extending from the brainstem to the cortex, is mostly responsible for sleep induction. Norepinephrine, serotonin, and acetylcholine are neurotransmitters that play a crucial role in inducing alertness and cognitive processes during wakefulness. At the same time, stimulation of certain areas in the brainstem induces sleep, illustrating the bimodal function of these structures in controlling sleeping and wakefulness. They work together to generate a tenuous balance that generates transitions between sleep stages and ensures restorative processes during sleep (Siwicki et al., 2018). Worth noting is the role of the thalamus, which acts as a relay point for sensory inputs and controls sleeping states. During NREM sleep, the thalamus is less sensitive to external stimuli, essentially cutting out sensory inputs and causing a resting state to be induced. Conversely, during REM sleep, increased activity is present in the thalamus, which is accompanied by enhanced dreaming and higher activity levels in the brain. The thalamic interaction with cortical sites also maintains the complex architecture of sleep, lending support to the belief that such brain regions form part of an integrated network responsible for maintaining circadian rhythms and sleep physiology as a whole. The brain sites as a whole highlight the interrelationship of neural circuits in sleep regulation, pointing to the precise balance of wakefulness and sleep (Figure 11.10).

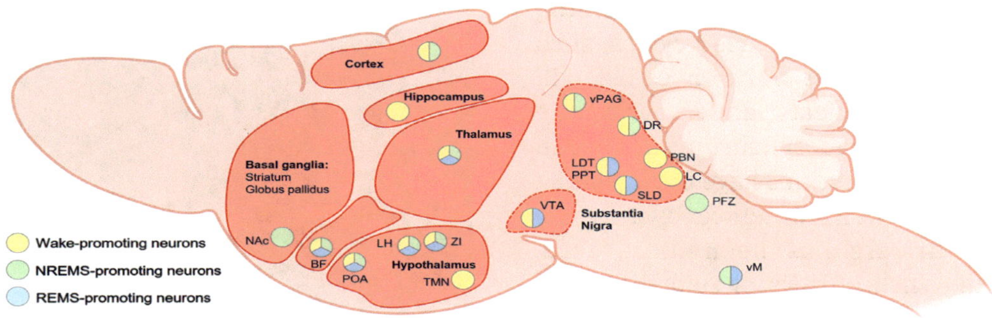

Figure 11.10. Understanding sleep regulation in normal and pathological conditions.

Source: https://journals.sagepub.com/cms/10.3233/JHD-230564/asset/25a30905-b9c3-4106-a960-8316cca182ad/assets/graphic/10.3233_jhd-230564-fig5.jpg.

Test Your Knowledge

1. What roles do neurotransmitters , such as serotonin, GABA, and acetylcholine play in sleep regulation?
2. How does the circadian rhythm influence the timing and quality of sleep?

11.3. Circadian Rhythms Explained

Learning Outcome

1. Explain the significance of circadian rhythms;
2. Define the role of the suprachiasmatic nucleus;
3. Describe the factors influencing circadian rhythms.

Our understanding of circadian rhythms has advanced significantly, revealing their profound impact on numerous physiological processes like sleep, metabolism, and behavior. Circadian rhythms are characterized by their about 24-hour periods, regulating functions of the body as it adapts to environmental cues, particularly light and darkness.

The central circadian clock is located in the suprachiasmatic nucleus (SCN) of the hypothalamus, orchestrating peripheral clocks found throughout the body. This intricate system allows the body to adapt to daily changes, maximizing energy usage and maintaining homeostasis. Disruptions of these cycles, such as, those induced by shift work or jet lag, will yield adverse health effects, underscoring the significance of circadian synchrony in overall well-being. Circadian rhythms have been studied scientifically, and their influence by internal and external drivers has been discovered. Environmental synchronizers, or zeitgebers, like light exposure, play a significant role in circadian stability, and they dictate sleep and alertness levels. Notably, literature is worried about the fact that changes in the stability of such rhythms tend to have negative consequences for human performance, particularly in high-risk situations like flying. For instance, tests of pilot physiology have shown how circadian misalignment can result in cognitive impairment and increased performance decline (Holley et al., 1981). This interaction between circadian rhythms and performance behavior persists in a broad variety of disciplines, and it underlines the need for methods improving synchronization and reducing the negative impact of rhythm disorders. Cross-coupling between circadian rhythms, sleep, and other cognitive processes has emerged as the core area of study in neurobiology. New findings suggest that circadian clock mechanisms not only control sleep but also play essential roles in modulating food intake and memory processes.

The discovery of central clock genes opened new avenues for investigation into how circadian biology maintains these coordinated physiological functions. Also, imaging technology advances allow for observation of rhythmic occurrences on cellular and systemic scales, and the growing knowledge of how circadian disruptions can lead to health risks (Boersma et al., 2009). This growing evidence establishes the significance of circadian rhythms in dealing with sleep disorders and other illnesses, moving towards an integrated approach to health that takes into consideration the rhythmical nature of biological systems (Figure 11.11).

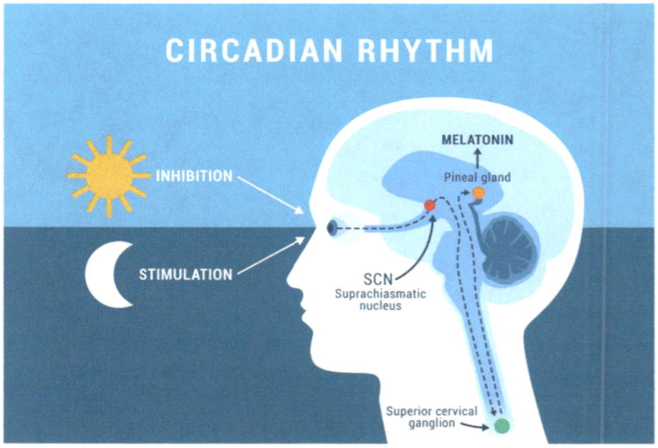

Figure 11.11. Circadian rhythm.

Source: https://images.squarespace-cdn.com/content/v1/5beb00a47e3c3abd688e43b4/1634632036472-PEDHEV4HX2APPZWLSG5L/Circadian+Rhythm+-+See+What+Is+It.png.

11.3.1. Definition and Significance of Circadian Rhythms

Circadian rhythms are innate biological oscillations that manifest in most physiological processes in a period of approximately 24 hours. These rhythms are a consequence of an intrinsic timing system that synchronizes with external environmental rhythms, primarily light and darkness. This synchronization is critical in the maintenance of homeostasis as well as in the optimization of body functions like sleep regulation, metabolism, and hormone secretion. The master clock, located in the suprachiasmatic nucleus of the hypothalamus, regulates the release of melatonin from the pineal gland, a hormone that plays a significant role in sleep and wakefulness. Circadian rhythm disruption has been linked to many ailments, such as, insomnia, mood disorders, and metabolic syndrome, further emphasizing its critical role in overall well-being and functioning in humans. The function of circadian rhythms in reproductive well-being goes beyond mere regulation of sleep; circadian rhythms have essential functions in other areas of reproductive well-being. Circadian rhythms have been implicated in regulating the cycle of estrus, hormonal spikes coinciding with ovulation, and the timing.

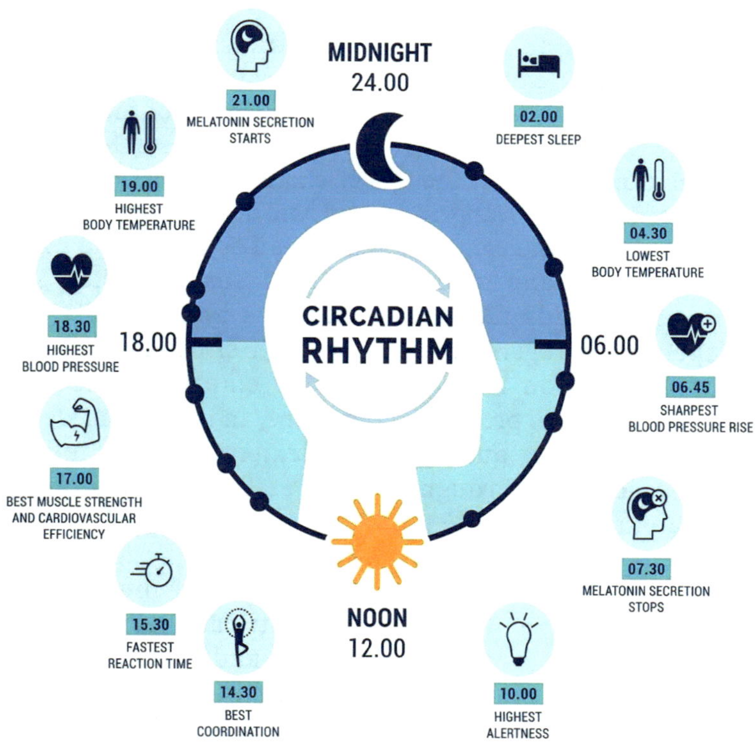

Figure 11.12. Significance of circadian rhythms.

Source: https://www.news-medical.net/image-handler/picture/2021/2/shutterstock_1742387510.jpg.

Circadian timing plays a key role in the proper coordination of all reproductive activities in this harmonious coordination. These rhythms also play roles in early preimplantation embryo development and parturition and postnatal care implications. Additional research on these circadian rhythmic processes can render interventions synchronizing reproductive health with circadian biology feasible, enhancing the success of fertility treatments and prenatal care, illustrating the unifying effect of circadian rhythms on multiple physiological systems (Boden et al., 2013). In addition, the association between circadian rhythms and illness underscores the complex interplay between daily physiological cycles and chronic illness. For example, disruption of circadian signals has been implicated in neurodegenerative illnesses like Huntington's disease, where patients undergo extensive sleep disturbance accompanied by progressive motor and cognitive deterioration. Research conducted on mouse models, like the Q175 mouse, has explained the therapeutic actions of treatment directed towards circadian regulation, with observations in locomotion, sleep modulation, and even the pathophysiology itself of such diseases (Wang et al., 2018). These findings accentuate the central interaction of circadian rhythms and sleep physiology, and the necessity to study further both in clinics and therapeutics to reverse the impact of circadian dysregulation on health. Such advances potentially have as much promise as to provide new tools for optimizing quality of life and altering disease course through circadian rhythm normalization (Figure 11.12).

11.3.2. The Role of the Suprachiasmatic Nucleus

The SCN is the mammalian master circadian clock, found within the hypothalamus. SCN, being the central regulator of circadian rhythms, samples the environmental light signals by direct photic input from retinal ganglion cells, thereby enabling it to synchronize physiological processes with the 24-hour day-night cycle. Not only is coordination vital for the regulation of sleep-wake cycles, but also vital for other behavioral and metabolic processes. The SCN synchronizes the timing of these complex operations by signaling with other neural and endocrine organs within the organism and thus can influence peripheral clocks. Being the master organ, disruptions to SCN function are capable of leading to an assortment of health issues, highlighting the necessity of circadian coherence in the context of external environmental cues. The interplay of SCNs with other physiological systems extends beyond the regulation of sleep and affects processes , such as metabolism and reproductive physiology. Evidence illustrates how the SCN controls energy expenditure, feeding rhythms, and the general metabolic well-being through the activation of peripheral circadian oscillators. These interactions are apparent through hormonal alterations and neurotransmitter function that establish food intake rhythms and energy consumption over a day, indicative of the SCNs' far-reaching control over homeostasis. Moreover, studies show that circadian SCN disturbances, either as a result of chronic desynchronization or photic stimulation, can lead to metabolic disorders and increased disease susceptibility, such as, obesity and diabetes, and indicate a strong relationship between circadian disruption and health. The results emphasize the importance of the SCN not only in regulating sleep patterns but also in implementing other fundamental mechanisms of metabolic control and health. In addition to its metabolic roles, the SCN plays a role in reproductive physiology by regulating the timing of reproductive processes via circadian rhythms. The intricate relationship between circadian timing and reproductive hormone regulation is facilitated through the SCN's regulation of the hypothalamic-pituitary-gonadal axis. This orchestration makes such events as the estrus cycle, ovulation, and insemination timing occur in synchrony with the external world, and this maximizes reproductive success. Interference with the SCN's regulatory functions can affect these processes and lead to fertility complications and gestation problems. Understanding the multi-faceted role of SCNs in reproductive health brings into focus the significance of circadian rhythm integrity within various biological systems, further validating that sleep physiology and circadian rhythms are closely associated and essential for overall well-being (Boden et al., 2013; Plano et al., 2017) (Figure 11.13).

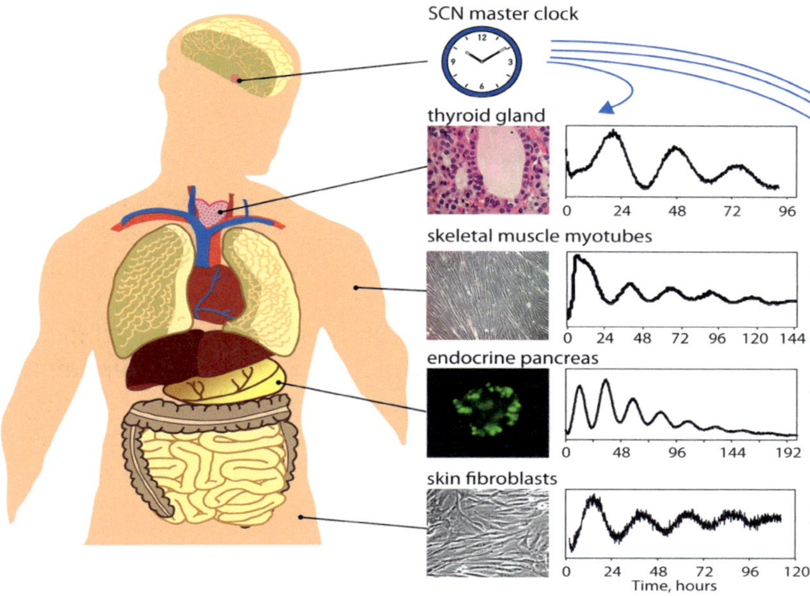

Figure 11.13. Applications for studying circadian phenotypes in physiology.

Source: https://www.frontiersin.org/files/Articles/144196/fneur-06-00095-HTML/image_m/fneur-06-00095-g001.jpg.

11.3.3. Factors Influencing Circadian Rhythms

There are several biological and environmental determinants involved in the control of circadian rhythms, the timing and quality of sleep being determined by them. One of the important biological determinants is the intrinsic genetic variation between humans, which decides the variability in circadian phenotypes, which are categorized as Early, Intermediate, or Late circadian phenotypes (ECPs, ICPs, LCPs). The phenotypes decide people's sleep-wake patterns, their alertness, and performance levels throughout the day. The significance of understanding these differences has arisen as increasingly crucial in a society that demands peak performance at all times, regardless of individual differences. To this end, innovative processes have been developed to measure sleep and circadian rhythm appropriately, combining subjective assessment with objective tracking processes , such as actigraphy, which captures movement, and laboratory analysis of biological samples. These strategies demonstrate how these differences in phenotypes can lead to huge variations in rest-activity patterns, reflecting the demand for individualized methods of optimizing performance and health (Facer-Childs et al., 2019). Environmental factors also have a central function in regulating circadian rhythms, particularly illumination and social information. Light is the primary zeitgeber, or time signal, responsible for synchronizing inner biological clocks with external conditions. Daytime sunlight exposure promotes alertness, while nighttime lack of sunlight signals the body to sleep, primarily through the secretion of melatonin. But the existing lifestyle tends to disrupt these signals, with more exposure to artificial light, especially in the evening, having a detrimental effect on the quality of sleep and synchrony of circadian rhythms. Also, social factors , such as work schedules, school schedules, and social engagements can further disrupt biological clocks and result in incongruence between internal and external requirements. Environmental determinants need to be studied in order to understand how their effects together might have an impact on sleep quality and health outcomes overall, particularly in settings where performance is of utmost importance (Bagshaw et al., 2019). In addition to environmental and biological aspects, psychological factors also have a strong influence on circadian rhythms, particularly within high-performance settings , such as competitive sport. Research has shown that mood states have circadian rhythms and, therefore, may impact psychological readiness and physical performance. For instance, a study with competitive child swimmers demonstrated various indicators of physiological preparedness, such as, handgrip strength and overall states of mood, based on time of day. These findings indicate non-trivial psychological effects on performance at different times and therefore, psychological preparedness must be monitored as well as physiological parameters. Interactions between circadian rhythms and psychological factors suggest the need to include mood and affective state in the optimization of training schedules and competition timing. Grasping this intricate relationship will allow coaches and players to personalize methods that incorporate sleep, performance, and mental health.

Test Your Knowledge

1. What are circadian rhythms, and which biological processes do they regulate in the human body?
2. Which structure in the brain acts as the master clock for circadian rhythms, and how is it synchronized?

11.4. Sleep Disorders

Learning Outcome

1. Identify the insomnia and its effects;
2. Define the sleep apnea and its implications;
3. Describe the circadian rhythm sleep disorders.

The intricate interaction between circadian rhythms and sleep disorders emphasizes the necessity for unimpaired sleep architecture to maintain physiological health. Sleep disorders, such as, insomnia, sleep apnea, and restless leg syndrome, disrupt the regular sleep-wake cycle, which in turn has a negative impact on numerous aspects of daily life. The circadian rhythms of the body, regulated by the suprachiasmatic nucleus (SCN) of the hypothalamus, adapt to the external world through light and other zeitgebers. This coordination is crucial to the release of melatonin, responsible for triggering sleep. Disturbances in circadian rhythms can result in poor secretion of melatonin, thus aggravating sleep disorders. Moreover, the increased use of technology has driven sleep quality issues, particularly in the younger population. Rising trends of the use of electronic media in late evenings have been documented, affecting sleep onset and duration, particularly among school children (Olteanu-Pascal & Lupuşor, 2020). The effects of sleep disorders go beyond fatigue; they have severe implications for metabolic health. Disturbance of sleep patterns and circadian rhythm results in hormonal imbalances affecting hunger control, and the risk of obesity and Type 2 diabetes is elevated. It has been found that sleep deprivation negatively impacts insulin sensitivity and glucose metabolism, suggesting a biological connection between desynchronization of the circadian rhythm and metabolic disease (Arble et al., 2015).

Therefore, sleep disorder patients are bound to be more susceptible to such chronic illnesses. This association implies the need not just to realize sleep problems as independent conditions but within the overall context of health. It will be imperative to have a multidisciplinary approach that includes the areas of sleep and metabolism to comprehend the complex processes and devise effective interventions. In the quest to enhance sleep disorders, education and lifestyle modifications cannot be overlooked. Public health campaigns for creating awareness regarding how technology affects sleep hygiene have the potential to educate individuals to make informed choices that better their sleeping behavior. Encouraging normal sleep habits, limiting screen time before sleep, and developing an environment that is conducive to sleep are simple strategies that can help contribute to the control of sleep disorders. Such measures are particularly important in this technology-driven era, where excessive exposure to blue light from screens has been shown to interfere with circadian control. Alliances between healthcare providers, educators, and families must be made to generate a culture of prioritizing healthy sleep practices. By targeting the causative factors of sleep disorders and focusing more on the significance of circadian entrainment, the prevalence of sleep disorders can be curtailed, leading to improved health outcomes (Olteanu-Pascal & Lupuşor, 2020) (Figure 11.14).

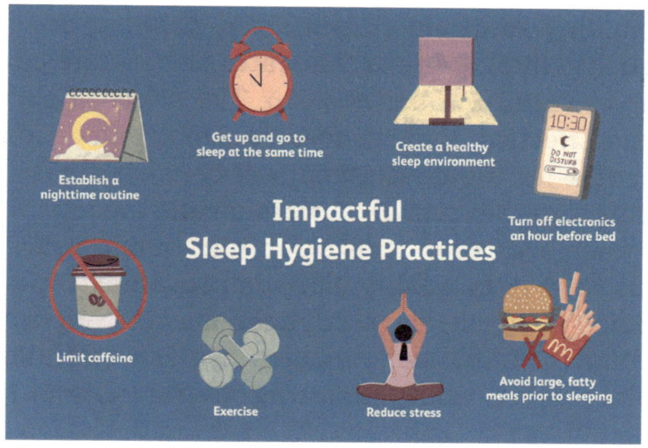
Impactful
Sleep Hygiene Practices
Establish a nighttime routine
Get up and go to sleep at the same time
Create a healthy sleep environment
Turn off electronics an hour before bed
Limit caffeine
Exercise
Reduce stress
Avoid large, fatty meals prior to sleeping

Figure 11.14. Sleep hygiene

Source: https://www.verywellmind.com/thmb/XTQmfLo6hR2Ho-TEFpjXEYuNpvs=/1500x0/filters:no_upscale():max_bytes(150000):strip_icc()/what-is-sleep-hygiene-5085887-FINAL-831b8421e75249f0952fbf4efb0adda7.png.

11.4.1. Insomnia and Its Effects

Insomnia, which involves trouble falling asleep or maintaining sleep, presents significant issues for patients across all age groups. Insomnia becomes more prevalent with age since most geriatric patients suffer from persistent sleep disturbances that hinder overall health and well-being. (Shochat, 2022) Insomnia, besides affecting the sleep quality, causes a variety of associated issues like daytime somnolence, irritability, and cognitive impairment. As insomnia disrupts restorative sleep, bodily recovery, both physically and psychologically, is hindered, impacting subsequent performance of daily tasks. Thus, understanding the consequences of insomnia is of great importance in preventing its broader health implications. Physiological mechanisms of insomnia suggest a complex interaction between neurobiological processes and circadian rhythm. Insomnia is established by disruption of the body's internal sleep-wake cycle, primarily governed by a variety of neuroanatomical and neurochemical systems, including monoaminergic and cholinergic transmission. (Rodríguez et al., 2019) Disturbance in these systems can lead to a vicious cycle where abnormal sleep makes stress and anxiety worse, and this contributes to the individual's inability to attain restful sleep. Notably, the neurobiological complexity reveals the necessity of quality interventions that cater to both the psychological and physiological aspects of insomnia so as to result in quality sleep. The effect of chronic insomnia extends beyond short-term cognitive and affective disturbances; it can also have long-term health consequences. Insomnia patients are at risk for the development of comorbidities , such as cardiovascular disease, obesity, and mental illness in the form of depression and anxiety. With statistics showing that older adults find it harder to achieve restorative sleep, the public health burden is substantial. Insomnia treatment is not just a case of quality sleep improvement; it is a case of resilience in overall health development. Being so extensive in implications, it is important to implement wide-ranging strategies, including behavior modification, sleep hygiene education, and potential pharmacotherapy, tailor-made for older adults, thus enhancing their quality of life and health status (Figure 11.15).

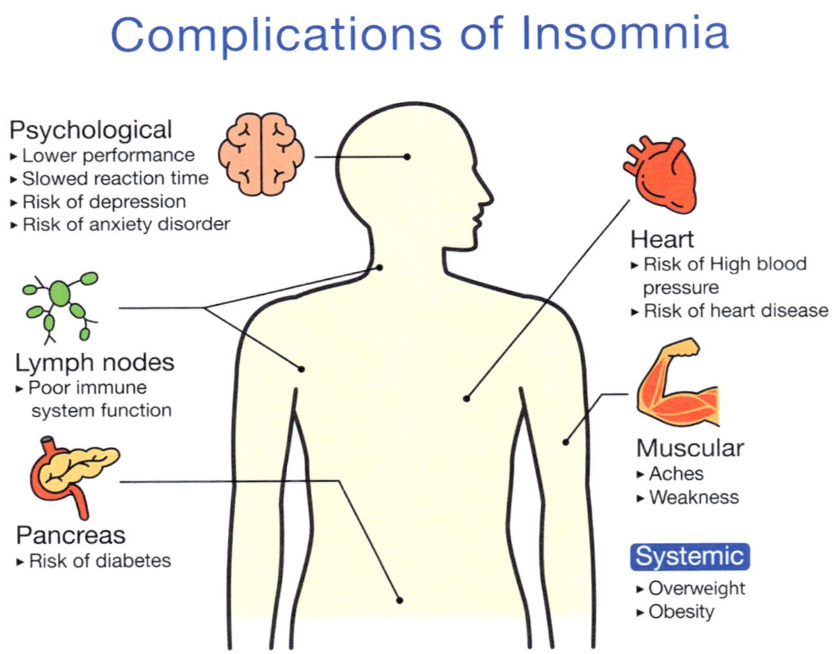

Figure 11.15. Complications-of-insomnia.

Source: https://www.amindfulway.com.au/wp-content/uploads/2018/06/complications-of-insomnia.jpeg.

11.4.2. Sleep Apnea and Its Implications

The occurrence of sleep apnea, but particularly obstructive sleep apnea (OSA), has been brought under more attention due to its impact on overall health and metabolic processes. Sleep apnea is the repeated disruption of breathing when asleep, and this will yield disturbed sleep patterns and significantly change circadian rhythms. An increasing number of studies link sleep apnea with higher risk for various health disorders , such as cardiovascular diseases, hypertension, and metabolic syndrome. It is worth noting that collaboration between sleep research and metabolic health studies, as emphasized in Arble et al., (2015), can enhance our understanding of the physiological relationships between sleep-disordered breathing and long-term health conditions. Understanding these relationships can inform interventions that target both normalization of sleep and enhancement of metabolism, with the long-term objective of advancing the quality of life of the affected. Furthermore, the effect of sleep apnea extends beyond its influence on cognition and psychiatric health. The disturbed sleep created by repeated apneic events disrupts the critical processes of memory consolidation and affect regulation. Chronic sleep loss can exacerbate depression and anxiety symptoms, thereby activating a cycle of decreasing sleep quality and heightened psychological distress. As further noted by Shochat (2022), age-related changes will nevertheless aggravate sleep patterns and advance the increased incidence of insomnia among the elderly, which can be coincidental with undiagnosed sleep apnea. Mental health and the quality of sleep together underpin the necessity of complete screening of sleep disorders in high-risk populations, in this instance the elderly, in order to limit cognitive as well as affective costs of untreated sleep apnea. Finally, treatment of sleep apnea, particularly with procedures like continuous positive airway pressure (CPAP), offers a window of opportunity to prevent its pathogenic influences on health. There is evidence from recent times that suggests that proper management can reduce the risk of developing other metabolic dysfunctions, as stated by Arble et al., (2015). This prophylactic approach is particularly relevant to patients with pre-diabetes combined with OSA, where the management of sleep apnea has the potential to postpone or even prevent the onset of diabetes. Furthermore, lifestyle changes, such as, temporal restricted feeding, have been shown to decrease obesity levels related to sleep disruption. Therefore, a multi-dimensional strategy, incorporating both lifestyle and medical intervention, is critical to controlling the broader effects of sleep apnea on health and quality of life, thus supporting the necessity of integrated treatment models in clinical practice (Figure 11.16).

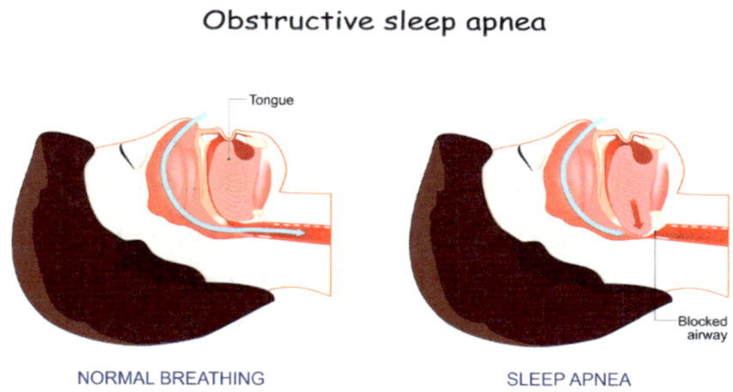

Figure 11.16. Obstructive sleep apnea (OSA) disease.

Source: https://www.birlahospital.com/wp-content/uploads/2022/08/Obstructive-Sleep-Apnea-OSA-Disease.jpg.

11.4.3. Circadian Rhythm Sleep Disorders

Circadian rhythm sleep disorders are a huge disruption of the regular sleep-wake cycle controlled by the internal clock of the body, which is primarily regulated by the SCN of the hypothalamus. Such disorders may present in the form of irregular sleep timing, impacting the quantity and quality of sleep individuals achieve. Of all the circadian rhythm disorders, advanced sleep-phase syndrome and delayed sleep-phase syndrome are the most prevalent. Individuals suffering from advanced sleep-phase syndrome sleep and wake up unusually early, while individuals suffering from delayed sleep-phase syndrome have problems falling asleep until late in the evening, often resulting in daytime functioning problems. As research indicates, the disorders can significantly interfere with daily life and well-being, and it is therefore important to research their mechanism and effects on human health. Research into circadian rhythm disorders has evolved, particularly as genetic studies have made clear the heritable nature of the disorders. Although familial cases of some circadian rhythm disorders have been reported, such as, the rare advanced sleep-phase syndrome, most of the information about their genetic basis at hand is incomplete. Recent findings in genetics have made it possible for scientists to discover specific genes that are involved in circadian regulation, and therefore decipher the structure and regulation of sleep-wake cycles (Jones et al., 2013). This innovation in genetics reveals potential mechanisms through which disruptions occur, and points to environmental factors and heredity as the combination that causes circadian rhythm disorders to develop. The importance of circadian rhythm sleep disorders extends beyond basic sleep disturbance, showing potential links to other illnesses. Circadian rhythm disturbance has been associated with metabolic syndromes, psychiatric disease, and cardiovascular disease, indicating a far-reaching effect on physical health (Jones et al., 1999). It is necessary to recognize these links to guide particular interventions and treatments. With the potential of advances in circadian biology and genetics, clinical practitioners are able to develop ways to restore normal circadian function and thereby enhance the health effects of these disorders. With the increasing prevalence of shift work and lifestyle elements influencing circadian rhythms, treatment for these disorders is paramount in order to achieve maximum individual and public health outcomes.

Test Your Knowledge

1. What are the common causes and symptoms of insomnia, and how is it typically managed?
2. How do conditions like obstructive sleep apnea and narcolepsy affect normal sleep architecture and daytime functioning?

11.5. The Impact of Light on Sleep

Learning Outcome

1. Describe the effects of natural light exposure;
2. Define the blue light and its consequences;
3. Discuss the strategies for managing light exposure.

The intricate dynamic between light and sleep depends on the processes that create circadian rhythms. Circadian rhythms are essentially biological processes that cycle on a roughly 24-hour rhythm, which have a profound impact on many physiological and behavioral processes, including the sleep-wake cycle. The master clock for these rhythms resides within the hypothalamus and employs environmental cues, primarily light, to stay in sync with the external environment. Particularly, exposure to light via the eyes communicates this internal clock, reaffirming ideal sleep-like and wake cycles. Interruption of this process, such as, in the case of shift work or travel across time zones, results in circadian desynchrony. Consequently, individuals may be affected by sleep disorders due to desynchronized biological rhythms to produce symptoms like insomnia or drowsiness during the day, highlighting the inherent function of light as a synchronizer of sleep cycles (Lockley et al., 2007). Furthermore, the influence of light on sleep is not merely synchronization but also directly impacts the production of melatonin, a hormone that has a significant function in the regulation of sleep. Melatonin is very closely related to exposure to light: it will typically peak in the evening when darkness arrives, causing drowsiness, and decline in the presence of morning light. This interdependent relationship is particularly critical in an era that is characterized by intense artificial light exposure. For instance, the blue light emitted by screens can inhibit melatonin synthesis, resulting in increased delays in sleep onset and disrupting the architecture of sleep. The most appropriate light exposure in intensity and timing is significant in aiding proper sleeping habits, and therefore, understanding the influence of light on the level of melatonin is an important way of learning about improved sleep management strategies, and the significance of using natural exposure to light as an approach to optimal sleep hygiene (Facer-Childs et al., 2019). There are also individual differences in circadian phenotypes that indicate variation in light influence on sleep among various individuals. Research indicates that individuals can be classified into Early, Intermediate, or Late circadian phenotypes based on their intrinsic sleep-wake preference and light responsiveness. These differences might indicate significantly different sleep behavior and general quality of sleep, and therefore, individualized practices in sleep health assume importance. Age phenotypes, lifestyle phenotypes, and genetic phenotypes all impact one's circadian phenotype about how much light functions as a sleep regulator. Interventions to optimize exposure to light may thus have to be modulated for these variations. By taking into account the heterogeneous response to light among circadian phenotype groups, researchers are able to better understand sleep physiology and design more effective interventions to improve sleep quality in various populations (Lockley et al., 2007) (Figure 11.17).

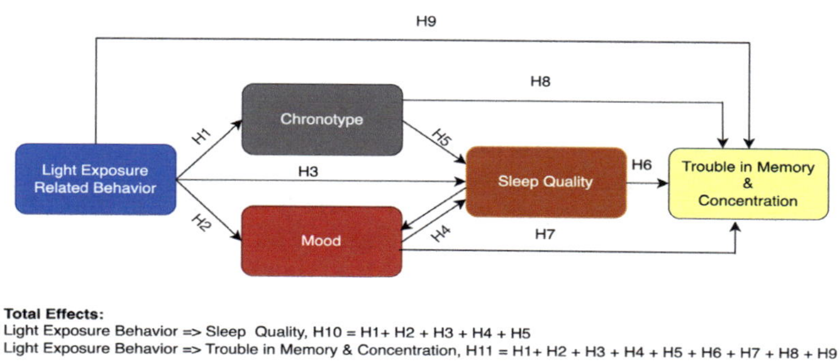

Figure 11.17. Light exposure behaviors predict mood, memory and sleep quality.

Source: https://media.springernature.com/full/springer-static/image/art%3A10.1038%2Fs41598-023-39636-y/MediaObjects/41598_2023_39636_Fig1_HTML.png.

11.5.1. Effects of Natural Light Exposure

Exposure to natural light has deep, far-reaching influences upon both sleep physiology and the circadian rhythms. Natural light is at the center of its power over the body's internal clock, largely through its impact on the suprachiasmatic nucleus (SCN) of the hypothalamus. The SCN is the master circadian clock, and it synchronizes many of the body's physiological processes to the environmental cycle of light and dark. Exposure to natural light during the daytime provokes alertness and mood, and signals the body that wake-up time is imminent. Dim light during the night enables the body to release melatonin, an important factor in inducing sleep. Every day exposure to sunlight, therefore, aids in firming up a healthy sleep-wake cycle, which is of central importance to overall health and metabolic well-being (Plano et al., 2017). Exposure to natural light is not only a wake-inducer; it has a significant impact on metabolic processes as well. The relationship between light and energy metabolism is intricate and is controlled by phase synchronization among peripheral circadian oscillators and the SCN. Research has indicated that phase coherence enforced by light-dark cycles dictates physiological processes , such as thermogenesis and energy expenditure. Further, disruptions of these cycles, through mechanisms like prolonged artificial light exposure or extended darkness, can lead to metabolic dysregulation, including weight gain and increased disease risk like diabetes. As light is a primary zeitgeber, or time cue, to the circadian system, daytime integration of light signals must occur to maintain energy balance and metabolic well-being (Plano et al., 2017). Also, the effects of altered light exposure patterns go beyond individual health to affect broader ecological and behavioral patterns. For instance, urban-adapted species typically experience extended artificial light exposure, which has been seen to hasten significant biological cycles, such as, reproduction and circadian activity cycles. In European blackbird research, scientists observed that birds kept in light-at-night conditions had lower melatonin levels than dark-conditioned birds, which was correlated with higher locomotor activity at early dawn. These findings point to the adaptive burden of urbanization and the pervasive influence of light on biological rhythms across the board. An understanding of these consequences illuminates the need for consideration of light exposure—natural and artificial—while navigating today's living environments and their effects on circadian health (Figure 11.18).

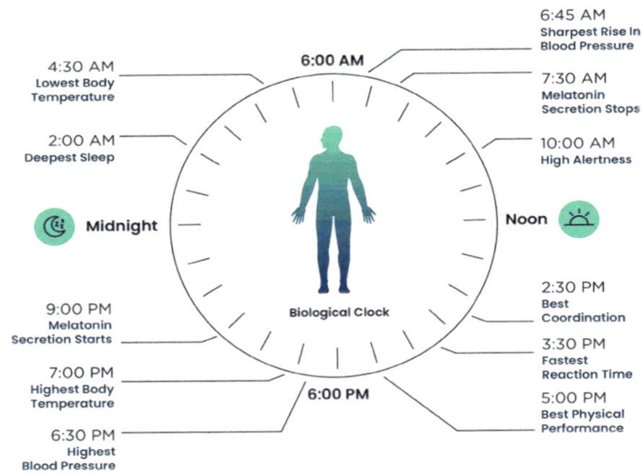

Figure 11.18. Effects of natural light exposure.

Source: https://a.storyblok.com/f/101818/1900x1478/31ef0e2dbd/lighting-tool-help-boost-productivity-1-delos.jpg.

11.5.2. Blue Light and Its Consequences

Its effect on sleep physiology and the circadian rhythm has been a lot of news in recent years. Blue light, which is primarily derived from electronic displays and light bulbs, significantly interferes with the natural cycle of sleeping and waking by suppressing the production of melatonin, the sleep hormone. Research indicates that being exposed to blue light in the evening can lead to a delay in sleeping and reduced sleep duration, ultimately affecting overall health. The impact of these disruptions extends beyond mere sleep loss; they can culminate in long-term consequences , such as mood disorders, obesity, and cardiovascular disease. These observations emphasize the need for individuals to monitor their exposure to blue light, particularly prior to bedtime, as the harmful impacts on sleep can pile up and create a vicious cycle that impacts daily function and overall health. Urban environments enhance the effect of blue light on biological timing by superimposing periodic artificial illumination, which can cause phase advancement of key physiological processes. Studies on urban bird species show profound alterations in activity and reproductive cycles after night-time lighting exposure, and it has been proposed that melatonin is a key mediator of these effects. For example, European blackbirds are highly influenced even by minimal amounts of light and show significant changes in their melatonin patterns, causing heightened activity before dawn. This pattern indicates that city birds experience longer daylight, which speeds up their circadian rhythms and is quite different from their rural counterparts, which still follow more conventional cycles. These different behaviors demonstrate the adaptability of circadian systems towards environmental pressure and signify potential environmental costs, where desynchronized natural rhythms can affect interspecific interactions and reproductive success in urban habitats (Dominoni et al., 2013). The overall biological generalization of biological clocks and circadian rhythms, backed by molecular data, demonstrates the significance of environmental cues like blue light. Existing studies demonstrate the pathways by which circadian rhythm disruption can cause physiological imbalance, like hormonal dysregulation and metabolic disturbances. The link between circadian rhythms and health illuminates a significant realm for possible remedies. For those affected by the adverse effects of blue light exposure, interventions , such as increasing awareness of light exposure can serve to re-advance circadian timing. As the widespread prevalence of blue lights in day-to-day life is an emerging issue, its effect becomes necessary to comprehend not only for individual health but also for greater implications in public health policy. Through increased awareness and setting standards for lowering exposure, society can foster general well-being and an equilibrium between modern lifestyles and healthy biological rhythms (Gnocchi & Bruscalupi, 2017).

11.5.3. Strategies for Managing Light Exposure

Therapeutic management of light exposure is required for optimizing sleep physiology and synchronization of circadian rhythms. The strategy employs light to modulate melatonin secretion and other hormonal responses that play a critical role in the regulation of sleep. Careful controlled bright light exposure during the day can enhance alertness and mood and aid in synchronizing the internal clock of the body. At the same time, decreasing exposure to evening light is also necessary because artificial light, particularly the blue light from the screen, is recognized to reduce melatonin release and delay the onset of sleep. Scientific studies emphasize that well-timed light exposure can alleviate sleep disorder symptoms and improve the quality of sleep overall, and therefore it is an elementary practice in the set of sleep management methods (Williams et al., 2017). Crossing time zones tends to exacerbate the issue of circadian rhythm control because individuals are susceptible to desynchronization. A common practice is to gradually change light exposure before traveling to align the internal clock of the body with the destination time zone. For example, increased morning light exposure when traveling east, or evening light exposure when traveling west, can allow for proper circadian phase shifting on time. Implementing such adaptations allows the body to acclimatize more effectively, reducing jet lag and subsequent negative impact on performance and health. Research has highlighted the effectiveness of these timed light exposure interventions not only in routine commuters but also in athletes, maximizing their recovery and performance following travel (Williams et al., 2017). In addition to pre-travel adaptation, ongoing regulation of light exposure while traveling is important to maintain circadian synchronization. This includes strategic application of light and darkness and, in effect, regulation of environmental inputs that influence sleep quality. For instance, the application of sleep masks and blackout curtains can enhance dark exposure in hotel rooms, while natural daylight exposure during the daytime ensures circadian rhythmicity. Of special note is evidence from studies on spaceflight environments, which finds that irregularly timed light exposure from operational schedules can lead to significant sleep loss and performance decrement. Addressing these factors, researchers note especially in high-impact circumstances like space missions where quality of sleep as well as cognitive performance is of utmost concern. Through such interventions, people can develop better quality sleep and align circadian rhythms, thus ensuring overall performance and improvement of health (Figure 11.19).

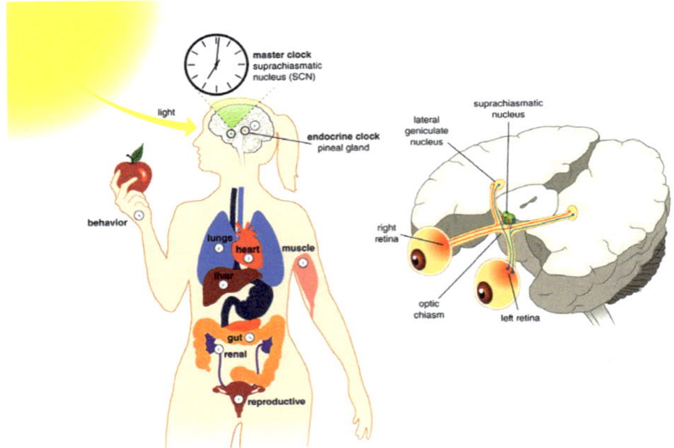

Figure 11.19. Synchronization of the body's internal clock.

Source: https://www.americanscientist.org/sites/americanscientist.org/files/2017-105-6-webb-2-natural.jpg.

Test Your Knowledge

1. How does exposure to natural and artificial light affect the regulation of melatonin and the sleep-wake cycle?
2. What role does the suprachiasmatic nucleus (SCN) play in processing light cues for circadian rhythm regulation?

11.6. Sleep and Health

Learning Outcome

1. Describe the relationship between sleep and mental health;
2. Define the sleep's impact on physical health;
3. Describe the consequences of sleep deprivation.

The intricate relationship between sleep and health is underlined by the importance of circadian rhythms, which regulate many bodily processes. These rhythms, driven by ambient light, choreograph daily fluctuation in behavior, metabolism, and immune response. Disturbance of these rhythms—by defective sleep habits or sleep deprivation—opens individuals to a wide array of health issues, including metabolic disease and heightened susceptibility to infection. There is evidence to suggest that circadian disruption can lead to microbiota shifts that are critical for the maintenance of metabolic health and immune function. There is a need to understand how circadian rhythms impact physiological well-being in the development of interventions that can reverse the adverse effects of sleep loss and improve the health profile among populations with chronic sleep disturbance (Pearson et al., 2020). Empirical studies have indicated a significant correlation between metabolic health and the quality of sleep, with specific reference to diabetes and obesity. A workshop sponsored by the National Institute for Diabetes and Digestive and Kidney Diseases highlighted the pressing need for exploring the interaction of sleep, circadian disruption, and energy balance. The findings highlighted the fact that insufficient emphasis is placed on translating core circadian studies into viable interventions to improve metabolic health. Researchers are encouraged to broaden their scope by incorporating multimodal sleep and circadian activity measurements as central components in existing research in diabetes care. This diversification of research approach can give rise to innovative preventive interventions that interact constructively with the complex biological substrates found to be associated with chronic sleep disruption and metabolic dysregulation (Arble et al., 2015). The bidirectional interaction between circadian rhythms and microbiota presents a fascinating frontier in the interaction between sleep and health. It has been demonstrated through research that microbial communities change in synchronization with host circadian rhythms, and these can feed back to affect host metabolism and immune function. Such interactions make understanding the role of the microbiome in disease and health of therapeutic interest. By working from this knowledge, researchers hope to create therapies that optimize both the health of the microbe and circadian activity. This approach would be particularly efficient in addressing the growth in the prevalence of conditions , such as prediabetes and obesity, where interventions , such as diet or lifestyle modification would enhance the quality of sleep as well as resynchronize circadian rhythms and thereby build a health-promoting environment. An integrated overview of such biological systems may yield valuable information about the etiology of sleep health issues as well as likely areas for intervention (Pearson et al., 2020) (Figure 11.20).

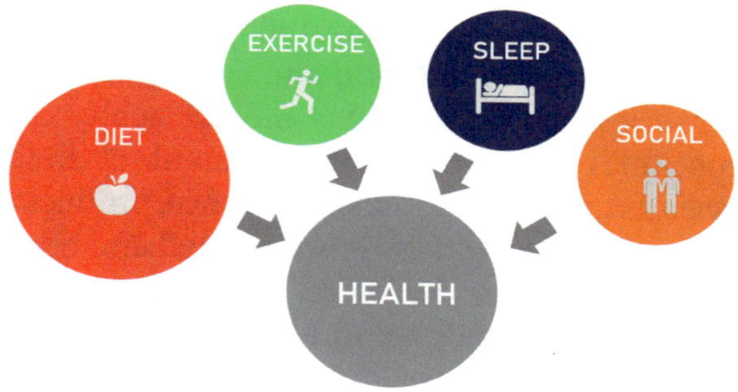

Figure 11.20. Sleep health.

Source: https://www.mdpi.com/ctn/ctn-08-00008/article_deploy/html/images/ctn-08-00008-g001.png.

11.6.1. Relationship Between Sleep and Mental Health

The mutually facilitating relationship between mental health and sleep has been of major interest to recent studies. Sleep, as a fundamental physiological process, wields great control over cognitive processing, emotion modulation, and overall psychological well-being. Sleep process abnormalities, most often catalyzed by life choices or illness states, have been shown to impart higher vulnerabilities toward the onset of mental illness, such as, depression and anxiety. For instance, sleep disorders like insomnia or sleep apnea have a propensity to co-exist with psychiatric disorders and exhibit a bidirectional relationship where poor sleep is revealed to cause the onset of mental disorders, while prevalent conditions are certain to compound sleep quality. Understanding these interactions is essential in constructing effective mental health interventions that address sleep hygiene as an inherent component of treatment interventions (Rutkowska et al., 2024). Apart from that, sleep architecture and sleep quality—characterized by distinct stages , such as NREM and REM) sleep—also play critical functions in emotional resilience and cognitive functioning. Both sleep stages exhibit distinct restorative functions necessary for psychological well-being. For instance, REM sleep is absolutely necessary for the processing of emotion and consolidation of memories, and thus yields mental acuity and emotional regulation. Derangement of these cycles may erode emotional resilience, producing hyper-responsive stress reactions and emotional dysregulation. Furthermore, alteration in sleep patterns that occurs alongside aging also serves to further complicate the sleep-mental health interface; as time passes, individuals increasingly experience less good sleep quality, alteration in type, and decreased duration, with increased vulnerability to mental health challenges. Emphasis on the value of healthy sleep hygiene may mitigate these aging effects and promote emotional well-being (Rutkowska et al., 2024). To improve mental health outcomes, developing an in-depth understanding of sleep hygiene and its application is necessary. Promoting routines centered on consistent sleep schedules, a restful sleeping environment, and cautious pre-sleep activities can significantly improve the quality of sleep, which consequently directly impacts mental health. Studies point out the significance of individuals embracing healthier lifestyle habits, such as, well-balanced dieting and exercising, that have been shown to improve the quality of sleep. Furthermore, public health initiatives in raising awareness regarding the significance of sleep can empower individuals to recognize the role that sleep takes as a mental health determinant. By these integrative approaches, society can optimize the overall quality of life, advocating for healthier sleeping patterns and positive mental health results, in turn promoting the important interdependence between the two (Rutkowska et al., 2024) (Figure 11.21).

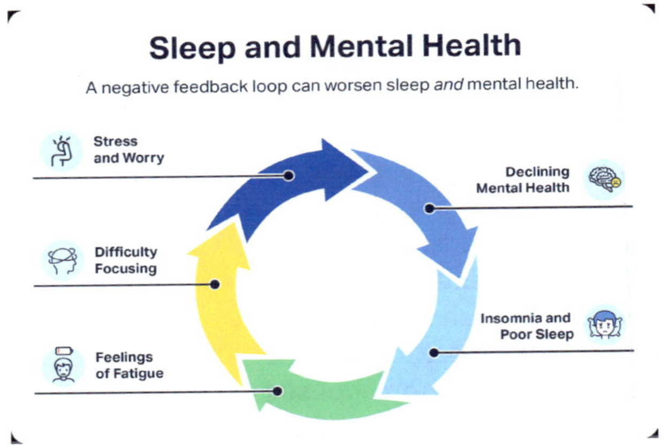

Figure 11.21. Mental health and sleep.

Source: https://www.sleepfoundation.org/wp-content/ uploads/2020/09/SF-23-234_SleepMentalHealth_Graphic-1024x717.png.

11.6.2. Sleep's Impact on Physical Health

The connection between sleep and health is significantly influenced by circadian rhythms, which regulate various body functions, including metabolism, hormone release, and body temperature. Sleep deprivation induces disturbances in these rhythms and leads to adverse physical health effects. Poor sleep has been linked with various physical health disorders, from obesity to cardiovascular diseases. Teenagers, for instance, typically have a disconnection of their biological clocks and societal clocks, which will likely impair daytime functioning and even exacerbate some diseases. Sleep requirements are typically overlooked at this age, leading to a sleep debt with deep impacts on mental and physical functioning, as highlighted by sleep science on adolescents and their altered chronotypes (Malik et al., 2021). Thus, it is crucial that the physiological mechanisms that regulate sleep's influence on health are comprehended to devise interventions to enhance sleep hygiene in all populations. Such work has further established the interaction between sleep disturbances and metabolic health, and particularly disease states , such as diabetes. Circadian disruption, either due to nonregular sleep patterns or through the environment, can impair metabolic processes , such as insulin sensitivity and glucose metabolism. One workshop conducted recently at the National Institute for Diabetes and Digestive and Kidney Diseases underlined the need to understand in depth the impact of sleep-wake cycles and circadian rhythms on energy balance and the likelihood of developing diabetes (Arble et al., 2015). The outcome of such workshops requires interdisciplinary collaboration between sleep researchers and metabolic health experts to develop interventions against the impact of sleep disorders. In addition, the inclusion of measures of sleep disturbance and quality within current cohort studies will further elucidate the impact of sleep on physical well-being. The consequences of inadequate sleep are not limited to acute cognitive impairment; they are inextricably linked with long-term health outcomes. Chronic sleep loss has been associated with elevated systemic inflammation, compromised immune function, and other physiological changes that foster chronic disease. Improving sleep interventions can significantly reduce such risks. For instance, intervention of sleep disorder breathing among patients with pre-diabetes using interventions , such as CPAP has been observed to delay or prevent the onset of diabetes (Arble et al., 2015). Moreover, exploring the effect of dietary habits, e.g., time-restricted feeding, coupled with good sleep, can offer healthy benefits in reducing obesity rates and in promoting of metabolic health. So, there should be an overall approach in which sleep health and nutrition come together to facilitate optimal physical welfare.

11.6.3. Consequences of Sleep Deprivation

Sleep deprivation has many consequences that extend way beyond mere fatigue, significantly affecting bodily functions and cognitive processes. The most significant consequence of sleep deprivation is the disruption of metabolic health, which has been the subject of much study. It has been documented that chronic sleep deprivation can lead to insulin resistance and increased risks of type 2 diabetes, citing the contribution of sleep to maintaining energy homeostasis—especially among groups of people with circadian rhythm desynchronizations (Arble et al., 2015). Such disturbances in metabolic functions can have negative impacts on overall well-being, leading to weight gain and other related conditions. It is important to know these disturbances in metabolism because they illustrate the intricate interconnection between diabetes, circadian rhythms, and sleep and, therefore, justifies the effectiveness of interventions aimed at enhancing the quality of sleep in order to enhance public health. Sleep deprivation also has adverse effects on cognition and memory consolidation. New findings from neuroscience have highlighted the critical function of sleep in memory consolidation of long-term memory, indicating that sleep deprivation can lead to severe cognitive deficits, including decreased attention, problem-solving, and decision-making (Samel et al., 1991). Most severely affected are challenging cognitive activities involving learned information. The interplay of social needs and circadian rhythms tends to amplify the effects of sleep loss, such that the mismatch between biological clock and social clock can lead to cognitive disturbance and inefficiency in academic and work settings. The determination of cognitive impacts of sleep loss is important for the creation of measures to improve cognitive function and sleep health. Social and health consequences are affected equally by sleep loss, affecting not just individual health but also societal dynamics as a whole. Sleep loss is also linked with increased occurrence of mood disorders, such as, depression and anxiety, thereby instigating mental illness in the population (Arble et al., 2015). Moreover, the effects spill into economic productivity at work since reduced judgment and less alertness lead to mistakes and accidents that increase the healthcare cost and limit economic production. Given that social demands and natural sleep patterns often conflict--through intense work schedules or educational pressures--the need for policies that reconcile social time with circadian biology is extremely urgent. By putting interventions that improve sleep quality and heighten the awareness of sleep's importance on their lists of priority, society can produce healthier citizens and increase community resilience to the ill effects of sleep deprivation (Figure 11.22).

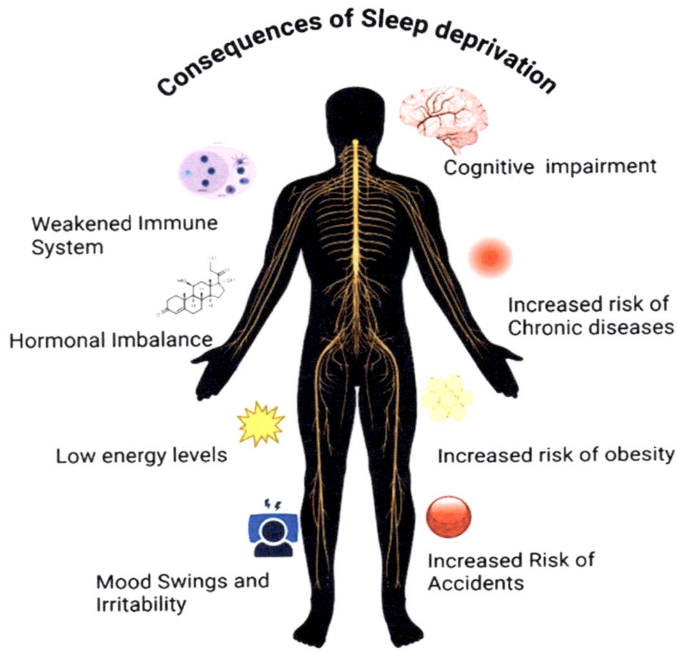

Figure 11.22. Consequences of sleep deprivation.

Source: https://ars.els-cdn.com/content/image/1-s2.0-S1568163724002757-gr5.jpg.

Test Your Knowledge

1. How does sleep contribute to physical health, including immune function, metabolism, and tissue repair?
2. What are the effects of chronic sleep deprivation on cognitive performance, mood, and mental health?

SUMMARY

In establishing the intricate relationship between circadian rhythms and sleep physiology, it is evident that a complete understanding of these phenomena is at the core of making sure to maintaining general health and well-being. Our circadian rhythms, which regulate most biological processes in synchrony with the natural day-night rhythm, are very closely linked with our physiological functions that regulate sleep. Habit disruption, which is common in modern society due to irregular sleep habits and various work schedules, can yield severe effects on metabolic well-being, mental function, and balance. An understanding of these relationships highlights the strong need for studies integrating fundamental scientific discoveries with relevance, as suggested at a seminal workshop on sleep and circadian disruption's impact on diabetes (Arble et al., 2015). In addition, circadian desynchronization consequences go beyond mere sleep deprivation; they also involve cognitive performance and memory consolidation. As recent gains in neuroscience show, adequately synchronized social time signals and individual circadian rhythms can enhance educational productivity and push forward public health initiatives. Adequate synchrony is particularly crucial among teenagers, who experience significant circadian rhythm differences, impacting learning capability and overall health. The results showing the health benefits of synchronizing social rhythms to individual circadian needs suggest a potential solution for the prevention of common diseases linked to sleep deprivation and circadian desynchronization (Samel et al., 1991). Overall, it is essential to develop an environment that honors intrinsic circadian clocks and promotes healthy sleep patterns for enhancing public and personal welfare. Policy makers, health workers, and teachers should collaborate to convert sleep and circadian research into policy-relevant strategies. These would include education initiatives, labor scheduling reforms, and overall awareness campaigns on the importance of sleep hygiene. Prioritizing sleep and circadian welfare would have much to offer society, including better cognitive functioning, improved mental health, and the avoidance of metabolic disease. Addressing these related factors can lead to a healthier, more productive workforce in the long term, indicative of the necessity of ongoing research and intervention in the science of sleep physiology and circadian rhythms.

Sleep physiology and circadian rhythms have a myriad of significant points that describe their pivotal roles in human health. Of utmost significance is the role of circadian rhythms, which are physiological processes with a loosely 24-hour cycle influencing the sleep-wake cycle, the release of hormones, and even metabolism. These rhythms are regulated primarily by the suprachiasmatic nucleus (SCN) of the hypothalamus, which further responds to environmental stimuli in the form of light and darkness. The effects of these rhythms range beyond sleep regulation to cognitive function, mood disorders, and overall well-being, highlighting the vital necessity for entrainment of environmental and biological clocks for optimal health, particularly under the condition of modern lifestyle pressures. The other very important area of exploring sleep physiology involves the differential impact of sleep quality and duration on physical health and mental function. Sleep disturbances have severe health consequences, including cardiovascular illness, weakened immune response, and even metabolic syndrome. Studies indicate that not getting enough sleep has been known to compromise insulin sensitivity and lead to weight gain, as well as affect one's psychological health by increasing depression and anxiety risks. Moreover, there are different phases of sleeping cycles, such as, non-REM and REM sleep, which serve definite functions like memory consolidation and body restoration. Understanding these phases is significant because a lack of appropriate, uninterrupted sleep can completely disrupt these restoration processes, leading to chronic disorders. The consequences of disrupted circadian rhythms are more relevant for the case of shift work, which has been associated with a range of unfavorable health conditions. As illustrated, the population working in shift work is growing, and it plays a critical role in disrupting sleep patterns and circadian rhythms. These disturbances affect not only global health but are also evidenced in specific physiological changes, e.g., in gut microbiota that may increase the vulnerability to metabolic disease. Altered food intakes accompany shift working and contribute to the detrimental effects on the gut. The combined impact of disrupted sleep and altered eating habits highlights the importance of further research into how these interact and impact the development of long-term illness, with a need for effective interventions in both sleep and gastrointestinal health (Lane et al., 2020).

KEY TERMS FROM THIS CHAPTER

- Adenosine
- Circadian rhythm
- Hypocretin/orexin
- Melatonin
- Pineal gland
- REM sleep
- Sleep deprivation
- Sleep homeostasis
- Sleep-wake cycle
- Chronotype
- Electroencephalogram (EEG)
- Light exposure
- Non-REM sleep (NREM)
- Polysomnography
- Sleep architecture
- Sleep disorders
- Sleep latency
- Suprachiasmatic nucleus (SCN)

CRITICAL THINKING QUESTIONS

1. **Which part of the brain is primarily responsible for regulating circadian rhythms?**
   a. Pineal gland
   b. Hypothalamus
   c. Suprachiasmatic nucleus (SCN)
   d. Brainstem
2. **What hormone is released by the pineal gland to promote sleep?**
   a. Serotonin
   b. Cortisol
   c. Melatonin
   d. Dopamine
3. **During which stage of sleep does most dreaming occur?**
   a. Stage 1
   b. Stage 2
   c. Stage 3 (Slow-wave sleep)
   d. REM sleep
4. **Which of the following best defines a circadian rhythm?**
   a. A 12-hour cycle of alertness and fatigue
   b. A 24-hour biological cycle regulating sleep, hormones, and body temperature
   c. A short-term cycle related to digestion
   d. A rhythm generated only during physical activity
5. **How does exposure to light affect circadian rhythms?**
   a. It reduces alertness and increases melatonin levels
   b. It synchronizes the SCN and suppresses melatonin production
   c. It increases REM sleep duration
   d. It initiates slow-wave sleep

Short Answer Questions

1. What are the two main types of sleep, and how do they differ?
2. Which part of the brain regulates circadian rhythms?
3. What is melatonin, and when is it typically secreted?
4. Define a circadian rhythm and provide one physiological example.
5. What role does the suprachiasmatic nucleus (SCN) play in sleep regulation?
6. Describe the function of REM (Rapid Eye Movement) sleep.
7. Describe the stages of the sleep cycle, including the physiological characteristics of each stage.
8. Explain the role of the suprachiasmatic nucleus (SCN) and melatonin in the regulation of circadian rhythms.
9. Discuss the effects of sleep deprivation on cognitive, immune, and metabolic functions.
10. Explain how circadian rhythms are synchronized with external environmental cues (zeitgebers).

Answers to Critical Thinking Questions

1. (c) 2. (c); 3. (d); 4. (b); 5. (b).

REFERENCES

1. Eric Murillo-Rodríguez, Tetsuya Yamamoto, André Barciela Veras, Nuno Barbosa Rocha, Diogo Telles-Correira, Sérgio Machado, Diogo Monteiro, Henning Budde, Pablo Torterolos(2019). Sleep disorders and genes. 2019, The Behavioral, Molecular, Pharmacological, and Clinical Basis of the Sleep-Wake Cycle, p. 143-158 (accessed on 28th June 2025).
2. Daniel C. Holleyet al. (1981). Effects of circadian rhythm phase alteration on physiological and psychological variables: Implications to pilot performance (including a partially annotated bibliography). NASA Technical Memorandum 81277 https://core.ac.uk/download/pdf/42860538.pdf (accessed on 28th June 2025).
3. Arble, D. M., Bass, J., Behn, C. D., Butler, M., et al. (2015). Impact of sleep and circadian disruption on energy balance and diabetes: A summary of workshop discussions. https://core.ac.uk/download/213087763.pdf (accessed on 28th June 2025).
4. Lockley, S. W., Arendt, J., & Skene, D. J. (2007). Visual impairment and circadian rhythm disorders. *Dialogues in clinical neuroscience*, *9*(3), 301–314. https://doi.org/10.31887/DCNS.2007.9.3/slockley (accessed on 28th June 2025).
5. Facer-Childs, E. R., Middleton, B., Bagshaw, A. P., & Skene, D. J. (2020). Human Circadian Phenotyping and Diurnal Performance Testing in the Real World. *Journal of visualized experiments : JoVE*, (158), 10.3791/60448. https://doi.org/10.3791/60448(accessed on 28th June 2025).
6. Bailly, L., Bailly, C., Bailly, F., Bailly, J., Botzung, A., Bourgine, P., Chaline, J., et al. (2011). A 2-dimensional geometry for biological time. https://core.ac.uk/download/231876541.pdf (accessed on 28th June 2025).
7. Williams, Biju BSc (Hons)[1]; Clarke, Richard MSc[1]; Aspe, Rodrigo MSc[1]; Cole, Matthew PhD[2]; Hughes, Jonathan PhD[1]. Managing Performance Throughout Periods of Travel. Strength and Conditioning Journal 39(4):p 22-29, August 2017. | DOI: 10.1519/SSC.0000000000000317(accessed on 28th June 2025).
8. Boden, M., Kennaway, D., & Varcoe, T. (2013). Circadian regulation of reproduction: From gamete to offspring. https://core.ac.uk/download/19445268.pdf (accessed on 28th June 2025).
9. Boersma, G. J., Hut, R. A., Zee, R. J., et al. (2009). The neurobiology of circadian rhythms. https://core.ac.uk/download/pdf/12961797.pdf (accessed on 28th June 2025).
10. Booth, V., & Diniz Behn, C. G. (2012). A fast-slow analysis of the dynamics of REM sleep. https://cupola.gettysburg.edu/cgi/viewcontent.cgi?article=1011&context=mathfac (accessed on 28th June 2025).
11. Albrecht U. (2012). Circadian rhythms and sleep--the metabolic connection. *Pflugers Archiv : European journal of physiology*, *463*(1), 23–30. https://doi.org/10.1007/s00424-011-0986-6(accessed on 28th June 2025).
12. Gnocchi, D., & Bruscalupi, G. (2017). Circadian Rhythms and Hormonal Homeostasis: Pathophysiological Implications. *Biology*, *6*(1), 10. https://doi.org/10.3390/biology6010010(accessed on 28th June 2025).
13. Jones, C. R., Campbell, S. S., Zone, S. E., Cooper, F., DeSano, A., Murphy, P. J., Jones, B., Czajkowski, L., & Ptácek, L. J. (1999). Familial advanced sleep-phase syndrome: A short-period circadian rhythm variant in humans. *Nature medicine*, *5*(9), 1062–1065. https://doi.org/10.1038/12502(accessed on 28th June 2025).

14. Wang, H. B., Loh, D. H., Whittaker, D. S., Cutler, T., Howland, D., & Colwell, C. S. (2018). Time-Restricted Feeding Improves Circadian Dysfunction as well as Motor Symptoms in the Q175 Mouse Model of Huntington's Disease. *eNeuro*, *5*(1), ENEURO.0431-17.2017. https://doi.org/10.1523/ENEURO.0431-17.2017(accessed on 28th June 2025).

15. Khalid MF, Lee C-Y, Doggett SL, Veera Singham G (2019) Circadian rhythms in insecticide susceptibility, metabolic enzyme activity, and gene expression in *Cimex lectularius* (Hemiptera: Cimicidae). PLoS ONE 14(6): e0218343. https://doi.org/10.1371/journal.pone.0218343(accessed on 28th June 2025).

16. Dominoni, D. M., Goymann, W., Helm, B., Partecke, J., et al. (2013). Urban-like night illumination reduces melatonin release in European blackbirds (*Turdus merula*): Implications of city life for biological time-keeping of songbirds. https://core.ac.uk/download/16458859.pdf (accessed on 28th June 2025).

17. Tamar Shochat(2022). Sleep, health, and aging. **2022**, Foundations of Sleep Health, p. 173-198 https://core.ac.uk/download/71356671.pdf (accessed on 28th June 2025).

18. Alexander Samel and Philippa Gander E(1991). Light as a chronobiologic countermeasure for long-duration space operations. NASA Technical Memorandum 103874 https://core.ac.uk/download/pdf/42811692.pdf (accessed on 28th June 2025).

19. Field, J., Lee, Y., & Sehgal, A. (2021). Circadian rhythms, disease and chronotherapy. https://core.ac.uk/download/614775571.pdf (accessed on 28th June 2025).

20. Jones, C. R., Huang, A. L., Ptáček, L. J., & Fu, Y. H. (2013). Genetic basis of human circadian rhythm disorders. *Experimental neurology*, *243*, 28–33. https://doi.org/10.1016/j.expneurol.2012.07.012(accessed on 28th June 2025).

21. Gerkema, M. P., Helm, B., & Schwartz, W. J. (2017). Wild clocks: Preface and glossary. https://core.ac.uk/download/96882813.pdf (accessed on 28th June 2025).

22. Marie Clare Grant and Jonathan Glen (2018). An investigation into sleep patterns and the effect of time of day on performance in youth swimmers. Taylor & Francis in Biological Rhythm Research on 15th January 2018, available online: wwww.tandfonline.com/10.1080/09291016.2018.1424774 https://core.ac.uk/download/228178255.pdf (accessed on 28th June 2025).

23. Plano, S. A., Casiraghi, L. P., García Moro, P., Paladino, N., Golombek, D. A., & Chiesa, J. J. (2017). Circadian and Metabolic Effects of Light: Implications in Weight Homeostasis and Health. *Frontiers in neurology*, *8*, 558. https://doi.org/10.3389/fneur.2017.00558(accessed on 28th June 2025).

24. Grossberg, S. (2017). Acetylcholine neuromodulation in normal and abnormal learning and memory: Vigilance control in waking, sleep, autism, amnesia, and Alzheimer's disease. https://core.ac.uk/download/215929174.pdf (accessed on 28th June 2025).

25. Siwicki, K. K., Hardin, P. E., & Price, J. L. (2018). Reflections on contributing to "big discoveries" about the fly clock: Our fortunate paths as post-docs with 2017 Nobel laureates Jeff Hall, Michael Rosbash, and Mike Young. *Neurobiology of sleep and circadian rhythms*, *5*, 58–67. https://doi.org/10.1016/j.nbscr.2018.02.004(accessed on 28th June 2025).

26. Lane, H. (2020). Shift work: Gut health and metabolic disease. https://core.ac.uk/download/322850892.pdf (accessed on 28th June 2025).

27. OLTEANU-PASCAL, Dina, LUPUȘOR, Nadejda. The influence of light from gadgets on circadian rhythm in children. In: MedEspera: the 8th Internat. Medical Congress for Students and Young Doctors: abstract book. Chișinău: S. n., 2020, p. 248-249.(accessed on 28th June 2025).

28. Malik, S., Rani, S., Verma, P., Yadav, P., et al. (2021). Biological clock vs social clock conflict in adolescents. https://core.ac.uk/download/390096541.pdf (accessed on 28th June 2025).

29. Overy, C., & Tansey, E. M. (2014). The recent history of seasonal affective disorder (SAD). https://core.ac.uk/download/30696938.pdf (accessed on 28th June 2025).

30. Pearson, J. A., Wen, L., & Wong, F. S. (2020). Crosstalk between circadian rhythms and the microbiota. https://core.ac.uk/download/337623172.pdf (accessed on 28th June 2025).

31. Rutkowska, M., Bieńko, M., Król, T., Toborek, M., Marchaj, M., Korta, K., ... Bednarz, K. (2024). Sleep Cycles and Health: Role of Sleep Stages, Circadian Rhythms, and Lifestyle Factors on Optimizing Physical Performance and Mental Well-Being – a literature review. *Quality in Sport*, *18*, 53398. https://doi.org/10.12775/QS.2024.18.53393(accessed on 28th June 2025).

DEVELOPMENTAL PHYSIOLOGY AND AGING

12

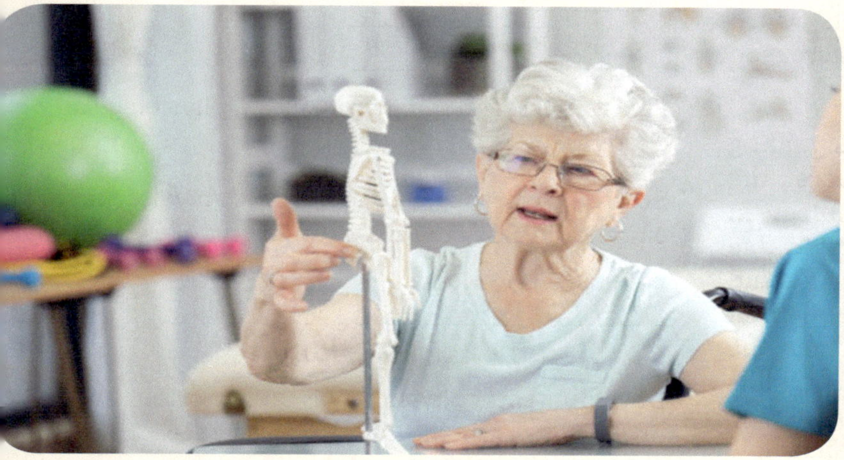

LEARNING OBJECTIVES

After studying this chapter, you will be able to:

1. Discuss the stages of human development.
2. Explain the cellular and molecular mechanisms of aging.
3. Discuss the physiological changes in aging.
4. Focus on hormonal changes and aging.
5. Learn about environmental influences on aging.
6. Evaluate the interventions to promote healthy aging.

Introduction

Developmental physiology is the examination of processes by which organisms mature and grow throughout the various stages of life. Developmental physiology is the physiological changes from birth to maturity, highlighting the intricate interaction between genetic and environmental factors. Developmental physiology is most pertinent when considering how such processes lead to aging. Through the understanding of cellular growth mechanisms, differentiation, and signaling pathways, researchers can deduce that developmental pathways dictate health in old age. The evidence to date is that interruptions during developmental windows can lead to lifelong diseases during aging, hence the need for an integrative approach that encompasses developmental and gerontological knowledge in physiological studies. This coming together of changes in lifespan remains at the heart of enhancing our understanding of health and disease across life. One of the unifying themes of developmental physiology is how cellular diversity sustains the maintenance of physiological function. New research has revealed that not only cell numbers but also their types and interactions are needed for the healthy development and function of organs. For instance, studies in special editions of high-impact factor journals have investigated the cellular dynamics in cardiovascular conditions to depict how cellular heterogeneity is involved in health and susceptibility to disease as a function of aging. By dismantling interactions amongst myocytes and non-myocyte cells, researchers can identify ways through which alterations in these cell milieus result in ailments , such as heart disease, occurring with increased frequency amongst aged populations.

With the understanding of cellular signaling networks in organs becoming ever clearer, the need to unravel developmental physiology in the context of aging cannot be overstated due to its implications for therapeutic control and prevention in geriatric care. Developmental physiology also seeks to understand how the environment, including nutrition and early life, influences physiological outcome throughout the lifespan. For example, human milk's bioactive molecules have been found to perform protective roles in infant development, as proof of the ways nutrition early in life affects long-term well-being. In publications, topical application of human milk has worked to promote healthy neonatal skin in neonatal intensive care units, revealing the importance of studying developmental components of neonatal care (Brodbeck et al., 2022). Such data reveal key associations between early interventions and adult health, indicating that the promotion of optimal developmental experiences may mitigate risks of aging. Continued study will further elucidate , such associations, and integrating concepts of developmental physiology into aging science will open doorways to novel healthcare strategies for enhancing quality of life in aging groups (Figure 12.1).

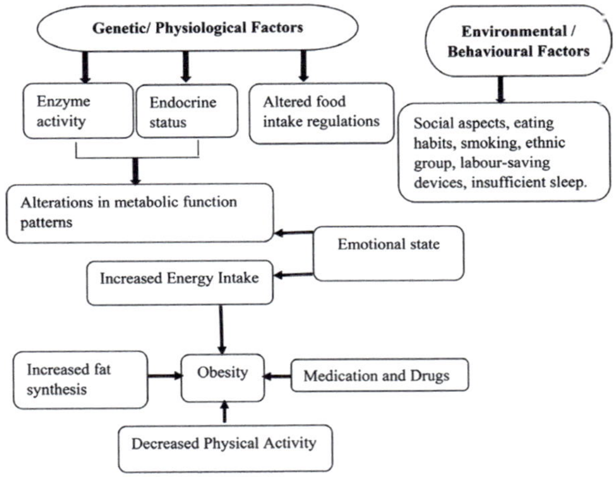

Figure 12.1. The aging process and physiological changes.

Source: https://cdnintech.com/media/chapter/60564/1512345123/media/F6.png.

Definition and Scope of Developmental Physiology

Developmental physiology is an important area of study within the biological sciences aimed at examining the physiological processes that take place during development and maturation throughout the lifetime of an organism. It is an interdisciplinary area of study encompassing areas like cellular differentiation, organogenesis, and the role of environmental and genetic influences on physiological transformation. As organisms progress from embryonic to adult organisms, developmental physiology attempts to understand how various cellular processes control this complex process. Understanding these physiological principles is essential to decipher not only the typical patterns of development but also the abnormalities that may develop during development. As such, researchers in this area often collaborate with geneticists, molecular biologists, and ecologists to better understand how physical and environmental stimuli influence development, thereby laying the groundwork for advances in regenerative medicine and gerontology. The field of developmental physiology goes beyond mere measurements of growth to encompass the wide-ranging effects of aging on physiological processes. Optimal development promotes maximum functional capacities, and disruption of developmental processes can lead to degenerative changes in physiological processes with age. As the population grays, the field of developmental physiology becomes increasingly relevant, particularly in the manner in which physiological systems change or degenerate over time. For instance, researchers are keenly interested in understanding how cellular processes and organ function evolve with age and lead to diseases that are prevalent among the elderly. In integrating data from developmental physiology, researchers can identify markers of biological aging and design interventions to enhance health span—the duration for which a person remains healthy—rather than solely extending lifespan. This focus underscores the applicability of developmental physiology to addressing the challenge posed by an aging population. Today, research places importance on the overlap of psychological health and physiological well-being as a person ages. Developmental physiology not just discusses the physical changes that occur during life but also focuses on resilience and psychological adjustment in sustaining these processes. According to research, proactive well-being can influence the aging process significantly, proving that psychological resilience is as much a prerequisite to physiological health in old age. Enhancing psychological well-being through purposeful activity, underscored by present evidence, indicates that it is equally important in extending life span and enhancing general health. As developmental physiology continues to develop, researchers are increasingly concentrating on the holistic interaction between emotional, psychological, and physiological factors in the process of aging. It is this interdisciplinarity that holds exciting prospects for improving quality of life and promoting healthier aging, thereby influencing society in general through personalized interventions for health (de Saussure, 2017; Ryff, 2013) (Figure 12.2).

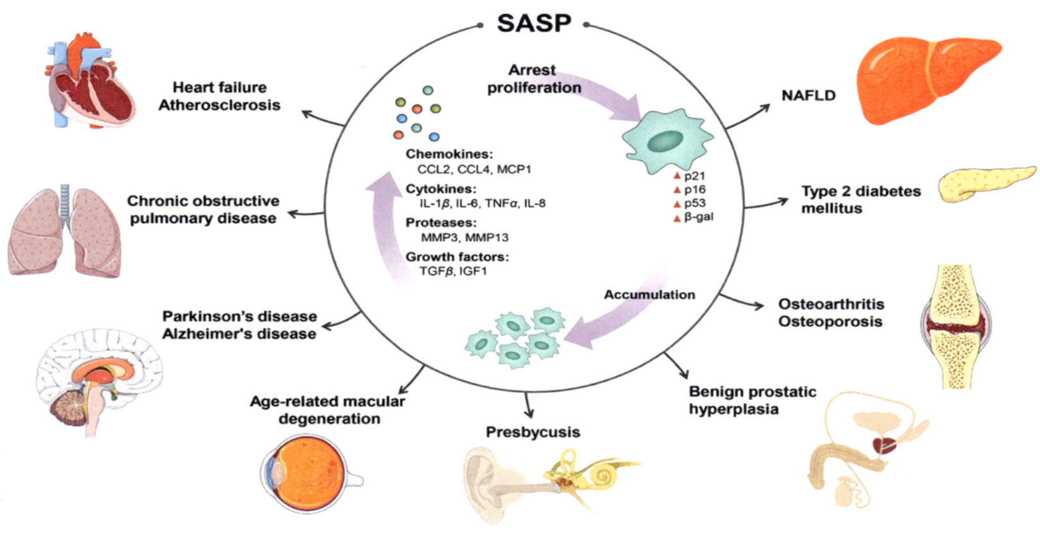

Figure 12.2. Aging and aging-related diseases.

Source: https://media.springernature.com/lw1200/springer-static/image/art%3A10.1038%2Fs41392-022-01251-0/MediaObjects/41392_2022_1251_Fig6_HTML.png.

Importance of Studying Developmental Physiology

Developmental physiology is important not only in deciphering mechanisms of growth and maturation but also in defining the biological processes that control aging. As individuals move along life cycles, physiological mechanisms can affect health, longevity, and overall quality of life. Insights gained from developmental physiology allow researchers to unravel the complex interdependencies of genetics, environment, and aging processes. For instance, knowledge of how early nutrition and exposure to stressors during developmental periods influence health trajectories can guide interventions leading to longevity as well as the prevention of age-related illness. Such background knowledge facilitates the generation of preventative and therapeutic paradigms for particular life phases, eventually culminating in healthier aging. The value of these physiological pathways is a reminder to incorporate developmental physiology into aging studies. A vital aspect of learning developmental physiology is its relevance to the determination of critical windows of intervention. Through research, certain stages of development have been found to be characterized by increased plasticity, under which considerable physiological adjustments to environmental influences can be made. Upon identifying these windows, it then becomes feasible to make interventions that can alter adverse health paths, thus improving developmental outcomes while counteracting the impact of senescence in later life. For example, understanding the intricate hormonal and metabolic changes that occur during adolescence may shed light on averting adult obesity as well as resultant chronic diseases. In addition, the role of epigenetics in controlling an individual's reaction to environmental stimuli during critical stages indicates that there exists a critical need for a developmental approach to public health policy. Thus, developmental physiology is a model for organizing intervention to exploit these sensitive periods in life and thereby foster resilience against decline with age. In addition, research on developmental physiology enriches our understanding of aging by providing context to age-related changes in the physiological systems. As individuals develop over time, physiological systems undergo changes that can lead to a decline in function and increased vulnerability to disease. From a developmental physiology point of view, researchers can investigate how life experiences and life's biological accommodations combine with aging. In more detail, cellular mechanism research, such as, apoptosis and senescence, reveals how such mechanisms are affected by life's developmental accommodations. For instance, developmental pathways governing inflammation can account for inflammatory diseases' rise with age among older adults. Lastly, the intersection of developmental milestones and aging puts a high value on the necessity of interdisciplinary investigation that synthesizes findings from several disciplines, such as, genetics and environmental science. Thus, a careful examination of developmental physiology not only illuminates aging mechanisms but also informs intervention strategies for increasing health span and life expectancy.

Overview of Aging as a Biological Process

Aging in the biological sense is a complex interaction of environmental, cellular, and genetic factors that together result in the gradual loss of physiological function. Cell by cell, aging results from a cascade of molecular changes in which telomeres shorten, oxidative damage happens, and gene expression is altered. These cellular changes initiate a cascade of metabolic changes that take place as the outward manifestations of aging, such as, diminished regenerative capacity and increased susceptibility to disease. These deteriorations with the passage of time accumulate and lead to the functional loss seen in aging organisms. This three-dimensional character of aging supplements the necessity for interdisciplinarity in research on its mechanisms and outcomes, which can be improved by dialogue among researchers with diverse areas of experience, suggested by the strong conceptual scheme of evolutionary biology and biodemography (Kaplan & Gurven, 2008). The influence of environmental factors on the process of aging cannot be overstated. Lifestyle, diet, and environmental stressor exposure differences all possess the potential to powerfully modulate biological aging. Organisms that live in low-gravity settings, such as, orbiting spaceflights, exhibit specific biological responses that complicate classical notions of aging and adaptation (Miquel et al., 2025). This intersection of environmental and biological processes makes clear the adaptive processes that organisms employ along the aging continuum.

Research on the effects of gravitational fluctuations provides significant insights into the fundamental rules governing aging in animals, demonstrating the significance of researching aging not just on the cellular level but also in a situational context that takes into consideration external influences. In recounting the aging process, there is a need to examine its impact on population dynamics and public health. With increasing life expectancy worldwide, insights into the biological mechanisms underlying aging will be crucial to engineer interventions that optimize healthspan, the duration of life lived in health. Translational research that connects cellular-level processes to outcomes at the population level is informative about how biological aging appears in health issues in daily life. Through highlighting teamwork in research on the continuum of biology, from molecular to demographic, scientists are able to address the multifaceted complexity of aging and open pathways to more beneficial effects of health on aging populations. Such integrative research may establish innovative solutions to society's age-related challenges (Kaplan & Gurven, 2008).

12.1. Stages of Human Development

Learning Outcome

1. Describe the prenatal development and its physiological changes;
2. Focus on childhood and adolescence: growth and maturation;
3. Learn about adulthood: physiological stability and peak performance.

The human development stages can be broken down into important phases, each with particular physiological and morphological changes. During infancy, an age ranging from birth to two years, human physiology changes quickly with significant neurological and physical development. Babies reach complete motor skills , such as reaching and crawling, that enable their intellectual development through interaction with the environment. It is during this stage that the foundation of social interaction is laid, with babies beginning to identify caregivers and respond to social stimuli. The achievement of milestones accomplished at this level determines the direction of later levels as they encourage reasoning, emotional regulation, and behavioral patterns that will persist throughout their lives. By examining the intricate interaction of the environment and biological development at this time, researchers can gain knowledge about the experiences that shape the long-term trajectory of health and susceptibility to disease. Childhood, succeeding infancy, takes place from age two to twelve and entails significant cognitive, emotional, and social milestones. This stage is characterized by fine-tuning motor skills and increased autonomy, allowing children to be more active in the world around them. Children learn language, problem-solving, and social skills through peer interactions and school experiences. Brain development in early childhood becomes increasingly influenced by external factors, such as, family life and schools, that have a strong impact on emotional and intellectual growth. Critical perspectives, including Vygotsky's sociocultural theory, emphasize the value of social interaction in cognitive development and propose that knowledge is created through transactions with more expert others. Overall, it is crucial to appreciate the complexity of child development to design settings that facilitate healthy development and learning. Coming into adolescence, lasting from roughly ages twelve to eighteen, the body and mind also undergo considerable transformation that helps in the transition from childhood to adulthood. Puberty occurs at this age, and it is brought about by a complex interaction of hormonal changes that initiates physical growth and sexual maturation. Adolescents have a tendency to grapple with identity formation, a process that is directed by both biology and society and culture. As intellectual abilities develop, individuals build more sophisticated reasoning and decision-making abilities, which create higher autonomy but higher susceptibility to risk behavior. At this level, physiological developments provide a foundational role in future health, as new evidence locates the influence of adolescent behavior on adult chronic illness. Thus, understanding the importance of the teenage period, as well as its risks and opportunities, leads to a further understanding of developmental physiology and its meaning in aging (Hoarau et al., 2024; Tang et al., 2024).

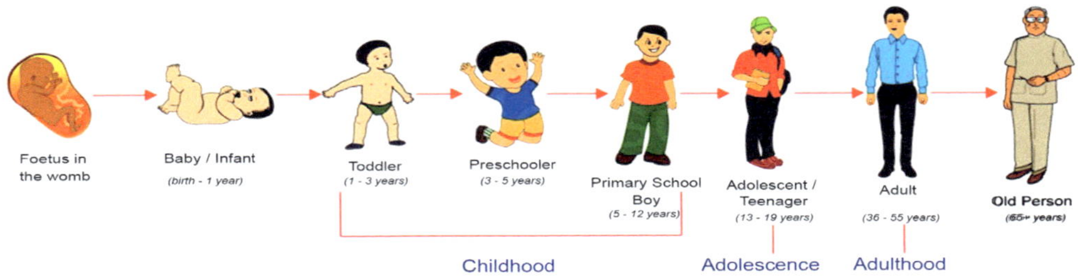

Figure 12.3. Stages of the human life cycle.

Source: https://k8schoollessons.com/wp-content/uploads/2013/05/human-life-cycle.jpg.

12.1.1. Prenatal Development and Its Physiological Changes

The intricate process of prenatal development involves a complex interplay of physiological changes that significantly influence the growth and maturation of the fetus. As gestation progresses, the mothers body adapts in various ways to support the developing fetus, including hormonal fluctuations and alterations in cardiovascular dynamics. These adaptations are critical for ensuring that essential nutrients and oxygen are delivered to the fetus, facilitating growth and the development of organs. Changes in maternal physiology, such as, increased blood volume and altered metabolism, reflect the increased energy demands required to sustain both maternal health and fetal development. Understanding these physiological transformations emphasizes the importance of maternal health during pregnancy, as compromised systems can lead to adverse outcomes affecting both the mother and the child's long-term health trajectory. Stress during pregnancy has been identified as a significant factor that may adversely impact prenatal development, prompting further investigation into its physiological implications. Chronic stress can elevate levels of cortisol and other stress hormones in the mother, disrupting the delicate hormonal balance necessary for healthy fetal growth. The phenomenon known as allostatic load refers to the cumulative strain on the body's systems due to prolonged exposure to stressors, which can increase the risk of complications , such as preterm birth. Research indicates that understanding the role of chronic stress in prenatal settings can enhance the assessment of individual risk factors, allowing for targeted interventions. Recognizing the relationship between maternal stress and prenatal outcomes is crucial, as it underscores the need for supportive healthcare measures to help mitigate the impact of stressors on both maternal and fetal well-being (McCreary et al., 2015). The impact of prenatal exposures extends beyond immediate outcomes, shaping long-term health trajectories through mechanisms of prenatal programming.

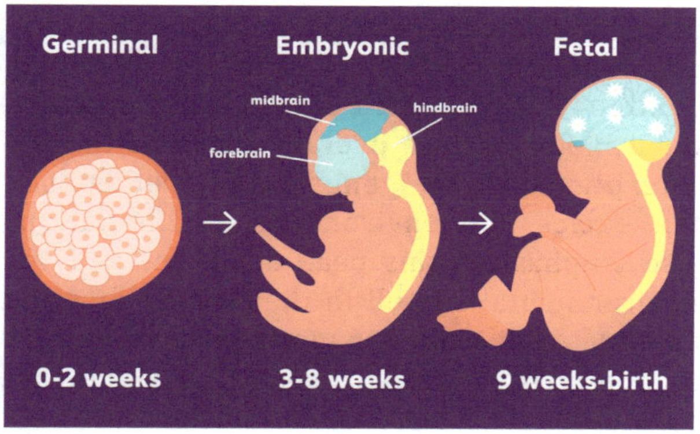

Figure 12.4. Prenatal development stages.

Source: https://www.verywellmind.com/thmb/bOGQenRSHLRpMRkpJ0e8PlM0-u4=/1500x0/filters:no_upscale():max_bytes(150000):strip_icc()/2795073-stages-of-prenatal-development-01-5a3040f6eb4d5200362d5553.png.

Research has shown that the gestational environment influences not only the health of the offspring but may also leave an epigenetic imprint that affects subsequent generations. Factors , such as maternal nutrition, stress, and exposure to environmental toxins can alter developmental pathways, particularly in neuroendocrine systems that govern reproductive health. In particular, the programming effects can disrupt the normal functioning of the hypothalamic-pituitary-gonadal axis, with potential implications for reproductive health in adulthood. By examining these critical interactions, researchers underscore the importance of a holistic approach to prenatal care, considering the lasting effects of maternal health and the environment on the development and future health of the offspring (Evans et al., 2016) (Figure 12.4).

12.1.2. Childhood and Adolescence: Growth and Maturation

Childhood and adolescence are characterized by widespread changes at the physiological level that influence the structure and function of the brain. As children develop into adolescents, neural development is particularly emergent, with imaging studies identifying critical changes in cortical circuits. These include a reduction in gray matter volume, increases in the myelination of critical connections, and overall reconfigurations to large-scale cortical networks. All these changes are required for cognitive development and form a linear developmental pattern that has an impact on global brain maturation. Specifically, the reduction of gyrification—associated with lower gyrification index scores—demonstrates that the cerebral cortex is under vast alterations during this stage. Understanding the complexity of such brain growth is extremely crucial in determining how specific alterations in the brain relate to cognitive advancement and behavior changes typical of adolescence (Klein et al., 2014). Conclusions, however, rest on more immediate evidence, e.g., biopsy studies or a longitudinal study of muscle development during sleep. Concurrently, musculoskeletal system growth from childhood through adolescence provides a special but complementary aspect of maturation. Muscle architecture research indicates enormous variability within developmental phases, particularly lower limb musculature. Research has examined how, as boys change from pre-peak height velocity to post-peak height velocity, there are increases in numerous muscle architecture parameters, such as, thickness and physiological dimensions. These findings illustrate the close relationship between maturation and optimization of muscle structure, which affects strength and functional capacity. This differentiation is crucial in that it provides perspective for the understanding of growth and training adaptation relative to normal developmental change. Thus, such muscle changes focus on the importance of recognizing maturation as a significant determinant of physical performance and preparedness to develop among adolescents (Radnor et al., 2020). Also, the interaction of neural and muscle growth features an intricate interaction that defines an adolescent's experience. The simultaneous development of the mind and physicality provides a dynamic in which learning and physical action are intertwined.

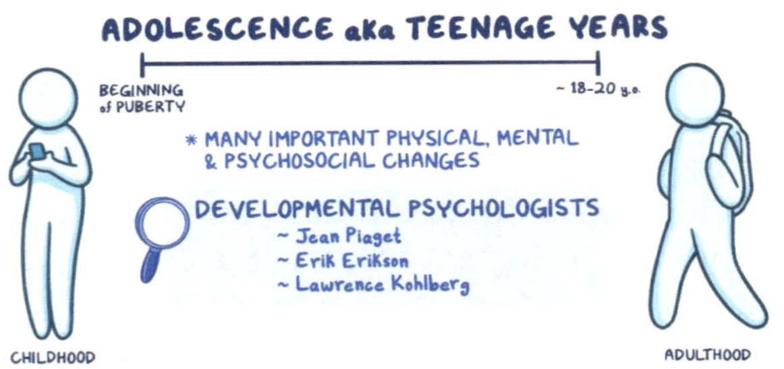

Figure 12.5. Childhood and adolescence: growth and maturation.

Source: https://d16qt3wv6xm098.cloudfront.net/JwgCRgqiSRK0XVPvTjOOEaWaTVqAxHXn/_.jpg.

Teenagers not only become better at employing their motor functions as their musculature gets stronger, but also carry out more advanced cognitive processes that capitalize on their higher brain function. Such diverse growth contributes to the development of greater self-knowledge and autonomy during a psychologically developmental phase. Thus, understanding how these trends of progress serve the principles of developmental physiology becomes crucial. Each of these areas can be addressed in developing education and sports programs that focus on youth development holistically, to create an environment that fosters cognitive and physical growth, and subsequently improved health as one grows into adulthood (Figure 12.5).

12.1.3. Adulthood: Physiological Stability and Peak Performance

At adulthood, physiological stability is the defining characteristic, being typically marked by peak performance in the various dimensions of health and fitness. This stage of life is marked by the maturation of organ systems, hormonal regulation, and capacity for work. Both muscle mass and cardiovascular capacity typically experience top levels of efficiency in young adulthood, from which stands the foundation for athleticism and overall body health. The interplay among genetically predisposed tendencies and environmental stimulations also emphasizes this peak achievement level. Environmental stimuli in the form of diet and exercise enable the enhancement or reduction of bodily functioning, prompting significant consideration toward ensuring health. Stress and its various forms also play central parts in this dynamic and affect both daily functioning and long-term health outcomes. Hence, understanding the multiform nature of adult physiological functioning is needed in order to foster optimal health trajectories. Physiological stability during adulthood also emanates from the intricate equilibrium between psychological health and bodily well-being. Research highlights that stress reactions vary widely between individuals, shaped by both genetic vulnerabilities and environmental challenges experienced during a lifetime (Epel et al., 2018). The individual's ability to cope with stress can play a robust role in influencing health behavior, which in turn shapes physiological stability. For instance, chronic stress can result in maladaptive coping, such as, an unhealthy diet or lack of exercise, that can erode health and performance. Conversely, individuals well experienced in the employment of adaptive stress-management techniques have increased vitality and resilience. These psychological processes further our understanding of how adults cope with health issues and maintain their best physiological functioning. Such an exchange emphasizes the importance of comprehensive health methods that handle both body and mind health management. Furthermore, the concept of behavioral stability across the life span serves to show how adult physiological characteristics are shaped by early experience. Over the course of early life, phenotypic expression of the individual is plastic, with important influence from both genotype and environmental circumstances the individual experiences (Brust et al., 2015). In adulthood, the accumulated behavioral trajectories are increasingly stable, influencing health and overall physical functioning. This fixity often signals an integration of prior life experience, genotype, and environmental adaptations through which individuals adjust to stressors. Hence, understanding this developmental perspective is crucial to the development of strategies for enhancing adult performance and health. It teaches us the profound impact that psychological, contextual, and historical factors have on physiological stability and requires an integrative perspective to aging and health, involving consideration of the former and consideration of the latter.

Test Your Knowledge

1. How do physical, cognitive, and emotional changes vary across the lifespan?
2. What are Erik Erikson's psychosocial stages of development, and how do they relate to personal growth?

12.2. Cellular and Molecular Mechanisms of Aging

Learning Outcome

1. Explain the telomere shortening and cellular senescence;
2. Define oxidative stress and its impact on cellular function;
3. Describe the genetic factors influencing aging processes.

The revelation of aging through the cellular and molecular mechanism paradigm reveals the delicate interaction of biological processes. Aging is not a deteriorating process in function but a multifaceted, complex process based on cellular signal transduction and genetic control. One theoretical model is grounded in the conceptualization that cellular aging is an incremental process of entropic development in biological systems that can be traced back to fundamental mechanisms of inter- and intracellular communication. From this perspective, while multicellular organisms evolve, their mechanisms of cell-to-cell communication must also evolve to maintain homeostasis and thus form the basis for explaining the dynamics responsible for aging. By systematic examination of these cell-cell interactions, it is possible to establish critical sites of failure leading to senescence, facilitating the creation of interventions that might be able to optimize health span and longevity, fulfilling an imperative in current medicine (Rehan et al., 2009). Central to the cellular events of aging lies the activity of the extracellular matrix (ECM) and its contribution to intercellular communication. The ECM is a functional and structural scaffold that, besides providing cells with physical support, participates in signaling processes that regulate growth, differentiation, and response to the environment. During aging of organisms, ECM structure and composition deteriorate, leading to abnormal cellular communication, ultimately causing tissue homeostasis disruption. This loss of ECM function could disrupt the highly regulated processes necessary for cellular organization and metabolic health. As detailed in recent studies, care for intercellular spaces organization illustrates how disruptions can initiate age-related dysfunctions and, with disease insight implications, as shown by cancer, where cellular cooperation is lost (Bich et al., 2019). Also, knowledge of molecular processes that control aging has profound implications for the formation of therapeutic interventions. Cellular senescence, which occurs when cells are no longer capable of dividing, is important in the process of aging as it accumulates in tissues and releases pro-inflammatory cytokines. This is a great illustration of how molecular cascades of signals affect aging-related pathology, thereby determining multicellular system functional capacity with increasing age. The convergence of proteomic and genomic methods is central to disentangling the complex regulatory loops that operate in aging cells. Full understanding not only contributes to elucidating the reason for physiological frailty but also underpins strategies for regenerative medicine aiming to reverse the consequences of aging. As researchers continue to investigate these molecular discoveries, the aim is to apply this to improve health in older ages and thus build a higher quality of life in older age (Rehan et al., 2009) (Figure 12.6).

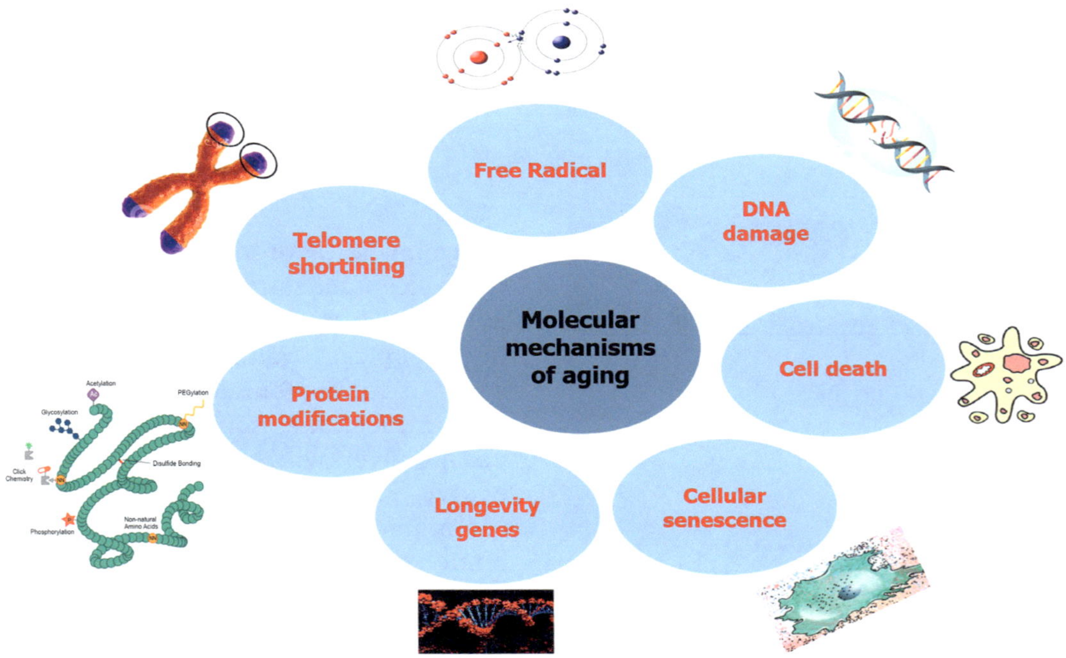

Figure 12.6. Aging and its molecular mechanism.

Source: https://encyclopedia.pub/media/item_content/202204/625e0491da2a8molecules-27-02316-g001.png.

12.2.1. Telomere Shortening and Cellular Senescence

The shortening of telomeres is a central biological aging and cellular senescence marker that links developmental physiology with the process of aging. Telomeres are repetitive nucleotide sequences found at chromosome ends that serve to guard genetic material throughout cell division. As cells divide, telomeres shorten progressively to the point where they ultimately reach the threshold length that causes cellular senescence—a state in which cells do not continue to divide but remain metabolically active. This aging process is not solely driven by chronological time; rather, it reflects cumulative cellular stressors like oxidative damage that may aid telomere loss. Decline in cellular proliferation allows room for the onset of age-related pathology, pointing to the importance of telomere dynamics research in developmental physiology and aging. Senescence of cells plays a pivotal role in numerous age-related diseases, especially organ system pathologies like the cardiovascular system.

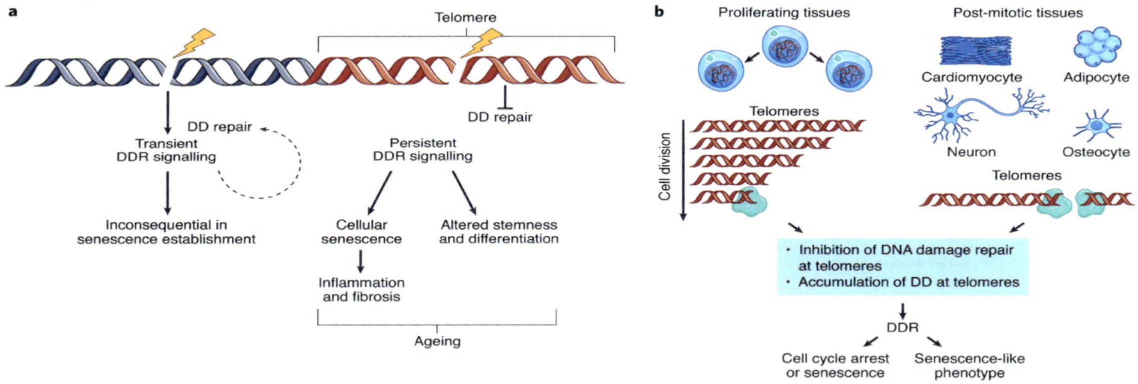

Figure 12.7. Telomere dysfunction in aging and age-related diseases.

Source: https://media.springernature.com/full/springer-static/image/art%3A10.1038%2Fs41556-022-00842-x/MediaObjects/41556_2022_842_Fig1_HTML.png.

As highlighted by studies, progressive decline of cardiovascular functions has its roots in the accumulation of senescent cells, which interfere with normal cellular function and result in tissue dysfunction. Senescent cells, for example, release inflammatory cytokines, growth factors, and extracellular matrix remodeling proteins into the milieu as a group referred to as the senescence-associated secretory phenotype (SASP). The SASP promotes the local tissue microenvironment, resulting in an inflammatory microenvironment that fuels age-related decline. The connection between telomere shortening and cellular senescence lies beyond the confines of cell function, emphasizing its role in the development and progression of cardiovascular disease and emphasizing the need for new strategies for rejuvenating old tissues by targeted interventions (Iop et al., 2017). Recent studies have established the impacts of environmental stresses on telomere shortening and biological aging, which yielded sensational findings on the impact of chronic stress exposure. For instance, in the Eurasian blackbird, studies have shown that repeatedly stressed subjects exhibit drastic declines in telomere lengths in concordance with increased biological aging. Based on such findings, one may infer that environmental factors play a major role in determining the telomere biology of organisms, with implications including raised cellular senescence and accompanying pathologies. Moreover, increases in oxidative damage brought about by stress have been shown to potentially contribute to the telomere erosion accelerated by stress, validating the intricate relationship between stress, telomere dynamics, and the consequences of aging. Thus, understanding the intricate interaction between telomere shortening, exposure to stress, and senescence at the cellular level is key to the development of effective interventions that seek to promote healthy aging and reverse the consequences of age-related diseases (Hau et al., 2015) (Figure 12.7).

12.2.2. Oxidative Stress and Its Impact on Cellular Function

The theory of oxidative stress is at the center of cellular complexity, particularly as organisms age. Cellular oxidative stress results from an imbalance between the generation of ROS and the cells ability to detoxify these harmful byproducts. This can generate extensive cellular damage like lipid peroxidation, protein oxidation, and DNA damage, which impair normal cellular function. With increasing age, the accumulation of oxidative damage may interfere with cellular communication and metabolic processes, ultimately affecting tissue homeostasis and organ function.

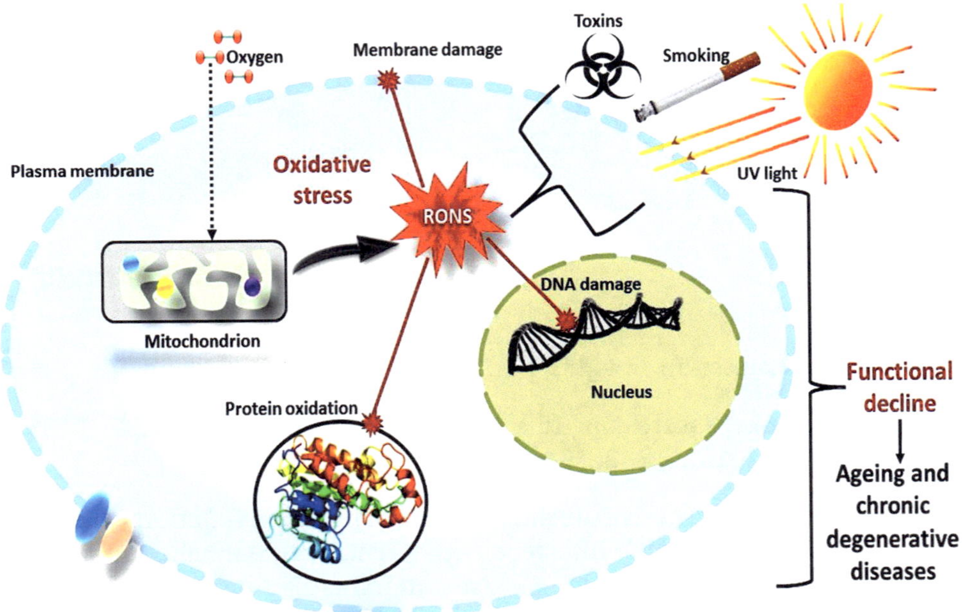

Figure 12.8. Oxidative stress and its impact on cellular function.

Source: https://pub.mdpi-res.com/ijms/ijms-23-07273/article_deploy/html/images/ijms-23-07273-g001.png?1656580779.

Mechanisms of oxidative stress are of relevance, as they may be responsible for elucidating the etiology of age-related disorders and facilitating the development of targeted therapies aimed at countering these events and preserving cellular integrity in elderly populations. One of the interesting fields of study includes the function of polyamines in cell function and how they interact with oxidative stress. Polyamines, which are key molecules involved in cellular homeostasis, have a broad spectrum of physiological functions , such as stimulating cell growth and redox status regulation. Changes in polyamine metabolism have been implicated in diseases, including age-related diseases, where reduced levels of polyamines are seen. Greater turnover of polyamines can enhance age-related oxidative stress, hence further conditioning the cell environment during aging.

Therefore, knowledge of the regulation of polyamines and their interaction with oxidative stress not only provides insight into the complexity of cellular aging but also therapeutic interventions. With the increased sophistication in our current understanding of polyamines, particularly their association with oxidative stress, novel methods of combating aging-associated dysfunction may be planned that hold potential for healthy old age.

The other crucial aspect that needs to be considered is the disruption of endoplasmic reticulum (ER) homeostasis due to oxidative stress. ER serves to fold proteins and undergo post-translational modification; however, increased oxidative stress can lead to ER stress, inducing an adaptive response known as the unfolded protein response (UPR). While activation of UPR initially serves a protective function, long-term ER stress can result in maladaptive cellular processes that ultimately contribute to aging. Research has confirmed that age-associated diseases, particularly in the lung, show signs of ER stress and deregulated proteostasis that are correlated with increased oxidative burdens. A comprehension of how oxidative stress, ER homeostasis, and the UPR are intricately interconnected can be a promising avenue toward the development of successful therapeutic interventions for age-related diseases, underscoring the significance of redress of oxidative stress as an aspect of developmental physiology and aging (Figure 12.8).

12.2.3. Genetic Factors Influencing Aging Processes

The intricate interdependence of genetic factors and aging processes has attracted considerable attention in recent scientific literature, particularly within the context of insulin/insulin-like growth factor 1 (IGF-1) signal transduction pathways. These are critical pathways involved in regulating various biological processes, from metabolic and growth functions to lifespan in various organisms, varying from yeast to mammals. One model organism that has been well described in this field is *Caenorhabditis elegans*, where reduced signaling through the insulin/IGF-1 pathway has been shown to enact a survival program that leads to substantially extended lifespan. In particular, the genetic alterations in *C. elegans*, i.e., the daf-2 gene, initiate a series of events that instigate metabolic modifications and increased stress tolerance and, thus, illustrate how genes can have a quiet yet measurable impact upon aging processes (Zečić & Braeckman, 2020). The transcription factor DAF-16 also plays a pivotal role in mediating the effect of the insulin/IGF-1 pathway on aging. Effectively, a longevity mechanism, DAF-16, regulates the transcription of various genes that correspond to development, immunity, and antioxidant activity in response to diminished IIS signaling. Interestingly, daf-2 mutants exhibit heterochronic activation of a dauer survival program during adulthood with elevated antioxidant defense and metabolic adjustments. The adjustments include trehalose and triglyceride accumulation, which are vital for survival and longevity. This sensitivity also highlights the complexity of genetic interactions that influence aging and the need to study these pathways between organisms to see the common mechanisms of longevity (Zečić & Braeckman, 2020). Not only is the impact of these genetic factors anecdotal, but rests on empirical evidence that demonstrates that alterations in some pathways are able to have a profound effect on aging. For instance, while upregulation of antioxidant activity is typically reported to be associated with increased lifespan, causality remains complex and, in some instances, unknown. Certain long-lived C. elegans mutants with reduced IIS have reduced oxidative damage rates, but the mechanism for this effect is multifarious and not entirely the result of increased macroautophagy. Additionally, differences in metabolic activity between organisms, namely, the production of trehalose and other carbohydrates, emphasize placing findings within evolutionary frameworks. Combining how different genetic pathways collaborate with one another across a variety of biological systems ultimately further clarifies mechanisms of aging and presents potential directions of therapeutic intervention (Braeckman & Dhondt, 2017).

Test Your Knowledge

1. How do free radicals and oxidative stress affect cellular aging and longevity?
2. What is the role of cellular senescence and apoptosis in tissue degeneration during aging?

12.3. Physiological Changes in Aging

Learning Outcome

1. Explain the changes in the cardiovascular system;
2. Define the alterations in the musculoskeletal system;
3. Describe the neurological changes and cognitive decline.

The physiological changes involved in the process of aging are multifaceted and encompass nearly all organ systems of the body. There is a natural diminution of the efficacy of most biological processes with age, and this has several apparent outcomes. A significant aspect of aging is the loss of regenerative capacity of tissues and organs, which undermines their ability to recover from injury or disease. For instance, cardiovascular function declines with increasing arterial stiffening, which contributes to hypertension and cardiovascular disease. Furthermore, the decline of muscular endurance and strength, or sarcopenia, exposes older individuals to higher risks of falls and fractures. These alterations are not only physiological disadvantages; they also can dramatically affect quality of life and health, which makes it important to actively be concerned with interventions that can reverse such change and allow for healthier aging. In addition, the interplay between personality and health becomes more relevant as individuals approach older age. Evidence is found to indicate that personality, as the Big Five measures it, can have a significant impact on health in older age. For example, higher conscientiousness has repeatedly been linked with healthier habits, such as, eating and exercise, which may be able to reverse some of the pathogenic physiological aspects of aging. Notably, studies have shown that personality and health indicators' correlations become intensified in middle adulthood and early late adulthood and show the developmental aspect of the relationship. However, as an individual reaches very old ages, the significance of these connections erodes, showing the complex dynamics of health through the aging process (Luo et al., 2023). This implies that recognizing personality's function in aging may help guide health promotion efforts for varying phases of life.

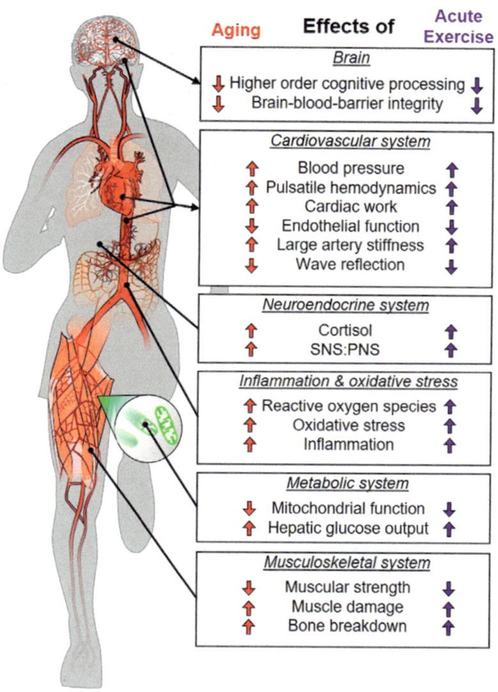

Figure 12.9. Exercise as an aging mimetic.

Source: https://www.frontiersin.org/files/Articles/866792/fphys-13-866792-HTML/image_m/fphys-13-866792-g001.jpg.

Also, research into biochemical alterations presents more information about the physiological terrain of aging. β-carboline alkaloids (βCBs), including harmine, have attracted attention for their involvement in neurodegenerative diseases, such as, Alzheimer's disease. Evidence shows that these compounds are not only extrinsic in nature but also have endogenous origins, being synthesized naturally in the body throughout various stages of life. With increasing age, tissue and plasma levels of harmine show dynamic variation, which is typically coordinated with that of neurotransmitters for cognitive function. The findings indicate that harmine levels decrease in the aging context, reflecting the complex relationship between physiological status and substance production (Cao et al., 2022). This emphasizes the potential for targeted interventions that could leverage these biochemical observations to combat the aging effect on neurological health (Figure 12.9).

12.3.1. Changes in the Cardiovascular System

With advancing age, there are extensive alterations in the cardiovascular system that influence health and function as a whole. These involve progressive decline in cardiac performance with structural changes within the heart itself, e.g., ventricular wall thickening and decrease in cardiac output. These changes have the propensity to augment vulnerability to cardiovascular disease, most prominently hypertension and heart failure. One of the prime determinants of these changes is the body's response to various stressors throughout the life course, as physiologic adaptations to stressors are at the heart of cardiovascular health. It has been proven that the overall exposure to stress can condition long-term cardiovascular responses, and hence the importance of measuring stress as a decontextualized event is lessened, while a series of interactions influencing heart health must be taken into consideration (Epel et al., 2018). The majority of age-related changes in the cardiovascular system are defined by alterations in vascular function and integrity. As age increases, the elastic properties of the arterial wall are lost, resulting in augmented stiffness of the arteries. Decreased flexibility impairs the capacity of the blood vessels to accommodate the changing flow of blood and elevates the levels of blood pressure and workload for the heart. Furthermore, aging is also associated with endothelial function changes that can compromise vascular health and increase cardiovascular risks further. The literature highlights the significance of a holistic consideration of such physiological changes, shedding light on how chronic psychological as well as physiological stressors over time cause adverse changes in cardiovascular health (Epel et al., 2018). In particular, the cardiovascular reaction to environmental change can also be seen as an adaptation to altered gravitational forces, particularly in spaceflight. Studies conducted in microgravity environments show that the cardiovascular system adapts with great magnitude, and researchers have looked to examine these effects as models for cardiovascular aging on Earth. The information gained from studying the response to hypo- and hyper gravity contains important information regarding the general mechanisms of adaptation in the elderly population. Not only does this question shed light on the physiological rationale for cardiovascular changes, but it also affords a deeper appreciation of body adaptability in the face of environmental stressors. Emphasizing these relationships is important in the development of effective interventions that will promote cardiovascular health throughout the aging process (Figure 12.10).

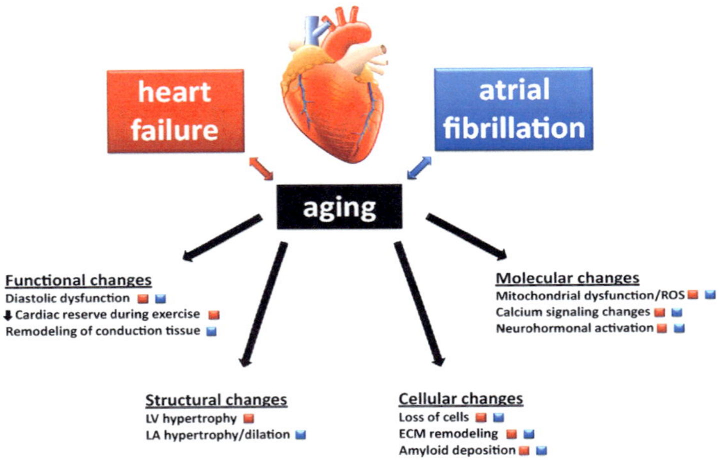

Figure 12.10. Age-related changes to the cardiovascular system.

Source: https://www.manipalhospitals.com/uploads/image_gallery/cardiac-changes-with-aging.png.

12.3.2. Alterations in the Musculoskeletal System

With advancing age, profound changes within the musculoskeletal system affect both structure and function. This intricate system of bones, muscles, tendons, and ligaments undergoes a continuum of alterations, such as, reduced bone mineral density, muscle mass, and joint flexibility. Osteopenia and osteoporosis that occur with advancing age manifest as a decline in bone mineral density, increasing the risk of fractures and mobility problems. Concurrently, sarcopenia, or loss of skeletal muscle mass with advancing age, weakens strength and endurance, makes everyday function more challenging, and enhances reliance on outside support. Such loss of musculoskeletal integrity is compounded by lifestyle factors , such as physical inactivity and malnutrition, which may accelerate the deterioration of muscle and bone tissues. Accordingly, it is critical to know how these alterations take place to create interventions for preserving musculoskeletal function during aging. The implications of gravitational changes, terrestrial and extraterrestrial, have significant implications for our understanding of musculoskeletal aging changes. Evidence indicates that exposure to microgravity conditions, as experienced by astronauts, provokes dramatic changes in the musculoskeletal system. The influence of prolonged weightlessness elicits muscle atrophy and decreased bone density due to lower mechanical loading, paralleling some geriatric changes observed on our planet. As research indicates, the plasticity inherent in the system allows the system to respond to stimuli, but episodes of extended disuse, such as, that which befalls older adults through sedentary behavior, replicate the unloading effects observed in space. This similarity underscores the need for proper countermeasures intended to preserve musculoskeletal function in both aging individuals and astronauts. Investigation of such responses provides invaluable insights into therapeutic interventions that might prevent deleterious effects of aging on the musculoskeletal system. As researchers delve further into the physiological changes that ensue following aging, it is increasingly apparent that comprehensive steps are required to maintain musculoskeletal integrity. Interventions consisting of goal-oriented exercise, nutritional supplementation, and drug therapy have reversed or delayed aging changes. Rehabilitation treatments, including resistance training, may enhance muscle strength and functional capacity, and adequate calcium and vitamin D nutrition must be ensured to preserve bone health. Additionally, the etiologic pathways of these alterations, including hormonal and inflammatory mechanisms, offer potential targets for innovative therapeutic interventions. Lastly, the incorporation of a combined multidisciplinary approach, including exercise, diet, and medication, will be critical. Through making a scientific understanding of musculoskeletal aging and tailoring evidence-based practices to achieve it, we can immensely improve the quality of life of the elderly and systemic physiological health (Figure 12.11).

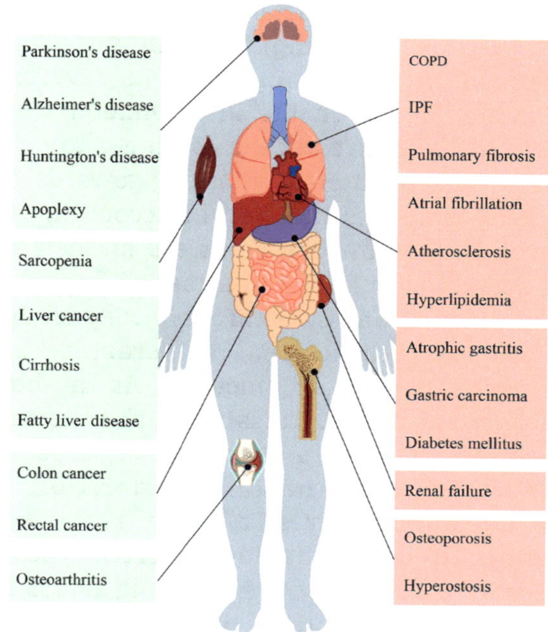

Figure 12.11. Aging in the human body organs will appear different degrees of pathological changes, thus causing a variety of diseases.

Source: https://www.frontiersin.org/journals/immunology/articles/10.3389/fimmu.2024.1405621/full

12.3.3. Neurological Changes and Cognitive Decline

As the aging process progresses, alterations in the neurological system are typically observed, with associated cognitive deterioration that can significantly impact daily functioning. Decline is characterized by a reduction in the volume of brain regions critical to information processing, such as, the hippocampus and prefrontal cortex. Neurological changes involve both structural, for example, loss of neural pathways and shrinkage of gray matter, and functional impairment of neurotransmission. These modifications enhance impairments in memory, attention, and executive functioning. In this way, cognitive impairment with increasing age is not just an age function; instead, it is a function of complex interactions between lifestyle, genetic susceptibility, and social environments, and this justifies adopting a multidimensional approach in accounting for and reversing the same. Moreover, the interconnectivity of stress and cognitive decline continues to be an area of related interest, pointing towards the complex dynamics involved in accounting for neurological health. Chronic stress, for instance, has been seen to have a detrimental impact on brain function and structure, typically leading to heightened emotional vulnerability and decreased intellectual functions. As the body is exposed to chronic stress, it is hit by allostatic overload that triggers physiological responses that might hasten neural deterioration. As illustrated within stress typology research, it is critical to determine how different types of stressors affect cognitive processing across the lifespan for interventions that may potentially enhance some of the aging-related cognitive impairments. By identifying the nuances of stress responses, one also better understands how psychological processes become intertwined with cognitive health with increasing age (Epel et al., 2018). Furthermore, cognitive decline in older age is highly linked with the loss of central, deliberative processes that support various linguistic and communicative activities. There is evidence to suggest that with increasing age, the efficiency of the central processes engaged in the more taxing deployment of language diminishes significantly. Decreased facility for metalanguage use, strategic planning, and inhibitory capability constitutes an obstacle to successful communication as well as to cognitive adaptability. Specifically, disturbances in these deliberative processes could underlie language disorders that interfere with social functioning and well-being among older adults. The vulnerability of these processes to age-related change sets the stage for the use of targeted treatment interventions that potentially enhance cognitive functioning and underscores the value of knowledge about neurological change with aging (Harley et al., 2011).

Test Your Knowledge

1. What are the major cardiovascular, respiratory, and musculoskeletal changes that occur with aging?
2. How does aging affect renal function, fluid balance, and electrolyte regulation?

12.4. Hormonal Changes and Aging

Learning Outcome

1. Identify the role of hormones in growth and development;
2. Define the age-related hormonal changes and their effects;
3. Describe the hormone replacement therapy and its implications.

Hormonal equilibrium in the human body is significantly affected by the process of aging, with almost every physiological function being deeply impacted. In middle and old age, there is a change in the endocrine system with the decrease in vital hormones , such as estrogen, testosterone, and growth hormone. The hormonal alterations are linked with various conditions of aging, like decreased muscle mass, increased fat gain, and loss of bone tissue. For instance, in women, the transition to menopause, marked by a dramatic reduction in estrogen, can make them prone to osteoporosis and cardiovascular disease. Similarly, men may develop low levels of testosterone, leading to weak libido, mood swings, and muscle malfunction. Combined, these hormonal alterations not only reflect the biological transformations of aging but also highlight the importance of taking the health of hormones into account in the general sense in geriatric practice. The interplay between hormones and microbiota is now a trendy field of research in the context of aging. Recent evidence focuses on the microbiota-gut-brain axis as a master regulator of hormonal homeostasis and overall physiologic regulation. With age, the variety of our gut microbiota decreases, impacting many of our metabolic processes, such as, those related to hormones like insulin and cortisol. Stress, particularly, exacerbates this, and we end up with a compromised microbiota that in turn can impact hormonal balance and be one of the contributing causes of conditions associated with age , such as obesity and diabetes. Moreover, microbial metabolites like short-chain fatty acids have been reported to exert significant effects on metabolic syndrome—a condition that is currently on the increase among elderly populations. Thus, learning the relationship between hormonal transformation and gut microbiota is crucial in order to establish mechanisms for controlling age-related differences in health, demonstrating the relationship of aging, hormone regulation, and microbiota composition (Cryan et al., 2019). Further, the impact of hormonal changes on cellular aging mechanisms should not be overlooked, as they are pivotal in determining longevity and health span. Growth factors and insulin are hormones that play a remarkable role in influencing senescence and apoptosis. With aging, decreased hormone signaling may lead to abnormal cellular functions and senescent cell accumulation, which also reinforces the aging phenotype. The Nomenclature Committee on Cell Death (NCCD) has categorized various forms of cell death, the majority of which are controlled by changes in hormones that can dictate whether cells in tissues live or are killed (Galluzzi et al., 2018). Understanding how these hormone changes correlate with shifts in mechanisms of cell death is important in establishing potential therapeutic options for degenerative disorders of aging. Therefore, the combination of hormonal research with cellular aging expertise provides a full paradigm to investigate the complexities of aging and cellular therapeutic frontiers (Figure 12.12).

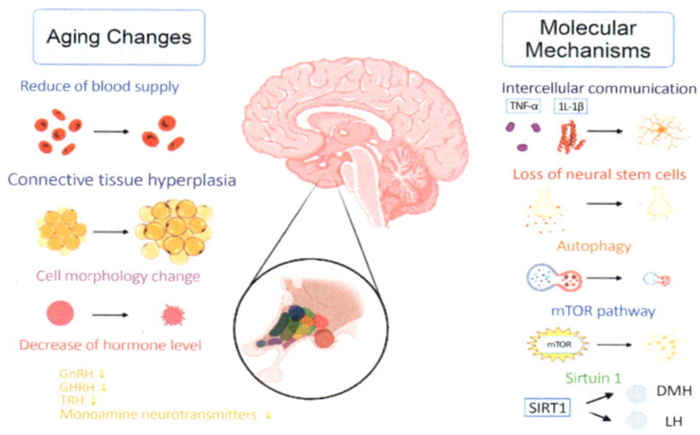

Figure 12.12. The timing sequence and mechanism of aging in endocrine organs.

Source: https://www.mdpi.com/cells/cells-12-00982/article_deploy/html/images/cells-12-00982-g006.png.

12.4.1. The role of Hormones in Growth and Development

Hormones play a vital role in the regulation of growth and development in most organisms as signaling molecules coordinating physiological processes essential for maturation. In primates, triiodothyronine (T3) is one of the thyroid hormones that are known to significantly influence developmental pathways. For instance, studies indicate that juvenile Assamese macaques present higher levels of fecal total triiodothyronine (IF-T3) than adults as evidence of the central role during early stages of development. This relationship suggests that the thyroid hormones are not just metabolic regulators but actually induce the physiological changes necessary for development and growth. In addition, variations in IF-T3 levels under the stresses of the environment suggest the sensitivity of the hormonal systems. These findings underscore the role played by hormones in modulating environmental stress and influencing developmental pathways, which in turn determine growth patterns among individuals within primate populations (Behringer et al., 2023). In plant physiology, hormones also play a crucial role in regulating plant development and growth processes, particularly senescence. The senescence process, through which plants grow old, is regulated by the fine balance of hormones and external regulation. When plants reach certain levels of development, senescence-inducing signaling molecules, like plant hormones like auxins and ethylene, cause cell components to break down. It is not an irreversible step; rather, it is recycling the nutrients, facilitating growth and additional development in the neighboring tissues. Reactive oxygen species (ROS) and other signaling molecules additionally orchestrate these physiological changes to render the plant adaptive in its environment. Information regarding hormonal regulation of senescence is paramount in maximizing crop yield and managing cycles of growth and growth regulation and highlights the complex interplay between hormones and environmental factors in managing plant development (Sharma, 2023).

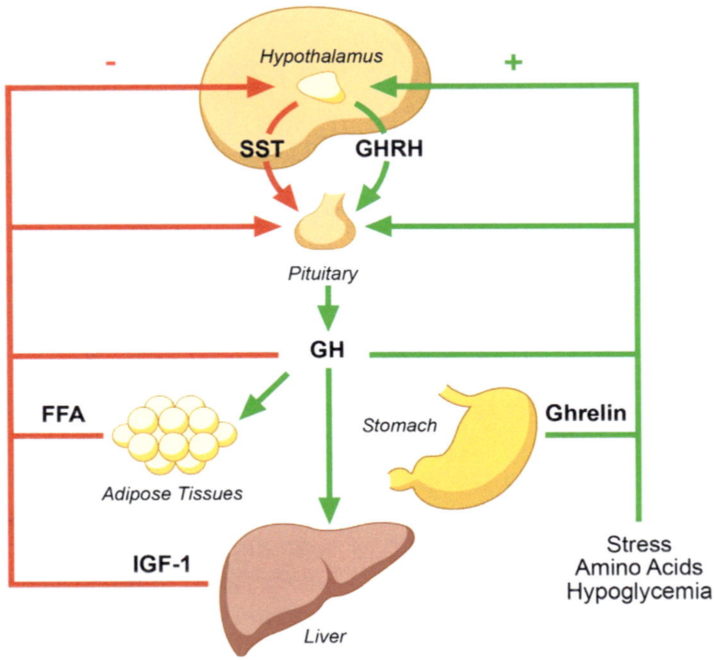

Figure 12.13. Role of hormones in growth and development.

Source: https://www.ncbi.nlm.nih.gov/books/NBK279163/bin/age-rel-chang-ghaght-Image003.jpg.

As organisms age, the role of hormones in the regulation of physiological balance becomes increasingly important. In animals and plants, alike, the interactions between growth hormones and senescent processes provoke information about the aging process. In mammals, the level of growth hormone (GH) typically declines with increasing age, facilitating reduced metabolism and body composition changes. On the other hand, senescence in plants is provoked or postponed through hormonal signals, influencing reproductive strategy and lifespan. The understanding of the action of hormones during aging provides valuable insights into developmental physiology. By explaining these processes, researchers can explore new ways of optimizing growth, enhancing tolerance to environmental stress components, and, perhaps, reverse the deteriorating effects of aging on performance and productivity in the natural environment as well as in agriculture, thus accentuating the central function of the hormones in development and aging (Behringer et al., 2023; Sharma, 2023) (Figure 12.13).

12.4.2. Age-Related Hormonal Changes and Their Effects

Aging is linked with generalized endocrine alterations that exert profound influences on several physiological systems of the body. Specific emphasis is placed on reductions in estrogen, testosterone, and growth hormone levels that affect not just reproduction but also musculoskeletal function and metabolic processes. The decline in estrogen levels, particularly post-menopause, can lead to an increased risk of osteoporosis and cardiovascular disease in women as bone density declines and lipid metabolism is altered. Similarly, the decline in testosterone levels in men is accompanied by decreased muscle mass, bone density, and fat distribution changes. These alterations broaden the aging process and illustrate the vital role played by hormones in providing health and vigor in the latter half of life. Furthermore, the effects of age-related hormonal change extend beyond reproductive and skeletal systems to have significant effects on cognition and the regulation of mood. It has been shown that declining levels of testosterone are correlated with increased rates of depression and cognitive impairment in older men.

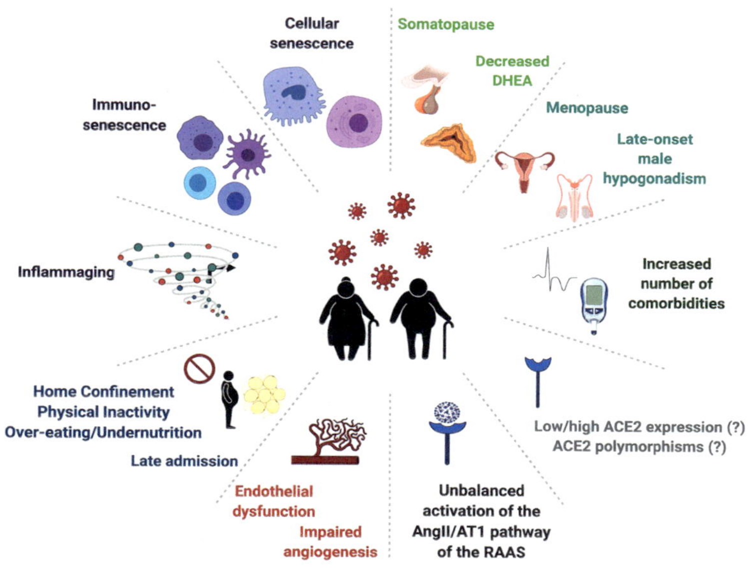

Figure 12.14. Age-related hormonal changes and their effects.

Source: https://media.springernature.com/lw685/springer-static/image/art%3A10.1007%2Fs11154-021-09656-y/MediaObjects/11154_2021_9656_Fig3_HTML.png.

Furthermore, in women and men, the reduction of hormone levels can influence stress response and emotional well-being, further complicating the aging process. Hormonal alterations, or more specifically, those involving adrenal hormones like cortisol, have been found to result in a dysregulation of stress response by the body, leaving older adults susceptible to mental illness. This interplay of hormonal change and psychological state emphasizes the need for an integrated philosophy of health comprising mental, emotional, and physical facets in aging. Of particular interest is how this comprehension of the influence of age-associated hormonal changes can be used to develop targeted interventions to reverse their impact. Interventions , such as hormone replacement therapy (HRT), dietary change, and exercise regimens have been tested to reverse declines observed in older populations. For instance, consistent physical exercise not only retains muscle mass but also has potential for positive impact on hormonal profiles. Resistance training stimulates testosterone release, thereby improving overall health outcomes. Lastly, the latest research identifies nutrition as a factor in hormone regulation, with certain nutrients having the potential to support maintenance of hormonal balance. Thus, managing hormonal changes through lifestyle modification is a good choice for enhancing the quality of life in the elderly, underscoring the significant connection between hormonal health and aging successfully (Figure 12.14).

12.4.3. Hormone Replacement Therapy and Its Implications

Hormone replacement therapy (HRT) is now a standard treatment for symptom control associated with aging, particularly in women going through menopause. Once these women attain this phase, typically between the ages of 45 and 55, they begin to experience a drastic reduction in estrogen levels, which generates various symptoms , such as night sweats, mood swings, and fatigue. Research has established that despite the fact that approximately 80% of women experience one or more of these symptoms during menopause, few people come near seeking medical relief, and thus they end up inflicting a very expensive toll on their quality of life (Doamekpor et al., 2025). HRT, usually prescribed in the form of estrogen with or without progestin, can alleviate these symptoms and also offer disease-protective benefits against osteoporosis and heart disease. Understanding the role of HRT in managing symptoms is critical because it has direct implications for women's health at a crucial point in their lives. As beneficial as it is, HRT is riddled with possible health consequences that need to be meticulously balanced. Long-term use of estrogen, in particular, has been associated with higher rates of some cancers, including breast cancer and thromboembolism. In the setting of specific disorders like Kallmann syndrome, where HRT can be prescribed to women, the impact of such treatment is potentially dramatic. In one study, it was determined that among women with Kallmann syndrome, those who did not take HRT had significantly higher risks for developing breast cancer, whereas those taking HRT had reduced risks for other conditions, including deep venous thrombosis and depression (Eidbo et al., 2025). This highlights the necessity for personalized medical approaches that consider individualized health profiles and potential oncological results, and thus offer patients safe and effective treatment modalities. Advances in hormone replacement therapies, such as, the development of innovative transdermal patches, provide a promising area for enhancing the safety and efficacy of HRT. These new patches are formulated to allow for hormone dosing to be individualized, enabling better management of menopausal symptoms with fewer side effects from the usual oral therapy with estrogen, such as, increased risk of venous thromboembolism (Bindra et al., 2025). The development of the MenoPatch, for instance, allows for sustained release and adjustment of hormone levels, thus promising not just improved symptom relief but also greater patient compliance. With more women seeking relief from menopausal symptoms, further research and development in HRT will become a key factor in formulating even better therapies and addressing the long-standing constraints involving states of hormone deficiency in aging populations.

Test Your Knowledge

1. Which hormones commonly decline with age, and how do these changes affect overall physiology?
2. How does aging impact the hypothalamic-pituitary axis and its hormonal outputs?

12.5. Environmental Influences on Aging

Learning Outcome

1. Describe the impact of nutrition on developmental physiology;
2. Define the role of physical activity in aging;
3. Discuss environmental toxins and their effects on aging.

Environmental factors play a significant role in the aging process, influencing aspects of health and longevity. Over the course of one's life, numerous stressors to which one is exposed have the potential to shape physiological results, including those of aging. Both acute and chronic experiences are among these stressors, demonstrating the active interaction between one's environment and individual responses. For instance, chronic stress has been linked with premature aging, as evident through its impact on telomere length and systemic inflammatory markers. The multidimensional aspect of stress, encompassing various dimensions and timing, underscores the need for a thorough understanding of environmental factors and how these drive health outcomes in older individuals. By embracing integrative models incorporating the stress complexities, researchers can gain important insights into how environmental factors modulate age-related physiological processes, and thereby inform potential interventions in facilitation of healthier aging (Epel et al., 2018). The environmental effects on aging also extend to the ways extrinsic conditions intersect with genetic and physiological compensations. Experiments have established that living organisms, including human beings, have a remarkable ability to accommodate altered conditions over time. These are frequently at the level of intricate interactions within a genome in which some traits enhance survival under altered conditions. As an illustration, in experiments on certain vertebrate organisms, this adaptation has been correlated with increased tolerance to climatic changes, indicating the role of the environment in shaping evolutionary processes. In understanding the functional genomic underpinnings of these adaptations, it is possible to unravel how individuals react to their environments, reinforcing the significance of environmental context in aging. Not only does this understanding better our understanding of developmental physiology, but it also offers a model for exploring gene-environment interactions, especially as global climate change threatens new obstacles to health outcomes across populations (Hamilton et al., 2017). By inserting environmental factors as an influencing concept to our understanding of aging, one can extend to investigating the health inequalities caused by varying environmental settings. Socioeconomic status, place, and access to healthcare can significantly impact how an individual is exposed to stressors and, thus, how aging mechanisms are influenced. Populations exposed to unhealthy environmental circumstances, i.e., excess pollution or socioeconomic disturbance, usually exhibit excess rates of age-related illness and poor health. Examining these differences can illustrate the critical areas in which intervention is required in both environmental determinants of health and policy supporting equal access to resources. As the science of aging proceeds, an advanced focus on environmental influences will be essential to informing global strategies aimed at encouraging health and long life across diverse populations, ultimately in the service of a larger understanding of developmental physiology and aging processes (Figure 12.15).

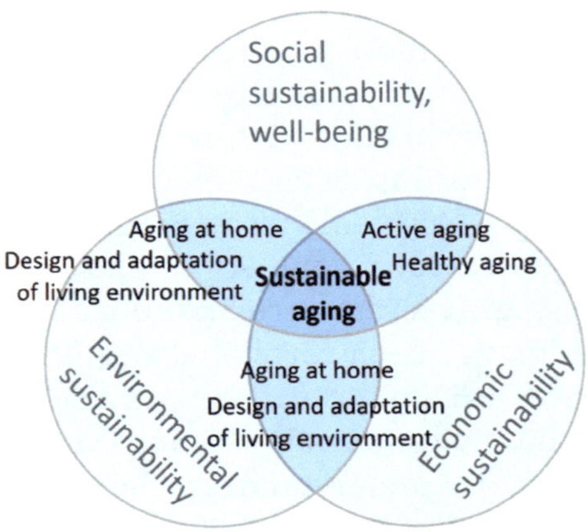

Figure 12.15. Environmental influences on aging.

Source: https://pub.mdpi-res.com/sustainability/sustainability-12-01853/article_deploy/html/images/sustainability-12-01853-g002.png?1583420551.

12.5.1. The Impact of Nutrition on Developmental Physiology

Nutrition plays a pivotal role in defining developmental physiology throughout life, impacting physical growth as well as mental ability. During the early stages of life, particularly prenatal and early childhood growth, the body is highly responsive to what it takes in. Adequate nutrition sets the course of neural pathways and promotes healthy brain development, something highly significant for mental ability as one reaches maturity. However, nutrient deficiencies during these initial years can result in lifelong developmental disorders, manifesting as physical stunting and compromised cognitive capacity that persists through adult life. For instance, malnutrition during early childhood has been linked to poor school performance and increased vulnerability to chronic disease in the future. This underscores the necessity to close nutritional gaps within vulnerable groups to optimize development and flow advantages throughout the life course, underlining the significance of anticipatory nutrition interventions rather than at specific developmental windows (Yoshikawa et al., 2020). The impact of nutrition continues far into early childhood, extending to developmental physiology throughout the life course, even into old age. As a person ages, the body undergoes various physiological changes, and changes in what one consumes lead to remaining healthy. Foods rich in nutrients may delay losses of muscle strength and mental function that accompany aging, supporting well-being. A diet rich in essential nutrients—, such as proteins, vitamins, and minerals—may boost the immune system, result in proper cell functioning, and reduce the risk of age-related diseases , such as osteoporosis and heart disease. In addition, certain dietary practices, such as, the Mediterranean diet, have been found to be protective of cognitive impairment and other physiological deficits typical of aging. Thus, the intersection of nutrition and aging highlights the necessity for adaptive dietary regimens to facilitate long-term health and enhance the quality of life among older persons, demonstrating how nutrition throughout the life course sets development pathways (Roberts et al., 2019). Furthermore, the effect of nutrition on developmental physiology can also be described by employing the context of recent attempts at farm mechanization towards food quality improvement.

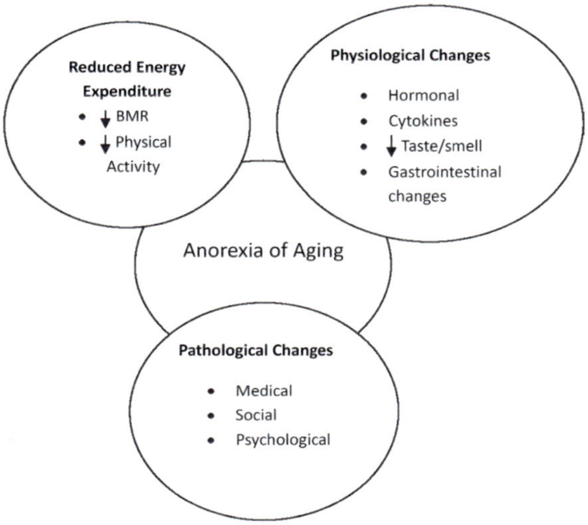

Figure 12.16. Nutrition on developmental physiology.

Source: https://www.mdpi.com/healthcare/healthcare-03-00648/article_deploy/html/images/healthcare-03-00648-g001-1024.png.

The utilization of cutting-edge genetic technologies in breeding adds the capability to enhance the nutritional content of staples, which is essential for addressing prevailing nutritional deficiencies among populations. Through the engineering of crops to include healthy bioactive constituents and essential nutrients, scientists are capable of amplifying overall intake in societies, particularly within low- and middle-income nations where malnutrition is elevated. In addition to solving acute nutritional needs, this method also enhances sustainable agricultural practices that strain the environment less. These food production innovations underscore the key role of nutrition to shape developmental trajectories throughout the life course, affirming a life course approach to the promotion of health and well-being (Yoshikawa et al., 2020) (Figure 12.16).

12.5.2. The Role of Physical Activity in Aging

Involvement in frequent physical exercise is also key in the aging process, having a large role to play in physical as well as emotional health. The body loses muscle mass, bone density, and cardiovascular ability with aging. Exercise, however, can keep these adverse effects at bay. Research indicates that active seniors are not only stronger than their sedentary counterparts but also experience improvements in strength, balance, and flexibility. This level of physical fitness is linked to greater independence and reduced risks for falls, which are a classic problem of geriatric medicine. Therefore, of primary concern is the role of physical activity in fostering longer, healthier lives, thereby enhancing the quality of aging and minimizing the physiological snares of old age. Additionally, the relationship between physical activity and mental function in aging populations cannot be overlooked. It is said that physical exercise enhances brain function and mental acuity, fostering neuroplasticity—brain capacity to reorganize through new neural pathways. This increasingly applies as mental decline poses a major challenge among the elderly. Engagement in aerobic or resistance training has been associated with improved memory and executive function, which may reduce the risk of neurodegenerative diseases , such as Alzheimer's. The position of physical exercise in the microbiota-gut-brain axis is used to further highlight this; the gut microbiome, which has an influence on cognitive health, is influenced by lifestyle, including diet and exercise. These findings underscore the need to integrate physical activity into a unified strategy for aging cognition, further elucidating how exercise, mental health, and aging interact (Cryan et al., 2019). Knowing the mechanisms of action through which physical activity influences aging is necessary for developing effective interventions as well. Physical exercise encourages cell adaptations like increased mitochondrial biogenesis and cellular stress resistance, which are critical for maintaining organismal homeostasis. Emerging forms of advances demonstrate how exercise modulates cell death and survival mechanisms, revealing potential therapeutic strategies against diseases of aging (Galluzzi et al., 2018). Also, exercise enhances the discharge of myokines, exercise-stimulated signaling molecules produced by muscle cells that play a role in inflammation and aging. These findings underscore the multi-dimensional worth of exercise not merely as an issue of lifestyle, but as a critical component of health programs for optimizing function and health in older adults. This holistic perspective on physical activity has the potential to redefine how we think about aging, no longer as a one-way decline, but as a phase that can be lived and mastered by taking initiative (Figure 12.17).

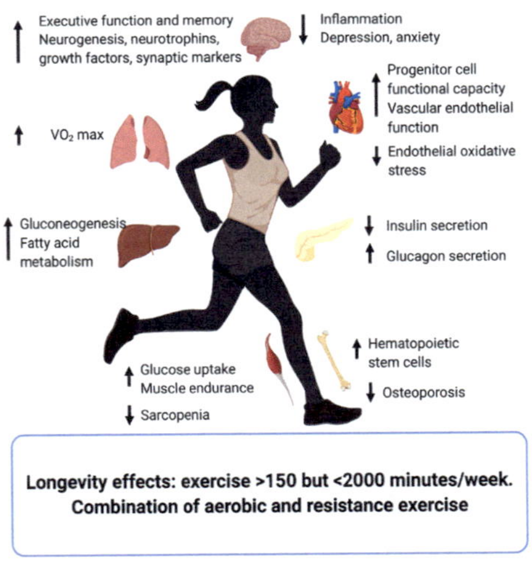

Figure 12.17. Role of physical activity in aging.

Source: https://www.aging-us.com/article/203051/figure/f1/large.

12.5.3. Environmental Toxins and Their Effects on Aging

The aging process has also been discovered to be influenced by a number of environmental factors, particularly by toxins that infest our environments. Toxins from industry, agriculture, and urban life can accumulate in human tissues and have adverse impacts on physiological processes involved in aging. For instance, heavy metal toxicity from exposure to lead and mercury has been discovered to directly cause cognitive impairment and neurodegenerative disease, both of which are prevalent among aging populations. These metals interfere with neuronal function and cause oxidative stress that destroys cells. Moreover, toxic chemicals in pesticides and pollutants have been shown to interfere with endocrine signaling and promote age-related diseases , such as diabetes and cardiovascular diseases. As a result, interaction between environmental toxins and the aging phenotype is something that must be explored more intensively because it presents an opportunity window for interventions that can limit the potential health hazards coming from aging individuals. Research indicates that not just the presence of environmental toxins but also their cumulative impact plays a central role in aging. There is overwhelming evidence to demonstrate that prolonged exposure to low levels of a variety of toxins leads to premature aging, a problem of great public health and regulatory importance. For example, agrochemical exposure not only kills detoxifying mechanisms but also potentially compromises immune systems, making the population progressively vulnerable to disease processes characteristic of aging. As explained in recent studies, synergism among various stressors can potentiate the acceleration of biological decay, rendering the diagnosis and treatment of aging-related disease problematic. In general, it is essential to recognize the cumulative impacts of environmental toxins in deciding on how lifestyle factors and control measures can be engineered to safeguard susceptible aging populations against the deleterious effects of these chemicals (Goulson et al., 2015). It cannot be ignored in academic discourse to address the multifaceted interplay between environmental toxins and aging. Interdisciplinary approaches, exemplified by studies in the field of biofilms, demonstrate the dynamic interactions between environmental determinants, microbial populations, and human health impacts. A good example is the manner in which toxin-induced modulation within the human microbiome will influence the regulation of systemic inflammation and immune responses, further exacerbating the process of aging. Likewise, as with biofilm-linked infections, constant exposure to toxins has the potential to result in heightened pathogen virulence, increasing the risks for elderly populations who tend to be more vulnerable to infection. Effective management programs would thus find it useful to tap into the knowledge acquired through biofilm investigations and other interdisciplinary fields, affirming the need for preventive measures against toxin exposure within aging populations (Römling et al., 2014). This convergence can guide future policies that will reduce environmental toxin exposure, ultimately resulting in healthier aging pathways.

Test Your Knowledge

1. How do lifestyle factors , such as diet, exercise, and sleep, influence the aging process?
2. What is the impact of chronic exposure to environmental toxins or pollutants on cellular aging and disease risk?

12.6. Interventions to Promote Healthy Aging

Learning Outcome

1. Describe the lifestyle modifications for better health outcomes;
2. Define the advances in medical technology and treatments;
3. Describe the role of social support and mental health.

Interventions to maximize healthy aging are ever more crucial as populations worldwide experience profound demographic transformation. Most interventions are likely to include a comprehensive program of physical, mental, and social dimensions of health. Physical activity is most crucial, and science has proven that exercise not only improves cardiovascular well-being but also enhances cognitive function and emotional well-being. Social relationships also have a vital role in the aging process. As age advances, it becomes easier to create families and friends' circles that make one happier and less lonely. Social programs that unite individuals in interaction and promote the choice of healthy lifestyles play a crucial role here, since they offer an environment where senior citizens feel confident and protected, which has a massive impact on their overall quality of life and longevity. Yet another vital component of healthy aging is addressing the specific social, cultural, and health-specific concerns of older adults. Among them is the very stigmatized issue of sexuality and intimacy.

Older adults are constantly beset with myths surrounding their sexuality that lead to under-addressed issues that have a detrimental impact on their quality of life. How to dispose of these problems requires sensitivity and awareness, driving physicians to start open talks on sexual health and its attendant expectations. Not only does it help reduce the impact of ageist ideology, but it might also encourage elderly adults to take advantage of interventions needed. A collaborative effort by healthcare providers to discuss, diagnose, and treat sexual dysfunction and intimacy disorders reinforces the need to maintain a healthy sex life as an integrated part of overall well-being, a focus emphasized in workshops to highlight these needs (Lindau, 2006). Healthy aging also appears to call for the implementation of evidence-based interventions aimed at enhancing psychosocial skills. As discussed when marketing resilience, interventions that focus on self-regulation, coping abilities, and social bonding are essential to prepare people for the transitions that accompany aging. Particularly for vulnerable populations, such as, those in foster care or those with major life transitions, establishing these abilities is crucial to encourage flexibility and active aging. The development of specialized programs that aid older individuals in the acquisition of necessary emotional and psychological competencies can lead to better successful aging experiences. Ultimately, the integration of these components into comprehensive geriatric care plans has the possibility to greatly improve outcomes and quality of life for older adults, enabling them to reach later life with dignity and contentment (Figure 12.18).

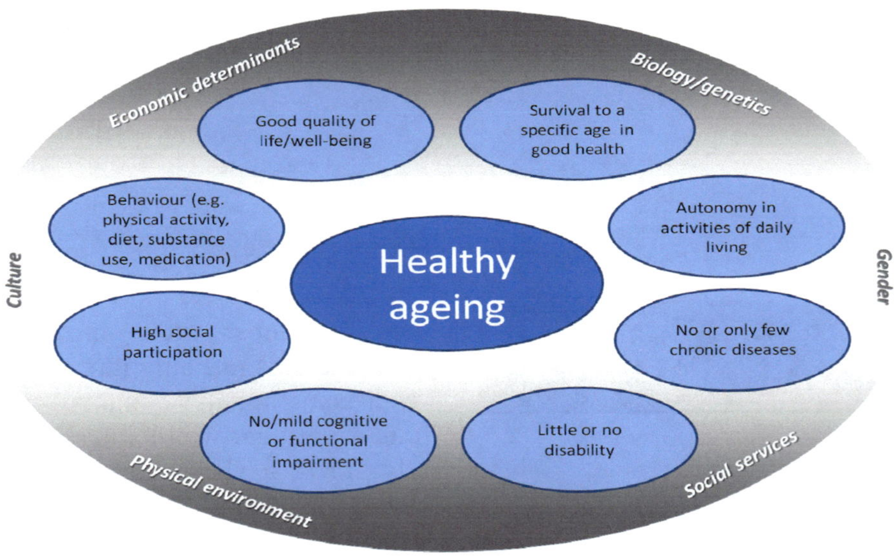

Figure 12.18. Indicators for healthy aging.

Source: https://www.mdpi.com/ijerph/ijerph-10-06630/article_deploy/html/images/ijerph-10-06630-g001-1024.png.

12.6.1. Lifestyle Modifications for Better Health Outcomes

Lifestyle modifications are critical to enhancing health outcomes, especially with the population aging and experiencing physiological change. Underlying these modifications are dietary modifications, physical exercise, and behavioral changes, all of which contribute to enhanced chronic disease control. A good example is a systematic strategy that involves regular exercise to assist in addressing obesity and its consequent health conditions like diabetes and cardiovascular disease. Studies have shown that moderate aerobic exercise not only leads to weight reduction but also enhances cardiovascular health and metabolic function. Through the adoption of lifestyle changes, older individuals can make a huge contribution to chronic disease incidence reduction, leading to a better quality of life in old age. Thus, embracing these changes for transformation is not only beneficial but imperative for aging populations in the face of the challenges brought about by developmental physiology. In addition, technology is increasingly taking a pivotal position in facilitating lifestyle change, particularly via telehealth programs. Technologies , such as telenursing offer a flexible mechanism of chronic disease management, where patients have access to healthcare services and education remotely. The effectiveness of these interventions has been evidenced by pilot studies of self-management treatment for conditions like diabetes. Participants demonstrated increased personal agency over their health outcomes through the use of telehealth measures to set personal goals and monitor progress toward healthier living. This electronic networking of patients and health workers can compensate for the space-related difficulties conventionally faced by old people, thereby enabling them to receive the needed care without the logistical burden of traditional healthcare provision. Thus, the integration of technology into lifestyle modification programs is transforming aging population healthcare provision with its potential to support their sustenance of health and wellness. Under the specific conditions, targeted therapy has also been effective in promoting better lifestyles among vulnerable groups. For example, studies among obese pregnant women have revealed the potential advantages of artificial intelligence and multidisciplinary team-directed lifestyle changes. These interventions target important elements , such as dietary modifications, increased physical activity, and behavior interventions based on individualized needs. According to research, using high-technology modalities for the promotion of health behavior change favors maternal weight control and pregnancy outcomes in order to impact long-term health in children and mothers. This is reflective of how lifestyle modification, supported by new health interventions, is imperative in enhancing health outcomes among different populations, even further supporting the notion that health management must be anticipatory in the aging process, particularly with the chronic disease and physiological deterioration associated with aging.

12.6.2. Advances in Medical Technology and Treatments

Medical technology has influenced profoundly the comprehension and management of diverse conditions associated with aging, outlining a critical intersection of developmental physiology and the aging process. Technologies , such as robotics, artificial intelligence, and telemedicine have revolutionized traditional health care to more sophisticated and accessible modalities. For instance, robot-assisted procedures not only improved the accuracy of surgical operations but also reduced the recovery time for elderly patients, a classic example of how this innovation has improved the quality of life. Telemedicine has also bridged the access gap so that the elderly are able to receive timely medical advice without interruption from mobility and transport challenges. These innovations outline a general trend whereby technology is being created to cater to the particular needs of an aging population, emphasizing the need to harmonize approaches to healthcare with the nuances of developmental physiology according to an individual's age. On top of this, the emergence of personalized medicine, where treatment is tailored to the individual genetic profile of a patient, is a massive development in medical technology. This approach enables doctors to predict what different therapies will do in individual patients, thereby maximizing therapeutic effectiveness with fewer side effects. Older individuals, with comorbidities in numbers, can have treatment schedules revolutionized by personalized medicine, allowing for more effective control of different conditions. As more is discovered about the genetic underpinnings of diseases common to aging individuals, clinicians can utilize targeted therapy that takes on these specific physiological challenges head-on. The convergence of genetics and technology to design personalized treatment plans not only represents an enormous step beyond the current practice of medicine but rewrites the story about aging as a journey marked by medical intervention, not inexorable deterioration. In addition to these technological advancements, regenerative medicine is also making way for a new age of treating age-related degeneration. Stem cell therapy and tissue engineering are promising to reverse the damage caused by aging and degenerative diseases. For instance, stem cell therapy can restore the lost organ and tissue function, making way for new modes of treatments in cardiovascular health and neural regeneration. As scientists further research the effectiveness of such treatments, the ways to enhance health span and lifespan become clearer. These breakthroughs not only reshape the trajectory of aging but also put a call for an overhaul of developmental physiology, underscoring the ability of the body to restore and renew itself long into old age. With these breakthroughs also spreading further, they paint a rosy picture of aging as one of resilience and accommodation held up by science and technology today (Figure 12.19).

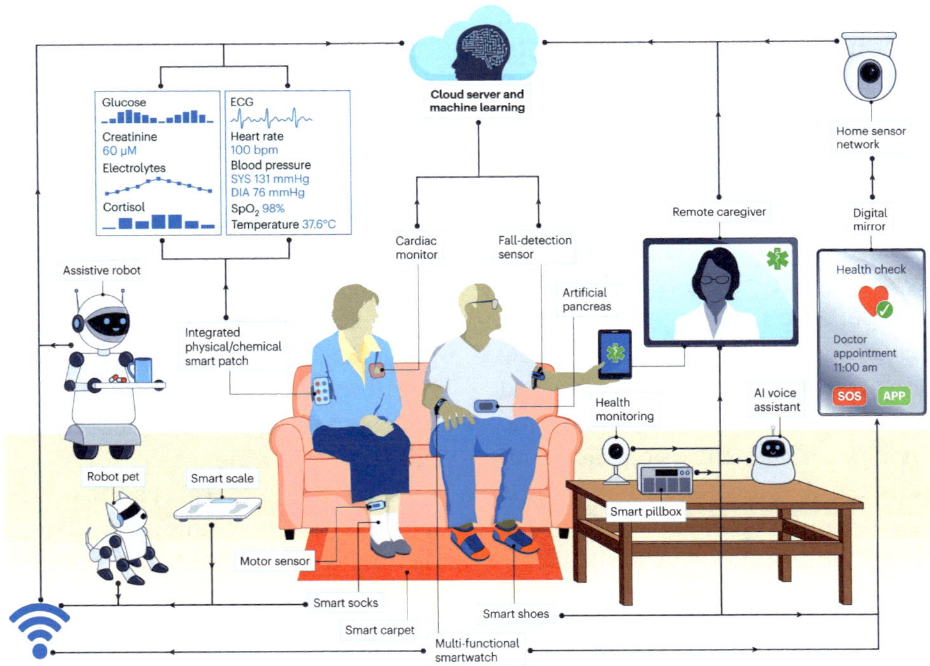

Figure 12.19. Digital health for aging populations.

Source: https://media.springernature.com/lw1200/springer-static/image/art%3A10.1038%2Fs41591-023-02391-8/MediaObjects/41591_2023_2391_Fig2_HTML.png.

12.6.3. The Role of Social Support and Mental Health

The intersection of social support and mental health is an essential component of the physiological and psychological development of the aged. With age, the complexity of social relationships in itself presents threat and opportunity to the mental well-being. Empirical findings confirm that strong social connections can mitigate the harmful impact of stress and boost resilience, hence the health status. Furthermore, individuals with stronger social support networks experience more life satisfaction and less depression and anxiety. This relation is particularly significant in older people who may experience increased loneliness with the loss of spouses and friends, thus providing increased relevance to community activities to create social relationships and influence broader mental health and well-being among older adults. In evaluating the empirical relationships among social support and mental health, it is apparent that the psychological benefits of social networks extend beyond companionship. Social interaction brings emotional stability, providing people with a sense of belongingness and guidance, which can reduce loneliness and hopelessness to a large degree. Furthermore, social support also can enhance cognitive ability and resilience among the elderly since healthy social interactions excite the brain. As considered in some research, older people who maintain close ties with their family members and friends do not exhibit cognitive impairment as much as their more secluded counterparts, showing social engagement as a protective psychological factor in the aging process (Cooper et al., 2010). Furthermore, the interrelation of social support with mental health is also complicated by environmental stresses, such as, exposure to lead or constant stress, which bear severe implications on cognitive function in the older adult. It has been established that those with heightened psychosocial stress exposure have decreased cognitive function regardless of their exposure to the environment. Of particular note is that the combination of mental stress and environmental stressors, including exposure to lead, increases the risk for cognitive impairment, indicating that systemic approaches to mental health will have to address both internal and external determinants. Therefore, the creation of social support systems is not only vital for emotional well-being but also a strategic public health objective to heighten cognitive resilience among the elderly, particularly against environmental stressors associated with old age (Peters et al., 2010).

Learning Outcome

1. What evidence-based lifestyle interventions can slow or mitigate age-related physiological decline?
2. How do caloric restriction and balanced nutrition influence longevity and metabolic health in older adults?

SUMMARY

In conclusion, the interactive character of developmental physiology and senescence indicates significant mechanisms determining the longevity and healthfulness of organisms. As development has shaped various physiological properties, it is evident that the understanding of these properties is critical to the interpretation of senescence. The intersection of developmental biology and functional genomics, as brought to the forefront in more current studies, illustrates genetic adaptation as it allows for responses to environmental stressors and can enlighten us on the resilience of species under aging. Everything stated regarding gene-environment interactions speaks volumes about the resilience of a robust paradigm for probing physiological systems' reaction to aging challenges that may end up providing more effective interventions in age-related loss (Hamilton et al., 2017). In addition, the implementation of a middle-out approach of evolutionary biology provides a profound insight into developmental processes in relation to aging. Using the model, researchers are able to identify parallelisms between physiological changes resulting from the process of aging and cell-to-cell communication. In particular, the observation that entropy decreases in living systems indicates that evolution is not a straightforward accumulation of adaptations but a complex, interwoven story of development and function across generations. This strategy facilitates the study of candidate genes responsible for aging phenotypes and thereby opens the door to predictive medicine beyond sole correlations between gene and disease (Rehan et al., 2009). Finally, careful examination of developmental physiology and aging identifies the necessity for interdisciplinary research integrating genetics, evolutionary biology, and medical practice. While considerable advances have been made, much remains to be discovered about the interplay of aging and physiological adaptation in its entirety. Clarifying the process by which they occur holds promise for revealing new therapeutic avenues for reducing age-related decline and enhancing quality of life. Future ventures will need to go to great lengths in designing approaches that leverage evolutionary understanding for biomedical applications, hence presenting an all-encompassing approach towards combating the diseases of aging in contemporary society.

This understanding of how living organisms adapt to various gravitational conditions is at the core of developmental physiology, and most particularly where it overlaps with aging. On board space vehicles, the near-zero gravity environment has provided significant insight into the influence of gravity on biological processes. This environment is an ideal model for studying adaptation mechanisms, such as, the physiological adjustment that occurs in hypo- and hyper gravity conditions. Studies indicate that gravity is a fundamental cause of the evolution of species and has an influence on not only development but even the health and happiness of the elderly. Through research on the adaptability of organisms to altered gravitational fields, it is possible for scientists to uncover the basis for phenomena that might be accountable for most of the changes with aging and thus contribute significantly to developmental physiology and its relevance to the aging process (Miquel et al., 2025). Moreover, the integration of systems biology into aging research has emerged as a very important component in demystifying the process of aging. The Rostock Symposium 2013 was centered on the use of computational models to dissect the aging process, with an interest in how ontologies can be applied in organizing and integrating cumbersome data in a structured way. This facilitates a better understanding of the mechanisms of aging by enabling researchers to make connections between different fragments of heterogeneous data. The symposium highlighted the potential of databases and data integration technologies for creating structures that enhance our understanding of aging disorders. Through computer-enabled simulation of the aging process, scientists can focus their attention on cellular stress, marker generation, and a few diseases that impact aged populations, hence contributing to the eventual goal of increased health span and longevity (Fuellen et al., 2013). Finally, the integration of concepts from gravitational biology and systems biology enables increased understanding of developmental physiology and senescence. By learning about how organisms react to gravitational stress and correlating this with computational models, scientists can design interventions aimed at aging-related disorders. The intersection of the two domains highlights the intricacies of the aging process and opens up new possibilities for mitigating its effects. This multi-disciplinary approach not only holds the prospect for the progress of biomedical research but also has direct relevance for enhancing the quality of life in aging populations. Lastly, combining outcomes from gravitational biology and systems biology embodies the innovative potential in developmental physiology that brings about subsequent investigations for investigating the intricate network of aging (Fuellen et al., 2013; Miquel et al., 2025).

KEY TERMS FROM THIS CHAPTER

- Apoptosis
- Cognitive decline
- Epigenetic changes
- Growth factors
- Hormonal regulation
- Neurodegeneration
- Organ maturation
- Puberty
- Senescence
- Cell differentiation
- Embryogenesis
- Fetal development
- Hormonal decline
- Mitochondrial dysfunction
- Neurodevelopment
- Oxidative stress
- Sarcopenia
- Stem cells

CRITICAL THINKING QUESTIONS

1. **Which hormone plays a crucial role in growth during childhood and adolescence?**
   a. Cortisol
   b. Insulin
   c. Growth hormone (GH)
   d. Thyroxine
2. **What is the primary physiological change in the cardiovascular system with aging?**
   a. Increased cardiac output
   b. Increased arterial elasticity
   c. Decreased heart rate variability
   d. Enhanced blood flow to tissues
3. **Which organ system shows the most significant decline in function with aging?**
   a. Nervous system
   b. Integumentary system
   c. Endocrine system
   d. Respiratory system
4. **What is sarcopenia, commonly seen in aging individuals?**
   a. Loss of bone density
   b. Loss of skin elasticity
   c. Loss of muscle mass and strength
   d. Loss of vision
5. **Which factor can slow down many age-related physiological changes?**
   a. High sugar diet
   b. Sedentary lifestyle
   c. Regular physical activity
   d. Chronic stress

Short Answer Questions

1. What is the role of growth hormone (GH) in early development?
2. How does the cardiovascular system change with age?
3. Define sarcopenia and its impact on mobility.
4. Name two changes in the endocrine system that occur with aging.
5. What is the typical pattern of bone density across the lifespan?
6. Describe the major physiological changes that occur during childhood, adolescence, and adulthood.
7. Discuss the structural and functional changes that occur in the nervous system with aging.
8. Explain the hormonal regulation of growth and development, and how it changes with age.
9. Describe age-related changes in the musculoskeletal system and their implications.
10. Discuss how lifestyle factors , such as exercise and diet, can influence the aging process and delay functional decline.

Answers to Critical Thinking Questions

1. (c); 2. (c); 3. (a); 4. (c); 5. (c).

REFERENCES

1. Hau, M., Haussmann, M. F., Greives, T. J., Matlack, C., Costantini, D., Quetting, M., Adelman, J. S., Miranda, A. C., & Partecke, J. (2015). Repeated stressors in adulthood increase the rate of biological ageing. *Frontiers in zoology, 12*, 4. https://doi.org/10.1186/s12983-015-0095-z(accessed on 28th June 2025).
2. Peters, J. L., Weisskopf, M. G., Spiro, A., 3rd, Schwartz, J., Sparrow, D., Nie, H., Hu, H., Wright, R. O., & Wright, R. J. (2010). Interaction of stress, lead burden, and age on cognition in older men: the VA Normative Aging Study. *Environmental health perspectives, 118*(4), 505–510. https://doi.org/10.1289/ehp.0901115(accessed on 28th June 2025).
3. Radnor, J. M., Oliver, J. L., Waugh, C. M., Myer, G. D., & Lloyd, R. S. (2020). The Influence of Maturity Status on Muscle Architecture in School-Aged Boys. *Pediatric exercise science, 32*(2), 89–96. https://doi.org/10.1123/pes.2019-0201s(accessed on 28th June 2025).
4. Behringer, V., Heistermann, M., Malaivijitnond, S., Schülke, O., & Ostner, J. (2023). Developmental and environmental modulation of fecal thyroid hormone levels in wild Assamese macaques (*Macaca assamensis*). *American Journal of Primatology, 85.* https://www.semanticscholar.org/paper/a130e799cd51a8105fc34771b8796697f9e0ac8e (accessed on 28th June 2025).
5. Evans, N. P., Bellingham, M., & Robinson, J. E. (2016). Prenatal programming of neuroendocrine reproductive function. *Theriogenology, 86*(1), 340–348. https://doi.org/10.1016/j.theriogenology.2016.04.047(accessed on 28th June 2025).
6. Bich, L., Moreau, J. F., & Pradeu, T. (2019). Understanding multicellularity: The functional organization of the intercellular space. https://core.ac.uk/download/228134961.pdf (accessed on 28th June 2025).
7. Bindra, A., Krist, D., Khalid, H., Abraskin, K., Gunya, D., Szeremeta, A., Guduri, S., et al. (2025). MenoPatch: Advancing transdermal hormone replacement therapy for menopausal symptom management. *North American Proceedings in Gynecology and Obstetrics–Supplemental.* https://www.semanticscholar.org/paper/246e3d107034b170bb8c1090468f2c957d00e54e (accessed on 28th June 2025).
8. Braeckman, B., & Dhondt, I. (2017). Lifespan extension in *Caenorhabditis elegans* insulin/IGF-1 signaling mutants is supported by non-vertebrate physiological traits. https://core.ac.uk/download/91390595.pdf (accessed on 28th June 2025).
9. Zečić, A., & Braeckman, B. P. (2020). DAF-16/FoxO in *Caenorhabditis elegans* and Its Role in Metabolic Remodeling. *Cells, 9*(1), 109. https://doi.org/10.3390/cells9010109(accessed on 28th June 2025).
10. Brodbeck, A., Helminak, G., Jacobson, E., Islas, D., Esser, M. S., Phelps, E. M., Streeton, A. C., et al. (2022). NANN Research Summit 2022. *Advances in Neonatal Care, 22*, E78–E85. https://www.semanticscholar.org/paper/067cac7462808f5dbbac8715ea18c595b53c6b18 (accessed on 28th June 2025).
11. Brust, V., Lewejohann, L., & Schindler, P. M. (2015). Lifetime development of behavioral phenotype in the house mouse (*Mus musculus*). https://core.ac.uk/download/211826121.pdf (accessed on 28th June 2025).
12. Fuellen, G., Boerries, M., Busch, H., de Grey, A., Hahn, U., Hiller, T., Hoeflich, A., Jansen, L., Janssens, G. E., Kaleta, C., Meinema, A. C., Schäuble, S., Simm, A., Schofield, P. N., Smith, B.,

Sühnel, J., Vera, J., Wagner, W., Wönne, E. C., & Wuttke, D. (2013). In silico approaches and the role of ontologies in aging research. *Rejuvenation research, 16*(6), 540–546. https://doi.org/10.1089/rej.2013.1517(accessed on 28th June 2025).

13. Cao, N., Li, S., Xu, A., Li, M., Zou, X., Ke, Z., Deng, G., et al. (2022). Dynamic changes of endogenic or exogenic β-carboline alkaloid harmine in different mammals and human *in vivo* at developmental and physiological states. *Frontiers in Aging Neuroscience, 13.* https://www.semanticscholar.org/paper/a24dcffd424d90225a90e3c8b695af52756d70ae (accessed on 28th June 2025).

14. Iop, L., Dal Sasso, E., Schirone, L., Forte, M., Peruzzi, M., Cavarretta, E., Palmerio, S., Gerosa, G., Sciarretta, S., & Frati, G. (2017). The Light and Shadow of Senescence and Inflammation in Cardiovascular Pathology and Regenerative Medicine. *Mediators of inflammation, 2017,* 7953486. https://doi.org/10.1155/2017/7953486(accessed on 28th June 2025).

15. Chen, L., Delville, C., Derous, D., Douglas, C., et al. (2016). The effects of graded levels of calorie restriction: V. Impact of short-term calorie and protein restriction on physical activity in the C57BL/6 mouse. https://core.ac.uk/download/77051829.pdf (accessed on 28th June 2025).

16. Cooper, R., Gale, C. R., Hardy, R., Kuh, D., et al. (2010). Objectively measured physical capability levels and mortality: Systematic review and meta-analysis. https://core.ac.uk/download/12182.pdf (accessed on 28th June 2025).

17. Epel, E. S., Crosswell, A. D., Mayer, S. E., Prather, A. A., Slavich, G. M., Puterman, E., & Mendes, W. B. (2018). More than a feeling: A unified view of stress measurement for population science. *Frontiers in neuroendocrinology, 49*, 146–169. https://doi.org/10.1016/j.yfrne.2018.03.001(accessed on 28th June 2025).

18. Cryan, J. F., O'Riordan, K. J., Cowan, C. S. M., Sandhu, K. V., Bastiaanssen, T. F. S., Boehme, M., Codagnone, M. G., et al. (2019). The microbiota-gut-brain axis. *Physiological Reviews, 99,* 1877–2013. https://doi.org/10.1152/physrev.00018.2018 (accessed on 28th June 2025).

19. de Saussure, F. (2017). *Course in General Linguistics.* Macat Library eBooks. https://doi.org/10.4324/9781912281732 (accessed on 28th June 2025).

20. Eidbo, S., Ratnani, A., Megiso, M., King, S., & Barnett, M. J. (2025). Long-term oncological implications of hormone-replacement therapy in women with Kallmann syndrome: A propensity-matched study from the Global Federated Health Research Network. *Journal of Clinical Oncology.* https://www.semanticscholar.org/paper/9fee5065ff66d11eba69f1956952d081de4f9785 (accessed on 28th June 2025).

21. Klein, D., Rotarska-Jagiela, A., Genc, E., Sritharan, S., Mohr, H., Roux, F., Han, C. E., Kaiser, M., Singer, W., & Uhlhaas, P. J. (2014). Adolescent brain maturation and cortical folding: evidence for reductions in gyrification. *PloS one, 9*(1), e84914. https://doi.org/10.1371/journal.pone.0084914(accessed on 28th June 2025).

22. Fu, Z., Wang, W., & Gao, Y. (2024). Understanding the impact of ER stress on lung physiology. *Frontiers in Cell and Developmental Biology, 12.* https://www.semanticscholar.org/paper/3130739b6809bde17dabc7eeeb24d753ba5ce9f4 (accessed on 28th June 2025).

23. Galluzzi, L., Vitale, I., Aaronson, S. A., Abrams, J., Adam, D., Agostinis, P., Alnemri, E. S., et al. (2018). Molecular mechanisms of cell death: Recommendations of the Nomenclature Committee on Cell Death 2018. *Cell Death and Differentiation, 25,* 486–541. https://doi.org/10.1038/s41418-017-0012-4 (accessed on 28th June 2025).

24. Goulson, D., Nicholls, E., Botías, C., & Rotheray, E. L. (2015). Bee declines driven by combined stress from parasites, pesticides, and lack of flowers. *Science, 347*. https://doi.org/10.1126/science.1255957 (accessed on 28th June 2025).

25. Grandi, E. (2023). Cell diversity and signaling in the cardiovascular system. *The Journal of Physiology, 601*. https://www.semanticscholar.org/paper/00d8d3ffe99eed948dec8e4eb634bd9b2010684b (accessed on 28th June 2025).

26. Hamilton, R., Holmes, L., Jordan, D., Rodríguez, C., et al. (2017). Genomic and phenotypic signatures of climate adaptation in an *Anolis* lizard. https://core.ac.uk/download/151161972.pdf (accessed on 28th June 2025).

27. Harley, T. A., Jessiman, L. J., & MacAndrew, S. B. G. (2011). Decline and fall: A biological, developmental, and psycholinguistic account of deliberative language processes and ageing. https://core.ac.uk/download/228176795.pdf (accessed on 28th June 2025).

28. Hoarau, A., Frauenpreis, A., Belgacemi, R., Glass, I., Al Alam, D., & Danopoulos, S. (2024). The effect of VEGF-A isoforms on capillary endothelial cell differentiation in human fetal lung development. *Physiology*. https://www.semanticscholar.org/paper/de1015809d85c01f03f124027f7a14ca0b660d21 (accessed on 28th June 2025).

29. Kaplan, H., & Gurven, M. (2008). Top-down and bottom-up research in biodemography. https://www.demographic-research.org/articles/volume/19/44(accessed on 28th June 2025).

30. Lester, B. M., & Boukydis, C. F. Z. (2011). *Infant Crying: Theoretical and Research Perspectives*. https://core.ac.uk/download/71356407.pdf (accessed on 28th June 2025).

31. Lindau, S. T. (2006). Intimacy and sexuality: Toward a lifespan perspective. https://core.ac.uk/download/71356407.pdf (accessed on 28th June 2025).

32. Luo, J., Zhang, B., Graham, E. K., & Mroczek, D. (2023). Does personality always matter for health? Examining the moderating effect of age on the personality-health link from life span developmental and aging perspectives. *Journal of Personality and Social Psychology, 125*(5), 1189–1206. https://www.semanticscholar.org/paper/dc0c44f9c12dc9db2b3bc01e3313afbbf78e1b07 (accessed on 28th June 2025).

33. McCreary, J. K., Metz, G. A. S., Ng, J. W. Y., Olson, D. M., et al. (2015). Allostatic load and preterm birth. https://core.ac.uk/download/74559442.pdf (accessed on 28th June 2025).

34. Miquel, J., & Souza, K. A. (2025). An overview of gravitational physiology. https://core.ac.uk/download/pdf/42810843.pdf (accessed on 28th June 2025).

35. Moriyama, M., Nahar, S., Shamsun Nahar, F. O., et al. (2025). Telenursing health education and lifestyle modification among patients with diabetes in Bangladesh: Protocol for a pilot study with a quasi-experimental pre- and postintervention design. *JMIR Research Protocols, 14*. https://www.semanticscholar.org/paper/e3b41dc61aab6cb0e23e1f038d1a775b5d2ada93 (accessed on 28th June 2025).

36. Naef-Daenzer, B., & Grüebler, M. U. (2016). Post-fledging survival of altricial birds: Ecological determinants and adaptation. *Journal of Field Ornithology, 87*, 227–250. https://doi.org/10.1111/jofo.12157 (accessed on 28th June 2025).

37. Rehan, V. K., & Torday, J. S. (2009). The evolution of cell communication: The road not taken. https://core.ac.uk/download/323077470.pdf (accessed on 28th June 2025).

38. Roberts, D. P., & Mattoo, A. K. (2019). Sustainable crop production systems and human

nutrition. *Frontiers in Sustainable Food Systems, 3.* https://doi.org/10.3389/fsufs.2019.00072 (accessed on 28th June 2025).

39. Römling, U., Kjelleberg, S., Normark, S., Nyman, L., Uhlin, B. E., & Åkerlund, B. (2014). Microbial biofilm formation: A need to act. *Journal of Internal Medicine, 276*, 98–110. https://doi.org/10.1111/joim.12242 (accessed on 28th June 2025).

40. Ryff, C. D. (2013). Psychological well-being revisited: Advances in the science and practice of eudaimonia. *Psychotherapy and Psychosomatics, 83*, 10–28. https://doi.org/10.1159/000353263 (accessed on 28th June 2025).

41. Schibalski, R. S., Shulha, A. S., Tsao, B., Palygin, O., & Ilatovskaya, D. V. (2024). The role of polyamine metabolism in cellular function and physiology. *American Journal of Physiology. Cell Physiology.* https://www.semanticscholar.org/paper/7071a2f2296009d20a5bed954be4aa61e7f5171a (accessed on 28th June 2025).

42. Sharma, M. K. (2023). Plant senescence: How plants choose, how and when to die. *International Journal of Biochemistry Research & Review.* https://www.semanticscholar.org/paper/9112d512413d203161d9891f27654970db01dfa8 (accessed on 28th June 2025).

43. Tang, S., Bridges, E., Davies, J., Lane, S., Wu, S., Lee, C., Mitchell, R., et al. (2024). O-132 A systematic spatial HiPlex proteomics exploration of human testicular tissues from birth to adulthood. *Human Reproduction.* https://www.semanticscholar.org/paper/ae55888f2879e20259928df8a12f6f64b22f0889 (accessed on 28th June 2025).

44. Wang, X., Bai, Y., Li, W., Yang, C., Zhang, L., Zhu, H., Bao, R., et al. (2025). Effect of artificial intelligence driven therapeutic lifestyle changes (AI-TLC) intervention on health behavior and health among obesity pregnant women in China: A randomized controlled trial protocol. *Frontiers in Public Health, 13.* https://www.semanticscholar.org/paper/884e93fe6c9b6974e5addb2b926b6fc3222bdbe3 (accessed on 28th June 2025).

45. Yoshikawa, H., Wuermli, A. J., Britto, P. R., Dreyer, B. P., Leckman, J. F., Lye, S. J., Ponguta, L. A., et al. (2020). Effects of the global coronavirus disease-2019 pandemic on early childhood development: Short- and long-term risks and mitigating program and policy actions. *The Journal of Pediatrics, 223*, 188–193. https://doi.org/10.1016/j.jpeds.2020.05.020 (accessed on 28th June 2025).

INDEX

D

E

F

G

H

I

R

S

T

U

V

W

Z